THYROID AUTOIMMUNITY

THYROID AUTOIMMUNITY

Edited by

A. Pinchera
University of Pisa
Pisa, Italy

S. H. Ingbar
Harvard Medical School
Boston, Massachusetts

J. M. McKenzie
University of Miami
Miami, Florida

and

G. F. Fenzi
University of Pisa
Pisa, Italy

PLENUM PRESS • NEW YORK AND LONDON

Library of Congress Cataloging in Publication Data

International Symposium on Thyroid Autoimmunity (1986: Pisa, Italy)
  Thyroid autoimmunity.

  "Proceedings of an International Symposium on Thyroid Autoimmunity...held
November 24–26, 1986, in Pisa, Italy"–T.p. verso.
  Includes bibliographies and index.
  1. Thyroid gland – Diseases – Immunological aspects – Congresses. 2. Autoimmune
diseases – Congresses. 3. Autoantibodies – Congresses. I. Pinchera, A. II. Title.
[DNLM: 1. Thyroid Diseases – immunology – congresses. 2. Thyroiditis, Autoimmune –
congresses. WK 200 I58t 1986]
RC655.49.I57 1986a   616.4′4079   87-29258
ISBN-13: 978-1-4612-8258-7   e-ISBN-13: 978-1-4613-0945-1
DOI: 10.1007/978-1-4613-0945-1

Proceedings of an International Symposium on Thyroid Autoimmunity,
Thirtieth Anniversary: Memories and Perspectives, held November 24–26, 1986,
in Pisa, Italy

© 1987 Plenum Press, New York
Softcover reprint of the hardcover 1st edition 1987
A Division of Plenum Publishing Corporation
233 Spring Street, New York, N.Y. 10013

PREFACE

In 1956, three groups independently reported evidence that some thyroid disease appearing spontaneously in humans or experimentally induced in animals are related to autoimmune processes. The interval between these landmark discoveries and the present has witnessed a remarkable and continuing growth of both knowledge and concepts concerning the mechanisms of immune regulation, the pathogenesis of autoimmune thyroid diseases, and their clinical and laboratory manifestations. More importantly knowledge of thyroid autoimmunity has, in many respects, comprised the vanguard of an ever increasing appreciation and understanding of autoimmune diseases in general.

On November 24-26 1986, an International Symposium on Thyroid Autoimmunity was held in Pisa. Its purpose was to commemorate the birth of thyroid autoimmunity as a scientific discipline, to summarize current knowledge and concepts in this area, and where possible, to anticipate areas of opportunity for the future — hence the theme of the Symposium, Memories and Perspectives. To open the meeting, the Magnifico Rettore (Chancellor) of the University of Pisa granted special Awards to Dr. Deborah Doniach, Dr. Ivan Roitt, and Dr. Noel R. Rose, who published the first fundamental studies in the field of thyroid autoimmunity, and to Dr. Duncan G. Adams, whose discovery of the long-acting thyroid stimulator (LATS) opened the door to our current understanding of the pathogenesis of Graves' disease. During the meeting thirty plenary lectures were presented. These covered the nature of thyroid autoantigens, TSH receptor antibodies, the cellular mechanisms of thyroid autoimmunity, the genetic control and animal models of autoimmune thyroid diseases, and finally the clinical aspects of these disorders. In addition, 112 free communications on related topics were accepted for presentation by poster. Some of these were aggregated into specific workshops to permit their discussion by experts in that particular subfield.

The meeting was attended by approximately 350 participants from throughout the world, most all of whom participated in what proved to be lively discussions of both the oral presentations and the posters. This volume is a collection of papers presented during the Symposium, and its intent is to provide, as promptly as possible, a comprehensive survey of current research progress, as well as a comprehensive source of references, in the field. We very much hope that it will fulfill those purpose, and in so doing, will stimulate further discussions and advances in our knowledge of thyroid autoimmunity.

The Editors are thankful to the speakers and attendees, all of whom contributed in diverse ways to the evident success of the Symposium. This productive meeting and the publication of this volume would not have been possible without the generous financial assistance of Becton Dickinson Laboratory Systems S.p.A. or without the invaluable collaboration of Dr. Stefano Mariotti, the secretarial assistance of IN.C.OR. organization, and the editorial help of Plenum Press.

We are deeply grateful to the University of Pisa for its sponsorship and to the City and Health Authorities of Pisa, who welcomed the participants in the gracious manner for which the city is famous. It seems appropriate, we hope, that this Symposium was held in the city of Galileo Galilei, which gave birth to critical advances in science that have benefitted mankind immeasurably.

A. Pinchera   J.M. McKenzie
S.H. Ingbar   G.F. Fenzi

CONTENTS

Graves' Disease:
A Paradigm for Autoimmunity 1
D.D. Adams, A. Knight, J.G. Knight and P. Laing

Nature of Thyroid Autoantigens:
The TSH Receptor.. 11
J. Chan, M. De Luca, P. Santisteban, O. Isozaki, S. Shifrin, S.M. Aloj,
E.F. Grollman and L.D. Kohn

Progress in Understanding the Thyroid Microsomal Antigen 27
L.J. DeGroot, L. Portmann and N. Hamada

A Possible Role of Bacterial Antigens in the
Pathogenesis of Autoimmune Thyroid Disease 35
S.H. Ingbar, M. Weiss, G.W. Cushing and D.L. Kasper

"ATRA I": A New Autoantigen in Autoimmune Thyroid Disease 45
B. Rapoport, H. Hirayu, P. Seto, R.P. Magnusson and S. Filetti

Monoclonal Antibodies in the Study of Thyroid
Autoantigens and Autoantibodies 53
J. Ruf, B. Czarnocka, M.E. Toubert, C. Alquier, C. De Micco, H. Henry,
C. Dutoit, Y. Malthiery, M. Ferrand and P. Carayon

LATS/TSAb: Then and Now 63
J.M. McKenzie

Pathogenic Roles of TSH Receptor Antibodies in Graves' Disease 69
S. Nagataki

Physiopathological Relevance of Thyroid Stimulating Antibody
(TSAb) Measurements in Graves' Disease 77
J. Orgiazzi, A.M. Madec and R. Mornex

TSH Receptor Autoantibodies Affecting Thyroid Cell Function 83
G.F. Fenzi, P. Vitti, C. Marcocci, L. Chiovato and E. Macchia

Heterogeneity of TSH Receptor-directed Antibodies (TRAb)
and Their Significance 91
M. Zakarija

Humoral Factors in Graves' Ophthalmopathy 99
R. Toccafondi, C.M. Rotella, R. Zonefrati and A. Tanini

Immunoregulatory Abnormalities in Autoimmune Thyroid Disease 109
R. Volpé and V.V. Row

Intrathyroidal Lymphocytes, Thyroid Autoantibodies and Thyroid
   Destruction 117
   S.M. McLachlan, C.A.S. Pegg, M.C. Atherton, S.L. Middleton,
   P. Rooke, C. Thompson, S. Dahabra, E.T. Young, F. Clark
   and B. Rees-Smith

Cellular Mechanisms for Autoimmune Damage in Thyroid-Associated 125
   Ophthalmopathy
   J. How, Y. Hiromatsu, P. Wang, M. Salvi and J.R. Wall

Thyroid Infiltrating T Lymphocytes in Hashimoto's Thyroiditis:
   Phenotypic and Functional Analysis at Single Cell Level 135
   G.F. Del Prete, A. Tiri, S. Mariotti, A. Pinchera, S. Romagnani and
   M. Ricci

An in Vitro Model for Thyroid Autoimmunity 145
   B.E. Wenzel, R. Gutekunst, S. Grammerstorf and P.C. Scriba

Genetic Aspects of Graves' Disease 153
   A.M. McGregor, S. Ratanachaiyavong, C. Gunn, K.W. Lee,
   P.S. Barnett, C. Darke and R. Hall

Thyroid and Related Autoimmune Disorders:
   Challenging the Dogmas 159
   G.F. Bottazzo, I. Todd, A. Belfiore, R. Mirakian and R. Pujol-Borrel

Molecular and Functional Characterization of Genes Encoding
   Anti-Thyroglobulin and Anti-TSH Receptor Antibodies 175
   M. Monestier and C.A. Bona

Autoantigenicity of Murine Thyroglobulin 181
   B. Champion, P. Hutchings, D. Rayner, K. Page, P. Byfield,
   J. Chan, I. Roitt and A.Cooke

IgG Subclass Distribution of Anti-Tg Antibodies among Thyroid
   Disease Patients and Their Relatives and in High and Low
   Responder Mouse Strains 189
   N.R. Rose, I.M. Outschoorn, C.L. Burek and R.C. Kuppers

Genetic Basis of Spontaneous Autoimmune Thyroiditis 199
   G. Wick, G. Krömer, H. Dietrich, K. Schauenstein and K. Hàla

Hetero-Transplantation of Autoimmune Human Thyroid to Nude
   Mice as a Tool for in Vivo Autoimmune Research 207
   K.H. Usadel, R. Paschke, J. Teuber and U. Schwedes

Post-Partum Thyroid Dysfunction 211
   R. Hall, H. Fung, M. Kologlu, K. Collison, J. Marco, A.B. Parkes,
   B.B. Harris, Darke, R. John, C.J. Richards and A.M. McGregor

Autoimmune and Autonomous Toxic Goiter: Differentiation
   and Clinical Outcome after Drug Treatment 221
   H. Schleusener, G. Holl, J. Schwander, K. Badenhoop, J. Hensen,
   R. Finke, G. Schernthaner, W.R. Mayr, P. Kotulla and R. Holle

Postpartum Onset of Graves' Disease 231
   N. Amino, H. Tamaki, M. Aozasa, Y. Iwatani, J. Tachi, K. Miyai,
   M. Mori and O. Tanizawa

Thyrotropin-Binding Inhibitor Immunoglobulins in Primary
    Hypothyroidism 241
    J. Konishi, K. Kasagi, Y. Iida and K. Torizuka

Thyroid Function Modulates Thymic Endocrine Activity 249
    A. Pinchera S. Mariotti, F. Pacini, N. Fabris and E. Moccheggiani

The BB/W Rat, a Model for "Tgl-associated Goitre" 257
    H.A.M. Voorbij, R.D. Van der Gaag and H.A. Drexhage

Non-Thyroidal Complications of Graves' Disease:
    Perspective on Pathogenesis and Treatment 263
    J.P. Kriss, I.R. McDougall, S.S. Donaldson and H.C. Kraemer

Cross Reactivity between Antibodies to Human Thyroglobulin and
    Torpedo Acetylcholinesterase in Patients with Graves'
    Ophthalmopathy 271
    M. Ludgate, C. Owada, R. Pope, P. Taylor and G. Vassart

Multiple Autoantigenic Determinants in Thyroid Autoimmunity 275
    A.P. Weetman, R. Smallridge, C. Hayslip and K.D. Burman

Further Characterization of the Thyroid Microsomal Antigen
    by Monoclonal Antibodies 279
    L. Portmann, N. Hamada, W.A. Franklin and L.J. DeGroot

Molecular Cloning of a Thyroid Peroxidase cDNA Fragment Encoding
    Epitopes Involved in Hashimoto's Thyroiditis (HT) 283
    C. Dinsart, F. Libert, J. Ruel, M. Ludgate, J. Pommier,
    J. Dussault and G. Vassart

Further Evidence that Thyroid Peroxidase and "Microsomal Antigen"
    Are the Same Entity 285
    B. Czarnocka, J. Ruf, C. Alquier, M.E. Toubert, C. Dutoit,
    M. Ferrand and P. Carayon

Competitive and Immunometric Radioassays for the Measurement of
    Anti-Thyroid Peroxidase Autoantibodies in Human Sera 289
    S. Mariotti, S. Anelli, J. Ruf, R. Bechi, A. Lombardi and P. Carayon

Thyroid Peroxidase and the "Microsomal Antigen", Cannot Be
    Distinguished by Immunofluorescence on Cultured Thyroid
    Cells 293
    L. Chiovato, P. Vitti, C. Mammoli, G. Lopez, P. Cucchi, S. Battiato,
    P. Carayon, G.F. Fenzi and A. Pinchera

Measurement of Anti-alpha-Galactosyl Antibodies in the Course of
    Various Thyroid Disorders and Isolation of an Antigenic
    Glycopeptide Fraction 297
    J. Etienne-Decerf, P. Mahieu, M. Malaise and R. Winand

The IgG Subclass Distribution on Thyroid Autoantibodies in
    Graves' Disease 301
    A.P. Weetman and S. Cohen

Thyroid Hormone Binding Autoantibodies (THBA) in Humans
    and Animals 305
    S. Benvenga and J. Robbins

High Frequency of Interferon-Gamma Producing T Cells in Thyroid
    Infiltrates of Patients with Hashimoto's Thyroiditis 309
    A. Tiri, G.F. Del Prete, S. Mariotti, A. Pinchera, S. Romagnani
    and M. Ricci

Lymphokine Production and Functional Activities of T Cell
    Clones from Thyroid Gland of Hashimoto's Thyroiditis 313
    M. Bagnasco, S. Ferrini, D. Venuti, I. Prigione, G. Giordano and
    G.W. Canonica

Circulatory Thyroglobulin Threshold in Suppressor Activation 315
    Y.M. Kong, M. Lewis, A.A. Giraldo and B.E. Fuller

Thyroglobulin Autoantibody IgG Subclasses; Regulation by T Cells 319
    N. Forouhi, S.M. McLachlan, S.L. Middleton, M. Atherton, P.H. Baylis,
    F. Clark and B. Rees Smith

Cellular Immunity and Specific Defects of T-cell Suppression in
    Patients with Autoimmune Thyroid Disorders 323
    S. Vento, C.J. O'Brien, T. Cundy, C. McSorley, E. Macchia and
    A.L.W.F. Eddleston

The Influence of Interleukin-1 on the Function of Human Thyroid
    Cells 327
    A. Krogh-Rasmussen, U. Feldt-Rasmussen, K. Bech, S. Poulsen
    and K. Bendtzen

Immunohistochemical Characterisation of Lymphocytes in
    Experimental Autoimmune Thyroiditis 331
    A.P. Weetman and S.B. Cohen

Lambda Light Chain Restriction in the Diffuse Thyroid Lymphoid
    Infiltrate in Untreated Graves' Disease 335
    C.A. Smith, B. Jasani, and E.D. Williams

Natural Killer Cell Activity in Hashimoto, Graves' Disease
    and Euthyroid Exophthalmos 339
    B.K. Pedersen, U. Feldt-Rasmussen, H. Perrild, J. Mølholm Hansen
    and T. Christensen

Interaction of Purified Graves' Immunoglobulins with the
    TSH-receptor 343
    P.G.H. Byfield and J. Worthington

Thyroid Stimulating Immunoglobulins without Evidence of in Vivo
    Thyroid Stimulation in Some Non-thyroid Autoimmune
    Disease 347
    K. Bech, U. Feldt-Rasmussen, H. Bliddal, C. Bregengaard, B.
    Danneskiold-Samsøe, S. Husby, K. Johansen, C. Kirkegaard,
    T. Friis, K. Siersbæk-Nielsen and H. Nielsen

The Effect of Thyroid Stimulating Immunoglobulins (TSI) on
    Thyroid cAMP: Comparison with TSH Activity 351
    S. Filetti, G. Damante, D. Foti, R. Catalfamo and R. Vigneri

Proliferation in Cultivated Follicles of Graves' Thyroids:
    Immunohistochemical Studies with Antibody Ki-67 355
    M. Derwahl, Ch. Sellschopp, H.M. Schulte and E.E. Ohnhaus

The Significance of Immunoglobulins Related to Stimulation of Thyroid Growth in Patients with Endemic Goiter 359
A. Halpern and G.A. Medeiros-Neto

Regulation of Growth of Thyroid Cells in Culture by TSH Receptor Antibodies and Other Humoral Factors 363

D. Tramontano, G.W. Cushing, M. Mine, A.C. Moses, F. Beguinot and S.H. Ingbar

Polyamine Modulation of Responses to Graves' IgG in Guinea Pig and Human Thyroid 367
P.P.A. Smyth and A.E. Corcoran

Evidence for Intrathyroidal Production of Thyroid Growth-Stimulating Immunoglobulins 371
H. Schatz, I. Ludwig, F. Wiss and P.E. Goretzki

Presence of Thyroid Growth Promoting Antibody in Patients with Graves' Disease in Remission: Medical versus Surgical Therapy 375
C.M. Rotella, C. Mavilia, E. Vallin, A. Lopponi and R. Toccafondi

Thyrotropin and Growth Promoting Immunoglobulin (TGI) of FRTL-5 Cells Have no Growth Stimulating Activity on Human Thyroid Epithelial Cell Cultures 379
B.E. Wenzel, M. Dwenger, T. Mansky, U. Engel, V. Bay and P.C. Scriba

Autoantibodies Stimulating Thyroid Growth and Adenylate Cyclase Cannot Be Separated in IgGs from Graves' Disease 385
C. Marcocci, P. Vitti, G. Lopez, C. Mammoli, L. Chiovato, G.F. Fenzi and A. Pinchera

Antiidiotypic Blocking of Graves' Disease Biologic Activity with Autologous Sera but not Consistently with Homologous Sera: Evidence for Polyclonality of Thyroid Receptor Antibodies (TRAb) 389
R. Paschke, J. Teuber, U. Schwedes and K.H. Usadel

Autoantibodies Blocking the TSH-induced Adenylate Cyclase Stimulation in Idiopathic Myxedema and Hashimoto's Thyroiditis 393
P. Vitti, Chiovato L., A. Lombardi, G. Lopez, F. Santini, P. Ceccarelli, C. Mammoli, L.F. Giusti, S. Battiato, G.F. Fenzi and A. Pinchera

Relevance of Maternal Thyroid Autoantibodies on the Development of Congenital Hypothyroidism 397
L. Giusti, C. Marcocci, L. Chiovato, M. Ciampi, F. Santini, P. Vitti, N. Formica and G.F. Fenzi

Ability of Immunoglobulins from Patients with Thyroid Disease to Stimulate Skin Fibroblasts 401
P. Wadeleux and R. Winand

Some Evidences that Thyrotropin and Autoantibodies Binding Sites are Located on Different Polypeptide Chains of Thyroid Plasma Membrane Proteins 405
A. Gardas and H. Domek

Presence of Thyroid Growth Promoting Antibody in Patients
with Hashimoto's Thyroiditis: Effect of Long-term
Thyroxine Treatment 409
A. Tanini, C.M. Rotella, L.D. Kohn and R. Toccafondi

Limited Clinical Value of TBII and TSAb for Prediction of the
Outcome of Patients with Graves' Disease 413
R. Hörmann, B. Saller and K. Mann

TSH Receptor Antibodies in Neonatal Hyperthyroidism 417
P.M. Hale, M. Liebert, N.J. Hopwood and J.C. Sisson

Thyroid Autoimmunity as a Major Cause for Congenital
Hypothyroidism 421
U. Bogner, A. Grueters, H. Peters, G. Holl, R. Finke and
H. Schleusener

Thyroid Growth Blocking Antibodies in Congenital Hypothyroidism 425
H. Peters, U. Bogner, G. Holl, A. Grueters, R. Finke and
H. Schleusener

Incidence of TSH Receptor Antibodies in Patients with Toxic
Diffuse Goiter 429
E. Macchia, R. Concetti, G. Carone, L. Gasperini, F. Borgoni,
G.F. Fenzi and A. Pinchera

Blocking Antibodies Apparently without Any Stimulatory Activity Are
Present in Sera of Patients with Graves' Disease 433
E. Macchia, R. Concetti, G. Carone, F. Borgoni, G.F. Fenzi
and A. Pinchera

Increased Frequency of HLA-DR5 in Metro Toronto Patients with
Goitrous Autoimmune Thyroiditis and Post-partum
Thyroiditis 437
P.G. Walfish, M.T. Vargas and D. Gladman

Post-partum Thyroid Dysfunction and HLA Status 441
M. Kologlu, H. Fung, C. Darke, C.J. Richards, R. Hall and A.M. McGregor

Methimazole, gamma-Interferon and Graves' Disease 445
M. Bagnasco, D. Venuti, M. Caria, C. Pizzorno, O. Ferrini and
G.W. Canonica

The Prognostic Value of Combined Measurement of Thyroid-stimulating
Antibody and Serum Thyroglobulin Levels during Graves' Disease
Long Term Thionamide Treatment 449
J.H. Romaldini, R.S. Werner, N. Bromberg, I.D. Pereira, R.P.
Dall'Antonia Jr. and C.S. Farah

Serum Thyroid Autoantibodies in a Long-term Study of Thyrostatic
Treatment of Graves' Disease 453
W. Meng, S. Meng, R. Hampel, M. Ventz and E. Männchen

The Effect of High Doses of Carbimazole in Patients with Graves'
Disease and in Subjects with Thyroid Antibodies 457
P. Tanzi, M. Vitillo, M. Mancuso, V. Fiore, P. Pozzilli, U. Di Mario
and D. Andreani

Thymulin Deficiency and Low T3 Syndrome in Infants with
Low-Birth-Weight Syndromes 461
E. Moccheggiani, N. Fabris, S. Mariotti, G. Caramia, T. Braccili,
F. Pacini and A. Pinchera

Constitutive Expression of HLA Class II Molecules in Human
    Thyroid Cells Transfected with SV-40 465
    A. Belfiore, T. Mauerhoff, R. Pujol-Borrel, R. Mirakian
    and G.F. Bottazzo

Specific DNA Polymorphism in the DQ Alpha Region of Patients
    with Graves' Disease and Hashimoto's Thyroiditis 469
    K. Badenhoop, V. Lewis, V. Drummond, V. Algar, G. Schwarz
    and G.F. Bottazzo

Survey of Post-partum Thyroid Antimicrosomal Autoantibody
    as a Marker for Thyroid Dysfunction 473
    P.G. Walfish, M.T. Vargas, J.P. Provias and F.R. Papsin

HLA Region Gene Involvement in Congenital Hypothyroidism 477
    M. Cisternino, M. Martinetti, R. Lorini, A. Gruppioni, D. Larizza,
    M. Cuccia Belvedere, M.R. Romano and F. Severi

Probability of a Beneficial, Dose-dependent, Immunosuppressive
    Action of Carbimazole in Graves' Disease 481
    J. Duprey, M.F. Louis, M. Sultan and E. Lifchitz

Evidence for DR-Ag-expression by RHS-cells and not by Thyroid
    Epithelial Cells 485
    J. Teuber, R. Paschke, V. Schwedes, M. Knoll, J. Christopher and K.H.
    Usadel

HLA-DR-ß Gene Analysis in Patients with Graves' Disease 489
    B.O. Boehm, E. Schifferdecker, P. Kuehnl, C. Rosak and K. Schöffling

Immune Signals Fail to Elicit Endocrine Responses in the Obese
    Strain (OS) of Chickens with Hashimoto-like Autoimmune
    Thyroiditis 493
    R. Faessler, K. Schauenstein, G. Krömer and G. Wick

Inappropriate HLA Class II Expression in a Wide Variety of
    Thyroid Diseases 497
    R. Pujol-Borrel, A. Lucas Martin, M. Foz, I. Todd and G.F. Bottazzo

Adverse Reactions Related to Methimazole and Propylthiouracil
    Doses 501
    M.C. Werner, J.H. Romaldini, N. Bromberg, M.T.A. Boesso
    and R.S. Werner

Thyroid Suppressibility in Graves' Disease: Relationship with Thyroid
    Stimulating Antibody and Serum Thyroglobulin Levels 505
    R.S. Werner, J.H. Romaldini, N. Bromberg, C.S. Farah, I.D. Pereira
    and R.P. Dall'Antonia Jr

Influence of Lymphokines and Thyroid Hormones on Natural Killer
    Activity 509
    M. Provinciali, M. Muzzioli and N. Fabris

Results of Thyrostatic Drug Treatment in Hyperthyroidism.
    A Clinical Long-term Study 513
    W. Meng, S. Meng, R. Hampel, M. Ventz, E. Männchen and
    B. Streckenbach

Predictive Use of TSH-receptor Antibodies Assay as a Prognostic
    Index in Graves' Patients Treated with Antithyroid Drugs or
    Radioactive-Iodine 517
    R. Concetti, E. Macchia, L. Gasperini, G. Carone, F. Borgoni,
    G.F. Fenzi and A. Pinchera

Affinity Purification of Orbital Antigens Using Human Monoclonal
    Antibodies in Graves' Ophthalmopathy 521
  M. Salvi and J..R. Wall

The Exophthalmos-related Eye Muscle Antigens Are not Related
    to Thyroid Antigens: Lack of Binding Inhibition Using
    Thyroid Microsomes and Thyroglobulin 525
  R. Moncayo, U. Bemetz and E.F. Pfeiffer

Humoral Immunity in Graves' Ophthalmopathy 529
  G. Adler, M. Faryna, A. Lewartowska, J. Nauman, A. Gardas
    and H. Domek

Autoantibodies of IgM and IgG Class against Eye Muscle Antigens in
    Patients with Graves' Ophthalmopathy 533
  G. Adler, A. Lewartowska, A. Gardas and J. Nauman

Endocrine Exophthalmos – Natural History and Results of
    Treatment 537
  E. Schifferdecker and K. Schöffling

Immunosuppressive Treatment of Graves' Ophthalmopathy with
    Cyclosporin A and Ciamexon 541
  C. Utech, M. Cordes, P. Pfannenstiel and K. Wulle

Treatment of Graves' Ophthalmopathy by Retrobulbar Corticosteroids
    Associated with Orbital Cobalt Radiotherapy 545
  C. Marcocci, L. Bartalena, M. Panicucci, G. Cavallacci, C. Marconcini,
    A. Lepri, M. Laddaga, F. Cartei and A. Pinchera

Immunological Features of Simple Endemic Goitre 549
  A. Costa, C. Ricci, V. Benedetto, P. Borelli, E. Fadda, N. Ravarino,
    B. Torchio, D. Urbano, P. Fragapane and G. Varvello

Thyroid Autoimmunity in Five Samples of General Population
    in Italy 551
  G.B. Salabé, H. Lotz, A. Menotti, S. Muntoni, G. Descovich,
    R. Antonini, E. Farinaro and G. Avellone

Prevalence of Hypothyroidism and Hashimoto's Thyroiditis in Two
    Elderly Populations at Different Dietary Iodine Intake 555
  E. Roti, M. Montermini, G. Robuschi, E. Gardini, D. Salvo, M. Gionet,
    C. Abreau, B. Meyers and L.E. Braverman

Evidence of the Influence of Iodine Intake on the Prevalence of
    Autoimmune Factors in Hyperthyroid Patients Living in an
    Endemic Goitre Area 559
  V. De Filippis, A. Balsamo, C. Danni, L. Mongardi, P.A. Merlin,
    O. Testori, R. Cerutti and R. Garberoglio

Further Data on Iodine-induced Autoimmunity 563
  D.A. Koutras, K. Evangelopoulou, K.S. Karaïskos, M.A. Boukis, G.D.
    Piperingos, J. Kitsopanides, D. Makriyannis, J. Mantzos,
    J. Sfontouris and A. Souvatzoglou

Study of Class I and Class II Antigen Expression and Lymphocytic
    Infiltrate on Thyroid Tumors 567
  C. Betterle, F. Presotto, A. Caretto, B. Pedini, A. Fassina,
    M.R. Pelizzo, M.E. Girelli and B. Busnardo

Incidence of Anti-thyroid Autoantibodies in Thyroid Cancer
Patients 571
F. Pacini, S. Mariotti, N. Formica, R. Elisei, S. Anelli, E. Capotorti,
L. Baschieri and A. Pinchera

Thyroid Autoantibodies in Thyroid Cancer 575
K. Bech, H. Bliddal, U. Andersen, A. Krogh Rasmussen, H. Sand
Hansen, U. Feldt-Rasmussen and J. Witten

Some Aspects of Cell Mediated Autoimmunity in Endemic Nodular
Goitre 579
A. Balsamo, F. Botto Micca, P.A. Merlin, V. De Filippis and
A. Stramignoni

Chronic Lymphocytic Thyroiditis in Endemic Goiter:
Local Ig Production and Deposition.................................. 583
H. Gao-sheng and L. Yan-fang

Autoimmune Thyroid Disease in the City of Graves 587
P.P.A. Smyth, T.J. McKenna and D.K. O'Donovan

A Retrospective Study of Thyroid Autoimmunity and Hypothyroidism
in a Random Obese Population 591
N. Lima, H. Cavaliere and G.A. Medeiros-Neto

Circulating Thyroid Autoantibodies in Children and Youngsters with
Insulin Dependent Diabetes Mellitus (IDDM) Are not Predictive
of Overt Autoimmune Thyroid Disease 595
F. De Luca, S. Bernasconi, M. Vanelli, M.F. Siracusano,
L. Di Geronimo, M.D. Finocchiaro and F. Trimarchi

Effects of Chronic Amiodarone Administration on Humoral Thyroid
Autoimmunity 599
E. Martino, F. Aghini-Lombardi, S. Mariotti, L. Bartalena, L. Grasso
and A. Pinchera

Serum Thyroid Autoantibodies in Patients with Breast Cancer 603
U. Feldt-Rasmussen, B. Rasmusson, K. Bech, L. Hegedüs,
M. Høier-Madsen and H. Perrild

Complement Activities and Circulating Immune Complexes in Sera
of Patients with Graves' Disease and Hashimoto's
Thyroiditis 607
K. Kaise, T. Sakurada, N. Kaise, K. Yoshida, T. Nomura, Y. Itagaki, M.
Yamamoto, S. Saito and K. Yoshinaga

Abnormalities of Thyroid Function in Sjögren's Syndrome 611
G. Villone, N. Panza, D. Tramontano, B. Merola, M. Columbo,
G. Lombardi, F.S. Ambesi-Impiombato and G. Marone

Thyroid and Renal Amyloidosis in Thyroglobulin Immunized
Rabbits 615
B.N. Premachandra and H.T. Blumenthal

Absence of Thyroglobulin in Kidney of Patients with Autoimmune
Thyroiditis and Nephropathies 619
F.X. Thierry, C. Burel, Ph. Caron, I. Vernier, G.J. Fournie,
J.P. Louvet and J.J. Conte

Persistence of Autoimmune Reactions During Recovering of Subacute
    Thyroiditis 623
  K. Bech, U. Feldt-Rasmussen, H. Bliddal, M. Høier-Madsen,
  B. Thomsen and H. Nielsen

Purified Protein Derivative Reaction and Urinary Immunosuppressive
    Acidic Protein in Patients with Subacute Thyroiditis 627
  H. Fukazawa, T. Sakurada, K. Tamura, K. Yoshida, M. Yamamoto
  and S. Saito

Interferences of Circulating Anti-TSH Antibodies in Methods for
    Thyrotropin Measurement 631
  P. Beck-Peccoz, G. Medri, C. Rossi and G. Faglia

Index 635

GRAVES' DISEASE

A PARADIGM FOR AUTOIMMUNITY

D.D. Adams, A. Knight, J.G. Knight, and P. Laing

Autoimmunity Research Unit
Medical Research Council of New Zealand
Otago University Medical School
Dunedin, New Zealand

INTRODUCTION

The presence of iodine atoms in thyroid hormone has proved to be fortunate for man in enabling him to understand great principles of the diseases which plague him. Dietary deficiency of iodine, leading to spectacular goitres, drew attention to the thyroid and the success of surgeons in extirpating goitres founded the study of endocrinology by showing that the thyroid secretes a product which is necessary for health and readily available from simple preparations of animal tissue[1].

Paul Ehrlich[2] discovered that our immunity system normally shuns reaction with our own antigens. He called this "horror autotoxicus". We now call it "immune tolerance". However, Ehrlich's awareness that failure of immune tolerance was a likely cause of disease[2] was lost sight of for over 50 years, until thyroidologists, personified by Deborah Doniach, Ivan Roitt, Ernest Witebsky and Noel Rose, brought autoimmunity into the medical armamentarium[3,4]. This ranks with Louis Pasteur's germ theory of disease in its importance for the advance of medicine.

Again because thyroid hormone contains iodine, it proved possible to devise technology with radioactive iodine which demonstrated that a long-acting thyroid stimulator (LATS), distinct form the pituitary gland's thyrotrophic hormone, exists in the blood of some patients with Graves' disease[5-7]. Soon LATS was shown to be an autoantibody by studies which included its being splitting into its constituent polypeptide chains, with loss of activity and recombination of the chains with recovery of activity[8,9]. No autoantibody has had its immunoglobulin nature more rigorously established. Developing radioreceptor assay technology, Manley and his colleagues[10] succeeded in demonstrating the mechanism of the thyroid-stimulating activity by showing, in vitro, that LATS competes with thyrotrophin for reaction with the hormone's receptor on the thyroid cell.

PATHOGENIC AUTOIMMUNITY

Many autoantibodies appear to be non-pathogenic. They include the widely prevalent autoantibodies against intra-cellular, microsomal antigens in thyroid, adrenal, gastric parietal and pancreatic islet cells. Noticing the unconvincing relationship of these autoantibodies to disease, many physicians formed the opinion that autoimmunity was merely a passive consequence of tissue damage and never actually caused disease. The first clear demonstration that an autoantibody can have a causative relationship to a disease came from the discovery of LATS protector (LATSP). While the stimulating action of LATS on guinea pig and mouse thyroids made it a very strong candidate for the causative role in the thyrotoxicosis of Graves' disease, the absence of LATS from more than half the patients, including many of the most severely affected ones was a puzzle. One of us (DDA) mistakenly ascribed the inconsistency to insufficient sensitivity of the LATS bioassay, together with variable degrees of impairment of thyroid efficiency in the patients, due to associated autoimmune thyroiditis[11]. The reality was revealed in a model interplay of ideas across the world.

LATS Protector

Trying to distinguish weak LATS responses from non-specific effects, T.H. Kennedy and one of us (DDA) applied Kriss's discovery[8] that the autoantibody can be neutralized by incubation with thyroid tissue preparations; a specific response would be one which was neutralizable in this fashion. However, LATS from different patients varied widely in its susceptibility to neutralization by thyroid tissue[12]. This was found to be due to the presence of variable amounts of a new thyroid autoantibody, which was inactive in the mouse bioassay, but protected LATS from neutralization by thyroid tissue extracts, in vitro. We named the new autoantibody LATS protector (LATSP) and were surprised to find it more prevalent in Graves' disease than LATS itself. Ivan Roitt saw why. He told Deborah Doniach, who wrote to us,

"London, May 5th., 1967.... I wonder why you assume the new LATS blocking antibody is not active in vivo? It could be more species specific and therefore, not show up in the mouse test, yet still have stimulating properties on the human thyroid".

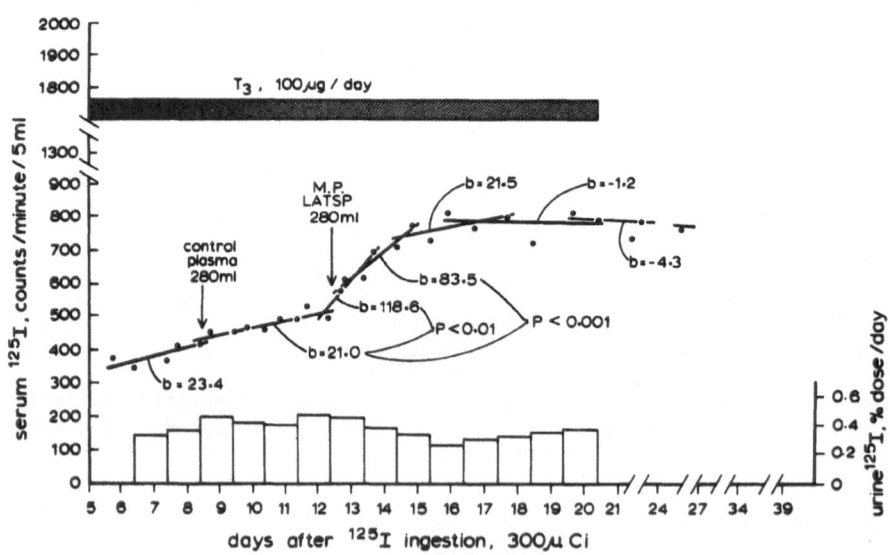

Fig. 1. Demonstration of the stimulating action of LATS protector on the human thyroid by infusion of a potent plasma into a volunteer. Reproduced with permission from the Journal of Clinical Endocrinology and Metabolism 1974; 39: 826.

2

The obvious test of this suggestion, that LATS protector is a human thyroid-stimulating autoantibody which does not cross-react with the mouse, was to see if the phenomenon still occurred when mouse thyroid tissue extracts were used instead of human ones. It did not[13]. Furthermore, bleeding patients 150ml. to obtain 40ml. of serum for ten-fold immunoglobulin concentration, Kennedy and I found significant LATS protector in all of the first twenty, clinically unequivocal patients we tested. Fig. 1 shows a direct demonstration of the thyroid-stimulating activity of LATS protector on the human thyroid, by infusion of 280ml. of our most potent LATS protector plasma (LATS negative) into one of ourselves[14]. Working with R.D.H. Stewart, we found 45 of 50 consecutive cases of Graves' disease, including all the severe and moderately - severe ones, to show LATS protector, whereas LATS was present in only 15[15]. Furthermore, the patients thyroid activities, as measured by ^{131}I uptake, showed a highly significant correlation with their LATS protector levels (P<0.001)[15]. The acme of precision in the measurement of any pathogenic autoantibody has been achieved by Munro and Dirmikis,[16] who established units of LATS protector and went on to show that maternal levels greater than 20U/ml. invariably result in neonatal thyrotoxicosis in the baby, that levels between 10 and 20U/ml. sometimes do and that levels below 10U/ml. do not (Fig. 2).

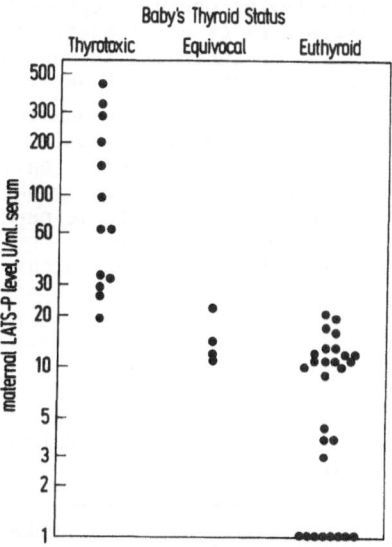

Fig. 2. Evidence for the pathogenic action of LATS protector by demonstration of the consistent relationship between maternal levels and occurrence of neonatal thyrotoxicosis in babies. Reproduced with permission from Munro et al., Brit. J. Obst and Gyn. 1978; 85: 837.

THE FORBIDDEN CLONE THEORY

Why does autoimmunity occur? The answer has its origin in what must rank as immunology's greatest conceptual advance — the realization by Niels Jerne[17] that antibodies are not built to fit an antigen (template theory) but are preformed in myriad diversity, awaiting the advent of an antigen which fits. Jerne's concept that antibodies are selected rather than induced has revolutionized understanding of the immunity system. Macfarlane Burnet[18], familiar with the multiplication and mutation of populations of bacterial cells, was able to understand the similar behaviour of populations of lymphocytes. Burnet defined the immunological <u>clone</u>, a set of lymphocytes with identical receptors for antigen, as the unit of immune specificity, hence the <u>clonal selection theory</u> of acquired immunity, now universally accepted. Burnet went on to postulate that forbidden (self-antigen's-reactive) clones are eliminated in foetal life, but may arise post-natally to cause autoimmune disease, through series of sequential somatic mutations in lymphocytes. This is the <u>forbidden clone theory</u> of autoimmune disease, at present remarkably overlooked,[19] to the detriment of medicine.

Evidence for Involvement of Somatic Mutation

The thyroid-stimulating autoantibodies (TSab) fulfill all the requirements of the forbidden clone theory. Their origin by somatic mutation, a random process, but limited by the specificity of the antigens providing the mitogenic drive, is shown by

(i) The variable, post-natal age of onset of Graves' disease, explained by the variable time taken for the necessary somatic mutations to occur.

(ii) The fine variation, from patient to patient, in the specificity of TSab paratopes (receptors for antigen), shown by variable cross-reactivity with murine, ovine and bovine thyrotrophin receptors[20]. This is explained by the variability of the sequences of point mutations which can produce a paratope with TSab activity. In contrast, thyrotrophin, coded for by a static, germline gene, tends to be the same in us all.

(iii) The presence of only one type of immunoglobulin light chain in thyroid-stimulating autoantibodies from individual patients. This was first noted by Zakarija and McKenzie[21,22], being confirmed by Knight et al,[23] for both LATS and LATSP, using affinity chromatography with monoclonal anti-κ and anti-λ antibodies. As each B lymphocyte is permanently committed to making antibodies containing only κ or λ light chains, this finding indicates that TSab clones arise from mutations occurring in a single cell, similarly to cancer.

Table 1. Light Chain Composition of Thyroid Autoantibodies from Individual Patients

| Autoantibodies | Assay Method | Number of Patients | | | |
		κ only	λ only	κ & λ	Total
a. Pathogenic:					
TSab	cAMP in vitro[22]	1	7	0	8
	LATS bioassay[23]	1	8	0	9
	LATSP bioassay[23]	0	2	0	2
		2*	17*	0	19
		$^{*}\chi^2 = 10.3$, P<0.005			
b. Non-pathogenic:					
TMab	ELISA[24]	0	0	10	10
TGab	ELISA[24]	0	0	10	10

Table 1 shows the combined data from a total of 19 thyrotoxic patients. In 17 of these the light chain type was λ, in 2 κ, a significant imbalance (P<0.005). In contrast, Table 1 also shows Laing's[24] data for thyroid microsomal (TMab) and thyroglobulin (TGab) autoantibodies, which contained both types of light chain in all patients tested. We think this reflects the non-pathogenic nature of TMab and TGab and the consequent lack of evolutionary pressure against their occurrence, on contrast to the TSab, whose presence, until recent years, was often fatal.

Invariance of the Autoantigen for TSab

Burnet's forbidden clone theory postulates reaction of mutant lymphocyte clones against unaltered host antigens. Again, the precise technology available to thyroidologists has enabled this to be tested[25]. In extensive tests of thyroid autoantigen preparations from 9 patients against LATS sera from 7 patients, there was no significant variation in the affinity of any individual thyroid preparation for any individual LATS serum. Similarly, tests with LATS protector sera from 55 patients showed an absence of allogeneic variation in thyroid preparations from 4 patients. Autologous reactions between thyroid preparations and LATS or LATSP showed no greater or lesser affinity than homologous ones.

These findings support Burnet's theory and, further, indicate that host histocompatibility antigens are not involved in the autoantigen for TSab.

Unlikely Concepts of Autoimmunity

A popular notion has been that autoimmunity occurs because of a loss of suppressor T cells, but purported evidence for this has not been confirmable[26,27].

Similarly, purported evidence that B cell clones for thyroglobulin autoantibodies (TGab) are universal, but held in check by lack of helper T cells, appears to have been a misinterpretation[26,28]. Stimulating peripheral blood lymphocytes with mitogens, Beall and Kruger[28], were able to demonstrate TGab - secreting B cells in people showing these autoantibodies, but not in other people. Further, these investigators found that T helper and T suppressor effects occurred with T cells from people with and without TGab. Beall and Kruger conclude that the abnormality responsible for autoantibody production does not lie in T cells[28].

AUTOIMMUNE COMPLICATIONS

With remarkable ingenuity, Frank Rundle and Eric Pochin demonstrated a precise correlation between Hertel exophthalmometer measurements of exophthalmos and degree of orbital filling in milligrams of orbital contents per millilitre of orbital volume[29]. Extracting fat with either, they showed that this component is increased in the extraocular muscles and orbital connective tissue of all thyrotoxic patients, accounting for the condition. Later Rundle was able to make post-mortem study of a patient with malignant exophthalmos, finding that in this condition the exophthalmos is entirely due to a gross increase in size of the extraocular muscles[30] as can be seen today by CAT scanning.

There is a highly significant relationship between the specificity of TSab and the occurrence of both exophthalmos[8,15,31] and pre-tibial myxoedema,[31,32] both conditions being associated with the more cross-reactive, LATS, variants (Table 2). As LATS is reactive with receptors on guinea pig adipocytes,[33] it seems probable that some variants of TSab

Table 2. Association of TSab Specificity (LATS,
Mouse Cross-Reactivity) with the
Thyrotoxicosis Complications,
Exophthalmos and Pretibial myxoedema

	Number of Patients LATS		
	+ve	-ve	Total
Thyrotoxicosis only[31]	3	26	29
Exophthalmos[31]	7	2	9
	χ^2=12.8, P<0.001		
Thyrotoxicosis only[15]	15	35	50
Pretibial myxoedema[31,32]	20	1	21
	χ^2=22.6, P<0.001		

cause the usual form of exophthalmos by reacting with orbital adipocytes to cause mitosis or increased fat storage[26].

The example of Graves' disease (Fig. 3) suggests that similar cross-tissue reactivity could be the cause of complications of other autoimmune diseases, including the retinopathy and nephropathy of insulin-dependent diabetes mellitus, which may be due to independent autoimmune reactivities rather than be metabolic consequences of insulin deficiency.

THE GENETICS OF AUTOIMMUNITY

It follows from the forbidden clone theory that autoimmunity has a somatic genetic component, the mutation of lymphocyte V (variable region of the receptor for antigen) genes, under mitogenic drive from environmental antigens. The randomness of somatic mutation accounts for the incomplete concordance of monozygous twins for Graves' and other autoimmune diseases[34]. Additionally, familial aggregation and the variation in risk imposed by sex and histocompatibility antigens indicate an influence of germline genes. What do these code for and how do they exert their influence?

The pioneering studies of Bartels[35] on inheritance of Graves' disease suggested recessive mode of inheritance, with incomplete penetrance, more incomplete in males than in females. However, frequent involvement of three successive generations suggested dominance. Uncertain mode of inheritance has been a characteristic feature of autoimmune diseases in general[36]. The explanation seems to be that the genes involved are multiple and co-dominant, with products (V genes and H genes) which have inconsistent influence on disease occurrence because of the somatic mutation involved[34].

V Gene Effect

When V genes coding for immune specificity were discovered they were at once attractive candidates for germline influence on autoimmunity, as they could account for the observed disease-specificity of the inheritance, e.g. Graves' disease runs in some families, insulin-dependent diabetes mellitus in others[34]. The preponderance of λ light chain type over κ in TSab (Table 1) suggests that immunoglobulin light chain V genes are genetic determinants for Graves' disease. In accord with this, using the κ chain allotypic marker Km(1) in unfinished family studies, we have found significantly (P<0.025) associated inheritance of κ chain V genes and Graves' disease.

Histocompatibility Antigen Effect

Following the discovery that histocompatibility antigen status influences immune response capacity for exotic antigens[37], Vladutiu and Rose[38] found that it also influences susceptibility of inbred mouse strains to induction of autoimmunity to thyroid antigens. In Graves' disease, the major histocompatibility complex (MHC) antigen, B8, was found to occur with increased frequency[39], carrying a relative risk of 3.26. Later it was found that the MHC D locus antigen, DR3, carries a relative risk of 3.77 [40] for Graves' disease. Various other suspected or established autoimmune diseases are associated with increased or decreased frequency of certain MHC alleles[40]. Why is this?

The H Gene Theory

As histocompatibility antigens appear never to be targets for autoimmune attack, they seem to be able to impose, unbreakable, life-long tolerance. Burnet postulated that tolerance induction was confined to foetal life, but Nossal and Pike[41] have shown that nascent lymphocytes from adult animals are tolerized by contact with antigen. This explains the absence of autoimmunity to H antigens, which, being on lymphocytes are always present during lymphocyte ontogeny.

The H gene theory[42] postulates that the association of H (histocompatibility) antigen status, including sex, with altered risk of autoimmune disease is due to the tolerance inductions of the H antigens. These alter the repertoire of immunological clones, which in turn alters the risk of development of forbidden clones by sequences of somatic mutations in lymphocyte V genes, as envisaged by Burnet. Tolerance inductions subtract from the immune repertoire, which readily accounts for protective H antigen effects, such as by DR2 for insulin-dependent diabetes mellitus and by male sex for Graves' disease, on the assumption that precursors of potential forbidden clones are deleted. However, increased risks, as by B27 and H-Y antigens for ankylosing spondylitis, require further explanation. The original H-gene theory[42] invoked Jernes' concept[43] that one clone frequently destroys another by paratope-idiotope reaction, so that an H antigen tolerance induction which removes an anti-idiotope clone would add a specificity to the repertoire. We now think that interclonal deletions may

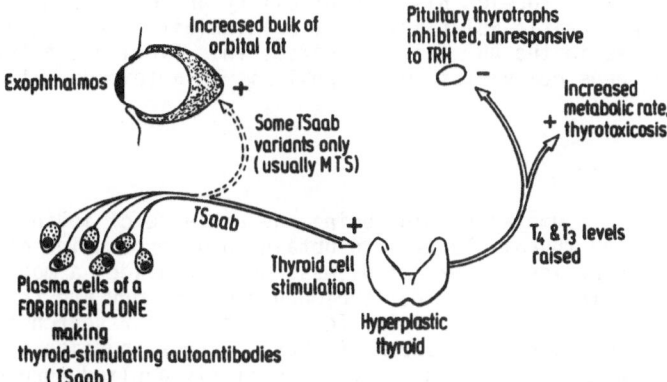

Fig. 3. The pathogenesis of the thyrotoxicosis and exophthalmos of Graves' disease. MTS is mouse thyroid-stimulator, another name for LATS. Reproduced with permission from Patient Management 1978; 7: no.11 : 11.

7

be rare. If so, the usual mechanism by which an H antigen tolerance induction predisposes to an autoimmune disease may be through alternative clonal development[44], based on competition between clones for antigenic contact, clones with lower affinities being shut out by ones with higher affinities. H antigen deletion of a high affinity clone for a microbial antigen may permit development and somatic diversification of a lower affinity clone for a related microbial antigen, and so provide different specificities, with increased risk of a particular autoimmunity[44].

It had been thought that H antigen influence on immune reactivity was mediated at the antigen presentation stage but there is now clear evidence that such effects can be based on tolerance induction[45]. The H antigen theory provides a much more comprehensive explanation of the genetic predisposition to autoimmune disease than does the previous concept, that MHC antigens are in linkage disequilibrium with undiscovered, disease-causing genes with unknown gene products and unknown mode of action[46].

FUTURE THERAPY AND PROPHYLAXIS

Burnet's forbidden clone theory focuses attention on the need to devise technology for the selective destruction of forbidden clones as the ideal therapy for autoimmune disease. Forbidden clones bear two potential targets, their paratopes and their idiotopes, both possibly utilizable for their destruction. Furthermore, Burnet's theory defines the objective for establishing the pathogenesis of suspected autoimmune diseases, namely to find the forbidden clone of T cells or B cells and its precise autoantigen.

Prophylaxis of autoimmune disease may prove easier to achieve than therapy. The decrease of in rheumatic fever[19] with decrease in epidemics of untreated streptococcal pharyngitis illustrates how autoimmune disease can be prevented by removal of a microbial antigenic trigger. Weiss, Ingbar et al[47] have shown that the gut bacterium, *Yersinia enterocolitica* has a saturable binding site for thyrotrophin. This suggests that B cell reactivity against this organism may be an essential step in the development of Graves' disease. Similar microbial antigenic triggering is likely to be the rule for autoimmune diseases. Multiple sclerosis is more common in people in cool climates than in genetically-similar people in warm climates,[19] again suggesting involvement of a microbial antigenic trigger, either predisposing in the cold climate or protective in the warm climate. Search for such antigenic triggers warrants intense effort, as their removal, by judicous vaccination or by other means, could provide very effective prophylaxis. Another approach is indicated by Naji et al's[48] finding that tolerance induction to foreign histocompatibility antigens (done in preparation for pancreatic islet allografting) inhibits development of autoimmune diabetes in the BB strain of rats. This finding confirms the H gene theory and opens new vistas for prophylaxis of autoimmune disease.

SUMMARY

A number of circumstances, including the presence of iodine in thyroid hormone,have enabled thyroidologists to obtain an understanding of the pathogenesis and genetics of Graves' disease which provides a model for autoimmune disease in general. The forbidden clone theory and the H gene theory provide badly-needed principles for direction of research towards therapeutic and prophylactic conquest of these distressing diseases. With our increasing technical competence more effectively applied through application of these two simple theories, we appear to be on the eve of a advance in medicine comparable to that which followed application of Pasteur's germ theory of disease.

REFERENCES

1. Harington CR. The Thyroid Gland. London, Oxford University Press, 1933.
2. Ehrlich P, Morgenroth J. In: The collected papers of Paul Ehrlich Himmelweit F, ed. Oxford: Pergamon, 1956.
3. Doniach D, Roitt IM. Autoimmunity in Hashimoto's disease and its implications. J Clin Endocrinol Metab 1957; 27: 1293-1304.
4. Witebsky E, Rose NR, Terplan K, Paine JR, Egan RW. Chronic thyroiditis and autoimmunisation. J Am Med Ass 1957; 164: 1439-1447.
5. Adams DD. The presence of an abnormal thyroid-stimulating hormone in the serum of some thyrotoxic patients. J Clin Endocrinol Metab 1958; 28: 699-712.
6. McKenzie JM. Delayed thyroid response to serum from thyrotoxic patients. Endocrinology 1958; 62: 865-868.
7. Munro DS. Observations on the discharge of radioiodine from the thyroid glands of mice injected with human sera. J Endocrinol 1959; 19: 64-73.
8. Kriss JP, Pleshakov V, Chien JR. Isolation and identification of the long-acting thyroid stimulator and its relation to hyperthyroidism and pretibial myxedema. J Clin Endocrinol Metab 1964; 24: 1005-1028.
9. Smith BR, Dorrington KJ, Munro DS. The thyroid-stimulating properties of long-acting thyroid stimulator γG-globulin subunits. Biochem Biophys Acta 1969; 192: 277-285.
10. Manley SW, Bourke JR, Hawker RW. The thyrotrophin receptor in guinea-pig homogenate: interaction with the long-acting thyroid stimulator. J Endocrinol 1974; 61: 437-445.
11. Adams DD. Pathogenesis of the hyperthyroidism of Graves' disease. Brit Med J 1965; 1: 1015-1019.
12. Adams DD, Kennedy TH. Occurrence in thyrotoxicosis of a gamma globulin which protects LATS from neutralization by an extract of thyroid gland. J Clin Endocrinol Metab 1967; 27: 173-177.
13. Adams DD, Kennedy TH. Evidence to suggest that LATS-P stimulates the human thyroid gland. J Clin Endocrinol Metab 1971; 33: 47-51.
14. Adams DD, Fastier FN, Howie JB, Kennedy TH, Kilpatrick JA, Stewart RDH. Stimulation of the human thyroid by infusions of plasma containing LATS protector. J Clin Endocrinol Metab 1974; 39: 826-832.
15. Adams DD, Kennedy TH, Stewart RDH. Correlation between long-acting thyroid stimulator protector level and thyroid ^{131}I uptake in thyrotoxicosis. Brit Med J 1974; 2: 199-201.
16. Munro DS, Dirmikis SM, Humphries H, Smith T, Broadhead GD. The role of thyroid stimulating immunoglobulins of Graves' disease in neonatal thyrotoxicosis. Brit J Obst & Gyn 1978; 85: 837-843.
17. Jerne NK. The natural selection theory of antibody formation. Proc Natl Acad Sci USA 1955; 41: 849-857.
18. Burnet FM. The Clonal Selection Theory of Acquired Immunity. Cambridge: University Press, 1959.
19. Wyngaarden JB, Smith LH, eds. Cecil Textbook of Medicine. 17th ed. Philadelphia: Saunders, 1985.
20. Knight A, Adams DD. Autoantibodies with intrinsic biological activity. Hormone Research 1980; 13: 69-80.
21. Zakarija M, McKenzie JM. Immunochemical characterization of TSab: evidence against its polyclonal nature. In: Thyroid Research VIII Canberra, Australian Academy of Science, 1980: 669-672.
22. Zakarija M. Immunochemical characterization of the thyroid-stimulating antibody of Graves' disease. J Clin Lab Immunol 1983; 10: 77-85.
23. Knight JG, et al. Thyroid stimulating autoantibodies usually contain only λ light chains: evidence for the forbidden clone theory. J Clin Endocrinol Metab 1986; 62: 342-347.
24. Laing P. Both κ and λ light chain types are present in thyroid microsomal and thyroglobulin autoantibodies. Proc Univ Otago Med Sch 1983; 61: 75-77.

25. Knight A, Adams DD. Absence of allotypic variation in the autoantigen for TSab. Clin Exp Immunol 1983; 52: 317-324.
26. Adams DD. Thyroid-stimulating autoantibodies. Vitamins and Hormones 1980; 38: 119-203.
27. Ludgate ME, et al. Failure to demonstrate cell-mediated immune responses to thyroid antigens in Graves' disease using in vitro assays of lymphokine-mediated migration inhibition. J Clin Endocrinol Metab 1985; 60: 98-102.
28. Beall GN, Kruger SR. Production of human antithyroglobulin in vitro. I Stimulation by mitogens. II Regulation by T cells. Clin Immunol Immunopathol 1980; 16: 485-497, 498-503.
29. Rundle F, Pochin E. The orbital tissues in thyrotoxicosis: a quantitative analysis relating to exophthalmos. Clin Sci 1944; 5: 51-74.
30. Rundle FF, Finlay-Jones LR, Noad KB. Malignant exophthalmos: a quantitative analysis of the orbital tissues. Australas Ann Med 1953; 2: 128-135.
31. Kriss JP, Pleshakov V, Rosenblum AL et al. Studies on the pathogenesis of the ophthalmopathy of Graves' disease. J Clin Endocrinol Metab 1967; 27: 582-593.
32. Hardisty CA, Fowles A, Munro DS. Serum long-acting thyroid stimulator (LATS and LATS-P) in Graves' disease associated with localized myxoedema. J Endocrinol Invest 1984; 7: 151-155.
33. Hart IR, McKenzie JM. Comparison of the effects of thyrotrophin and the long-acting thyroid stimulator on guinea-pig adipose tissue. Endocrinology 1971; 88: 26-30.
34. Knight JG, Adams DD. The genetic basis of autoimmune disease. Ciba Foundation Symposium 1982; 90: 35-56.
35. Bartels ED. Heredity in Graves'disease. Copenhagen: Munksgaard, 1941.
36. McKusick VA. Mendelian Inheritance in Man. 6th ed. Baltimore: Johns Hopkins, 1983.
37. McDevitt HO, Chinitz A. Genetic control of the antibody response: relationship between immune response and histocompatibility (H-2) type. Science 1969; 163: 1207-1208.
38. Vladutiu AO, Rose NR. Autoimmune murine thyroiditis. Relation to histocompatibility (H-2) type. Science 1971; 174: 1137-1138.
39. Grumet FC, Payne RD, Konishi J, Kriss JP. HL-A antigens as markers for disease susceptibility and autoimmunity in Graves' disease. J Clin Endocrinol Metab 1974; 39: 1115-1119.
40. Tiwari JL, Terasaki PI. HLA and Disease Associations. Berlin: Springer-Verlag, 1985.
41. Nossal JGV, Pike B. Evidence for the clonal abortion theory of B-lymphocyte tolerance. J Exp Med 1975; 141: 904-917.
42. Adams DD, Knight JG. H gene theory of inherited autoimmune disease. Lancet 1980; 1: 396-398.
43. Jerne NK. Towards a network theory of the immune system. Ann Inst Pasteur (Paris); 1974; 125C: 373-389.
44. Adams DD, Adams YJ, Knight JG, McCall J, White P, Horrocks R, van Loghem E. A solution to the genetic and environmental puzzles of insulin-dependent diabetes mellitus. Lancet 1984; 1: 420-424.
45. Dos Reis GA, Shevach EM. Antigen-presenting cells from non-responder strain 2 guinea pigs are fully competent to present bovine insulin B chain to responder strain 13 T cells. J Exp Med 1983; 157: 1287-1299.
46. Adams DD. Autoimmune mechanisms. In: Davies TF, ed. Autoimmune Endocrine Disease, New York: Wiley, 1983: 1-39.
47. Weiss M, Ingbar SH, Winblad S, Kasper DL. Demonstration of a saturable binding site for thyrotrophin in Yersinia enterocolitica. Science 1983; 219: 1331-1333.
48. Naji A, Silvers WK, Bellgrau D, Barker CF. Spontaneous diabetes in rats: destruction of islets is prevented by immunological tolerance. Science 1981; 213: 1390-1392.

NATURE OF THYROID AUTOANTIGENS: THE TSH RECEPTOR

John Chan, Michele De Luca, Pilar Santisteban,
Osamu Isozaki, Sid Shifrin, Salvatore M. Aloj,
Evelyn F. Grollman, and Leonard D. Kohn

National Institute of Diabetes Digestive and Kidney Diseases
National Institute of Health, Bethesda, MD 20892

INTRODUCTION

Graves' disease is an autoimmune disorder of the thyroid (Adams, 1981) characterized by a goiter and hyperthyroidism. The concept that the signs and symptoms of Graves' disease reflected the action of circulating antibodies to the TSH receptor evolved because thyroid stimulating antibodies (TSAbs) increased adenylate cyclase activity as did TSH (McKenzie and Zakarija, 1977; Zakarija and McKenzie, 1980; Adams, 1981; Kasagi, et al., 1982) and because IgG preparations from Graves' patients could inhibit TSH binding to thyroid membrane preparations (TBIAb activity) (Smith and Hall, 1974; Manley et al. 1974; Mehdi and Nussey, 1975). It was argued the two activities were exhibited by the same antibody. Unfortunately the concept ran into several problems. Thus, in most studies, assays measuring thyroid stimulating antibodies (TSAbs) and thyrotropin binding inhibiting antibodies (TBIAbs) did not correlate in a significant number of patients. (Ozawa et al, 1979; Sugenoya et al, 1979; Pinchera et al, 1980; Zakarija and McKenzie, 1980; Macchia et al, 1981). Further several studies indicated that the growth stimulating activity of Graves' IgG preparations did not correlate with the thyroid stimulating activity in all cases (Doniach et al, 1980; Drexhage et al, 1980, 1981; Valente et al, 1983).

MONOCLONAL ANTIBODY STUDIES RESOLVE QUESTIONS

Studies which isolated and characterized monoclonal antibodies to the TSH receptor were able to resolve these questions (Yavin et al, 1981; Valente et al, 1982a,b, 1983; Kohn et al, 1983b, 1984, 1985a,b, 1986a,b; Ealey et al, 1984, 1985). Thus, these studies identified several types antibodies to the TSH receptor, each with different activities but all of which were specific, competitive agonists or antagonists of TSH (Table 1). One group, representative of TBIAbs, inhibited TSH binding and TSH stimulated adenylate cyclase activity; none of this group exhibited an ability to increase adenylate cyclase activity but some had growth action. A second group were TSAbs able to increase adenylate cyclase activity, iodide uptake, and iodide release from prelabeled glands in vivo; all were poor inhibitors of TSH binding and all could induce the

growth of thyroid cells. A third group with both TBIAb and TSAb
properties, therefore termed mixed antibodies, were extremely potent
growth stimulators, better than TSAbs relative to their adenylate cyclase
stimulatory activity.

In sum, there was a multiplicity of antibodies to the TSH receptor,
each with a different spectrum of TSH binding-inhibition activity,
adenylate cyclase stimulatory action, and growth potential (Table 1).
These observations reconciled the clinical discrepancies and established
that all the signs and symptoms of Graves' disease could indeed be
related to antibodies to the TSH receptor.

TSH RECEPTOR STRUCTURE AND SIGNAL TRANSDUCTION

The monoclonal antibodies have now been used to define the TSH
receptor structure and to examine the nature of the signal transduction
systems used by the antibodies to initiate their activities.

Previous studies have defined two membrane components on thyroid
membranes which interact with TSH with some degree of specificity (Kohn,
1978; Kohn and Shifrin, 1982; Kohn et al, 1980, 1982, 1983a, 1984,
1985a,b; Laccetti et al, 1984). The first, a membrane glycoprotein, was
generally agreed to be the component of the TSH receptor that bound TSH
to the cell with high affinity; its loss, for example, when cells were
exposed to trypsin, resulted in a loss in both TSH-binding and
TSH-stimulated functions. The role of the second component, a membrane
ganglioside, was more controversial. The evidence for its physiologic
importance derived mainly from the observations that (i) higher order
gangliosides, with the ability to interact with TSH, were absent in a
thyroid tumor that had lost its functional TSH receptor; (ii) resynthesis
or reconstitution of gangliosides in membranes from this tumor could
cause both a return of the ability of TSH to stimulate adenylate-cyclase
activity; (iii) this reconstitution was effected by a thyroid-specific
ganglioside. The ganglioside was also suggested to modulate the apparent
specificity, affinity, and capacity of the glycoprotein receptor
component and induce a conformational change in the hormone believed to
be necessary for subsequent message transmission. It appeared to couple
the high affinity binding site to the adenylate-cyclase signal system by
acting as an emulsifying agent to allow the hormone and receptor to
interact with other membrane components within the hydrophobic
environment of the lipid bilayer.

Using monoclonal antibodies to the TSH receptor (Yavin et al, 1981;
Valente et al, 1982a,b, 1983; Kohn et al., 1983b, 1984, 1985a,b, 1986a,b)
the relationship of both membrane components to the physiologic TSH
receptor has been confirmed (Fig. 1). Thus, the glycoprotein receptor
component was shown to react with the thyrotropin binding inhibiting
antibodies and be the high affinity TSH binding site. The ganglioside
component was the primary thyroid stimulating antibody (TSAb) binding
site and exhibited low affinity binding to TSH. The TSH binding to the
glycoprotein is relatively salt insensitive (Meldolesi et al, 1977) and
that to the ganglioside is salt sensitive (Aloj et al, 1979). Expression
of the salt sensitive site in cell culture systems used to measure TSH
and TSAb action causes enhanced expression of bioactivity as measured by
increases in cAMP levels and membrane potential (Grollman et al, 1977;
Kasagi et al, 1983; Ambesi-Impiombato, 1986).

Solubilization studies of the glycoprotein component of the TSH
receptor have defined components of approximately 300K (Tate 1975; Kohn
1978; Kohn et al, 1983a, 1985a,b; Czarnocka et al, 1981; Iida et al,
1983; Drummond et al, 1982; Kress et al, 1986). Our cross-linking
studies have also defined a receptor component which is a 70K structure

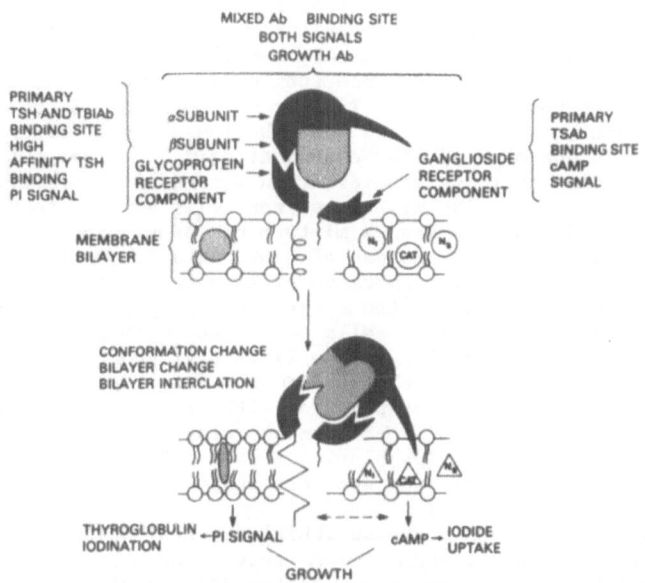

Figure 1. Model of TSH receptor based on binding studies with ^{125}I-TSH and on studies involving monoclonal antibodies to the TSH receptor. The evidence indicates that the glycoprotein receptor component is linked to a Ca^+/IP_3/arachidonate (PI) signal system, whereas the ganglioside is linked to cAMP signaling. The PI function identified is iodide transport into the follicular lumen and iodination of thyroglobulin. A cAMP function is iodide uptake into the cell from the bloodstream. It is presumed that the beta subunit of TSH has the primary recognition determinants based on reconstitution experiments; the alpha subunit does, however, contribute more than a conformational constraint on the beta subunit. The alpha-subunit portion that intercalates within the bilayer is presumed to include that region with nonapeptide hormone sequence analogies.

composed of ~50K and ~20K pieces (Kohn et al, 1983, 1985a,b). The same picture has emerged in cross-linking studies by Smith and his colleagues (Buckland et al, 1985). Radiation inactivation has defined both a >250K and a ~70K TSH binding component (Nielsen et al, 1984). There are, however, numerous oher reports of TSH binding membrane components, i.e., components of ~200K, ~175K, 130K, 90K, 30K, etc. (Heyma et al, 1984; Islam et al, 1985; Eggo et al, 1985). The reality of the physiologic TSH receptor has thus been an enigma. To try and resolve this, we used FRTL-5 thyroid cells labeled with [^{35}S]methionine and/or [^{3}H]glucosamine and ^{125}I-surface-labeled bovine thyroid membranes. We purified the TSH binding components by sequential chromatography of detergent solubilized membrane preparations on TSH affinity columns followed by immunopurification using our monoclonal antibodies.

Whether membrane preparations were from cells treated with TSH or those which had not been exposed to TSH for over 5 days, two peaks of radiolabeled protein could be eluted from the TSH-affinity column, the first at high salt and high pH, the second at acid pH values. Both peaks were further purified by immunoprecipitation with a TBIAb monoclonal, 11E8. In the experiment using membranes from cells exposed to TSH, the first peak contained a heterogeneous mixture of TSH binding proteins, the second only two, one of ~300K and one of ~70K. Studies with the surface-labeled bovine thyroid membranes yielded the same data. The data were very different if, however, the experiment was performed using solubilized membranes from FRTL-5 cells maintained without TSH. One then saw the 70K protein predominating in the first peak and the ~300K TSH binding protein nearly alone in the second peak (Fig. 2A) of the TSH affinity columns after immunoprecipitation with the 11E8 antibody. The ~300K protein behaves as a single homogeneous protein when subjected to gel filtration on guanidine-hydrochloride, has a molecular weight of ~310K on the guanidine column, and does not react with antibodies to thyroglobulin.

If, however, one removes protease inhibitors from the buffers, the ~300K protein breaks down to form a ~70K protein which has the same amino acid composition and tryptic map as the 70K protein isolated in the first peak (Fig. 2B).

TSH causes the thyroid cell to increase both the synthesis and degradation of the glycoprotein receptor component (Fig. 3). This apparently results in further fragmentation of the 70K receptor derivative to ~50K and ~20K fragments (Fig. 3), which were seen in the cross-linking studies and in immunoprecipitation studies using solubilized membranes from thyroid tissues removed from different animal species (Kohn et al, 1983a, 1985a,b).

Incorporation of [^{35}S]methionine into the TSH receptor in FRTL-5 cells as a function of time indicates that there is progressive incorporation of label into the ~300K protein over 36 hrs but a turnover of the 70K protein suggesting a 6-12 hr half life. These data also raise the possibility that there are two ~70K receptor pieces which are nonidentical.

The ~300K protein reacts with the autoimmune TBIAbs such as 122G3 or 129H8 (Fig. 2C). Surprisingly, it also reacts with the TSAbs whose predominant in vitro reaction was with the ganglioside (Fig. 3C). This last observation is explained by the fact that the ganglioside is tightly bound to the glycoprotein. Thus, when the immunoprecipitates of the glycoprotein receptor component, obtained with either a TSAb or TBIAb, are Folch extracted, thin-layer chromatography of the aqueous soluble lipid extract shows that the glycoprotein contains a specific ganglioside distinct from the total ganglioside pool (Fig. 4). In bovine thyroid glycoprotein receptor component preparations, this ganglioside is the

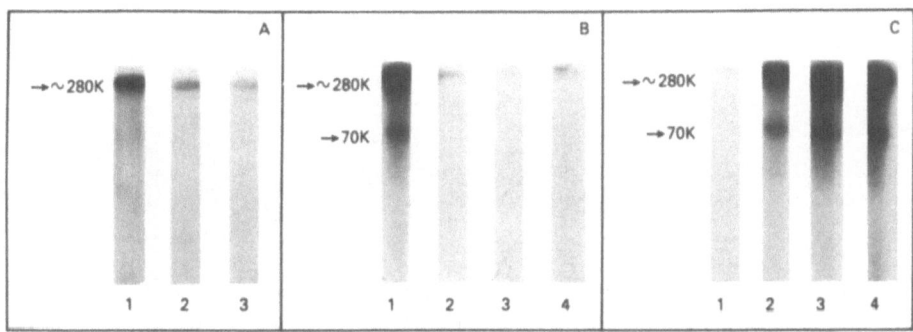

Figure 2. (A) Autoradiograph of analytic slab gels containing a [^{35}S]-methionine-labeled ~280K TSH receptor from FRTL-5 rat thyroid cells maintained for 3 days with no TSH. The gels depict results after sequential purification (12,000-fold) by TSH affinity chromatography and 11E8 monoclonal anti-TSH receptor immunopurification. Gel 1: Purified receptor eluted from 11E8 antibody bound to Sepharose. Gel 2: Decreased amount of receptor is bound to 11E8-Sepharose-coupled antibody when it is coincubated with 1 x 10^{-10}M TSH. Gel 3: No significant 280K receptor is bound to normal mouse IgG coupled to Sepharose when eluted as per Gel 1. Gels are 5% acrylamide and are run using a sodium dodecyl sulfate - 0.1M mercaptoethanol buffer system. (B) Autoradiography of a [^{35}S]-methionine-labeled TSH receptor purified from FRTL-5 thyroid cells (as noted in Figure 2A), and then incubated 24 hours in buffers wherein the aprotinin protease inhibitor used in purification buffers was removed. Gel 1: Material from Gel 1, Fig. 2A incubated without aprotinin, then reimmunoprecipitated with 11E8-Sepharose antibody to TSH receptor. Gel 2: The same material as used in the Gel 1 experiment, but incubated with 1 x 10^{-10}M TSH during the second immunoprecipitation. Neither the ~280K receptor glycoprotein nor the 70K fragment now bind to 11E8. Gel 3 and 4, respectively: No receptor binds or elutes if 11E8-Sepharose is replaced with normal mouse IgG-Sepharose or with Sepharose coupled to a "normal" mouse monoclonal that binds to thyroid membranes, but is not directed against the TSH receptor. (C) Immunoprecipitation of TSH receptor by normal human IgG coupled to Sepharose (Gel 1) by human IgG monoclonal TBIAb, 129H8 (Gel 2) or 122G3 (Gel 3); or by a human monoclonal TSAb, 307H6 (Gel 4).

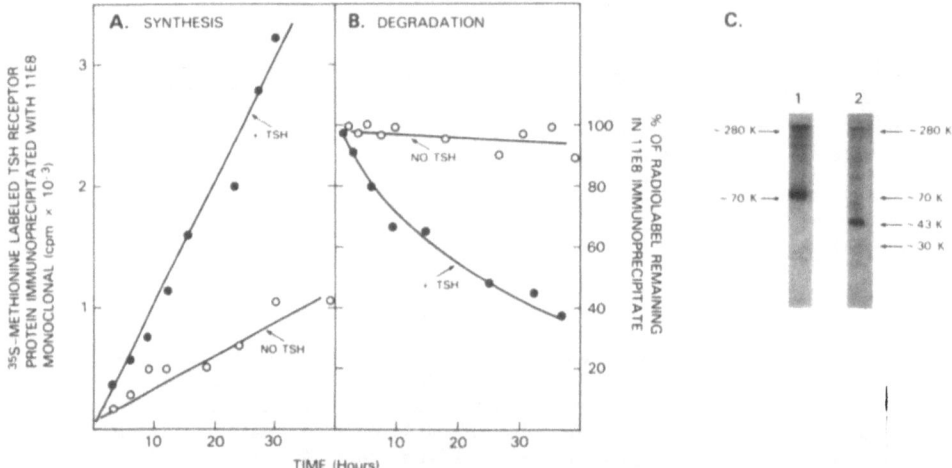

Figure 3. TSH regulation of the synthesis (A) and degradation (B) of the
TSH receptor glycoprotein in FRTL-5 cells as measured by
[^{35}S]-methionine incorporation into 11E8 monoclonal (TBIAb)
immunoprecipitable receptor material after pulsing cells with
[^{35}S]-methionine (A) or after an equilibrium labeling period followed
by a "chase" with medium without radiolabeled methionine (B). In A,
FRTL-5 cells were grown in the presence of TSH to near confluency. At
zero time, [^{35}S]-methionine was added and the cells maintained in the
presence or absence of TSH. At the times noted, cells were washed,
solubilized with a triton/deoxycholate/ sodium-dodecyl-sulfate mixture,
and immunoprecipitated with 11E8 coupled to Sepharose or normal IgG
coupled to Sepharose. The 11E8-specific, immunoprecipitable radiolabel
was plotted as a function of time. In (B), the cells were equilibrium
labeled by incubating them in the absence of TSH and in
[^{35}S]-methionine for four days, at which time fresh media with
unlabeled methionine and with TSH (+) or without TSH (NO) was added. The
cells were solubilized at the times noted and the 11E8-bound radiolabel
was measured. In (C), the autoradiography of 11E8 immunoprecipitable
material from a [^{35}S]-methionine equilibrium labeled FRTL-5 cell not
exposed to TSH for five days is compared with that from a comparably
labeled FRTL-5 cell exposed to TSH for one day. The TSH causes a
dramatic decrease in the ~70K 11E8 binding component and an increase in
the components having molecular weights of approximately 50K and 20K.

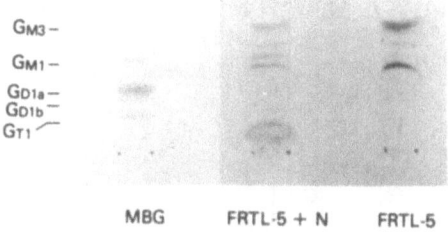

A. TOTAL FRTL-5 GANGLIOSIDES

G_{M3} –
G_{M1} –
G_{D1a} –
G_{D1b} –
G_{T1}

MBG   FRTL-5 + N   FRTL-5

B. EXTRACTED FROM RECEPTOR GLYCOPROTEIN

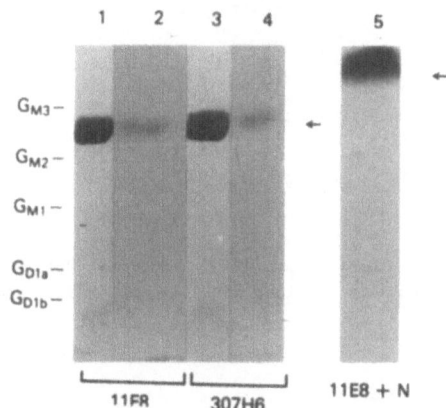

1   2   3   4   5

G_{M3} –
G_{M2} –
G_{M1} –
G_{D1a} –
G_{D1b} –

11FR   307H6   11E8 + N

Figure 4. (A) Thin layer chromatogram of gangliosides extracted from
FRTL–5 cell membranes before (FRTL–5) and after (FRTL–5 + N)
neuraminidase treatment. A mixed brain ganglioside mixtue (MBG) is
presented as a control. Detection is by resorcinol staining. (B)
Thin–layer chromatography of the gangliosides extracted from the
12,000–fold purified ~280K TSH receptor glycoprotein from FRTL–5 cells
after it was immunopurified by 11E8 (lanes 1, 2 and 5) or after it was
immunopurified by 307H6 (Gels 3 and 4). The ~280K protein was from
FRTL–5 cells labeled with [³H]–N–acetyl glucosamine. The thin–layer
plates were cut in strips and they either were resorcinol stained (lanes
2 and 4) or subjected to autoradiography (lanes 3 and 5). Gangliosides
were extracted and purified after the ~280K receptor glycoprotein
preparation was sonicated (Ultrasonics, Inc., Model W185 D cell
disrupter; 3 min; output 3) under a stream of nitrogen. The final
fraction was obtained using a sep Pak™ cartridge. The purified
fractions, dried under a stream of nitrogen and dissolved in methanol,
were chromatographed on silica gel 60 HP–TLC plates (E. Merck, Darmstadt,
Germany). The running buffer was chloroform: methanol:KCl 2.5 mg/ml
(120:70:16 by vol). Neuraminidase treatment (+N) of a ganglioside
preparation was for 24 hours with a cholera vibrio enzyme; reactions were
terminated by 10–fold dilution with methanol; the gangliosides were
reconstituted in buffer after drying with a stream of nitrogen.
Gangliosides were chromatographed with authentic standards, each of whose
migration is noted.

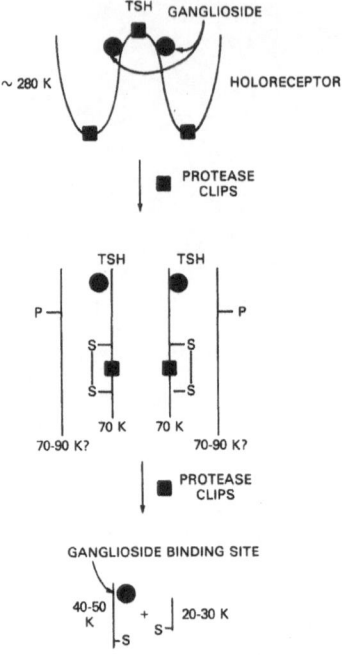

TSH RECEPTOR STRUCTURE

Figure 5. Tentative model of TSH receptor structure. The possibility of non TSH binding subunits analogous to the insulin or IGF-I receptor structure cannot be excluded.

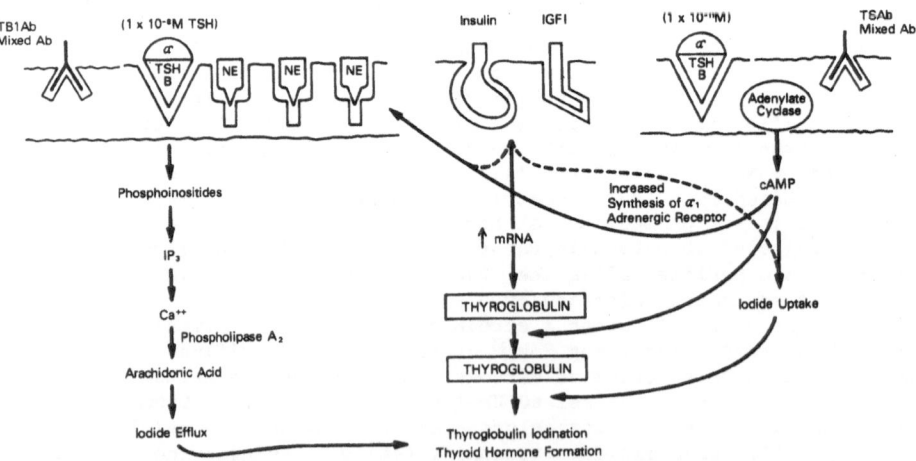

Figure 6. Signal induction systems important for thyroid hormone formation and their regulation by TSH, TSAbs, TBIAbs, and mixed antibodies.

Table 1. Representative Monoclonal Antibodies to the TSH Receptor[a]

Clone No.	TSH Receptor Source	Primary Classification[d]	Growth Activity (degree)[e]	Exophthalmogenic Activity[f]
13D11	bovine	TBIAb	no	yes
11E8	bovine	TBIAb	no	yes
59C9	human	TBIAb	no	no
60F5	human	TBIAb	yes(++)	no
129H8[b]	human	TBIAb	yes(+)	weak
122G3[b]	human	TBIAb	no	weak
22A6	bovine	TSAb	yes(+)	no
206H3[b]	human	TSAb	yes(++)	no
307H6[b,c]	human	TSAb	yes(++)	yes
304D3[b,c]	human	TSAb	yes(+)	no
308L2[b,c]	human	TSAb	yes(+)	no
410F9[b]	human	TSAb	yes(+)	no
52A8	human	mixed	yes(++++)	no
208F7[b]	human	mixed	yes(+++)	no

[a]Each monoclonal had the ability to be competitively and specifically inhibited from binding to thyroid membranes, i.e., it was inhibited by TSH but not by luteinizing hormone, human chorionic gonadotropin, insulin, glucagon, or albumin. Each was a competitive antagonist or competitive agonist of TSH in assays measuring adenylate cyclase activity.
[b] Heterohybridomas derived from lymphocytes of Graves' patients
[c] From the same patient.
[d] A TBIAb is an antibody which competitively inhibits TSH binding and TSH activity in assays of adenylate cyclase action, iodide uptake, or thyroid hormone release in vivo. None has significant stimulatory activity in these assays. A TSAb is a stimulator of activity in assays of adenylate cyclase action, iodide uptake, and thyroid hormone release in vivo; although they are inhibited from binding to thyroid membranes by TSH, they are weak inhibitors of TSH binding. Mixed antibodies have properties of a TSAb and TBIAb but can be distinguished in mixing experiments and in asays of growth activity in FRTL-5 thyroid cells, i.e., per unit of adenylate cyclase stimulatory action they are significantly more potent in stimulating growth than TSAbs, whether measuring cell number or thymidine uptake activity.
[e]Measured as increases in cell number or thymidine uptake in FRTL-5 cells.
[f]Ability to act like IgG preparations from exophthalmos patients in increasing collagen synthesis but not cAMP levels or growth in fibroblasts (Rotella et al 1986).

Table 2. Effect of Monoclonal Antibodies to the TSH Receptor
on the Growth of FRTL-5 Thyroid Cells as Measured by Radiolabeled
Thymidine Uptake into DNA

Monoclonal Antibody	[^{3}H]-Thymidine Uptake[a] Alone	(cpm/μg DNA) +Indomethacin
None	1600	1400
N1 IgG	1450	1510
TSH 1 x 10^{-10}M	6800	3500
1 x 10^{-9} M	31,000	14,000
"Stimulating" TSAbs[b]		
22A6	6800	6900
307H6	8700	9200
"Mixed" Antibodies[b]		
52A8	28,600	7400
208F7	24,700	6500
"Inhibiting" TBIAbs		
122G3	9350	1460
129H8	5600	1480

[a]Seventy-two-hour thymidine uptake (Valente et al, 1983).
[b]Tested at concentrations of IgG that increased cAMP levels in FRTL-5
thyroid cells to exactly the same extent.

same as a thyroid-specific ganglioside (Mullin et al, 1978) identified in earlier experiments to have the highest ability to inhibit TSH binding to thyroid membranes. Little is known about the ganglioside. It fractionates on DEAE as a disialoglycolipid; it probably has a G_{DIb} rather than a G_{DIa} configuration; it is sensitive to neuraminidase treatment, which destroys its reactivity with the TSAbs; and it appears to contain a fucose residue.

The sum of these data supports a TSH receptor structure as depicted in Fig. 5. The ~300K glycoprotein is a primary synthetic structure; at least two ~70K units are derived from the ~300K structure by protease action. The ~50K and ~20K units are formed from the ~70K unit by protease action; the ~50K unit has bound ganglioside. Whereas the ~300K and ~70K pieces predominate under conditions where TSH increases cAMP levels; the ~50K fragment is linked to a growth action of TSH separate from cAMP.

Monoclonal antibodies studies support the idea that both the growth and function of the FRTL-5 thyroid cell appears to involve both a cAMP signal and a signal involving phosphoinositides/IP_3/Ca^{++}/ phospholipase A2/ and arachidonate (Fig. 1) (Kohn et al, 1986c, Philp and Grollman, 1986; Bone et al, 1986; Corda and Kohn, 1985; Corda et al, 1985; Burch et al, 1986; Santisteban et al 1987; Marcocci et al, 1987). Studies with monoclonal antibodies indicate that the ganglioside is the receptor component coupled to the adenylate cyclase complex whereas the glycoprotein receptor component is more linked to the IP_3/Ca^{++}/ arachidonate signal system (Fig. 1). The difference in a growth as opposed to a functional response, when either TSH or a monoclonal antibody interact with the glycoprotein component of the TSH receptor and initiate the Ca^{++}/arachidonate transduction signal, seems to be whether an indomethacin sensitive, cycloxygenase derivative of arachidonic acid is involved as an intermediate (growth) or a ETYA sensitive lipoxygenase derivative of arachidonate is the intermediate (function) (Kohn et al, 1986c; Marcocci et al, 1987; Burch et al 1986; Santisteban et al, 1987).

Thus TSAbs stimulate growth via an indomethacin insensitive cAMP signal; some TBIAbs stimulate growth via an indomethacin-sensitive IP_3/Ca^{++}/arachidonate signal; the mixed antibodies or TSH invoke both (Table 2). Thyroid hormone formation is a complex process involving iodide uptake, iodide efflux into the follicular lumen, thyroglobulin synthesis, vectorial transport of thyroglobulin to the follicular lumen, and iodination of thyroglobulin. TSAbs stimulate iodide uptake via the cAMP signal (Fig. 6) (Weiss et al 1984a; Marcocci et al 1985). TSAbs do not stimulate iodide efflux or iodination of thyroglobulin whereas some TBIAbs and mixed monoclonal antibodies do (Fig. 6) (Weiss et al 1985b, Santisteban, 1987a). TSAbs and cAMP can increase thyroglobulin synthesis but full expression requires insulin and/or IGF-I (Santisteban 1986, 1987b) (Fig. 6).

SUMMARY

Studies of monoclonal antibodies to the TSH receptor show that different autoantibodies to the TSH receptor can exist in the same patient and can cause different effects on growth and thyroid hormone formation. These different efects appear to be caused by interactions with different determinants of the TSH receptor which, in turn, can be coupled to different transduction signals. It thus is not surprising that the spectrum of TSH receptor autoantibodies in Graves' causes a varied phenotypic expression rather than a uniform well defined clinical syndrome.

REFERENCES

Adams, D. D., 1981, Thyroid stimulating autoantibodies, in: "Vitamins and Hormones," E. Diczfalusy and R. E. Olson, eds., Academic Press, New York, p 119.

Aloj, S. M, Lee, G., Consiglio, E., Formisano, S., Minton, A. P., and Kohn, L. D., 1979, Dansylated thyrotropin as a probe of hormone-receptor interactions, J. Biol. Chem., 254:9030.

Ambesi-Impiombato, F. S., 1986, Living, fast growing thyroid cell strain, FRTL-5. United States Patent No. 4,608,341.

Bone, E. A., Alling, D. W., and Grollman, E. F., 1986, Norepinephrine and thyroid stimulating hormone induce inositol phosphate accumulation in FRTL-5 cells. Endocrinology 119, in press.

Burch, R. M., Luini, A., Mais, D. E., Corda, D., Vanderhoek, J. Y., Kohn, L. D., and Axelrod, J., 1986, α_1 Adrenergic stimulation of arachidonic acid release and metabolism in a rat thyroid cell line. Mediation of cell replication by prostaglandin E_2. J. Biol. Chem. 261:11236.

Buckland, P. R., Howells, R. D., Richards, C. R., and Rees Smith, B., 1985, Affinity-labeling of the thyrotropin receptor. Characterization of the photoactive ligand, Biochem J. 225:753.

Corda, D., and Kohn, L. D., 1985, TSH upregulates α_1 adrenergic receptors in rat FRTL-5 thyroid cells. Proc. Natl. Acad. Sci., USA 82:8677

Corda, D., Marcocci, C., Kohn, L. D., Axelrod, J., and Luini, A., 1985, Association of the changes in cytosolic Ca^{++} and iodide efflux induced by thyrotropin and by the stimulation of α_1 adrenergic receptors in cultured rat thyroid cells. J. Biol. Chem., 260:9230.

Corda, D., and Kohn, L. D., 1987, Phorbol myristate acetate inhibits α_1 adrenergic but not TSH regulated functions in FRTL-5 thyroid cells, Endocrinology, in press.

Czarnocka, B., Gardas, A., and Nauman, J., 1981, Thyrotropin binding glycoprotein isolated from bovine thyroid, Acta Endocrinol (Copenh), 96:335.

Doniach, D., Bottazzo, G. F., and Khoury, E. L., 1980, Prospects in human autoimmune thyroiditis, in: "Autoimmune Aspects of Endocrine Disorders", A. Pinchera, D. Doniach, G. F. Fenzi, and L. Baschieri, eds., Academic Press, London, p 25.

Drexhage, H. A., Bottazzo, G. F., and Doniach, D., 1980, Evidence for thyroid growth-stimulating immunoglobulins in some goitrous thyroid diseases, Lancet, 2:287.

Drexhage, H. A., Bottazzo, G. F., Bitensky, L., Chayen, J., and Doniach, D., 1981, Thyroid growth-blocking antibodies in primary myxedema, Nature, 289:594.

Drummond, R. W., McQuade R., Grunwald, R., Thomas, Jr., C. J., Nayfeh, S. N., 1982, Separation of two thyrotropin binding components from porcine thyroid tissue by affinity chromatography: characterization of high and low affinity sites. Proc. Natl. Acad. Sci., USA, 79:2202.

Ealey, P. A., Kohn, L. D., Ekins, R. P., and Marshall, N. J., 1984, Characterization of monoclonal antibodies derived from lymphocytes from Graves' disease patients in a cytochemical bioassay for thyroid stimulators, J. Clin. Endocrinol. Metab., 58:909.

Ealey, P. A., Valente, W. A., Ekins, R. P., Kohn, L. D., and Marshall, N. J., 1985, Characterization of monoclonal antibodies raised against solubilized thyrotropin receptors in a cytochemical bioassay for thyroid stimulators, Endocrinology 116:124.

Eggo, M. C., and Burrow, G. N., 1985, Cross-linking techniques in the isolation of TSH receptor proteins, in: "Thyroglobulin-the prothyroid hormone," M. C. Eggo, and G. N. Burrow, eds., Raven Press, New York, p 191.

Grollman, E. F., Lee, G. Ambesi-Impiombato, F. S., Meldolesi, M. F., Aloj, S. M., Coon, H. G., Kaback, H. R., and Kohn, L. D., 1977, Effects of thyrotropin on the thyroid cell membrane: hyperpolarization induced by hormone-receptor interactions, Proc. Natl. Acad. Sci., USA, 74:2352.

Heyma, P., and Harrison, L. C., 1984, Immunoprecipitation of the thyrotropin receptor and identification of thyroid autoantigens using Graves' disease immunoglobulins, J. Clin. Invest., 74:1090.

Iida, Y., Konishi, J., K. Kasagi, K., Endo, K., Misaki, T., Kuma, K., and Torizuka, K., 1983, Partial purification and properties of the TSH receptors from human thyroid plasma membranes, Acta Endocrinol (Copenh) 103:198.

Islam, M. N., and Farid, N. R., 1985, Structure of the porcine thyrotropin receptor: a 200 kilodalton glycoprotein heterocomplex, Experientia, 41:18.

Kasagi, R., Konishi, J., Iida, Y., Ikekubo, K., Mori, T., Kuma, K., and Torizuka, K., 1982, A new in vitro assay for human thyroid stimulator using cultured thyroid cells: effect of sodium chloride on adenosine 3', 5'-monophosphate increase, J. Clin. Endocrinol. Metab. 54:108.

Kohn, L. D., 1978, Relationships in the structure and function of receptors for glycoprotein hormones, bacterial toxins, and interferon. in "Receptors and Recognition," P. Cuatrecasas and M. F. Greaves, eds., Chapman and Hall, London, England, Series A, Vol. 5, p 133.

Kohn, L. D., and Shifrin, S., 1982, Receptor structure and function an exploratory approach using the thyrotropin receptor as a vehicle, in: "Horizons in Biochemistry and Biophysics," L. D. Kohn, ed., John Wiley & Sons, New York p 1.

Kohn, L. D., Consiglio, E., De Wolf, M. J. S., Grollman, E. F., Ledley, F. D., Lee, G., and Morris, N. P., 1980, Thyrotropin receptors and gangliosides, in: "Structure and Function of Gangliosides," L. Svennerholm, P. Mandel, H. Dreyfus, and P. F. Urban, eds., Adv. Exp. Med. Biol. 125:487 Plenum Press, New York.

Kohn, L. D., Aloj, S. M., Beguinot, F., Vitti, P., Yavin, E., Yavin, Z.,Laccetti, P., Grollman, E. F., and Valente, W. A., 1982, Molecular interactions at the cell surface: role of glycoconjugates and membrane lipids in receptor recognition processes, in: "Membranes and Genetic Diseases," J. Shepard, V. E. Anderson, and J. Eaton, eds., Alan R. Liss, New York, p 55.

Kohn, L. D., Valente, W. A., Laccetti, F., Cohen, J. L., Aloj, S. M., and Grollman, E. F., 1983a, Multicomonent structure of the thyrotropin receptor: relationship to Graves' disease, in: "Life Sciences," vol. 32, S. Werner, eds., Pergamon Press, Elmsford, New York, p 15.

Kohn, L. D., Yavin, E., Yavin, Z., Laccetti, P., Vitti, P., Grollman, E. F., and Valente, W. A., 1983, Autoimmune thyroid disease studied with monoclonal antibodies to the thyrotropin receptor, in: "Monoclonal Antibodies: Probes for the Study of Autoimmunity and Immunodeficiency," B. F. Haynes, and G. S. Eisenbarth, eds., Academic Press, New York, p 221.

Kohn, L. D., Tombaccini, D., De Luca, M. L., Bifulco, M., Grollman,
E. F., and Valente, W. A., 1984, Monoclonal antibodies to the
thyrotropin receptor, in: "Antibodies to Receptors; Receptors and
Recognition series," M. F. Greaves, ed., Chapman and Hall, Ltd.,
London, p 201.
Kohn, L. D., Aloj, S. M., Shifrin, S., Valente, W. A., Weiss, S.
J., Vitti, P., Laccetti, P., Cohen, J. L., Rotella, C. M., and
Grollman, E. F., 1985a, The thytropin receptor, in: Receptors for
Polypeptide Hormones, B. T. Posner, ed., Marcel Dekker, New York,
p 299.
Kohn, L. D., Aloj, S. M., Tombaccini, D., Rotella, C. M.,
Toccafondi, R., Marcocci, C., Corda, D., and Grollman, E. F., 1985b,
The thyrotropin receptor, in: "Biochemical Actions of Hormones," G.
Litwak, ed., Marcel Dekker, New York p 457.
Kohn, L. D., Alvarez, F., Marcocci, C., Kohn, A. D., Chen, A.,
Hoffman, W. E., Tombaccini, D., Valente, W. A., De Luca, M.,
Santisteban, P., and Grollman, E. F., 1986, Monoclonal antibody
studies defining the origin and properties of autoantibodies in
Graves' disease, in: "Autoimmunity: Experimental and Clinical
Aspects," R. Schwartz, and N. Rose, eds., Ann NY Acad Sci., New York
p 157.
Kohn, L. D., Valente, W. A., Cheng, A., Tombaccini, D., Chan, J.,
Corda, D., Kohn, A., Rotella, C., Santisteban, P., De Luca, M., Bone,
E., and Grollman, E. F., 1986b, Monoclonal antibodies to the TSH
receptor in the study of Graves' disease, in: "Serono Symposium on
Monoclonal Antibodies: Basic Principles, Experimental and Clinical
Applications in Endocrinology," G. Forti, M. Serio, and M. B.
Lipsett, eds., Raven Press, New York p 232.
Kohn, L. D., Bone, E., Chan, J., Corda, D., Isozaki, O., Luini, A.,
Marcocci, C., Santisteban, P., and Grollman, E. F., 1986c,
Interactions of peptinergic and biogenic amine signals in the
regulation of thyroid function and growth, in: Signal transmission
systems of the nervous system, F. Bloom, and P. Magister, eds.,
Foundation for the Study of Central and Peripheral Nervous System,"
Switzerland, in press.
Kress, B. C., and Spiro, R. G., 1986, Studies on the glycoprotein
nature of the thyrotropin receptor: Interaction with lectins and
purification of the bovine protein with the use of Bandeiraea
(griffonia) simplicifolia I affinity chromatography, Endocrinology,
118:974.
Laccetti, P., Tombaccini, D., Aloj, S. M., Grollman, E. F., and
Kohn, L., 1984, Gangliosides, the thyrotropin receptor, and
autoimmune thyroid disease, in: "Ganglioside Structure, Function, and
Biomedical Potential," R. W. Leeden, R. K. Yu, M. M. Rapport, and K.
Suzuki, eds., Plenum Press, New York p 355.
Macchia, E., Fenzi, G. F., Monzani, F., Lippi, F., Vitti, P.,
Grasso, L., Bartalena, L., Baschieri, L., and Pinchera, L, 1981,
Comparison between thyroid-stimulating and TSH binding inhibiting
immunoglobulins of Graves' disease, Clin. Endocrinol, 15:175
Manley, S. W., Bourke, J. R., and Hawker, R. W., 1974, The
thyrotropin receptor in guinea-pig thyroid homogenate: interaction
with long-acting thyroid stimulator, J. Endocrinol., 61:437.
Marcocci, C., Luini, A., Santisteban, P., and E. F. Grollman, 1987,
Norepinephrine and TSH stimulation of iodide efflux in FRTL-5 thyroid
cells involves metabolites of arachidonic acid and is association
with the iodination of thyroglobulin. Endocrinology, in press.

McKenzie, J. M., and Zakarija, M., 1977, LATS in Graves' disease. Recent Prog. Horm. Res., 33:29.

Mehdi, S. Q., and Nussey, S. S., 1975, A radio-ligand receptor assay for the long acting thyroid stimulator, Biochem J., 145:105.

Meldolesi, M. F., Fishman, P. H., Aloj, S. M., Ledley, F. D., Lee, G., Bradley, R. M., Brady, R. O., and Kohn, L. D., 1977, Separation of the glycoprotein and ganglioside components of thyrotropin receptor activity in plasma membranes. Biochem. Biophys. Res. Commun., 75:581.

Mullin, B. R., Pacuszka, T., Lee, G., Kohn, L. D., Brady, R. O., and Fishman, P. H., 1978, Thyroid gangliosides with high affinity for thyrotropin: potential role in thyroid regulation. Science, 199:77.

Nielsen, T. B., Totsuka, Y., Kempner, S. S., and Field, J. B., 1984, Structure of the thyrotropin receptor and thyroid adenylate cyclase system as determined by target analysis. Biochemistry, 23:6009.

Ozawa, Y., Maciel, R. M. B., Chopra, I. J., Solomon, D. H., and Beall, G. N., 1979, Relationships among immunoglobulin markers in Graves' disease, J. Clin. Endocrinol. Metab., 48:381.

Philp, N. J., and Grollman, E. F., 1986, Thyrotropin and norepinephrine stimulate the metabolism of phosphoinositides in FRTL-5 thyroid cells, FEBS Letts., 202:193.

Pinchera, A., Fenzi, G., Bartalena, L., Chiovato, L., Marcocci, C., Toccafondi, R., Rotella, C., Aterini, S., and Zonefrati, R., 1980, Thyroid cell-surface and thyroid-stimulating antibodies in patients with thyroid autoimmune disorders, in: "Thyroid Research, VIII," J. R. Stockight, and S. Nagataki, eds., Australian Academy of Science, Canberra p 707.

Santisteban, P., Kohn, L. D., and Di Lauro, R., 1986, Thyroglobulin mRNA is regulated by insulin and IGF-I as well as by thyrotropin in the FRTL-5 cell line, in: "Advances in Gene Technology: Molecular Biology of the Endocrine System", "Proceedings of the 18th Miami Winter Symposium. D. Puett, et al, eds. ICSU press, Cambridge, P. 322.

Santisteban, P., De Luca, M., Corda, D., Grollman, E. F., and Kohn, L. D., 1987a, Regulation of thyroglobulin iodination and thyroid hormone formation in FRTL-5 cells, in: "Proceedings of International Thyroid Association," G. Mederos-Nieto, ed., Sao Paulo, Brazil, in press.

Santisteban, P., Kohn, L. D., and Di Lauro, R., 1987, Thyroglobulin gene expression is regulated by insulin and IGF-I, as well as thyrotropin, in FRTL-5 thyroid cells. J. Biol. Chem., in press.

Smith, B. R., and Hall, R., 1974, Thyroid-stimulating immunoglobulins in Graves' disease. Lancet, 24:427.

Smith, B. R., Richards, C. R., Daires Jones, E., Kajita, Y., Buckland, P. R., Creagh, F. M., Howells, R. D., Hashim, F., Parkes, A. B., and Petersen, V. B., 1985, The thyrotropin receptor and its role in Graves' disease. J. Endocrinol. Invest., 8:175.

Sugenoya, A., Kidd, A, Row, V. V., and Volpe, R., 1979, Correlation between thyrotropin-displacing activity and human thyroid stimulating activity by immunoglobulins from patients with Graves' disease and other thyroid disorders. J. Clin. Endocrinol. Metab., 48:398.

Tate, R. L., Schwartz, H. I., Holmes, J. A., Kohn, L. D., and Winand, R. J., 1975, Thyrotropin receptors in thyroid plasma membranes. J. Biol. Chem., 250:6509.

Valente, W. A., Vitti, P., Yavin, Z., Yavin, E., Rotella, C. M.,
Grollman, E. F., Toccafondi, R. S., and Kohn, L. D., 1982, Monoclonal
antibodies to the thyrotropin receptor: stimulating and blocking
antibodies derived from the lymphocytes of patients with Graves'
disease. Proc. Natl. Acad. Sci., USA, 79:6680.

Valente, W. A., Yavin, Z., Yavin, E., Grollman, E. F., Schneider,
M., Rotella, C. M., Zonefrati, R., Toccafondi, R. S., and Kohn, L. D.
(1982b) Monoclonal antibodies to the thyrotropin receptor: the
identification of blocking and stimulating antibodies. J.
Endocrinol. Invest., 5:293.

Valente, W. A., Vitti, P., Rotella, C. M., Vaughan, M. M., Aloj, S.
M., Grollman, E. F., Ambesi-Impiombato, F. S., and Kohn, L. D., 1983,
Antibodies that promote thyroid growth: a distinct population of
thyroid-stimulating autoantibodies. N. Engl. J. Med., 309:1028.

Weiss, S. J., Philp, N. J., Ambesi-Impiombato, F. S., and Grollman,
E. F., 1984, Thyrotropin-stimulated iodide transport mediated by
adenosine 3', 5'-monophosphate and dependent on protein synthesis.
Endocrinology, 114:1099.

Weiss, S. J., Philp, N. J., and Grollman, E. F., 1984, Effect of
thyrotropin on iodide efflux in FRTL-5 cells mediated by Ca^{2+},
Endocrinology, 114:1108.

Yavin, E., Yavin, Z., Schneider, M. D., and Kohn, L. D., 1981,
Monoclonal antibodies to the thyrotropin receptor: implications for
receptor structure and the action of autoantibodies in Graves'
disease. Proc. Natl. Acad. Sci., USA, 78:3180.

Zakarija, M., and McKenzie, J. M., 1980, The thyroid stimulating
antibody of Graves' disease: its assay, some physiochemical
characteristics and clinical significance, in: "Autoimmune Aspects of
Endocrine Disorders," A. Pinchera, D. Doniach, G. F. Fenzi, and L.
Baschieri, eds., Academic Press, New York p. 83.

PROGRESS IN UNDERSTANDING THE THYROID MICROSOMAL ANTIGEN

Leslie J. Degroot, Luc Portmann, and Noboru Hamada

Thyroid Study Unit, Department of Medicine,
University of Chicago, IL 60637

Microsomal antigen has been recognized for nearly three decades as a component of the thyroid cell apical membrane and intracellular membranes reactive with sera from most patients with Hashimoto's thyroiditis and Graves' disease. Although antibodies to thyroglobulin have been much more thoroughly investigated because of the readily available thyroglobulin antigen, there is considerable doubt that this antibody plays a pathogenic role in autoimmune disease. In contrast, antibody dependent cytotoxic reactions have been described using antibodies to the microsomal antigen, suggesting that this antibody-antigen system may be important in destruction of thyroid cells.[1] Several attempts have been made to solubilize and analyze the antigen in the past, usually using detergents, sonication, proteolysis, or high concentrations of salt. It was suggested that the antigen might be a lipoprotein.[2]

Identification of Microsomal Antigen by Western Blot

Three years ago Hamada et al[3,4] applied to this problem newer techniques for analysis of antigens. Human thyroid tissue was homogenized, the "microsomal fraction" recovered by differential centrifugation, and solubilized partially by sonication. This material was subjected to polyacrylamide gel electrophoresis without denaturation, in the "native" antigen condition, in denaturing conditions using urea and SDS, and in denaturing plus reducing conditions, with the addition of mercaptoethanol. The proteins were electrophoretically transferred to nitrocellulose paper, incubated with human polyclonal antisera positive in the microsomal antigen tanned red cell agglutination test, and lacking thyroglobulin or thyroid stimulating antibodies, and the bound immunoglobulin was detected using protein A or peroxidase coupled second antibody. The results were dramatic (Fig. 1). In the native condition, antibodies bound to a smear of heavy weight proteins ranging in size from over 300,000 kD down to approximately 100,000 kD. Denatured proteins also presented a smear, although with several more discrete large molecular weight bands of approximately 200 - 100 kD. The results in reducing-denatured conditions were most interesting in that some antisera did not recognize any antigen, whereas 20% of antisera bound strongly to proteins at 101 and 107 kD. This antigen was found to exist only in the thyroid. Polyvalent human antisera were found to precipitate the antigen from solubilized microsomal tissue, and were found to bind it when the antibodies were coupled to Sepharose 4B. When high molecular weight proteins observed in non-denaturing conditions were

27

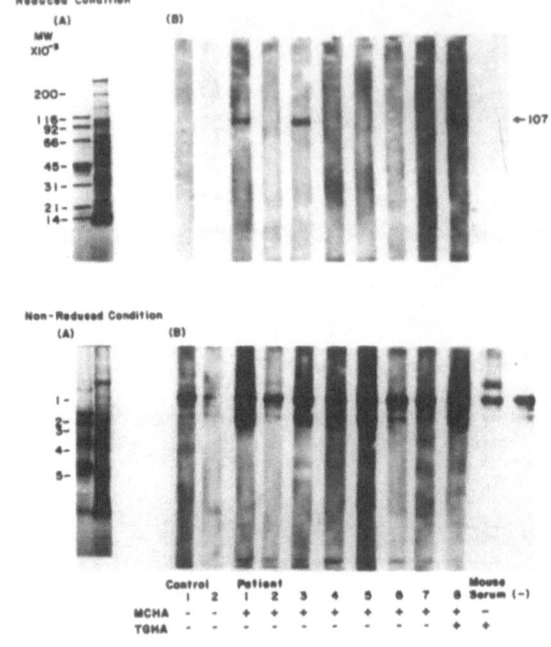

Fig. 1. SDS-PAGE and Western blot using thyroid microsomes. Each lane
contained 40 μg microsomal proteins heated for 15 min at 65 C in 0.009 M
Tris-HCl buffer, pH 8.0, containing 2.5% SDS and 2.25 M urea with (1) or
without (2) 5% 2-mercaptoethanol. Bands were resolved in a 3.3 - 20%
linear gradient gel. A, SDS-PAGE stained with Coomassie blue; B, Western
blot against various sera [a and b, control; c-j, patient sera (c, 1; d, 2;
e, 3; f, 4; g, 5; h, 6; i, 7; j, 8); k, mouse Tg antibody; l, no serum].
Sera were diluted 1:400. *, Mol wt (MW) markers. These do not run correctly
under nonreducing conditions. 1) Myosin (mol wt, 200,000); 2) β-galactosidase
(mol wt 92,500); 4) BSA (mol wt, 66,200); 5) ovalbumin (mol wt, 45,000).

electroeluted from gels, and then rerun in denaturing-reducing conditions,
they could be identified only as 101 and 107 kD peptides (Fig. 2). Further,
when 101 and 107 kD peptides were electroeluted, dialyzed extensively, and
run in denaturing but non-reducing conditions, large molecular weight
complexes were identified by antisera. On two dimensional polyacrylamide
gel-isoelectric focusing studies, one protein with a kD of approximately
107 and a pI of 7 was identified.

Relationship to Peroxidase

At the same time the above studies were ongoing, Portmann et al[5]
studied the relationship of the antigen to thyroid peroxidase. Human
thyroid peroxidase was prepared from Graves' disease tissue using
established techniques, and the solubilized protein was incubated with
sera having potent antimicrosomal antibody titers. On secondary incubation
with protein A, some of the sera precipitated the thyroid peroxidase. The
precipitating activity paralleled microsomal antibody titer, although
there was not a perfect relationship (Figures 3, 4). Some sera were
highly potent in precipitating peroxidase.

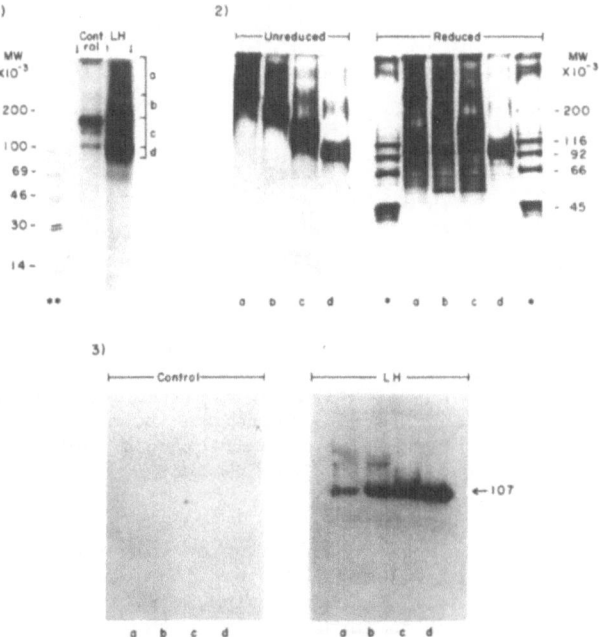

Fig. 2. Poorly defined large molecular weight proteins visualized in Western blot run under non-reducing conditions contain 107 kD protein. (1) Fifty micrograms of microsomal proteins were electrophoresed in SDS-PAGE (3.3 - 20%, linear gradient gel) in non-reducing condition, and transferred onto NC sheets, incubated with control and patient LH sera. Bound antibody was visualized with ^{125}I-protein A followed by auto-radiography. (2) Proteins correspond to a, b, c, and d in 1) were electroeluted from 3.0 mg of microsomal proteins run on 6% preparatory SDS-PAGE. Each fraction was analyzed in SDS-PAGE (3.3 - 20%) under reducing or non-reducing conditions. Gel was stained with silver staining. (3) Proteins electrophoresed in reduced condition were analyzed by Western blot against control or patient LH sera. One-tenth and one-fourth of each protein fraction were used for silver staining and Western blot, respectively. * = Mol wt (MW) markers. ** = Radioactive Mol wt (MW) markers.

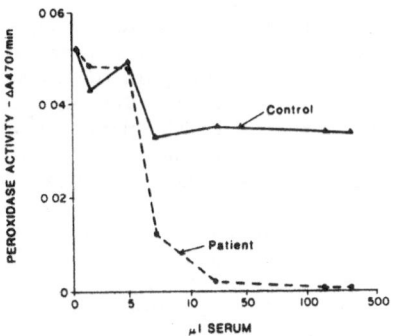

Fig. 3. Effect of graded amount of serum on peroxidase. 190 µg TPO was added to various amounts of serum (0 - 500 µl). Peroxidase activity was assayed in the supernatant after incubation of TPO with serum and Protein A Sepharose CL-4B. A control serum (▲——▲) and serum (●-----●) from one of the four patients' sera causing complete precipitation of peroxidase were used. Each point is the mean of duplicate assays.

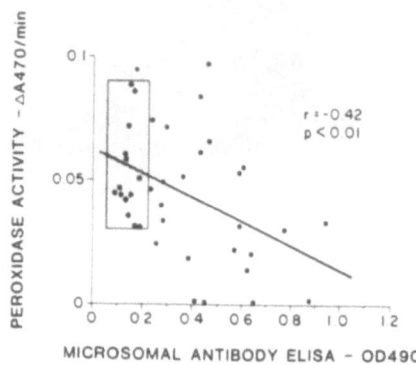

Fig. 4. Correlation between peroxidase activity (remaining after incubation of TPO with controls or patients' sera + Protein A-Sepharose CL-4B) and microsomal antibodies measured by ELISA. The rectangle includes the mean ± 2 SD of results using control sera in both assays.

These studies led our group to the conclusion that the microsomal antigen existed as a duplex of 101 and 107 k peptides which had similar antigenicity, although obviously different molecular structure. These peptides apparently could exist in larger forms, either as multimers or in association with other peptides, probably through formation of disulfide bonds. Further, the microsomal antigen was specific to thyroid, and was possibly identical with thyroid peroxidase.

Coincident with this work, Philippe Carayon and collaborators were proceeding along similar lines.[6] This group purified human thyroid peroxidase (TPO) by a novel chromatographic method and made monoclonal antibodies to it. These were used for further purification of TPO, which was found to consist of two peptides of approximately 98 and 105 kD. These peptides were reactive with sera that contained microsomal antibodies in Western blots. This group also reached the conclusion that the microsomal antigen and peroxidase were probably identical.[7] Kotani et al have also identified antibodies reacting with TPO in patients with AITD.[8]

Monoclonal Antibodies to the Microsomal Antigen

More recently, Portmann et al[9] have electroeluted protein from the 107 kD band in preparative polyacrylamide gels, and developed monoclonal antibodies using conventional fusion techniques with SP2/O myeloma cells. Six monoclonal antibodies were recovered which reacted specifically with the 101 and 107 kD bands present in PAGE gels of microsomal antigen done in denatured-reducing conditions (Fig. 5). The antibodies reacted weakly with large molecular weight proteins in the native state. These observations confirmed even more specifically that the 101 and 107 kD proteins were immunologically very similar. Further, the monoclonal anti-microsomal antibodies reacted with 101 and 107 kD proteins immuno-precipitated by polyvalent human antisera, and vice versa. Most interesting were reactions of the monoclonal antibodies with purified TPO. Alvin Taurog kindly provided a sample of purified pig thyroid peroxidase, and five of the six monoclonal antibodies reacted vigorously with a ∿ 54 kD broad band of protein. Carayon kindly provided a sample of purified human thyroid peroxidase, and in confirmation of the identity of the two proteins, the monoclonal antibodies identified approximately 94 and 105 kD duplex bands in this preparation. In collaboration with Carayon, we have shown

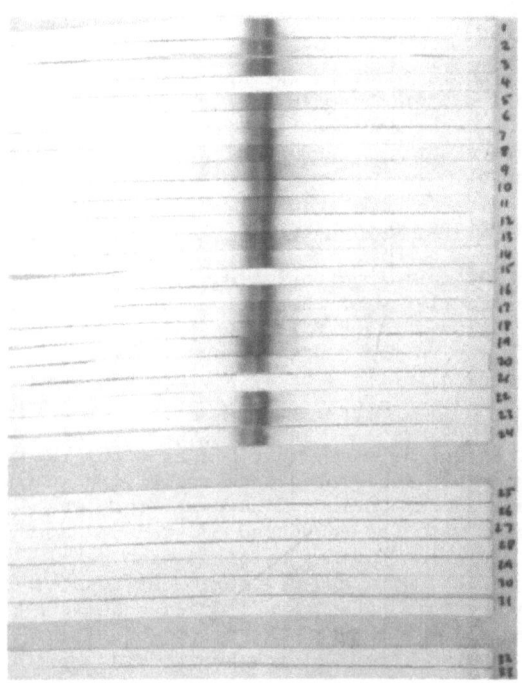

Fig. 5. 107 kD microsomal antigen was eluted from SDS-PAGE and used to
immunize mice. Spleen cells were fused to SP2-0 myeloma cells. Several
monoclonal antibodies were recovered. All reacted only with the 107 kD
and 101 kD forms of the antigen on Western blot of microsomes - as shown
above. There was no cross-reactivity with other tissues. The monoclonals
also reacted with purified human and porcine TPO.

that our monoclonal antibodies react extensively and completely with his
purified peroxidase, and that 1 of 16 monoclonal antibodies that he
developed against TPO reacts in Western blot to the same protein bands
as do our monoclonal antibodies. Thus it seems impossible that there can
be anything less than identity between "microsomal antigen" and "thyroid
peroxidase".

Structure of the Microsomal Antigen as Determined By A Proteolytic Digestion

Digestion of the microsomal antigen with trypsin leads to development
of two smaller 84 and 88 kD bands which react with all of the monoclonal
antibodies. Interestingly, these bands represent the commonly reported
sizes of human and animal thyroid peroxidase, prepared using trypsin.[10]
Thus trypsin must cut off a portion of the microsomal antigen making the
protein more soluble, and leaving the catalytic function intact. Most
polyvalent human antisera do not react with this smaller antigen, although
some do react vigorously. Thus the monoclonal antibodies recognize
different epitopes present in the denatured condition of the antigen and
largely distinct from those recognized by most polyvalent human antisera.

Incubation with V8 protease destroys the 107 kD band, but not the 101
kD peptide. Thus the 101 kD peptide must lack a peptide domain present in
the 107 kD form. An explanation for this could be that two forms of
protein are determined from the same gene, possibly from differential
splicing of the hnRNA, leaving out one or more exon.

A Model of the Microsomal Antigen

Putting the data above together, we can suggest a model for the function of the microsomal antigen, which would include domains having epitopes recognized only in the denatured condition, domains having epitopes recognized in the native antigen, and specific trypsin and V8 protease sensitive sites (Fig. 6).

Clinical Studies on Antisera Detecting Different Forms of the Antigen

We have studied 197 sera from patients with autoimmune thyroid disease and determined their reactivity to the native antigen in the tanned red cell agglutination, native antigen ELISA, or native antigen Western blot techniques.[11] Reactivity to the denatured antigen was determined using an ELISA based on a denatured antigen, or by Western blot, and antibodies reacting with the reduced and denatured antigen were determined by semi-quantitative Western blotting. In general, reactivity in all these systems ran in parallel in the sense that higher titer reactivity to the native antigen was commonly associated with reactivity in the denatured or the denatured plus reduced antigen. However, this was not always the case; some sera reacted with the denatured and reduced antigen and much less to other forms. Eleven - 30% of patients with Hashimoto's thyroiditis and Graves' disease reacted with the denatured and reduced antigen. There was a correlation in patients with Graves' disease between reactivity to the denatured and reduced antigen and the period of illness, and also with the onset of hypothyroidism after RAI treatment (Fig. 7).

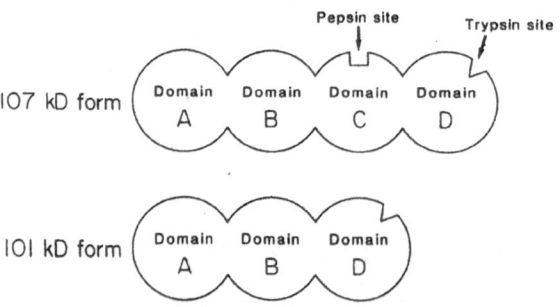

Hypothetical model of mirosomal antigen –TPO

Fig. 6. The 107 kD and 101 kD forms of the antigen must be closely related since both forms react with polyvalent antisera and monoclonal antibodies, thus having in common domains labeled A and B. The 107 kD form lacks a Pepsin sensitive domain present in the 101 kD form. Both are split by trypsin (domain D) producing two smaller peptides.

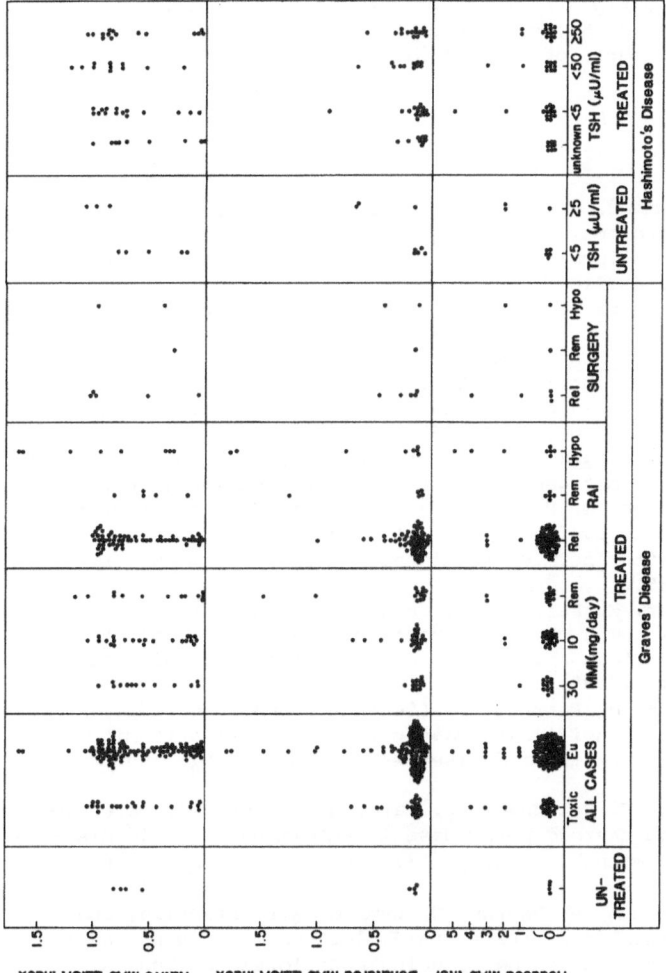

Fig. 7. Native MAb ELISA Index, denatured MAb ELISA Index, and denatured and reduced (reduced) MAb titer in 134 patients with Graves' disease and 59 patients with Hashimoto's disease. The patients with Graves' disease were first divided into untreated and treated patients. The patients with Graves' disease were further classified according to the thyroid function or type and result of the treatments (MMI: Methimazole, RAI: Radioactive iodine treatment, Rem: Remission, Rel: Relapse). Patients in "Remission" were euthyroid for more than six months after antithyroid drug treatment. The patients with Hashimoto's disease were also divided into untreated and treated patients, and than classified according to the level of serum TSH before treatment.

33

The Future

We are just beginning to understand the microsomal antigen. It is most fascinating that it is related to thyroid peroxidase. Possibly thyroid antibodies can inhibit peroxidase function in vivo, although this has yet to be proved. Cloning of the microsomal antigen is probably just around the corner and will lead to interesting studies on the expression of the gene and its structure. Definition of the epitopes of the antigen, and correlations of reactivity of antisera from patients with different epitopes and the clinical features of their disease may prove most interesting. One fascinating idea is that antibody reactivity to the denatured form of the antigen could be related to cross reactivity in other tissues, such as in the eye or elsewhere, and produce some of the clinically important aspects of Graves' disease.

REFERENCES

1. E.L. Khoury, L. Hammond, G.F. Bottazo, and D. Doniach, Presence of the organ specific "microsomal" autoantigen on the surface of human thyroid cells in culture: its involvement in complement-mediated cytotoxicity, Clin. Exp. Immunol. 45:316 (1981).

2. S. Mariotti, A. Pinchera, C. Marcocci, P. Vitti, C. Urbano, L. Chiovato, M. Tosi, and L. Baschieri, Solubilization of human thyroid microsomal antigen, J. Clin. Endocrinol. Metab. 48:207 (1979).

3. N. Hamada, C. Grimm, H. Mori, and L.J. DeGroot, Identification of a thyroid microsomal antigen by Western blot and immunoprecipitation, J. Clin. Endocrinol. Metab. 61:120 (1985).

4. N. Hamada, L. Portmann, and L.J. DeGroot, Characterization and isolation of thyroid microsomal antigen, Submitted for publication (1986).

5. L. Portmann, N. Hamada, G. Heinrich, and L.J. DeGroot, Antithyroid peroxidase antibody in patients with autoimmune thyroid disease: possible identity with antimicrosomal antibody, J. Clin. Endocrinol. Metab. 61:1001 (1985).

6. B. Czarnocka, J. Ruf, M. Ferrand, P. Carayon, and S. Lissitzky, Purification of the human thyroid peroxidase and its identification as the microsomal antigen involved in autoimmune thyroid diseases, FEBS Letters 190:147 (1985).

7. B. Czarnocka, J. Ruf, M. Ferrand, S. Lissitzky, and P. Carayon, Interaction of highly purified thyroid peroxidase with anti-microsomal antibodies in autoimmune thyroid diseases, J. Endocrinol. Invest. 9:135 (1986).

8. T. Kotani, K. Umeki, S. Matsunaga, E. Kato, and S. Ohtaki, Detection of autoantibodies to thyroid peroxidase in autoimmune thyroid diseases by micro-ELISA and immunoblottin, J. Clin. Endocrinol. Metab. 62:928 (1986).

9. L. Portmann, F.W. Fitch, W. Havran, N. Hamada, W.A. Franklin, and L.J. DeGroot, Characterization of the thyroid microsomal antigen, and its relationship to thyroid peroxidase, using monoclonal antibodies, Submitted for publication (1986).

10. D.S. Cooper, F. Maloof, and E.W. Ridgway, Rat thyroid peroxidase biosynthesis in vitro: studies using antisera to porcine thyroid peroxidase, Annual Meeting of the American Thyroid Association, New York, NY (1984). (Abstract No. 26)

11. N. Hamada, N. Jaeduck, L. Portmann, K. Ito, and L.J. DeGroot, Antibodies against denatured and reduced thyroid microsomal antigen in autoimmune thyroid disease. J. Clin. Endocrinol. Metab. (in press for 1987).

A POSSIBLE ROLE OF BACTERIAL ANTIGENS IN THE

PATHOGENESIS OF AUTOIMMUNE THYROID DISEASE

Sidney H. Ingbar, Mordechai Weiss, Gary W. Cushing,
and Dennis L. Kasper

Charles A. Dana Research Institute and the Harvard-
Thorndike Laboratory at Beth Israel Hospital,
Department of Medicine, Beth Israel Hospital and
Harvard Medical School, Boston, MA 02215, U.S.A.

This discussion concerns the possible relationship between bacterial antigens and the pathogenesis of autoimmune thyroid disease (AITD), with emphasis on the human pathogen Yersinia enterocolitica (Y.e.) and on Graves' disease. It is divided into three parts: a description of the fascinating background information that prompted us to investigate this topic; a brief description of our findings to date; and a consideration of their possible significance with respect to the pathogenesis of AITD.

BACKGROUND

Y.e. is a gram-negative coccobacillus of the family Enterobacteri-aceae. The species is not homogeneous, comprising a group of organisms that are separable on the basis of 33 O- and 19 H-antigens, 5 biotypes, and 5 phage types. Three O-antigen types, O:3, O:8, and O:9, account for the majority of infections with Y.e. A puzzling feature is the wide variation in the frequency with which yersinial infection is encountered in differing parts of the world, as well as the predominance of differing serotypes in different areas, some close by to one another (see review, Ref. 1). In Scandinavia, for example, Y.e. is a common cause of enteric infection, and agglutinating Y.e. antibodies occur in approximately 17% of normal healthy subjects (2). In the U.S., in contrast, clinical infection with Y.e. is uncommon, Y.e. antibodies being found in <8% of a normal population in New York City (3,4). In Denmark, serotype O:3 is the most common cause of yersinial infection, whereas both O:3 and O:8 are evidently important in the U.S. (1,3).

Diarrhea is the cardinal feature of infection with Y.e., but of particular interest and possible relevance to the present discussion are the occurrence, during the acute disease or subsequently, of various abnormalities that suggest autoimmune disease, as described by Gripenberg et al. (5). Among them are erythema nodosum, carditis, glomerulonephritis and iritis. Arthralgias, arthritis, and Reiter's syndrome are also seen, and are strongly associated with haplotype HLA-B27. Further, studies of sera obtained within three months after the onset of symptoms, all with a diagnostic titer of Yersinia agglutinins, provided evidence of a diffuse stimulation of humoral immunity, including an increase in isohem-agglutinin titers, a high frequency of antinuclear and smooth muscle

antibodies (SMA), and a high frequency by indirect immunofluorescence
assay (IFL), of antibodies against gastric parietal cells, renal tubular
epithelium, and human thyroid epithelium (5).

In the mid-1970s and over the next several years there developed two
separate, but converging, lines of evidence linking Y.e. to thyroid disease. One line of evidence, already cited, was the appearance of antibodies that bind to human thyroid epithilium in sera of patients recovering from infection with Y.e. (5). Earlier, Lidman and co-workers had reported that among 100 sera that contained agglutinins against Y.e. serotype 0:3., 74% were positive by IFL for antibodies binding to the membranes of thyroid glands removed from patients with hyperthyroidism (6).
In a later study, the same group found that 26/96 of sera showing marginal staining of the membrane region of thyroid cells were from patients
acutely infected with Y.e. serotype 0:3. In addition, approximately 80%
of 63 sera with agglutinins against serotype 0:9 reacted with thyroid
epithelium by IFL (7). In contrast to the IFL-reacting antibodies found
by Gripenberg et al, these could not be absorbed by treating sera with a
source of SMA. Of particular interest was the dependence of the IFL reaction on the nature and mode of preparation of the thyroid tissue. Negligible reactions were seen with live human thyroid cells, indicating
that the antigen was cytoplasmic. Similarly, clear-cut IFL reactions
were not seen in "atoxic" human thyroid tissue or in thyroids from the
monkey or the rat. Absorption of sera with heat-killed Y.e. removed agglutinins, but not IFL reactions, indicating that the IFL-reactive antibody was not directed toward the O antigen. Further, IFL-reactivity was
partly or completely abolished, respectively, by absorption of sera with
formalinized or sonicated bacteria, indicating that the reactive antigens are only poorly represented on the bacterial surface. These findings are mainly consonant with our own (v.i.). Also relevant is the
finding, that by conventional techniques, positive tests for antimicrosomal antibodies, in titers as high as $1/10^5$, were present in the sera
of 18% of patients convalescing from Y.e. infections, whereas tests were
positive in only 6.5% of normal blood donors (5). In patients followed
serially, positive tests for antibodies proved to be transitory.

A second line of evidence, developing concurrently, comprised data
that revealed an inordinately high frequency of agglutinating antibodies
against Y.e. among patients with various thyroid diseases who were not
known to have suffered infection with this organism. A remarkably close
concordance of the data was seen in studies conducted in the laborabora-
tories of Beck (8,9), Weiss (10) and Shenkman (3,4) and their colleagues
in Denmark, Israel, and the United States, respectively. Among patients
with various thyroid disorders, variously comprising in the several studies Graves' disease, Hashimoto's disease, diffuse and nodular nontoxic
goiter, toxic adenoma, idiopathic myxedema, and a few cases of subacute
thyroiditis and of thyroid carcinoma, significant agglutinin titers were
found in approximately 50-90%. What makes the data all the more remarkable is that this concordance was seen in the face of wide variations in
the frequency of Y.e. agglutinins in the control population (17% in Denmark; 0/77 in Israel; and <8% in the U.S.). In the studies of Shenkman
and co-workers (3,4), Y.e. agglutinins were demonstrated with the following frequencies: Graves' disease, 24/36; autonomous adenoma, 5/6;
Hashimoto's thyroiditis, 7/7; primary myxedema, 3/5; nontoxic nodular
goiter, 4/11: thyroid carcinoma 1/2. Antibodies against serotype 0:3
were the most prevalent, particularly in sera from patients with Grave's
disease, in whom titers tended to be the highest. No correlation was
evident between the state of thyroid function or titers of antithyroid
antibodies and those against Y.e.
Even more important to this line of evidence are the data of Beck
and colleagues, who employed the migration-inhibition assay to study the

frequency and characteristics of cell-mediated immune responses to Y.e. and human thyroid extracts in patients with various thyroid disease (11). Lymphocytes from 64 patients with nodular or diffuse nontoxic goiter, toxic adenoma, or Graves' disease were compared with those from 25 normal controls. For the entire group of patients, and for those with Graves' disease or diffuse nontoxic goiter, significantly positive tests in response to Y.e. antigen were observed. Further, in controls, the migration index was unrelated to the presence or absence of Yersinia antibodies, but in patients, the migration index was lower (i.e., more strongly positive) in those with Yersinia antibodies than those without. Most interestingly, significant inhibition of leucocyte migration in response to thyroid antigen was evident only in Graves' disease, and here, unlike in controls, a significant correlation between the inhibition of migration produced by thyroid extract and that produced by Y.e. was evident.

Several possible explanations for the foregoing constellation of findings have been suggested, and certain of these will be discussed below, but the explanation most commonly offered is that Y.e., particularlarly serotype 0:3, contains one or more antigens that cross-react immunologically with antigens in human thyroid tissue. We were greatly intrigued by this possibility and its potential ramifications, and several years ago set out to study the problem in a somewhat different manner.

EXPERIMENTAL FINDINGS

Our initial efforts were directed to detecting functional, and by inference stuctural, homology between components in the thyroid membrane and in Y.e. Initial studies were therefore directed to a search for a a saturable binding site for TSH in Y.e. Studies were conducted with Y.e. serotype 0:3 (12). Organisms stored in the frozen state were thawed, cultured in blood agar, and then subcultured overnight in brain-heart infusion broth at room temperature, rather than 37 C. Binding of tracer concentrations (approx. 10^{-11}M) of ^{125}I-labeled bovine TSH (bTSH) was studied by conventional techniques (12), and various methods of treating the bacteria in order to maximize binding were tested. Specific binding of tracer concentrations of ^{125}I-bTSH was evident in all, but was greatest in a particulate prepared by treating the whole organism with EDTA and lysozyme (Fig. 1). Hence, the latter method of extracting the organism was used in all subsequent binding experiments.

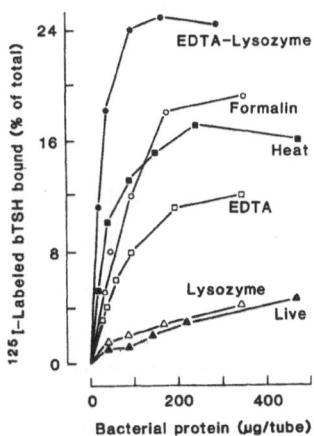

Fig. 1. Binding of ^{125}I-bTSH to Yersinia enterocolitica treated by various methods. Reprinted, with permission, from Ref. 12.

Binding of ^{125}I-bTSH was time- and temperature-dependent. Binding was most rapid at 37 C, peaking in 30 min, but declining thereafter. Steady-state binding was greatest at 4 C, but was achieved too slowly for practical use, whereas binding at 22 C was nearly as high, and steady-state was maintained between 1-6 hr. This temperature was therefore selected for further studies.

Binding of bTSH to the EDTA-lysozyme extract of Y.e. was saturable, saturation being achieved at a bTSH concentration of about 0.5U/ml (12). Scatchard analysis of these data revealed the presence of a single apparent binding site with a binding maximum (B_{max}) of 2.9 x 10^{-8} mole/mg bacterial protein and dissociation constant (K_d) of 4.2 x 10^{-8}M (Fig. 2). Hence, the affinity of the TSH binding site in Y.e. is less than that of of the high affinity site in human thyroid membranes, but greater than that of the low affinity site (13).

Additional studies revealed a concordance of the major properties of the TSH-binding site in Y.e. with those of the TSH receptor in human and bovine thyroid membranes. As in thyroid membranes (14), a dose dependent inhibition of ^{125}I-bTSH binding was produced by the other glycopeptide hormones, in order of decreasing potency: bLH, hCG, and bFSH. All were far less potent than bTSH itself, and porcine insulin and glucagon, as well as ACTH (1-24) and bovine serum albumin, were inactive at high concentrations (12).

Further, as in mammalian thyroid membranes (13,14), enrichment of the medium with the monovalent cations Na$^+$ and K$^+$ produced a dose dependent inhibition of binding (half-maximum at approximately 12mM), and a much more potent inhibition, half maximum at approximately 1mM, was produced by the divalent cations Ca^{2+} and Mg^{2+} (15).

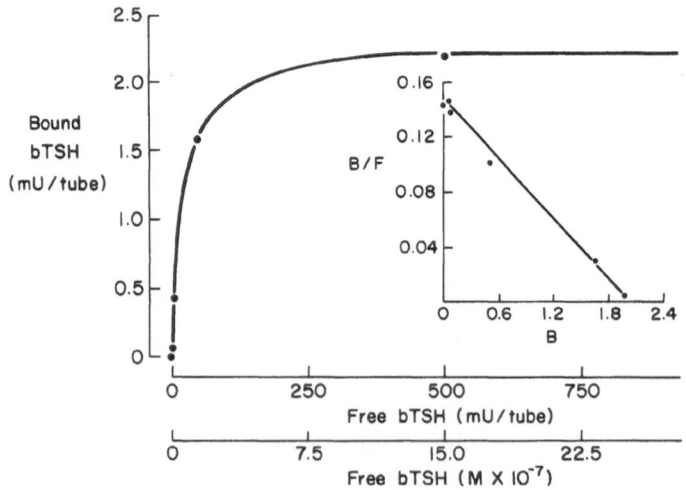

Fig. 2. Saturable binding of bovine TSH to an EDTA-lysozyme extract of <u>Yersinia enterocolitica</u>. Reprinted, with permission, from Reference 12.

The localization of the TSH binding site within the cell wall of Y.e. was then determined. Spheroplasts were subjected to osmotic lysis and were then sedimented through a sucrose density gradient. Three major protein peaks were obtained, and these were analyzed for ^{125}I-bTSH binding and lactic dehydrogenase (LDH) activity. As seen in Table 1, both activities were least in the densest fraction, Fraction I, and greatest in the least dense fraction, Fraction III (15). Since LDH is principally localized in the inner bacterial membrane, this seems to be the locale of the TSH-binding site, as well. This would appear to explain the lesser binding of bTSH in heat- or formalin-treated organisms than in the EDTA-lysozyme extract and could explain the only partial removal of IFL-reactive antibodies by heat-killed or formalinized Y.e., as seen in the studies of Lidman and co-workers (7).

A limited survey of organisms other than Y.e. for the presence of TSH-binding sites revealed high levels of binding (approximately 10-12%) in EDTA-lysozyme extracts of clinical isolates of Escherichia coli (E.c.) pseudomonas aeruginosa, and Neisseria meningitides, though binding was less than that in extracts of Y.e. (approximately 24%). Little, if any, binding (<3%) was observed in extracts of Group A or Group B Streptococcus (15).

In view of the demonstration of a saturable binding site for TSH in the inner bacterial membranes of Y.e. serotype 0:3, akin in many of its properties to the TSH receptor in human and other mammalian TSH receptors, and in other gram-negative bacteria as well, it seemed imperative to obtain evidence as to whether these TSH binding sites would also react with the TSH receptor antibodies of Graves' disease. To examine this question, we exploited the receptor-purification technique developed in our laboratory that employs the guinea pig fat cell membrane to provide, from crude IgG, preparations very highly enriched in TSH receptor antibodies, but apparently devoid of antibodies against other thyroid antigens (16). Preparations of normal and Graves'-IgG were subjected to the receptor-purification technique, and both the original IgG and receptor-purified products were tested in a TSH-binding inhibition (TBI) assay. EDTA-lysozyme extracts of Y.e., rather than thyroid membranes, were employed as a source of TSH-binding sites. At the very low concentrations purposely employed (up to 100 ug/tube), neither the crude normal or Graves'-IgG produced significant inhibition of TSH binding, and this was also true of the "receptor-purified" preparation of normal IgG. Receptor-purified Graves-IgG, in contrast, produced a potent dose-related inhibition of TSH binding (approximately 80% inhibition at 20 ug/tube) (15).

The foregoing studies suggested that antibodies in Graves'-IgG bind to Y.e., that in so doing they interfere with binding of TSH to its binding site, and that their potency in this respect is greatly increased when they are enriched in TSH receptor antibodies. These antibodies must, therefore, recognize the bacterial TSH binding site. More direct evidence of this association was provided by experiments in which the

Table 1. Localization of the bTSH binding site in EDTA lysozyme extracts of Yersinia enterocolitica.

Fraction	LDH Activity (umol/min/mg protein)	^{125}I-bTSH binding (%/100 ug protein)
I	2	10
II	20	12
III	80	48

binding of crude and receptor-purified normal and Graves'-IgG to Y.e.,
E.c., and Group G Streptococcus coated on microtiter plates was measured
by ELISA. Antibodies that bound to all three organisms were detected in
crude IgG preparations from both normal controls and patients with
Graves' disease. In the case of normal IgG, titers were completely unaffected by "receptor-purification." In contrast, receptor-purified
Graves'-IgG displayed greatly increased binding to Y.e. and E.c., organisms that contain TSH binding sites in significant number, but not to
Group B Streptococcus, in which binding of bTSH was negligible. Further,
in studies with E.c., binding of both crude and "receptor-purified" normal IgG, as well as crude Graves'-IgG, was negligibly affected by the
addition of bTSH, whereas binding of receptor-purified Graves'-IgG was
markedly inhibited (15). These findings provide powerful evidence, we
believe, that the TSH receptor antibodies in the serum of patients with
Graves'-disease bind to antigens in Y.e. and E.c., and that the epitopes
in the bacteria to which they bind are their TSH binding sites.

In view of the foregoing evidence of functional and immunological
cross-reactivity between the TSH receptors of the human thyroid membrane
and the TSH binding site of the bacterial membrane, we have initiated
attempts to induce the formation of TSH receptor antibodies, i.e., to
develop an animal model of Graves' disease by immunizing rabbits with
extracts of Y.e. Among 5 rabbits, one displayed, in a serum obtained in
an early bleeding, IgG that had consistent and pronounced TBI activity in
guinea pig fat cell membranes, but strangely, not in human or rabbit thyroid membranes; this activity was gone from sera obtained in subsequent
bleedings. Compared with pre-immunization specimens, IgG also displayed
increased binding to human thyroid membranes in ELISA (17). These results, though quite preliminary, suggest that it is possible to raise TSH
receptor antibodies by immunizing animals with Y.e., and further studies
to this point are proceeding.

DISCUSSION

The findings described, we believe, leave no room for doubt that
Y.e. serotype 0:3 contains a saturable, hormone-specific binding site
for mammalian TSH that resembles in many of its properties the receptor
for TSH in the human thyroid gland. Further, we have identified similar,
though less well-characterized, binding sites in several other gram-
negative bacteria, including at least some strains of the ubiquitous E.c.
It appears, moreover, that such TSH binding sites are more widely distributed in lower life forms than even our data would indicate, since
Sack and co-workers have recently reported the presence of saturable,
specific binding sites for TSH in membranes of Leishmania and Mycoplasma
(18,19). To date, it is unclear whether there exists within these organisms a corresponding ligand. A TSH-like factor has been isolated from
the culture medium of Clostridium refringens (20), but a complementary
binding site evidently has not been sought for in this organism. Neither
is there information as to what function any interaction between TSH
binding sites and their putative ligands in these organisms may subserve,
but the broad biologic distribution and apparent evolutionary conservation of TSH binding sites suggest that an interaction with a ligand of
either endogenous origin, or perhaps native to their host, may be important to their survival or infectivity. There is now overwhelming evidence for the presence of a variety of peptide hormones and/or their receptors in unicellular eukaryotes and prokaryotes (21,22). Though their
function therein is still uncertain, cytosolic receptors for estrogenic
steroids have been detected in Saccharomyces cerevisiae and Paracoccidioides brasiliensis, and a biologic response to estradiol has been observed in the latter (23,24). These findings are outside of the realm
of conventional endocrinology, but answers to the questions they raise

are deserving of vigorous pursuit because of their intrinsic interest and almost certain biological significance.

To return to Y.e. and E.c., the organisms in which we have been particularly interested, our data seem clearly to confirm the widely-postulated cross-reactivity between antigens in the human thyroid and antigens in Y.e., and they clearly identify one of the cross-reacting antigens as the thyroid's TSH receptor. The functional similarity of the bacterial binding site to that in the thyroid, the ability of the IgG from the serum of patients with Graves' disease to bind to Y.e. and E.c., the enhanced binding of Graves'-IgG, but not normal IgG, after purification by the TSH receptor in guinea pig fat, as well as the ability of TSH to inhibit such binding, all indicate that this is the case. Nonetheless, it appears that there are other antigens in human thyroid that cross-react with antigens in Y.e. Thus, antibodies against thyroid microsomes, as measured by conventional techniques, appear transiently in an inordinately high percentage of patients recovering from yersinial infections (5). In addition, antibodies to Y.e. that interact with human thyroid, as judged by IFL, do so in cryostat sections, but not in live cells. This suggests that, unlike the TSH receptor, they are not localized on the cell membrane, but rather are cytoplasmic (7). Further, they do not react with rat or monkey thyroid (7). Although this might imply that there are important structural differences between the human TSH receptor and that in the rat and monkey, the receptor in rat thyroid is sufficiently homologous to that in man to make possible use of rat thyroid in TBI assays of Graves'-IgG. Further, some reports indicate that an interaction with human thyroid can be detected by IFL in the case of the SMA that appear in the serum in patients recovering from infection with Y.e. (25). It seems likely, therefore, that Y.e. contains multiple antigens that cross-react with those in human thyroid, and this may have some bearing on the most important and interesting question of all, whether bacterial antigens could possibly play a role in the pathogenesis of AITD.

The concept that immunological cross-reactions between heterophilic antigens in micro-organisms and antigens in the tissues of the host, one form of "molecular mimicry," may lead to autoimmune disease is one that has received increasing attention, and several mechanisms by which this may occur have been suggested (26,27). Certainly, many micro-organisms, including Y.e. (5) and the Mycoplasma mentioned above, are capable of eliciting antibodies that interact with a variety of tissues, though these do not necessarily cause disease. More to the point is the accepted role of heterophilic antibodies in explaining the relationship between beta-hemolytic streptococcus and rheumatic fever (28), as well as that between infection with Mycoplasma and cold agglutinin-mediated hemolytic disease (29). More recently, sharing of antigen determinants among proteins in E.c., Proteus vulgaris, Klebsiella pneumoniae and those in the nicotinic acetylcholine receptor has been suggested to play a role in the pathogenesis of myasthenia gravis (30).

Could a similar relationship apply in the case of Y.e. and AITD? The possibility that it may currently rests on the remarkable frequency of antibodies to Y.e. in the serum of patients with AITD, and conversely, the frequency of antibodies that react with various thyroid antigens in the serum of patients who have been infected with Y.e. Several explanations for these findings have been suggested (4). First, the relationship might be merely coincidental, resting on the chance occurrence of cross-reacting antigens in human thyroid and Y.e. In support of this explanation is the fact that evidence of prior infection with Y.e. is lacking in most or all patients with thyroid disease whose serum contains antibodies against Y.e. Also in favor of this interpretation is the similar frequency of Y.e. antibodies in the sera of patients with AITD reported from diverse parts of the world, in which the frequency of yersinial disease varies widely (4,8-10). Similarly, it seems most unlikely that those patients with AITD who live on the eastern seaboard of the U.S., and whose sera contain antibodies that interact with Leishmania antigens (18), have actually been exposed to that organism. All these considerations would support the contention that a coincidental occurrence of cross-reacting antigens would account for the presence of antibodies that interact with bacterial and parasitic proteins in patients with AITD. The strength of this argument is diminished, however, by the demonstration of TSH binding sites not only in Y.e., but also in other micro-organisms, and it is possible, if not likely, that these organisms share other antigens as well. Therefore, a single organism could elicit antibodies that both would be involved in the pathogenesis of AITD and would cross-react with antigens in organisms to which the patient had never been exposed.

Another consideration that militates against the suggestion that the association of AITD with antibodies against Y.e. is merely coincidental stems from the fact that, in all studies of the frequency of Y.e. antibodies in patients with thyroid disease cited thus far, the tests employed have measured antibodies against the O-antigen. Yet, it is clear from studies of patients recovering from Y.e. infection, that antibodies against the O-antigen are not those which interact with human thyroid. This consideration would lend support to the idea that patients with AITD who possess antibodies against Y.e. have previously been infected with Y.e. or some other cross-reacting organism. As is demonstrable by immunoelectrophoresis, patients and animals infected with Y.e. develop antibodies against both the O-antigen and a bacterial protein(s) (31). Evidently, the frequency of antibodies of the latter type in patients with AITD has not been examined, but such studies could prove rewarding, since the protein is much more likely than the O-antigen to contain the antigens that cross-react with antigens in the thyroid.

A finding that seems quite inconsistent with the role of bacterial antigens in the pathogenesis of AITD is the frequency with which Y.e. agglutinins are found in the sera of patients with thyroid diseases, such as toxic adenoma and carcinoma, that are not considered to be autoimmune in nature. It is true that in most studies, antibodies against Y.e. are found with greatest frequency in patients with AITD in general and Graves' disease in particular. Nonetheless, if thyroid diseases such as toxic adenoma and carcinoma do indeed lack an autoimmune basis, then one would expect patients with these diseases to display antibodies against Y.e. only in a frequency which matches that of the normal, healthy population, and this is clearly not the case.

For the present, the question of whether bacterial antigens contribute to the pathogenesis of AITD, or its perpetuation or exacerbation once established, remains unanswered. The TSH binding site in Y.e., which interacts with Graves'-IgG, exemplifies one type of bacterial antigen that could play a role in the development of AITD, but the diversity of organisms that share this site with the human thyroid complicates the issue greatly and makes it unlikely that a causative relationship can be proven by the type of epidemiological data applied to the question thus far. Development of an animal model of Graves' disease by immunization with bacterial antigen would fulfill another of Koch's postulates, but would not in itself be conclusive. Studies of the thyroid bioactivity of antibodies present in the serum of patients recovering from infection with Y.e. would likely illuminate their functional significance, if any, and a careful search for other well-defined thyroid antigens, such as the microsomal antigen, in Y.e. and other micro-organisms that contain a TSH binding site would provide critical information. Further, a study of the frequency of various histocompatability antigens among those patients with AITD who display antibodies against Y.e. and those who do not might reveal important associations, like that of HLA-B27 and Yersinia-related arthropathies (32). Although studies of this type may not conclusively prove or disprove a role of bacterial antigens in the pathogenesis of AITD, they are certain to provide information of interest and importance.

REFERENCES

1. G. P. Wormser and G. T. Kensch, Yersinia enterocolitica: clinical observations, in: "Yersinia Enterocolitica," E. J. Bottone, ed., CRC Press, Boca Raton (1981).

2. K. Bech J. H. Larsen, J. M. Hansen, and J. Nerup, Yersinia enterocolitica infection and thyroid disorders (letter), Lancet 2:951 (1974).

3. L. Shenkman and E. J. Bottone, Antibodies to Yersinia enterocolitica in thyroid disease, Ann. Int. Med. 85:735 (1976).

4. L. Shenkman and E. J. Bottone, The occurrence of antibodies to Yersinia enterocolitica in thyroid diseases, in: "Yersinia Enterocolitica," E. J. Bottone, ed., CRC Press, Boca Raton (1981).

5. M. Gripenberg, A. Miettinen, P. Kurki, and E. Linder, Humoral immune stimulation and antiepithelial antibodies in yersinia infections, Arthr. Rheum. 21:904 (1978).

6. K. Lidman, U. Eriksson, A. Fagraeus, and R. Norberg, Antibodies against thyroid cells in Yersinia enterocolitica infection, Lancet 2:1449 (1974).

7. K. Lidman, U. Eriksson, R. Norberg, and A. Fagraeus, Indirect immunofluorescence staining of human thyroid by antibodies occuring in Yersinia enterocolitica infections, Clin. Exp. Immunol. 23:429 (1976).

8. K. Bech, J. Nerup, J. H. Larsen, Yersinia enterocolitica infection and thyroid diseases, Acta Endocrinol. 84:87 (1977).

9. K. Bech, O. Clemmensen, J. H. Larsen, and G. Bendixen, Thyroid disease and yersinia, Lancet 1:1060 (1977).

10. M. Weiss, E. Rubinstein, E. J. Bottone, L. Shenkman, and H. Bank, Yersinia enterocolitica antibodies in thyroid disorders, Israel J. Med. Sc. 15:553 (1983).

11. K. Bech, O. Clemmensen, J. H. Larsen, S. Thyme, and G. Bendixen, Cell-mediated immunity to Yersinia enterocolitica serotype 3 in patients with thyroid diseases, Allergy 33:82 (1978).

12. M. Weiss, S. H. Ingbar, S. Winblad, and D. L. Kasper, Demonstration of a saturable binding site for thyrotropin in Yersinia enterocolitica, Science 219:1331 (1983).

13. F. Pekonen and B. D. Weintraub, Thyrotropin receptors on bovine thyroid membranes: two types with different affinities and specificities, Endocrinology 105:352 (1979).

14. S. M. Amir, H. Uchimura, and S. H. Ingbar, Interactions of bovine thyrotropin and preparations of human chorionic gonadotropin with bovine thyroid membranes, J. Clin. Endocrinol. Metab. 45:280 (1977).

15. M. Weiss, D. L. Kasper, and S. H. Ingbar. Unpublished observations.

16. K. Endo, S. M. Amir, and S. H. Ingbar, Development and evaluation of a method for the partial purification of immunoglobulins specific for Graves' disease, J. Clin. Endocrinol Metab. 52:1113 (1981).

17. G. W. Cushing, D. L. Kasper, and S. H. Ingbar. Unpublished observations.

18. J. Sack, K. D. Burman, D. Dwyer, and D. Zilberstein. Thyrotropin binding proteins in Leishmania; serum antibodies in patients with auto-immune thyroid disease directed against specific parasitic membrane antigens. Clin. Res. 34:433A (1986) (abstract).

19. J. Sack, D. Zilberstein, M. F. Barile, L. Wartofsky, D. Dwyer, and K. D. Burman, Characterization of thyrotropin binding proteins in mycoplasma: Serum antibodies directed against a specific mycoplasma membrane determinant in patients with auto-immune thyroid disease, Program of the 68th Annual Meeting of the Endocrine Society, Anaheim, CA, June 25-27, 1986 (abstract).

20. V. Machia, R. W. Bates, and I. Pastan, Purification and properties of a thyroid stimulating factor isolated from Clostridium perfringens, J. Biol. Chem. 242:3726 (1967).

21. D. LeRoith, C. Roberts, Jr., M. A. Lesniak, and J. Roth, Receptors for intracellular messenget molecules in microbes: similarities to vertebrate receptors and possible implications for diseases in man, Experientia 42:782 (1986).

22. D. LeRoith, G. Delahunty, G. L. Wilson, C. T. Roberts, Jr., J. Shemer, C. Hart, M. S. Lesniak, J. Shiloach, and J. Roth, Evolutionary aspects of the endocrine and nervous systems, Recent Progr. Horm. Res. 42:549 (1986).

23. A. Burshell, P. A. Stathis, Y. Do, S. C. Miller, and D. J. Feldman, Characterization of an estrogen-binding protein in the yeast saccharomyces cerevisiae, J. Biol. Chem. 259:3450 (1984).

24. D. S. Loos, E. P. Stover, A. Restrepo, D. A. Stevens, and D. Feldman, Estradiol binds to a receptor-like cytosol binding protein and initiates a biological response in Paracoccidioides brasiliensis, Proc. Natl. Acad. Sci. (U.S.A.) 80:7659 (1983).

25. G. Biberfeld, A. Fagraeus, and R. Lenkai, Reaction of human smooth muscle antibody with thyroid cells, Clin. Exp. Immunol. 18:371 (1974).

26. Editorial, Lancet 1:734 (1977).

27. I. M. Roitt, Prevailing theories in autoimmune disorders, Triangle 23:67 (1984).

28. R. C. Williams, Jr., Rheumatic fever and the stroptococcus. Another look at molecular mimicry, Amer. J. Med. 75:727 (1983).

29. J. E. Deas, F. A. Janney, L. T. Lee, and C. Howe, Immune electron microscopy of cross-reactions between Mycoplasma pneumoniae and human erythrocytes, Infect. Immunol. 24:211 (1979).

30. K. Stefansson, M. E. Dieperink, D. P. Richman, C. M. Gomez, and L. S. Marton, Sharing of antigenic determinants between the nicotinic acetylcholine receptor and proteins in Escherichia coli, Proteus vulgaris, and Klebsiella pneumoniae: possible role in the pathogenesis of myasthenia gravis, N. Engl. J. Med. 312:221 (1985).

31. S. Ogata, M. Kanamori, and K. Miyashita, Antigenicity of protein and lipopolysaccharide from Yersinia enterocolitica, in: "Yersinia Enterocolitica. Biology, Epidemiology, and Pathology," P. B. Carter, L. LaFleur, and S Thoma, eds., Karger, Basel (1977).

32. K. Aho, P Ahvonen, O. Laitinen, and M. Leirisalo, Arthritis associated with Yersinia enterocolitica infection, in: "Yersinia Enterocolitica," E. J. Bottone, ed., CRC Press, Boca Raton (1981).

"ATRA 1": A NEW AUTOANTIGEN IN AUTOIMMUNE THYROID DISEASE

B. Rapoport, H. Hirayu, P. Seto, R.P. Magnusson, and
S. Filetti

Departments of Medicine, Metabolism 111F, V.A. Medical
Center, San Francisco, CA 94121 and the University of
San Francisco, San Francisco, CA 94143

INTRODUCTION

With the exception of thyroglobulin (1), autoantigens in autoimmune
thyroid disease are poorly defined. Molecular cloning of some of these
antigens would contribute greatly toward their characterization. We have
used serum from a patient with Hashimoto's thyroiditis to screen a human
thyroid cDNA library in the expression bacteriophage vector lambda gt11
(2). We report the molecular cloning and partial nucleotide sequence of
part of a gene that does not have significant homology with any human
gene previously described. The thyroid protein expressed by this gene
therefore represents a new autoimmune thyroid disease-related antigen
(ATRA).

METHODS AND MATERIALS

Human thyroid cDNA library

A lambda gt11 cDNA library (2) was constructed using mRNA prepared
from Graves' thyroid tissue. The library was screened (3) using serum
from a patient with Hashimoto's thyroiditis with a microsomal antibody
titer of $1:10^6$ and no detectable anti-thyroglobulin antibody. Positive
plaques selected by the antiserum were cloned to homogeneity.

Western blots

Lysogens of selected lambda gt11 clones were made in Y1089 cells
for generation of fusion proteins (3). Aliquots of bacterial lysates
were applied to 7.5% polyacrylamide gels and were transferred onto
nitrocellulose paper, followed by the same protocol used to screen the
library (3).

Northern blots

Human thyroid and human liver poly(A)+ mRNA were electrophoresed
in 1.5% agarose and transferred by electroblotting to Nytran paper
(Schleicher and Schuell, Inc., Keene, NH). The paper was probed with
the nick-translated 0.6 kb Eco R1-Eco R1 clone 1 (IL-28) fragment.

Miscellaneous

Human thyroid microsomes were prepared from Graves' thyroid tissue by the method of Hamada et al. (4). Nucleotide sequencing was performed by the dideoxynucleotide method of Sanger (5).

RESULTS

Clone selection

Initial screening of the human thyroid gt11 cDNA library yielded 5 plaques that could be cloned to homogeneity. In order to determine the specificity of these 5 clones as antigens in autoimmune thyroid disease they were tested against the serum of different patients. None of the 17 normal sera reacted with clones 1 and 2, but 7 of 17 normal samples and 11 of 24 samples from patients with autoimmune thyroid disease reacted with clones 3, 4, and 5 (Table I). In contrast to clones 3, 4, and 5, clones 1 and 2 only reacted with serum from patients with auto-immune thyroid disease (Table I). In particular, clone 1 reacted with serum from 4 of 15 (27%) patients with Hashimoto's thyroiditis and 1 of 9 (11%) patients with Graves' disease. Clone 2 only reacted with serum from 2 patients (sisters) with Hashimoto's thyroiditis. Because it reacted with more serum samples, we focused on clone 1.

Three known antigens in autoimmune thyroid disease are the micro-somal antigen, thyroglobulin and the TSH receptor. In order to determine whether clone 1 represented a fragment of one of these antigens we attempted to competitively inhibit antibody binding to the proteins pro-duced by these clones. Neither 100 mU/ml bTSH, 10^{-7} M thyroglobulin nor human thyroid microsomes (150 µg protein/ml) inhibited antiserum binding to clones 1 and 2 (Figure 1). There was no correlation between anti-microsomal antibody titer and the reactivity of various serum samples with clones 1 and 2 (data not shown).

Proof of the specificity of the reaction of serum from a Hashimoto's disease patient with the fusion protein in clone 1 was obtained by Western blot analysis (Figure 2). This figure also indicates more specifically that the fusion protein in clone 1 does not contain thyroglobulin or microsomal antigen, in that these 2 antigens did not inhibit antibody binding.

Northern blot analysis of mRNA from human thyroid and human liver tissue was performed using the 0.6 kb Eco R1 - Eco R1 cDNA insert in clone 1 as a probe. A single band of 3.3 kb was evident in the lane containing thyroid mRNA (Figure 3). The absence of a corresponding mRNA species in liver indicates that clone 1 expresses a thyroid specific protein fragment.

The nucleotide sequence of the clone 1 cDNA insert was determined in both directions (Figure 4). In the sequence of 572 bp, the longest open reading frame from the 5'-end was 117 bp (39 amino acids) with an untranslated 3'-end of greater than 455 bp. The full extent of this untranslated region could not be estimated because the clone does not contain the 3'-end of the gene. The orientation of the nucleotide sequence, as shown in Figure 4, is also uncertain, and was chosen because the longest open reading frame in the opposite orientation was for only 20 amino acid residues. No significant homology was found between this thyroid cDNA fragment and any known sequence in the Gen-Bank and Dayhoff gene banks.

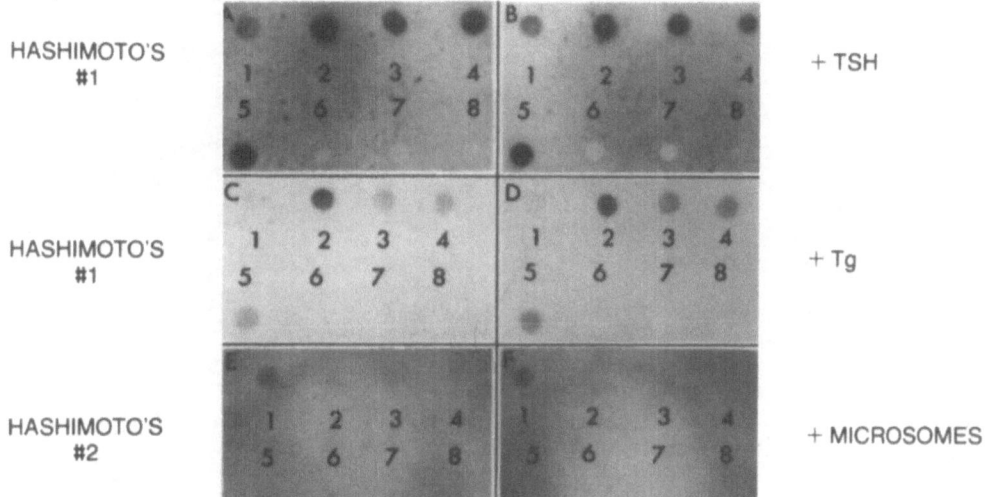

HASHIMOTO'S #1   + TSH

HASHIMOTO'S #1   + Tg

HASHIMOTO'S #2   + MICROSOMES

Figure 1. Specificity of antigens. TSH, thyroglobulin (Tg) and human thyroid microsomes did not prevent binding of Hashimoto's antiserum to the proteins generated by clones 1-5. Each panel represents 1 Petri dish spotted with approximately 1000 pfu each of clones 1-5. Spots 6 and 7 are two different concentrations of wild type lambda gt11, and 8 represents a non-specific clone. In panels A, C and E the filters were exposed to antiserum without the added antigen. In panels B, D and F the same antiserum contained, in addition, 100 mU/ml TSH, 10^{-7} M thyroglobulin. (Tg) and 150 µg protein/ml human thyroid microsomes, respectively.

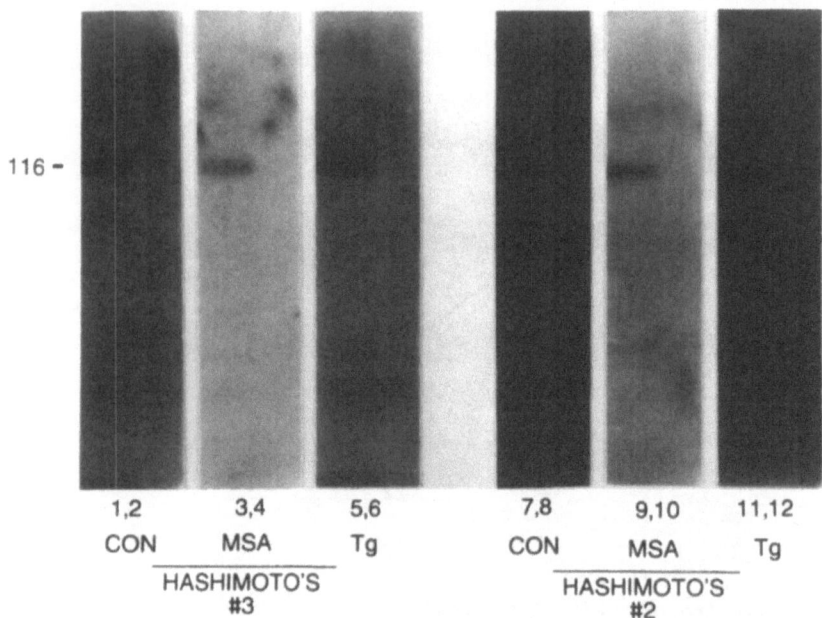

116 −

| 1,2 | 3,4 | 5,6 | 7,8 | 9,10 | 11,12 |
| CON | MSA | Tg | CON | MSA | Tg |

HASHIMOTO'S #3   HASHIMOTO'S #2

Figure 2. Specificity of binding of Hashimoto's antiserum to the fusion protein. Aliquots (approximately 50 μg protein) of the clone 1 (IL-28) bacterial lysate were applied to lanes 1, 3, 5, 7, 8 and 11 in a 7.5% polyacrylamide gel. Lanes 2, 4, 6, 8, 10 and 12 contained BNN97 lysate, a lysogen containing wild type lambda gt11. The proteins transferred to nitrocellulose paper were probed using serum from two Hashimoto's patients (#3 and #2). In control (con) lanes the filter was incubated in antiserum without any additives. Other strips were exposed to the same antibody with the addition of 150 μg protein/ml human thyroid microsomes (MSA) or 10^{-7} M thyroglobulin (Tg). The fusion protein is indicated by the β-galactosidase molecular weight marker of 116,000 Daltons.

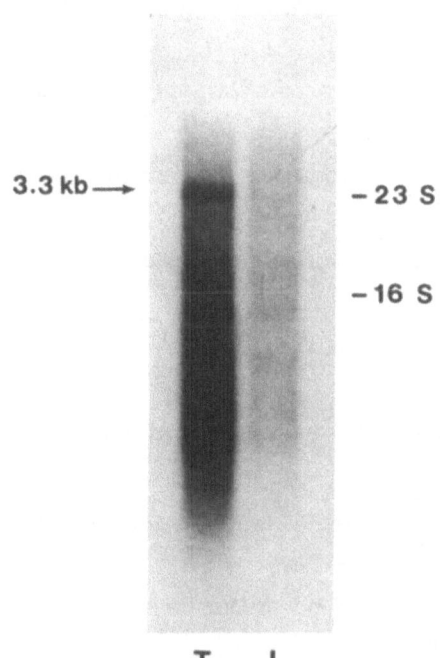

3.3 kb ⟶

−23 S

−16 S

T L

Figure 3: Northern blot analysis of thyroid mRNA (T) and human liver mRNA (L) using the clone 1 (IL-28) cDNA probe. The single band indicated by the arrow was of approximately 3.3 kb, based on molecular weight markers of 16S and 23S ribosomal RNA, and tRNA.

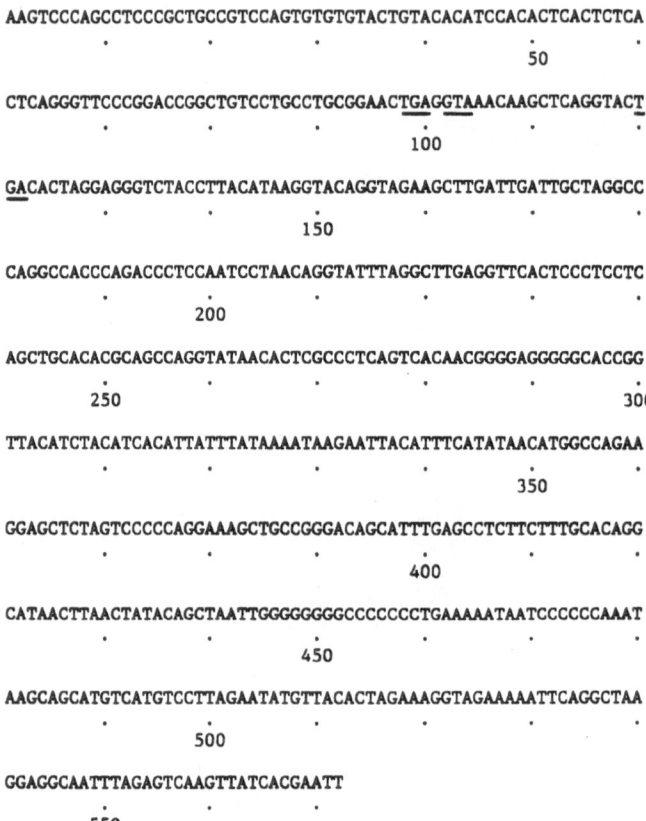

AAGTCCCAGCCTCCCGCTGCCGTCCAGTGTGTGTACTGTACACATCCACACTCACTCTCA
      .   .   .   .   .   .
                                 50

CTCAGGGTTCCCGGACCGGCTGTCCTGCCTGCGGAACTGAGGTAAACAAGCTCAGGTACT
      .   .   .   .   .   .
                             100

GACACTAGGAGGGTCTACCTTACATAAGGTACAGGTAGAAGCTTGATTGATTGCTAGGCC
      .   .   .   .   .   .
                        150

CAGGCCACCCAGACCCTCCAATCCTAACAGGTATTTAGGCTTGAGGTTCACTCCCTCCTC
      .   .   .   .   .   .
            200

AGCTGCACACGCAGCCAGGTATAACACTCGCCCTCAGTCACAACGGGGAGGGGGCACCGG
      .   .   .   .   .   .
   250   300

TTACATCTACATCACATTATTTATAAAATAAGAATTACATTTCATATAACATGGCCAGAA
      .   .   .   .   .   .
                             350

GGAGCTCTAGTCCCCCAGGAAAGCTGCCGGGACAGCATTTGAGCCTCTTCTTTGCACAGG
      .   .   .   .   .   .
                             400

CATAACTTAACTATACAGCTAATTGGGGGGGGCCCCCCCTGAAAAATAATCCCCCCAAAT
      .   .   .   .   .   .
                             450

AAGCAGCATGTCATGTCCTTAGAATATGTTACACTAGAAAGGTAGAAAAATTCAGGCTAA
      .   .   .   .   .   .
                         500

GGAGGCAATTTAGAGTCAAGTTATCACGAATT
      .   .   .
   550

Figure 4. Nucleotide sequence of the 0.6 kb clone 1 cDNA insert (IL-28). The 5' end is depicted on the left, and is so assigned because this orientation provided the longest open reading frame. The solid underlines indicate the initial stop codons in each of the three different reading frames.

DISCUSSION

We describe the identification and partial characterization of a new autoimmune thyroid disease-related antigen (ATRA). This antigen is not thyroglobulin, the microsomal antigen, or the TSH binding site of the TSH receptor. The Northern blot of human thyroid and human liver mRNA indicates that ATRA 1 is thyroid tissue specific. In anticipation that other such antigens will be described, and until the exact nature of the present antigen is determined, we suggest the term ATRA 1 to describe this protein. The functional relevance and pathological significance of ATRA 1 remains to be determined.

Because the cDNA in clone 1 contains only a part of the structural gene, it follows that there must be fewer epitopes on the protein expressed by the fragment than on the entire protein. This, together with the polyclonicity of the microsomal antibody, as well as the hetero-geneity of the epitopes of the microsomal antigen, makes it reasonable that ATRA 1 reacts with only 27% of the Hashimoto's serum samples tested. Even though this incidence could conceivably be higher if the entire ATRA 1 molecule were available for testing, the results with the intact microsomal antigen suggest that this would not be the case (4).

Table I. Reactivity of selected clones with serum from normal subjects and patients with Hashimoto's disease or Graves' disease.

Clone	1[a]	2[b]	3	4	5
Normal[c] (n=17)	0 (0%)	0 (0%)	7 (41%)	7 (41%)	7 (41%)
Hashimoto's disease[d] (n=15)	4 (27%)	2 (13%)	7 (47%)	7 (47%)	7 (47%)
Graves' disease[e] (n=9)	1 (11%)	0 (0%)	4 (44%)	4 (44%)	4 (44%)

[a]IL-28

[b]IL-33

[c]Antimicrosomal antibody titers < 1:100.

[d]Antimicrosomal antibody titers 1:6400 - >1:10^6 (before absorption with BNN97 lysate)

[e]Antimicrosomal antibody titers of < 1:100 - 1:6400 (before absorption with BNN97 lysate)

REFERENCES

1. L. Mercken, M-J Simons, S. Swillens, M. Massaer and G. Vassart,
    Primary structure of bovine thyroglobulin deduced from the
    sequence of its 8,431-base complementary DNA. Nature 316:647
    (1985).
2. R.A. Young and R.W. Davis, Efficient isolation of genes by using
    antibody probes. Proc. Natl. Acad. Sci. USA 80:1194 (1983).
3. T.V.Hunyh, R.A. Young and R.W. Davis, Constructing and screening
    cDNA libraries in lambda gt10 and lambda gt11. in: "DNA
    Cloning Techniques: A Practical Approach" D. Glover, ed.,
    IRL Press, Oxford (1984).
4. N. Hamada, C. Grimm, H. Mori and L.J. DeGroot, Identification of a
    thyroid microsomal antigen by western blot and immunoprecipi-
    tation. J. Clin. End. and Metab. 61(1):120 (1985).
5. F. Sanger, S. Nicklen and A.R. Coulson, DNA sequencing with chain
    terminating inhibitors. Proc. Natl. Acad. Sci. USA 74:5463
    (1977).

MONOCLONAL ANTIBODIES IN THE STUDY OF THYROID AUTOANTIGENS AND AUTOANTIBODIES

J. Ruf, B. Czarnocka, M.E. Toubert, C. Alquier*, C. De Micco§,
M. Henry, C. Dutoit, Y. Malthiery, M. Ferrand and P. Carayon

U 38 INSERM - UA 178 CNRS,*U172 INSERM - UA 1179 CNRS and
§Neuropathology
University of Aix-Marseille Medical School, Marseille, France

INTRODUCTION

Autoimmune disorders of the thyroid gland are associated with the presence of autoantibodies (aAb) specific for antigens localized to the cell cytoplasm, surface membranes and colloid space[1-3]. While some thyroid autoantigens such as thyroglobulin (Tg), the thyroid hormones and, more recently, the thyroid peroxidase (TPO) have been already identified[1-5], the nature of other thyroid autoantigens such as the second colloid antigen, remains unknown[1,2] The main evidence for the involvment of the TSH receptor in autoimmune thyroid diseases is the ability of autoantibodies to inhibit the binding of TSH to thyroid membrane preparations[1,2] Still, the exact role of the TSH receptor in the alterations of thyroid function observed in patients with autoimmune thyroid diseases remains a matter of controversy[1,2]. Assay of aAb to Tg, the microsomal antigen and, in a lesser extent, to the TSH receptor are currently performed[1,2]. However, information on the characteristics of these autoantibodies are rather scarce. The advent of the hybridoma technology offered a new approach to decipher the pathophysiological mechanisms of autoimmunity. Monoclonal antibodies (mAb) are currently in use in numerous laboratories to study the cellular and molecular aspects of autoimmune diseases. We will review here several applications of mAb in thyroid autoimmunity currently in progress in our laboratory.

1- ANTIGEN LOCALIZATION

Numerous mAb directed against thyroid membrane antigens were produced in our laboratory. Nineteen mAb were screened for cross-reactivity with anti-microsomal aAb. One of these mAb appeared to be directed against the microsomal antigen. Optical microscopic examination of human thyroid tissue sections revealed that staining with the mAb was almost identical to that observed with anti-microsomal aAb[4]. Complete extinction of mAb staining was obtained after preincubating thyroid tissue sections with aAb[6]. We

---

Address Correspondence to Dr Pierre Carayon, U 38 INSERM, Faculté de Médecine, F-13385 Marseille Cedex 5, France.

also noted that the localization of the microsomal antigen was closely related to that of TPO which first suggested that TPO and the microsomal antigen were identical. Electron microscopic examination of thyroid tissue sections further showed that both TPO and the microsomal antigen were found in the apical microvillar membranes and also in the endoplasmic reticulum, the perinuclear cisternae and the exocytic vesicles of the follicular cells[7] (Fig. 1, upper part). Preincubation of human thyroid follicles with anti-TPO mAb and anti-microsomal aAb indicated that both antigens were equally submitted to a process of endocytosis (Fig. 1, lower part).

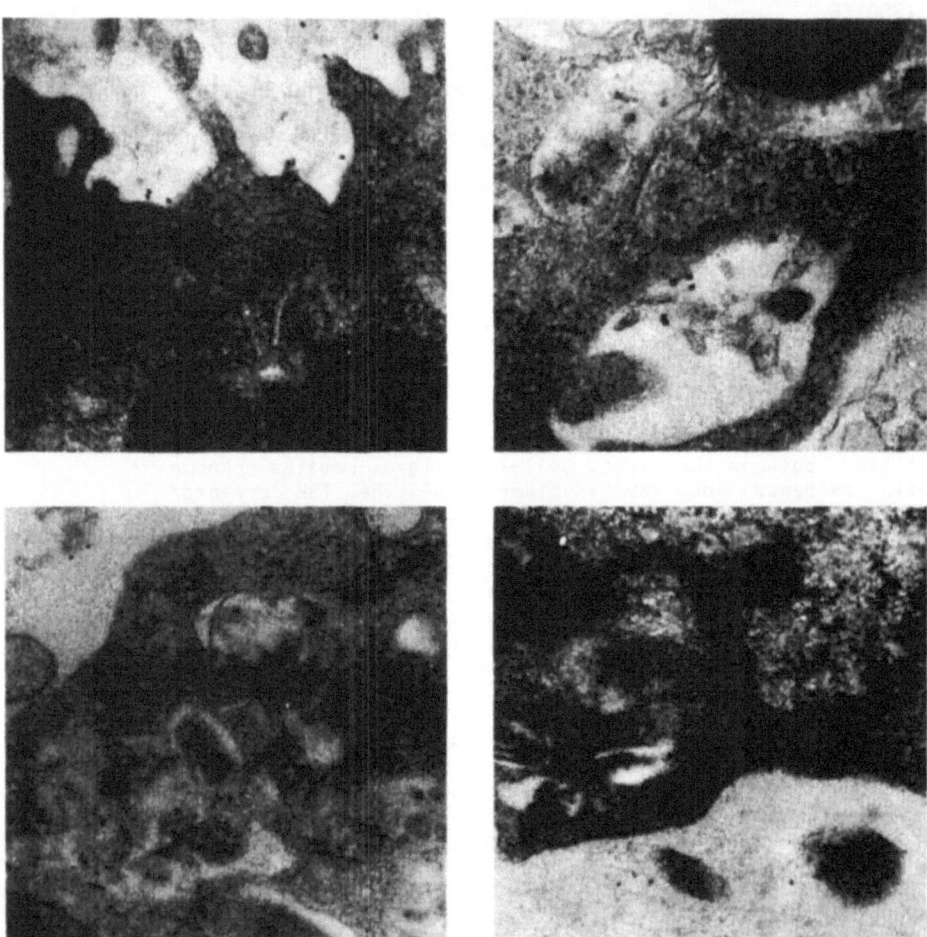

Fig.1. Localization of binding sites for anti-TPO mAb (left part) and anti-microsomal aAb (right part) on human thyroid tissue sections (upper part) and sections of isolated human thyroid follicles (lower part).

Table 1 Activity of thyroid peroxidase at various stages of purification

Stage of purification	Total protein	Total units	Specific activity	Purification factor
	(mg)	(U/mg)	(U/mg)	
Microsomes	791	915	1.1	1
Solubilizate	383	861	2.2	2
Affinity chromatography	1.6	610	381	331

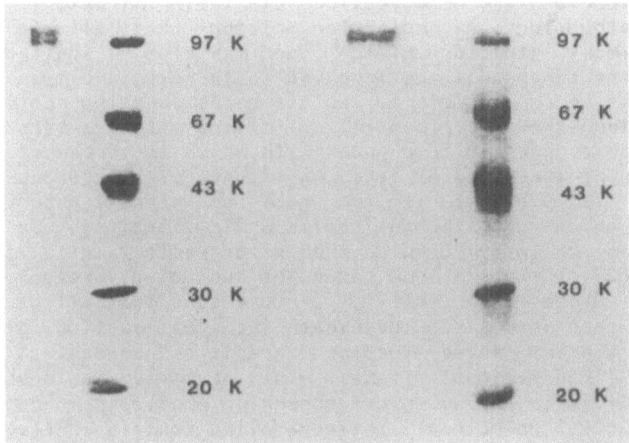

Fig 2 Polyacrylamide gel electrophoresis of affinity purified TPO in reducing (left panel) and non reducing conditions (right panel).

2 - ANTIGEN PURIFICATION

Polyclonal aAb assisted affinity chromatography has been carried out in order to purify the microsomal antigen and the TSH receptor. All the attempts failed to yield pure antigens due to the polyspecificity of the antibodies present in the aAb preparations. Using the anti-TPO mAb previously shown to cross-react with anti-microsomal aAb, we undertook the purification of the microsomal antigen from surgical specimens of human thyroid glands[5]. The purification procedure was monitored by measuring TPO activity. In initial thyroid homogenates and particulate fractions, the TPO activity was found to vary widely from batch to batch. This fluctuation could be accounted for by the origin of the thyroid specimens which were from patients with various diseases and interference with the guaiacol assay in crude preparations. On the basis of previous papers from other groups[8,9], a purification of about 10-fold over the starting material to microsomes might be assumed. In the microsomal fraction, the specific activity of TPO ranges from 1.0 to 2.0 U/mg and increased to 300 to 400 U/mg in the purified material eluted from the mAb affinity column. Therefore, it was estimated that TPO was purified 3000 to 3500 fold over the starting thyroid homogenate (Table 1). The physico-chemical characteristics of the affinity-purified TPO were extensively studied. Electrophoresis in sodium dodecylsulfate polyacrylamide slab gels showed two contiguous bands of apparent molecular weight 95 and 105 KDa (Fig.2 left panel) ; in non-reducing conditions, TPO resolved in one band migrating in the same region (Fig.2, right panel).

3 - ANTIGEN PRIMARY STRUCTURE

Determination of the amino acid sequence of proteins is an important step towards the elucidation of their structure and function. The methodology of molecular biology has allowed to decipher the primary structure of Tg[10,11] and may also be applied to the study of the other antigens involved in thyroid autoimmunity. Several strategies are possible to isolate genes encoding proteins of interest. Often the experimentally limiting step has been the lack of a suitable nucleic acid probe with which to screen clones for those containing the relevant gene. An immunological approach to screening clones is possible if the gene of interest encodes a polypeptide for which specific antibodies are available[12]. Genomic DNA fragments can be inserted in an expression vector, gt11, that expresses the foreign insert DNA under the control of prokaryotic gene signals in Escherichia coli [13,14]. To ensure that all of the coding sequences are expressed requires the construction of a recombinant DNA library whose foreign inserts are present in all orientations and translational frames. The next step is to use a specific and efficient immunological screening procedure to detect translation products. Polyclonal antisera often contain irrelevant antibodies which could react with unwanted antigens. This is generally the case with antisera to thyroid antigens which present at least anti-Tg antibodies due either to contamination of the antigens by Tg or to an autoimmune reaction of the recipient. The use of a mixture of carefully selected mAb ensures a very specific survey of the antigens expressed by recombinant clones.

This approach has been undertaken in our and other laboratories to disclose the structure of thyroid autoantigens. As a

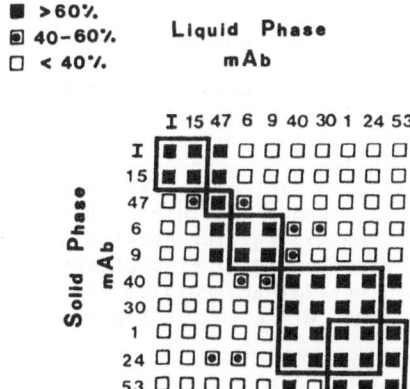

¹²⁵I LABELED mAb

	J7C 9.3	J7C 76.20	J8B 45.5	J8B 6.12	J8B 89.5	J7C 44.6	J8A 32.13	J7C 73.7	J7B 49.15	J8A 53.9
J7C 9.3	■ᵛ	□	□	□	□	□	□	□	□	□
J7C 76.20	□	■ᵛᴵ	□	□	□	□	▨	▨	▨	▨
J8B 45.5	□	□	■	■ᴵᴵ	▨	□	▨	▨	▨	▨
J8B 6.12	□	□	■	■	▨	▨	▨	▨	▨	▨
J8B 89.5	□	□	▨	▨	■ᴵᴵᴵ	□	□	□	□	□
J7C 44.6	□	□	□	▨	□	■	■	■	■ᴵⱽ	■ᴵ
J8A 32.13	▨	□	□	▨	□	■	■	■	■	■
J7C 73.7	□	□	□	▨	▨	□	■	■	■	■
J7B 49.15	□	□	▨	▨	▨	□	■	■	■	■
J8A 53.9	□	□	□	□	▨	□	■	■	■	■

(rows labelled **UNLABELED mAb**)

Fig.3 Schematic representation of the Tg binding inhibition curves of the 10 radioiodinated mAb by the 10 unlabelled mAb. ■ indicates a complete inhibition, ▨ indicates a partial inhibition, and □ indicates no inhibition. Reactivity with identical antigenic regions are suggested by mAb which reciprocally achieved complete inhibition and accordingly are grouped in cluster (numbered solid line).

■ >60%.
▣ 40-60%.
□ < 40%.

Liquid Phase mAb

	I	15	47	6	9	40	30	1	24	53
I	■	■	■	□	□	□	□	□	□	□
15	■	■	■	□	□	□	□	□	□	□
47	□	▣	■	▣	□	□	□	□	□	□
6	□	□	■	■	▣	▣	□	□	□	□
9	□	□	▣	■	■	▣	□	□	□	□
40	□	□	□	▣	□	■	■	■	■	■
30	□	□	□	□	▣	■	■	■	■	■
1	□	□	□	□	□	■	■	■	■	■
24	□	□	▣	▣	□	■	■	■	■	■
53	□	□	□	□	□	■	□	■	■	■

(rows labelled **Solid Phase mAb**)

Fig 4. Relationship among the epitopes recognized by 10 anti-TPO mAb investigated by cross-inhibition experiment. Each MAb was tested for its ability in solution (Liquid Phase) to inhibit the binding of labelled TPO to microtiter plate coated mAb (solid Phase).

matter of example, informations about the gene of TPO are expected very soon.

4 - ANTIGEN THREE DIMENSIONAL STRUCTURE

Major advances in the elucidation of the primary structure of proteins have been made possible by molecular biology techniques. However, information about the higher order structures of these molecules is not abundant. An approach to examine the three dimensional structure of proteins is to use antibodies for mapping their antigenic surface [15].

Among the numerous anti-Tg mAb produced in our laboratory, 10 were purified and characterized [16]. To define the topology of the antigenic sites recognized by the mAb we established the Tg binding inhibition curves of each of the 10 radiolabelled mAb by each of the 10 unlabelled mAb [17]. Three patterns of inhibition were distinguished : complete inhibition observed with 1 to 10 ug/ml unlabelled mAb, partial inhibition and no inhibition. The results of the cross-inhibition experiments are summarized Fig.3. Reactivity with identical antigenic regions was suggested by mAb which reciprocally achieved complete inhibition and were accordingly grouped in clusters. Six distinct regions might be delineated. Taking into account not only complete but also partial inhibitions nine patterns of cross-inhibition might be observed. Only two mAb (J7C73.7 and J7B49.15) interacted identically. The enumeration of Tg epitopes was further studied using more mAb kindly made available to us by several research groups. 56 mAb were used, 29 were labelled with alkaline phosphatase and their binding to Tg was measured in the absence or presence of various concentration of the 56 unlabelled mAb. We thus obtained more than 1600 dose-response curves. Analysis of the data indicated that 18 mAb did not cross-react with the 29 labelled mAb. The remaining 38 mAb inhibited the binding to Tg of one to 13 labelled mAb and delineated 18 patterns of reactivity. From these data it emerges that Tg presents an extraordinary antigenic diversity. This suggests that the number of antigenic determinants presented by Tg far exceeds the number of 40 previously proposed by another group [18].

The same approach has been taken for studying the immunological structure of TPO [6]. Ten out of 66 anti-TPO mAb were selected for their ability after coating to microtiter plates to efficiently bind radioiodinated TPO. Preincubation of labelled TPO with mAb in solution resulted in various degree of inhibition of TPO binding to the coated mAb. Converted into qualitative terms i.e. complete, partial or no inhibition, the results were incorporated into an 10 x 10 matrix. As shown Fig.4, five clusters of reactivity were distinguished. These preliminary results indicated that human TPO expressed at least five different antigenic domains on its surface.

5 - AUTOANTIBODY HETEROGENEITY

It is generally accepted that the repertoire of aAb is restricted as compared to heterologous antibodies [18]. It has been shown that human Tg presented at least 40 antigenic sites in heterologous system but only two or three in homologous system [2,18]. No information were available for anti-microsomal aAb.

Affinity-purified anti-Tg aAb were assayed for their ability to inhibit the binding to Tg of the 10 radioiodinated mAb previously used for criss-cross experiments (see Fig 3). Typical results are presented in Fig. 5. aAb from patients with Graves'disease generally exhibited strong inhibition of mAb directed against the same antigenic domain and weak but significant inhibition of all other mAb (Fig.5 upper part).

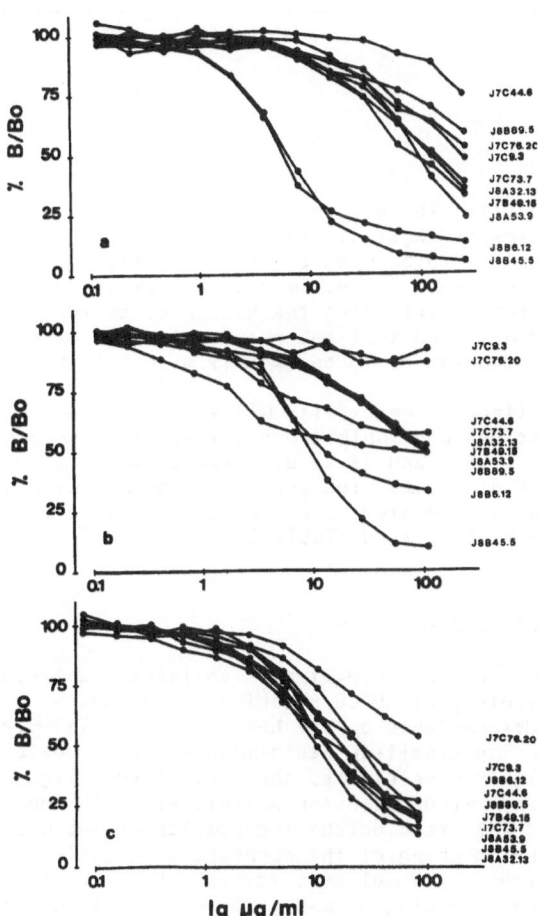

Fig 5. Inhibition curves of 10 radioiodinated mAb binding to Tg by affinity purified anti-Tg aAb from patients with Graves'disease (upper part), Hashimoto's thyroiditis (middle part) and thyroid cancer (lower part).

Table 2 Inhibition of mAb binding to TPO by pools of 5 sera from patients with Graves'disase and Hashimoto's thyroiditis

	Pool dilution	I	15	47	6	9	40	30	1	24	53
						mAb					
Graves' disease	1/3000	7[a)]	20	0	10	0	0	5	0	0	0
	1/200	94	48	30	95	100	3	19	11	28	0
	1/100	100	83	51	100	100	25	34	15	28	0
	1/20	100	100	58	100	100	51	36	50	50	16
Hashimoto's thyroiditis	1/3000	0	9	0	13	9	0	0	0	20	3
	1/200	66	42	40	89	100	0	2	0	22	0
	1/100	95	72	50	100	100	0	20	0	24	4
	1/20	95	100	71	100	100	44	28	40	50	11

a) % inhibition

In Hashimoto's thyroiditis the pattern of mAb binding inhibition was more complex. mAb directed against several domains of Tg were often found inhibited by aAb (Fig.5, middle). By contrast, anti-Tg aAb in some patients with thyroid carcinoma might inhibit the whole set of mAb (Fig.5 lower part). Extending the number of antigenic domains and patients studied we found that aAb reacted strongly with several reccurent antigenic domains of Tg and weakly with all the remaining antigenic domains [19].

The same pattern of reactivity was found with anti-TPO aAb [20]. At low concentration aAb inhibited significantly the binding of two pairs of mAb (I-15 and 6-9) directed against two different domains of TPO (see Fig. 4). At high concentration the binding sites for these mAb appeared saturated by aAb which displayed significant inhibition of the other mAb tested (Table 2).

6 - AUTOANTIBODY IDIOTYPIC ANALYSIS

Five xenogeneic anti-idiotypic antisera (anti-id) were produced against individual BALB/c-derived mAb which bound to different peptidic determinants on the human Tg molecule [21]. Idiotypic analysis performed using sensitive radioimmunoassays revealed that : (1) the anti-id highly precipitated their homologous ligands : (2) two anti-id displayed minor cross-reactivities with one or two heterologous mAb ; (3) each unlabelled homologous mAb was able to inhibit the idiotype binding of the corresponding anti-id ; (4) no significant inhibition of homologous idiotype binding was observed with large excess of heterologous mAb ; (5) efficient inhibition of mAb binding to Tg was observed only when homologous anti-id served as inhibitor. These data supported the conclusion that xenogeneic anti-id might detect on their corresponding ligands individual idiotypic specificities that could be located at the mAb-combining site. Such reagents may constitute appropriate probes for further studies on anti-Tg autoimmunity.

CONCLUSION

The monoclonal antibody technology appears instrumental in the elucidation of the mechanisms involved in autoimmune thyroid diseases. Associated with methods used in biochemistry, cell biology and molecular biology, monoclonal antibodies may allow a quantum leap in our understanding of thyroid autoimmunity.

ACKNOWLEDGMENTS

This work was supported in part by grants from the Association pour la Recherche contre le Cancer and the Association pour la Recherche en Biologie Cellulaire.

REFERENCES

1. R. Volpé, "Auto-Immunity in the endocrine System", Springer-Verlag, New-York (1981)
2. A. Pinchera, G.F. Fenzi, P. Vitti, L. Chiovato, L. Bartalena, E. Macchia, and S. Mariotti, Significance of thyroid auto antibodies in autoimmune thyroid diseases, in : "Autoimmunity and the Thyroid", P.G. Walfish, J.R. Wall and R. Volpé, eds., Academic Press, Orlando pp 139-152 (1985)
3. E.L. Khoury, G.F. Bottazzo and I.M. Roitt, The thyroid microsomal antibody revisited, J. Exp. Med. 159 : 577 (1984)
4. B.Czarnocka, J. Ruf, M. Ferrand and P. Carayon, Antigenic relationship between thyroid peroxidase and the microsomal antigen involved in auto-immune thyroid diseases, C.R. Acad. Sci (Paris) 300 : 577 (1985)
5. B. Czarnocka, J. Ruf,, M. Ferrand, P. Carayon and S. Lissitzky, Purification of the human thyroid peroxidase and its identification as the microsomal antigen involved in autoimmune thyroid diseases, FEBS Lett. 190 : 147 (1985)
6. J. Ruf, B. Czarnocka, C. De Micco, C. Dutoit, M. Ferrand and P. Carayon, Thyroid peroxidase is the organ-specific "microsomal" autoantigen involved in thyroid autoimmunity, Acta Endocrinol., accepted for publication
7. C. Alquier, J. Ruf and P. Carayon, Co-localization of thyroid peroxidase and the binding sites for anti-microsomal and anti-peroxidase antibodies, Submitted for publication.
8. T. Hosoya and M. Morrison, The isolation and purification of thyroid peroxidase, J. Biol. Chem. 242 : 2828 (1967)
9. N.M. Alexander, Purification of bovine thyroid peroxidase, Endocrinology 100 : 1610 (1977)
10. L. Mercken, M.J. Simons, M. Massaer and G. Vassart, Primary structure of bovine thyroglobulin deduced form the sequence of its 8,431-base complementary DNA, Nature, 316 : 647 (1985)
11. Y. Malthiery and S. Lissitzky, Primary structure of human thyroglobulin deduced from the sequence of its 8,448 base complementary DNA, Submitted for publication
12. H.A. Erlich, S.N. Cohen and H.O Mc Devitt, Immunological detection and characterization of products translated from cloned DNA fragments, Methods in Enzymology, 68 : 443 (1979)
13. R.A. Young and R.W. Davis, Efficient isolation of genes by using antibody probes, Proc. Natl. Acad. Sci. USA 80 : 1194 (1983)
14. B. Lapeyre and F. Amalric, A powerful method for the preparation of cDNA libraries : isolation of cDNA encoding a 100 kDal nucleolar protein, Gene 37 : 215 (1985)

15. W.R. Moyle, P.H. Ehrlich and R.E. Canfield, Use of monoclonal antibodies to subunits of hCG to examine the orientation in its complex with receptor, Proc Natl Acad Sci USA, 79 : 2245 (1982)
16. J. Ruf, P. Carayon, N. Sarles-Philip, F. Kourilsky and S. Lissitzky, Specificity of monoclonal antibodies against human thyroglobulin ; comparison with autoimmune antibodies, EMBO J. 2 : 1821 (1983)
17. J. Ruf, P. Carayon and S. Lissitzky, An approach to human thyroglobulin structure by immunological methods using monoclonal antibodies, in : "Thyroglobulin. The Prothyroid Hormone", M.C. Eggo and G.N. Burrow eds, Raven Press, New-York, pp 13-20 (1985)
18. I.M. Roitt, L. De Carvalho, L. Nye and G. Wick, Some general aspects of organ-specific autoimmunity in "Autoimmune Aspects of Endocrine Disorders", A. Pinchera, D. Doniach, G.F. Fenzi and L. Baschieri eds, Academic Press, London, pp 3-10 (1980)
19. J. Ruf, M. Henry, C. De Micco and P. Carayon, characterization of monoclonal and autoimmune antibodies to thyroglobulin ; applications to clinical investigation, in : "Thyroglobulin and Thyroglobulin Antibodies", C. Reiners ed, Thieme Verlag-Stratton, New-York, in press
20. J. Ruf, B. Czarnocka, M.E. Toubert, M. Ferrand and P. Carayon, Characterization of monoclonal, polyclonal and autoimmune antibodies to human thyroid peroxidase, Submitted for publication.
21. J. Ruf, P. Carayon and S. Lissitzky, Idiotypic analysis of five xenogeneic antisera to anti-human thyroglobulin monoclonal antibodies, Immunology Lett. 13 : 39 (1986)

LATS/TSAb: THEN AND NOW

J.M. McKenzie

Department of Medicine
University of Miami School of Medicine
Miami, FL

Thirty years ago a description of the clinical syndrome of Graves' disease was similar to that which would be written today. There has been some increased understanding of specific situations such as "euthyroid ophthalmopathy" and the expected consequences of a given mode of therapy; by and large, however, the clinician today is different from the 1956 physician primarily in the technology that is available to facilitate (or obfuscate) patient-management.

On the other hand, when one considers understanding of pathogenesis, there are major advances in these 3 decades, even although much remains to be elucidated. Back then, TSH was generally seen to be the pathogenetic agent, certainly of hyperthyroidism, and even of ophthalmopathy, although the difficulty of accepting the thesis was regularly debated. One of the major negative influences on the acquisition of new knowledge was the available technology for measuring TSH. There was no radioimmunoasay, no clear knowledge of the chemical nature of TSH and certainly no understanding of the mode of action of the hormone. The bases on which one could expect progress in research, considering theories of the time, were more sensitive assays to quantitate TSH bioactivity in pituitary, blood and urine, as had been the approach for the previous 25 years. By 1956, bioassay data had accumulated, such as in the work of D'Angelo (1), Gilliland and Strudwick (2) and Querido and his colleages (3), that seemed to give major support to the importance of TSH in Graves' disease. This was despite recognition that TSH ought to be suppressed by the excess thyroid hormone. Arguments to accommodate this difficulty included the following: TSH secretion by the pituitary was controlled by a "higher setting of the thyrostat", i.e. suppression occurred only with a supra-normal concentration of thyroid hormone [as is, indeed, now accepted in the rare syndrome of pituitary-resistance to the hormone (4)]; the thyroid gland in Graves' disease was ultra-sensitive, so that sub-normal concentrations of TSH were stimulatory; TSH was indeed the thyroid-stimulator but the well-recognized lymphoid tissue hyperplasia in Graves' disease was responsible for metabolism of the hormone so that it was not in high concentration in the peripheral blood. With these and other arguments being raised to reconcile the frequent failure to measure TSH in the blood of the Graves' disease patient, the emphasis of research was to develop more sensitive procedures to prove the generally accepted tenet that TSH was circulating and causing the syndrome.

In this environment, Adams and Purves in New Zealand developed a sensitive procedure for the bioassay of TSH. This entailed the in vivo labelling of thyroid iodine of a guinea pig with 131I, suppression of endogenous TSH, and the measurement of thyroid-stimulation by identifying an increase in blood radioactivity following the injection of test material. Part of the initial assay design was a "cross-over" component whereby the same guinea pig was used on the following day to assess the responsiveness of the animal to standard TSH. With the injection of serum from a patient with Graves' disease it was noted that the blood radioactivity on the second morning was unexpectedly high. Rather than discard the data, and animal, Adams and Purves had the perspicacity to explore further the cause of this irritating anomaly, and so came to the recognition of an "abnormal TSH" in Graves' disease (5). Unfortunately for the sake of confirmation of these findings, apparently only Adams was adept at bleeding a guinea pig that "should be quietly dozing at this stage" (6) (Purves, personal communication) and therefore an alternate animal, the mouse, was tested (7) and was found to be more generally useful. Thus began the period of research into what by 1960 (at the 4th International Thyroid Congress) became known as the long-acting thyroid stimulator (LATS).

By 1964 LATS activity was known to reside in an IgG molecule (8) and the thought that it might be an antibody began to develop. However the low frequency of its occurrence in Graves' disease ($\simeq$20%) led to the concept of LATS causing hyperthyroidism to fall into disfavor. One circumstance that persuaded some to retain a central role for LATS was the finding that neonatal hyperthyroidism was associated with the transplacental passage of LATS (9,10). Now that it is recognized that LATS activity represents a cross-reaction in the mouse of the most potent preparations of TSAb-IgG (11), the low frequency of positive LATS assay and the association with neonatal Graves' disease become readily interpretable.

Further advances in our understanding of LATS/TSAb arose from the realization that a human antibody ought to be- and indeed is - most effectively identified by a system based upon the use of a human thyroid preparation. The earliest use of human thyroid was the development of the LATS-protector assay (12). This, in effect, although not initially viewed as such, was the first assay in this field designed on the basis of a competition of ligands for a receptor. That is, TSAb in a LATS-negative serum prevented the absorption of a standard LATS by the TSH receptor in human thyroid membranes. The technique was taken up particularly by Munro and his colleagues who contributed important observations as a result (reviewed in 13). Some time later other assays were reported in which colloid droplet formation in human thyroid slices (14) or an increase in cAMP concentration in such tissue (14,15) were the end-points. On a similar conceptual basis, direct stimulation of adenylate cyclase in human thyroid membranes was assessed as an index of LATS/TSAb activity (16,17). From the use of these techniques much relevant data were accumulated. However, it has been the assay with human thyroid cells in primary monolayer culture, originally reported by Rapoport and his colleagues (18), and now available commercially, that has made it possible for many laboratories to study TSAb, leading to general acceptance of the concept that it is the cause of hyperthyroidism in Graves' disease.

An alternate principle for the assay of TSAb is the inhibition of the binding of radio-labelled TSH to its receptor. The original relevant reports were by Manley and colleagues (19) and Mehdi and Nussey (20), but most of the credit for efficient exploitation of the system goes to Smith and Hall and their colleagues (21,22,23). This TSH-binding inhibition (TBI) assay is convenient and is available to any laboratory that has the interest to set it up and, indeed, is marketed as a commercial kit. The latter is based upon the TSH receptor prepared from solubilized porcine thyroid membranes.

Although TSAb may be accepted as inhibiting TSH binding, so too do other antibodies that are not stimulatory. Furthermore, it is now recognized (see Zakarija, this symposium) that multiple thyroid receptor antibodies may be present in patients with autoimmune thyroid disease, variably influencing thyroid function. Consequently, since inhibition of TSH-binding is clearly not synonymous with thyroid-stimulation, care has to be taken in interpreting data obtained with this type of assay.

Current status of TSAb

To cull the data reported from many laboratories the following is offered as a summary of the current status of TSAb.

1. It is best measured with human thyroid cells in culture. A more convenient, but less sensitive, alternative is the continuous culture line of functioning rat thyroid (FRTL-5) cells (24); unfortunately, as might be expected, there are instances when this non-human system apparently fails to respond to the human antibody.

2. It causes hyperthyroidism but is of little special use in patient management, except as a prognosticator of relapse if TSAb is found to remain in the blood at the end of a course of antithyroid drugs (25).

3. A specific clinical circumstance where TSAb data are most useful is in forecasting neonatal Graves' disease. A high level (an operational definition that, as yet, varies from one laboratory to another) of TSAb in the pregnant woman in the third trimester indicates that the child will have hyperthyroidism in the neonatal period (26). A variant of this syndrome is where multiple antibodies occur, influencing thyroid function by enhancement or inhibition of TSAb (27,28).

These statements would, I believe, meet a general consensus but it is clear that there are areas of disagreement in the field, some of which will now be reviewed.

The TBI assay, as referred to above certainly has produced "false negative" results, in that it is not always positive despite the presence of TSAb; this may be seen as a reflection of less sensitivity. However, what of the reported high incidence of TBI-positive IgG in patients who have goiter that would otherwise be considered to be of a non-immune origin? For instance, Brown et al reported such data with sera from patients with non-toxic nodular goiter (29). Cytochemical bioassays have been developed, characterized by extreme sensitivity, but with undoubted operational problems (30). Proponents of these procedures have reported that TSAb occurs in the blood in non-toxic goiter and toxic adenoma (31,32). Perhaps more disturbing to the view that TSAb is an antibody specifically related to Graves' disease, is the use of a technique based upon direct stimulation of thyroid membrane adenylate cyclase, that led to identification of TSAb in other autoimmune disorders such as rheumatoid arthritis and type I diabetes mellitus (33,34). These are all reports in which data appear to refute the specificity of TSAb and that fact has to be acknowledged. While I do not wish to be seen as an apologist in these matters, the following points are offered in favor of retaining the view that TSAb is pathogenetic in only Graves' disease and in seeing its true occurrence in such as Hashimoto's disease as reflecting overlap of autoimmune thyroid disorder.

First, there are the simple facts that Graves' disease is an autoimmune disturbance and TSAb is an autoantibody. Recognition of stigmata of involvement of the immune system in the syndrome antedates the LATS/TSAb era and came before even the development of understanding of the significance of the observations. That is, in 1928, Warthin referred to the "constitutional entity of exophthalmic goiter" by way of allusion to thymic and lymphoid hyperplasia (35). Indeed Halsted was so impressed by the relationship that he advocated, and practised, thymectomy for Graves' disease (36) (with results that would not encourage a return to that approach). Currently, lymphoid infiltration of the thyroid is recognized as such a prominent feature of Graves' disease that some argue for the thyroid as being the major site of production of TSAb (37). In other words, although this may be seen as arguing "ad hoc , propter hoc", the production of an autoantibody, by our current understanding of immune regulation, should be accompanied by associated anatomical and histological features - localized or generalized - of immune reactivity. In Graves' disease this concept is supported beyond thyroid involvement in that there is well-accepted co-incidence of other autoimmune disorders in the patient and in family members. The general lack of such features of autoimmunity in patients with non-toxic goiter or toxic adenoma necessitates rigour in accepting data that would enfold them into a category of autoimmune pathogenesis.

So what of the various reports, referred to above, that would damage the Graves'- specific status of TSAb? Regarding TBI assays, it may be relevant to emphasize that not only does normal IgG influence TSH-binding, but that the fraction characterized by a high pI, as separated by isoelectric focussing, is especially potent in this regard (38). This may relate to the low pI of the TSH receptor (39) that presumably facilitates non-specific binding to a molecule of complementary charge. There are no data that identify the variability of the proportion of high pI IgG in serum and, using a pool of normal serum as a control preparation, would mask this variability.

The sensitivity of cytochemical assays has already been referred to. This not only necessitates strict criteria for assay design including double-blind determinations (that is now largely routine), but leaves open the question of thyroid-stimulators other than TSAb influencing the preparations. More and more stimulators of many metabolic pathways - in the thyroid and other organs - are being identified (40). It may be worthy of emphasis that inhibition of a given effect by the addition of antibody to IgG does not exclude the possibility of the co-precipitation of a non-IgG; anti-TSH was shown some time ago to be a potent thyroid stimulator because of associated TSH (41).

One approach to determining the relevance of in vitro assay

data is to make the assumption that a putative activity ought to have an effect _in vivo_, and test accordingly. This has been done, as reported at this symposium, by Feldt-Rasmussen and colleagues, who identified stimulation of thyroid membrane adenylate cyclase by IgG from patients with rheumatoid arthritis or diabetes mellitus. Their findings indicate that the _in vitro_ assay data did not correlate with _in vivo_ results that would be expected if TSAb were circulating and stimulating the patient's thyroid gland.

To summarize this polemic in favor of the Graves'- specificity of TSAb, there are undoubtedly many reports contrary to that view. Nonetheless, after consideration of autoimmune disorders in general, the occurrence of TSAb in what otherwise appears to be non-immune disease ought to be bolstered with more than _in vitro_ assay data. Specifically, in conditions such as sporadic goiter and toxic adenoma, the apparent existence of TSAb as evidenced by assay results, that are usually marginally positive, should not necessarily be taken as an indication that the "TSAb" is causing the disease. Longitudinal studies and _in vivo_ correlations with the _in vitro_ measurements will be required to establish that TSAb truly occurs in these conditions.

Finally, to end a review of the status of TSAb in Graves' disease, one should touch on the current exciting developments in related research and advances in immunology that have caused research in the field of thyroid autoimmunity to explode (although it may be a problem that we as thyroidologists often make shaky immunologists – and vice versa!). Presumably, the underlying disorder is of cellular control mechanisms; but is the primary source of TSAb the thyroid or other organ such as bone marrow or lymph nodes? With recognition of DR expression on thyroid epithelial cells (41), the question of its relevance to maintenance of TSAb-production arises. And is it possible a cross-reacting antigen for the TSH receptor, as identified in Yersinia enterocolitica (43), enters into pathogenesis? Is stress involved in initiating or maintaining production of TSAb? The magnitude of the questions, certainly combined, makes it highly likely that there will be good reason to repeat this symposium in the decades ahead.

Acknowledgements

The author is the Kathleen and Stanley Glaser Professor of Medicine. Thanks are expressed to Mrs. Gilda Manicourt for expert typing of the manuscript.

References

1. D'Angelo SA, Paschkis KE, Gordon AS, Cantarrow A 1951 J Clin Endocrinol Metab 11:1237
2. Gilliland ID, Strudwick JL 1956 Brit Med J 1:378
3. Querido A, Lameijer LDF 1856 Proc Roy Soc Med 49:209
4. Weintraub BD, Gershengorn MC, Kourides IA, Fein H 1981 Ann Intern Med 95:339
5. Adams DD, Purves HD 1956 Proc Univ Otago Med Sch 34:11
6. Adams DD, Purves HD 1955 Endocrinology 57:17
7. McKenzie JM 1958 Endocrinology 62:865
8. Kriss JP, Pleshakov V, Chien JR 1964 J Clin Endocrinol Metab 24:1005
9. McKenzie JM 1964 J Clin Endocrinol Metab 24:660
10. Sunshine P, Kusumolo H, Kriss JP 1965 Pediatrics 36:869
11. Zakarija M, McKenzie JM 1978 J Clin Endocrinol Metab 47:249
12. Adams DD, Kennedy TH 1967 J Clin Endocrinol Metab 27:173

13. Kendall-Taylor P, Dirmikis S, Munro DS 1974 Quart J Med 43:619
14. Onaya T, Kotani M, Yamada T, Ochi Y 1973 J Clin Endocrinol Metab 36:859
15. McKenzie JM, Zakarija M 1985 Methods in Enzymology 109:677
16. Orgiazzi J, Williams DE, Chapra IJ, Solomon DH 1976 J Clin Endocrinol Metab 42:341
17. Bech K, Madsen SN 1979 Clin Endocrinol (Oxford) 11:47
18. Rapoport B, Filetti S, Takai N, Seto P, Halverson G 1982 Metabolism 31:1159
19. Manley SW, Bourke JR, Hawker RW 1974 J Endocrinol 61:437
20. Mehdi SQ, Nussey SS, Gibbons CP, El Kabir DJ 1973 Biochem Soc Trans 1:1005
21. Smith BR, Hall R 1974 Lancet 2:427
22. Mukhtar ED, Smith BR, Pyle GA, Hall R, Vice P 1975 Lancet 1:713
23. McGregor AM, Dewar PJ, Petersen MM, Miller M, Smith BR, Hall R 1980 Lancet 2:1101
24. Vitti P, Rotella CM, Valente WA, Cohen J, Aloj SM, Laccetti P, Ambesi-Impiombato FS, Grollman EF, Pinchera A, Toccafondi R, Kohn LD 1983 J Clin Endocrinol Metab 57:782
25. Zakarija M, McKenzie JM, Banovac K 1980 Ann Intern Med 93:28
26. Zakarija M, McKenzie JM 1983 J Clin Endocrinol Metab 57:1036
27. Zakarija M, McKenzie JM, Munro DS 1983 J Clin Invest 72:1352
28. Zakarija M, Garcia A, McKenzie JM 1985 J Clin Invest 76:1885
29. Brown RS, Pohl SL, Jackson IMD, Reichlin S 1978 Lancet 1:904
30. Loveridge N, Zakarija M, Bitensky L, McKenzie JM 1979 J Clin Endocrinol Metab 49:610
31. Smyth PPA, Neylan D, O'Donovan DK 1982 J Clin Endocrinol Metab 54:357
32. McMullan NM, Smyth PPA 1984 Clin Endocrinol 20:269
33. Bliddal H, Bech K, Johansen K, Nerup J 1984 Eur J Clin Invest 14:1984
34. Feldt-Rasmussen U, Bech K, Bliddal H, Bregengaard C, Danneskiold-Samsoe B, Husby S, Johansen K, Kirkegaard C, Friis T, Siersboek-Nielsen K, Nielsen H This symposium
35. Warthin AS 1928 Ann Intern Med 2:553
36. Halsted WS 1914 Bull Johns Hopkins Hosp 25:223
37. Weetman AP, McGregor AM 1984 Endocr Rev 5:309
38. Zakarija M 1980 Hormone Res 13:1
39. Smith BR 1976 Immunol Commun 5:345
40. James R, Bradshaw RA 1984 Ann Rev Biochem 53:259
41. Meek JC 1970 J Clin Endocrinol Metab 31:48
42. Bottazzo GF, Pujol-Borrell R, Hanafusa T, Feldmann M 1983 Lancet 2:1115
43. Weiss M, Ingbar SH, Winblad S, Kasper DL 1983 Science 219:1331

PATHOGENIC ROLES OF TSH-RECEPTOR ANTIBODIES IN GRAVES' DISEASE

Shigenobu Nagataki

The First Department of Internal Medicine
Nagasaki University School of Medicine
Nagasaki 852, Japan

INTRODUCTION

Since the discovery of long acting thyroid stimulator, the significance of circulating abnormal thyroid stimulators or TSH-receptor antibodies in untreated patients with Graves' disease has been investigated extensively by numerous investigators. However, the pathogenic roles of TSH-receptor antibodies for thyrotoxicosis of Graves' disease are still not completely elucidated.

In this symposium, I would like to present at first our data on the stimulation of thyroids by circulating antibodies and on the cellular interactions within the thyroids in producing antibodies and in affecting functions of thyrocytes and then on the immunogenetics of Graves' disease. Finally, considering the presented data, pathogenic roles of TSH-receptor antibodies in Graves' disease will be discussed.

STIMULATION OF THYROIDS BY CIRCULATING ANTIBODIES

There have been reported many methods to determine TSH-receptor antibodies in sera of Graves' patients. Table 1 shows the results in our laboratory on the incidence of TSH-receptor antibodies in untreated patients with Graves' disease.

Table 1   Incidence of TSH-Receptor Antibodies in
Untreated Patients with Graves' Disease

Tests		Incidence
TBIAb		
human thyroid membrane		70%
solubilized porcine thyroid membrane		85%
TSAb		
human thyroid membrane	(HTACS)	60%
human thyroid slice	(TSAb)	80%
porcine thyroid membrane	(PTACS)	40%
FRTL-5 cell line		85%
porcine thyroid cells		95%

Although the incidence is very high in many methods, there exists a dissociation of values among some methods. Fig. 1 depicts the correlations among TBIAb, TSAb and T_3-suppressibility in untreated patients and in patients during thionamide therapy. Values for TBIAb and TSAb did not correlate significantly in both untreated and treated patients, and TSAb did not correlate with T_3-suppressibility[1]. Similar results were reported from various laboratories and studies on monoclonal antibodies developed from lymphocytes of Graves' patients revealed that in addition to monoclonals with TBIAb and TSAb activities, some had only TBIAb activity and the others had only TSAb activity.

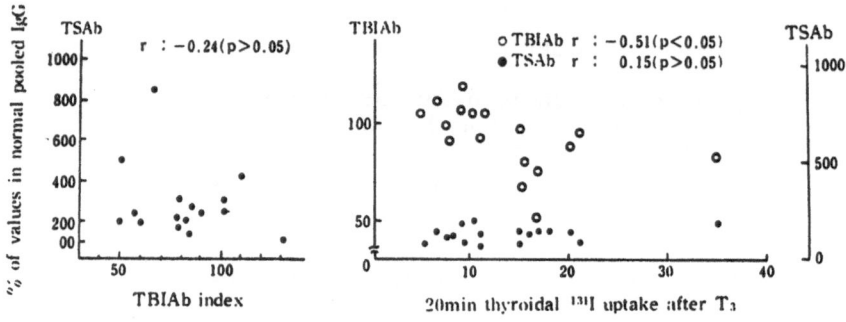

Fig. 1   Correlations among TBIAb, TSAb and T_3-suppressibility

In an attempt to clarify the incidence of these various monoclonal antibodies in sera of untreated patients with Graves' disease, lymphocytes from 8 untreated patients were transformed by Epstein-Barr virus and were distributed into many wells. After the first culture for 4 weeks, the cells in each well positive for TBIAb and/or TSAb were further distributed and cultured for additional 2 weeks. TBIAb and TSAb activity were then determined in the supernatants of 372 wells of the 2nd culture in 8 patients. As shown in Table 2, 31 wells had only TBIAb and 41 wells only TSAb, and 4 wells showed both TBIAb and TSAb, indicating that most of TSH-receptor antibodies are being produced from clones with a single function[2]. A dissociation among values for TSH-receptor antibodies determined by different methods is due to

Table 2.   TSH-Receptor Antibodies Produced in Supernatants of Cultured Lymphocytes Obtained from Untreated Graves' Patients and Transformed by EBV Infection

	TBIAb only	TSAb only	TBIAb & TSAb
Patients 1	6	8	2
2	3	3	0
3	2	9	0
4	6	3	0
5	3	4	0
6	7	7	1
7	2	6	1
8	2	1	0
Total	31	41	4
	94.7%		5.3%

multiple antibodies with a single function. These results raise the question of which one of these TSH-receptor antibodies is pathogenic for thyrotoxicosis of Graves' disease and it would be impossible to decide whether TBIAb or TSAb is the sole pathogenic factor.

In order to determine the stimulatory effects of circulating antibodies, it seemed to us that the ideal method would be to use human thyroid tissues, to observe an end-product of stimulation, such as thyroid hormone release as an index, and to observe chronic stimulatory effects since thyroids of Graves' patients are being chronically stimulated. For this purpose, we have developed a technique of organ culture of human thyroids to measure the release of thyroid hormones while being stimulated chronically by TSH[3],[4]. With this method, TSH stimulated the T_3-release as well as thyroidal cAMP concentrations in a dose dependent manner and the sensitivity to TSH was as sensitive as the McKenzie's mouse bioassay. However, in spite of a significant increase in thyroidal cAMP concentrations, the release of thyroid hormones from normal thyroid tissues was not stimulated by IgG obtained from untreated patients[3]. Since the release of thyroid hormones from thyroids of patients with Graves' disease must be stimulated by their own IgG, we felt that the stimulatory effects of IgG could be observed if it were incubated with autologous thyroids in this organ culture system. Therefore, the release of thyroid hormones from cultured thyroid slices of untreated Graves' patients in response to their own IgG and to IgG from other untreated patients was investigated in 11 untreated patients with Graves' disease.

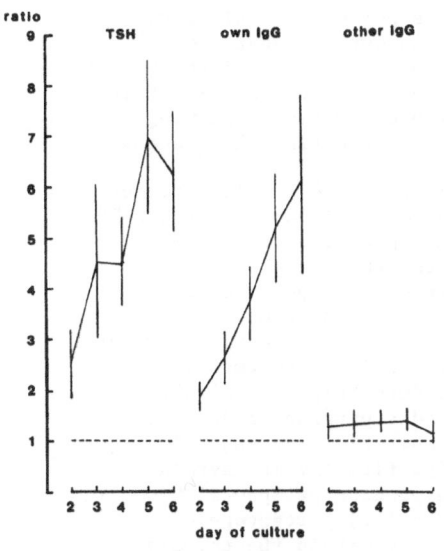

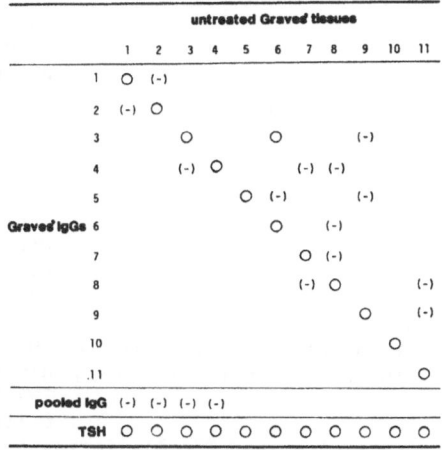

o : Increase in T_3
(-): No increase in T_3

Fig 2. Ratio of T_3-Concentrations in Media with or without Stimulator

Fig. 3 Specificity of Graves' IgGs for their own Thyroids

As shown in Fig. 2, the release of T_3 was stimulated by TSH, and autologous IgG stimulated the release of T_3 3 to 10 fold above controls on the 5th day. However, when slices were incubated with IgG obtained from other untreated patients, the concentrations of T_3 in media did not differ from that in controls.

In Fig. 3, thyroid tissues from 11 untreated Graves' patients are listed along the abscessa, and stimulators (Graves' IgG and TSH) are listed along the ordinate. When IgG of 11 patients were incubated with autologous thyroid slices, notable increase in T_3 in the media were invariably observed. However, when the same IgG were incubated with allogeneic slices, no increase in medium T_3 was noted, with one exception.

These results strongly suggest that thyroid hormone releasing activity of circulating IgG in Graves' patients is highly specific for autologous thyroids[5]. Specific recognition of autologous thyroid cells by T cells was also demonstrated by other investigators[6]. Although results are not shown, the self recognition observed in organ culture system was not observed in cell culture. Interactions among circulating IgG, thyrocytes and lymphocytes within thyroid tissues appears to be very important in the self recognition.

CELLULAR INTERACTIONS WITHIN THYROID GLANDS

Recently Hanafusa et al[7] have shown that the HLA–DR antigens are expressed on the surface of thyroid epithelial cells (thyrocytes) from patients with autoimmune thyroid disease[8]. In our previous studies, it was shown that interferon γ induces HLA–DR antigen expression on thyrocytes from patients with Graves' disease, and these cells induce proliferation of autologous T cells, which may, in turn, act on thyrocytes to perpetuate the immune process within the thyroid glands.

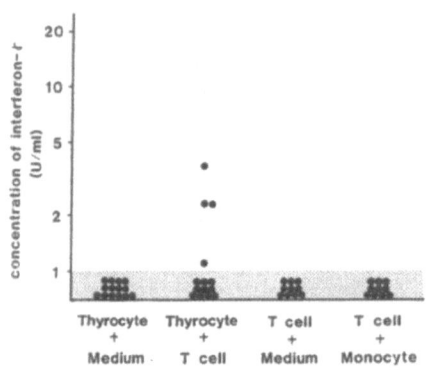

Fig. 4   Production of Interferon γ
          in Culture Supernatants

Furthermore, as shown in Fig. 4, interferon γ was detected in culture supernatants only when thyrocytes were incubated with autologous T cells, indicating that production of interferon γ within the thyroids is really playing a role in perpetuating the process.

Although the results are not shown here, the increase of HLA–DR antigen expression on T cells within the thyroid glands were found in both helper/inducer T cells ($CD4^+$) and suppressor/cytotoxic T cells ($CD8^+$). However, when $CD4^+$ cells were further divided into helper T cells ($CD4^+$ $2H4^-$) and suppressor inducer T cells ($CD4^+$ $2H4^+$) as shown in Fig. 5, percentage of helper T cells increased significantly in thyroid tissues when compared to values in the corresponding peripheral blood T cells (left panel). In contrast to helper T cells, percentage of suppressor inducer T cells decreased remarkabley within the thyroid glands as shown in the right panel.

In addition to the study on T cell subsets, function of suppressor T cells within the thyroids was compared to that in peripheral blood. Lymphocytes obtained from thyroid glands (TG) and from peripheral blood (PB) were separated into $CD4^+$, $CD8^+$ and B cells and IgG production in the supernatants of coculture of $CD4^+$ and B cells with PWM for 7 days was determined with or without $CD8^+$ cells. In the left panel of Fig. 6, IgG production by TG-B and TG-$CD4^+$ from 13 patients with Graves' disease are shown in the middle. When autologous PB-$CD8^+$ cells were added in the coculture of TG-B and TG-CD4[+], IgG production was significantly inhibited as shown in the left, whereas when autologous TG-CD8[+] cells were added, IgG production was not affected as shown in the right.

The right panel of Fig. 6 shows the results with regard to the production of IgG by PB-B and PB-CD4[+] cells. Here again, autologous

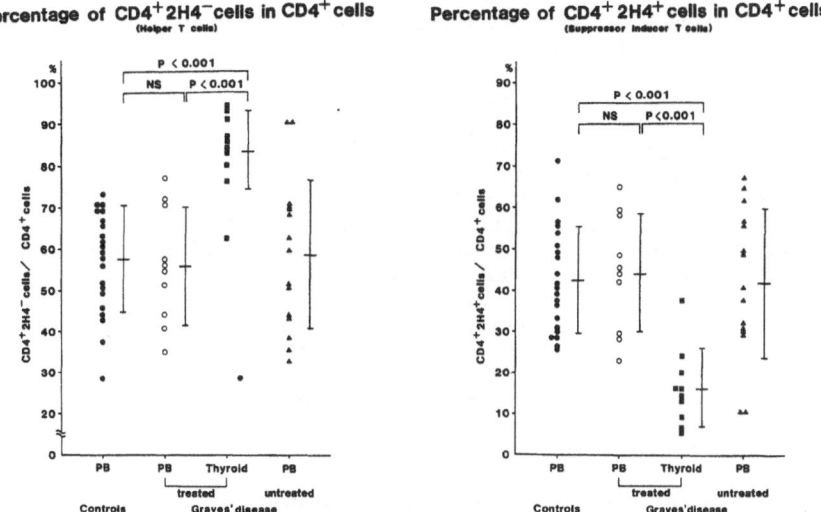

Fig. 5   Percentage of Helper T Cells and Suppressor Inducer T Cells

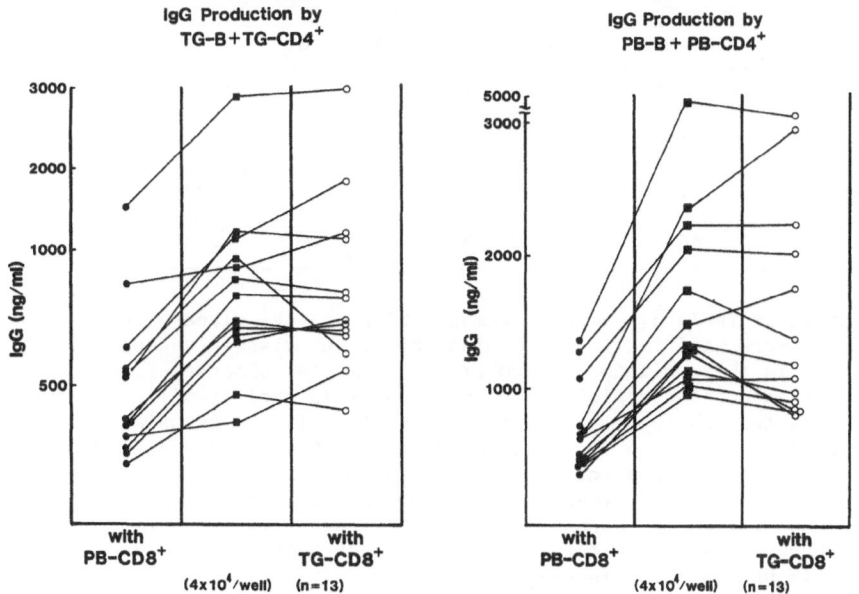

Fig. 6   Comparison of Suppressor Function of T Cells in Thyroids and in Peripheral Blood

PB–CD8$^+$ cells suppressed IgG production significantly, but TG–CD8$^+$ did not affect IgG production by PB–B and PB–CD4$^+$ cells. These results clearly indicate that suppressor function of intrathyroidal T cells is decreased when compared to that in peripheral blood T cells. Although the results are not shown, ratios of CD4$^+$/CD8$^+$ cells were not different between T cells in thyroids and those in peripheral blood.

From these results on cellular interactions within the thyroids, it is suggested that the expression of HLA-DR antigen on thyrocytes is very important to perpetuate the immune process, and cellular interactions within thyroid glands may play an important role in producing antibodies and in affecting functions of thyrocytes.

IMMUNOGENETICS OF GRAVES' DISEASE

It has been reported that Graves' disease occurs frequently within one genealogical family and consanguineous occurrence of Graves' disease suggests the possibility that hereditary factors are important in its pathogenesis. Recent many reports have demonstrated that the susceptibility to autoimmune thyroid disease is real linkage to certain immunogenetic factors, such as HLA antigens.

In the study on immunogenetics of Graves' disease, haplotypes of HLA and the immunoglobulin allotype (Gm) were analyzed in 243 members of 37 families in which 2 or more first degree relatives had Graves' disease. The disease associated haplotypes of HLA and Gm for each family were identified by determining the haplotypes concordant in 2 members with Graves' disease.

Table 3.   Association among Graves' and Hashimoto's Disease;
           HLA and Gm Haplotypes in 37 Families (243 Subjects)
           in which 2 or More First Degree Relatives were
           Affected with Graves' Disease

	Concordance of disease-associated haplotypes of				
	Both HLA and Gm	HLA only	Gm only	Neither HLA nor Gm	Total
Graves' disease	95 (74+21)	0	1	0	96 (74+22)
Hashimoto's disease	14	0	0	0	14
Others	37	16	38	42	133
Total	146	16	39	42	243

As shown in Table 3, among 96 members with Graves' disease in 37 families, 74 were used for the determination of the disease-associated haplotypes. In the remaining 22 members with Graves' disease, 21 had both disease-associated haplotypes of HLA and Gm in their families. All 14 patients with Hashimoto's disease had the same disease-associated haplotypes of both HLA and Gm as had members with Graves' disease in each family. Among 55 subjects who had haplotypes of only HLA or only Gm, only one was Graves' disease and none of 42 subjects who had neither HLA nor Gm had Graves' or Hashimoto's disease. However, among 146 subjects who had disease-associated haplotypes of both HLA and Gm, 37 had no autoimmune thyroid diseases.

The findings in these families suggest that two genes linked to HLA and Gm, respectively, control the susceptibility of Graves' or

Hashimoto's diseases and those who do not have immunogenetic factors are very unlikely to develop Graves' or Hashimoto's disease. However, since one fourth of subjects who had both disease-associated haplotypes were not affected by autoimmune thyroid diseases, environmental factors or unknown immunogenetic factors may be important to develop clinical Graves' or Hashimoto's disease.

CONCLUSIONS

In Table 4, the results of the present studies are summarized. Thyroid slices from untreated patients with Graves' disease are stimulated by their own IgG but not IgG from the other untreated patients. Circulating antibodies recognize the autologous thyroids. In studies on cellular interactions, relationship between thyrocytes and infiltrated mononuclear cells appears to be very important in perpetuating the process and finally two genes linked to human major histocompatibility complex and to immunoglobulin allotype control the susceptibility to Graves' disease.

Table 4   Pathogenesis of Graves' disease

1. Stimulation of thyroids by circulating antibodies:

    Thyroid glands are stimulated only by their own IgG

        THYROID   IgG

2. Cellular interactions within thyroid glands:

    Intrathyroidal cellular interactions important
    in perpetuating the process

        THYROCYTES   LYMPHOCYTES

3. Immunogenetics:

    Two genes control the susceptibility of Graves' disease

        HLA   Gm

These results appear to be correlated among each other and may suggest the direction of the future studies on the pathogenesis of Graves' disease. TSH-receptor antibodies determined by the present method may be one of the important pathogenic factors of Graves' disease, but are not the goal of the study on the pathogenesis of Graves' disease.

ACKNOWLEDGEMENTS

The author would like to express cordial thanks to Misses K. Hakugawa and Y. Takahara for their excellent secretarial assistance and to the following scientists for their cooperations.

University of Tokyo: H. Uchimura, K. Kubota, T. Mitsuhashi,
                                 M. Chiu
Saitama Medical School: H. Ikeda
Tsukuba University: N. Kuzuya
Kyushu University: H. Tamai, S. Matsubayashi
Tokyo Womens' Medical College: M. Maeda
Osaka City Medical School: N. Hamada
Harvard Medical School: C. Morimoto

Ito Hospital: K. Ito
Kuma Hospital: K. Kuma
Noguchi Hospital: A. Noguchi, S. Noguchi
Nagasaki University:
(Endocrine Group)
    M. Izumi, S. Okamoto, I. Morimoto, K. Sato, M. Taura, K. Ohta,
    S. Ohtakara, I. Kubo, S. Hirayu, S. Yamashita, S. Morita,
    N. Yokoyama, F. Kakezono, T. Kiriyama, H. Nanba, S. Inoue,
    Y. Nagayama, K. Ashizawa, S. Harakawa
(Immunology Group)
    K. Eguchi, M. Mine, T. Fukuda, N. Ikari, A. Kurata, H. Kanazawa,
    M. Matsunaga, H. Tezuka, Y. Ueki, Y. Kawabe, T. Ohtsubo,
    C. Shimomura, H. Nakao, N. Ishikawa

REFERENCES

1. N. Kuzuya, S.C. Chiu, H. Ikeda, H. Ikeda, H. Uchimura, K. Ito, and
    S. Nagataki, Correlation between Thyroid Stimulators and 3, 5, 3'-
    Triiodothyronine Suppressibility in Patients during Treatment for
    Hyperthyroidism with Thionamide Drugs: Comparison of Assays by
    Thyroid-Stimulating and Thyrotropin-Displacing Activities, J Clin
    Endocrinol Metab. 48: 706 (1979).
2. N. Yokoyama, M. Izumi, and S. Nagataki, Heterogeneity of Graves'
    IgG: Comparison of TSH Receptor Antibodies in Serum and in Culture
    Supernatants of Lymphocytes Transformed by EB Virus Infection, J
    Clin Endocrinol Metab. (in press).
3. S. Nagataki, Pathogenic Factors of Graves' disease, in: "Current
    problems in Thyroid reseach," N. Ui, K. Torizuka, S. Nagataki, and
    K. Miyai, ed., Excerpta Medica, Amsterdam-Oxford-Princeton (1982).
4. N. Hamada, T. Okabe, K. Kubota, S.C. Chiu, H. Uchimura, T. Mimura,
    K. Ito, and S. Nagataki, Chronic Effect of TSH on Human Thyroid
    Tissue in Organ Culture, Proc Soc Exp Biol Med. 172: 153 (1983).
5. S. Yamashita, M. Izumi, and S. Nagataki, Specific stimulatory
    effects of Graves' IgG on the release of triiodothyronine from the
    patients' own thyroids, Acta Endocrinol. 112: 204 (1986).
6. M. Londei, G.F. Bottazzo, and M. Feldman, Human T-Cell Clones from
    Autoimmune Thyroid Glands: Specific Recognition of Autologous
    Thyroid Cells, Science. 228: 85 (1985).
7. T. Hanafusa, L. Chiovato, D. Doniach, R. Pujol-Borrell,
    R.C.G. Russell, G.F.Bottazzo, Aberrant expression of HLA-DR antigen
    on thyrocytes in Graves' disease : relevance for autoimmunity,
    Lancet. 2: 1111 (1983).
8. M. Matsunaga, K. Eguchi, T. Fukuda, A. Kurata, H. Tezuka,
    C. Shimomura, T. Otsubo, N. Ishikawa, K. Ito, and S. Nagataki,
    Class II Major Histocompatibility Complex Antigen Expression and
    Cellular Interaction in Thyroid Glands of Graves' Disease, J Clin
    Endocrinol Metab. 62: 723 (1986).
9. H. Tamai. H. Uno, Y. Hirota, S. Matsubayashi, K. Kuma,
    H. Matsumoto, L.F. Kumagai, T. Sasazuki, and S. Nagataki,
    Immunogenetics of Hashimoto's and Graves' Diseases, J Clin
    Endocrinol Metab. 60: 62 (1985).

PHYSIOPATHOLOGICAL RELEVANCE OF THYROID STIMULATING ANTIBODY (TSAb)

MEASUREMENTS IN GRAVES' DISEASE

Jacques Orgiazzi, Anne-Marie Madec and René Mornex

INSERM U.197
Faculté de Médecine Alexis Carrel
69008 Lyon, France

It is paradoxical that TSAb measurement, although this antibody is responsible for the hyperthyroidism of Graves' disease, appears to have only an ancillary role in the management of the patients. Using several approaches we have therefore sought to elucidate whether TSAb levels correlated with the severity of Graves' disease. More than 150 patients have been studied in various clinical situations. In most cases, severity of the disease was evaluated in chronological term in prospective studies with extended follow-up. In addition, we tested the appropriateness of TSAb determination in ascribing apparently isolated ophthalmopathy to Graves' disease.

Patients and protocols

Groups of patients with Graves' disease were studied according to different therapeutic protocols :

A/ 26 patients were treated with propranolol only. These had been selected for mild Graves' disease ; they were given, after informed consent, 160-320 mg propranolol daily. Patients in whom any delay in onset of conventional treatment of hyperthyroidism could have been deleterious were meticulously excluded from the study as well as those who could not adhere to a very strict follow-up. The status of the patients was evaluated regularly after the beginning of the treatment both clinically and biologically[1].

B/ In 27 unselected patients we compared initial and on-carbimazole treatment values of the early thyroid radioiodine uptake (ERU) and of TSAb. On the average, 3 determinations were performed in each patient during a mean 11 month treatment period. Treatment of these patients combined carbimazole at a constant dose of 30 mg per day and L-T3 50-75 µg per day[2].

C/ A series of 135 patients prospectively studied were systematically treated with carbimazole. A subgroup of these was randomly allocated to a short-term (6 months ; 48 patients) or a long-term (18 months ; 46 patients) treatment regimen[3]. The remaining patients were treated for 18 months[4]. Carbimazole was prescribed in decreasing doses in order to maintain euthyroidism and was not combined to replacement therapy. After cessation of treatment, patients were regularly examined ; in those apparently remaining euthyroid, follow-up after the end of the treatment was ⩾ 2 years.

D/ 29 patients with euthyroid Graves' ophthalmopathy were also studied and followed up in order to determine the diagnostic potency of TSAb as compared to that of the TRH/T3-suppression test or of the antithyroid antibody measurement.

Methods

TSAb was determined as previously reported [5] by a cAMP stimulation assay using cultured human thyroid cells incubated with whole serum. Based on 12 different experiments, reproducibilities were : intraassay = 10 % ; interassay = 19 %, 17 % and 13 % for basal values, 0.1 mU/ml b-TSH and our in-house standard TSAb at 1 %, respectively. Fig. 1 shows the average (m+SD) dose-response curve for our standard TSAb ; cAMP production stimulation Is expressed in percent of basal values measured in the presence of normal serum. In sequential studies, the various serum samples from the same patient were assayed in the same experiment.

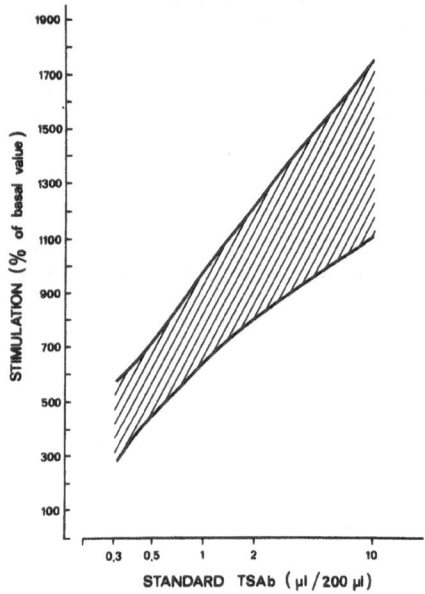

Fig. 1. Dose-response curve of cAMP production stimulation by a standard TSAb preparation made from a pool of potent sera.

Other laboratory determinations used routine or previously reported methods[2,5].

Results and comments

A. Among the whole group of 150 patients, no correlation was found between TSAb levels on our hand and any clinical (estimated pretreatment duration of Graves' disease, apparent severity of disease, goiter size, presence of ophthalmopathy) or biological (thyroid hormone levels) characteristics of the disease. A barely significant correlation was observed between TSAb levels and the T3/T4 ratio [6]. Also, no correlation was found between TSAb levels and presence of HLA-DR3 determinant or the pretreatment OKT4/OKT8 lymphocyte subset ratio [5]. This lack of concordance is of general observation although earlier studies reported some correlations.

On the average, TSAb was initially present in more than 75 % of the patients. However, interestingly enough, we noticed that prevalence of TSAb was uneven between groups of patients from various french centers, ranging from 60 to more than 90 %. A more systematic study of a possible geographical distribution within this country of the frequency of TSAb in untreated Graves' disease patients is under way. If confirmed, this could suggest a population effect on the expression of this autoantibody.

B. Relationship between ERU and TSAb was studied before and during treatment. ERU is considered as a sensitive index of thyroid stimulation in vivo, even during antithyroid drug treatment. It is therefore appropriate to study in parallel this parameter and TSAb circulating levels. Before treatment, ERU ranging from 15 to 54 % of the injected dose of radioactivity was significantly correlated with TSAb values ($p < 0.01$). During treatment, of an average 11 months duration, among the 21 patients sequentially studied several evolution patterns were observed : in 5 patients, TSAb remained negative throughout the study and ERU decreased by 57 % of its initial value (Group A); in 9 patients, TSAb became undetectable and ERU decreased by 56 % (Group B) ; in 7 other patients, TSAb remained detectable and ERU decreased by 8 % only (Group C). Moreover, serial values of TSAb and ERU varied in parallel in Group B, but were discordant in Group C. These studies suggest that in a majority of patients ERU value reflects reasonably well the level of TSAb both before and during treatment. In some patients however, the two parameters were not correlated, which suggests either that circulating TSAb may not be the more relevant estimate of thyroid stimulatory activity or that expression of stimulation by the gland is variable. The ERU-TSAb patterns described above were not related to any clinical or biological peculiarities of the patients. It has been suggested that the main source of thyroid-stimulating antibodies was the thyroid gland itself[7]. In addition, Gossage et al. using a binding assay have also described instances of variability in the character of thyrotropin receptor antibodies in Graves' disease [8]. It is therefore likely that heterogeneity of thyrotropin receptor antibodies contributes also to non-parallelism between circulating titers and level of thyroid function.

C. In a study of the spontaneous evolution of the disease, selected patients were treated only with propranolol. 27 % went into long-lasting remission $\geqslant$ 18 months, 23 % into temporary remission ($<$ 18 months), and 50 % with no improvement had to be treated conventionnally[1]. The question arises as to whether initial TSAb values are predictive of the disease outcome. When patients were subgrouped according to the above-mentionned evolution types, it appeared that no simple clinical or biological characteristic was significantly indicative. We observed, however, that FT4, FT3 as well as TSAb, tended to be higher, in the patients in whom the disease did not improve. For instance, TSAb values were 12.4 + 4.6 µl-equivalent/ml, 7.12 + 2.8 and 5.16 + 1.7 (m+SEM) in the no-improvement, temporary remission and long-lasting remission group, respectively. Previous studies had similarly failed to predict prospectively those patients who will remit on medical therapy [9] . In 8 patients, TSAb levels were sequentially studied during 4-36 months propranolol treatment or follow-up. Fluctuations in the TSAb levels were observed, not always concordant with the clinical status. In some cases, presence of inhibitory anti-TSH receptor antibodies was excluded by co-incubation experiments. In this clinical situation, therefore, TSAb levels did not appear useful for the practical management of the patients.

D. In the prospective study of the patients systematically treated with carbimazole, initial TSAb levels appeared to be only weak predictors of post-treatment outcome. Level was 775 + 103 (% of basal production of cAMP) in the relapse group and 453 + 55 in the remission group ; these values were significantly different ($p < 0.01$), but because of their wide

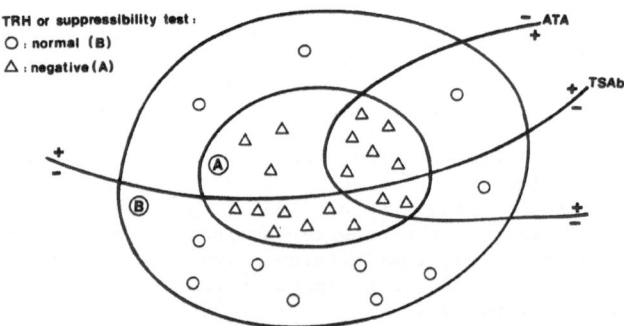

Fig. 2. Various combinations of results of thyroid
stimulating antibody, antithyroid antibody TRH
and/or suppressibility test determinations in
29 patients with Euthyroid Graves' Ophthalmopathy

scattering they were not indicative for a given patient. However, when patients were sub-grouped according to duration of treatment, a highly significant difference was observed in initial TSAb levels between the patients who went into remission after a short treatment (6 months ; stimulation index : 354 % + 57) and those who relapsed after a long treatment (18 months ; 859 % + 169 ; p < 0.01). Pre-treatment TSAb measurement could therefore be of some help, among other characteristics, in determining the duration of the carbimazole treatment. In an other study [6] , we had confirmed previous observations indicating that after a drug course of 6 months or more, only elevated TSAb levels (> 350 %) had a prognostic significance. In this condition, nearly 100 % of the patients relapsed. On the contrary, relapse rate approximated 50 % in the patients in whom TSAb was undetectable or weakly positive. These results suggest that TSAb does not discriminate between response to treatment and true remission of the disease. In that line, we had also searched for a correlation between TSAb and the T lymphocyte subsets determined as the OKT4/OKT8 ratio in patients treated with carbimazole[5] . Sequential studies showed no concordant evolution of these two parameters. Clearly, studies of this type await for determinations of immuno-competent cells more specifically linked to thyroid auto-immunity.

We also questionned the role of circulating TSAb in the emergence of relapsing hyperthyroidism in patients previously treated with carbimazole. 16 patients were studied sequentially ; they all had a 18-month carbimazole course ; 70 % of these relapsed within 2 years after drug withdrawal, 15 % at 3 and 15 % at 4 years. TSAb levels, determined in the same assay for each patient, were 850 % + 116 and 230 % + 48 prior to and at the end of the treatment, respectively ; however, at relapse time, their TSAb averaged 150 % + 34.

E. Finally, in a different perspective, in patients with euthyroid Graves' ophthalmopathy, we have compared the diagnostic usefulness of TSAb with that of the TRH/T3-suppression test or of the antithyroid antibody measurement. Clinical diagnosis of Graves' ophthalmopathy was based on examination and exclusion of a tumoral etiology by CT scan and/or extended follow-up. TSAb was detectable in 12/29 patients studied, 7 of whom had also detectable antithyroid antibodies and 6 an abnormal TRH/suppression test. TSAb was undetectable in 50 % of the patients with abnormal TRH/suppression test. In 2/29 patients was TSAb the only marker of autoimmune thyroid disease ; however, 7/29 patients were free from any of the abovementionned abnormalities.

Conclusion : There is not direct link between circulating TSAb levels as determined by stimulation assay and intensity or severity of Graves' disease. Since the presence of blocking antibodies in the samples tested has been ruled out, it is likely that in some patients, immunological thyroid stimulation is not accurately reflected by circulating TSAb titers.*

REFERENCES

1. P. Blanc, R. Roulier, M. Pugeat, J. Orgiazzi, P. Carayon, and J.L. Codaccioni, Follow-up of patients with Graves' disease under long-term propranolol therapy, in : Proceedings of the 9th International Thyroid Congress, G. Medeiros-Neto and E. Gaitan ed., Plenum Press, New York (1986).
2. L. Baldet, A.M. Madec, C. Papachristou, A. Stefanutti, J. Orgiazzi, and C. Jaffiol, Thyroid-stimulating antibody : an index of thyroid stimulation in Graves'disease ? Submitted for publication (1986).

*Data presented in this work have been obtained in collaboration with Drs H. Allannic, L. Baldet, P. Carayon, J.L. Codaccioni and C. Jaffiol.

3. H. Allannic, J. Orgiazzi, Y. Lorcy, A.M. Leguerrier, R. Fauchet, and B. Genetet, 15th Annual meeting of the european thyroid association, Ann. Endocrinol. 47:20 (1986).
4. C. Delambre, A.M. Madec, N. Massart, B. Hody, M.C. Roumieux, A. Colobert, and H. Allannic, 15th Annuel meeting of the european thyroid association, Ann. Endocrinol. 47:74 (1986).
5. A.M. Madec, H. Allannic, N. Genetet, M. Gueguen, G. Genetet, R. Fauchet, A. Stefanutti, and J. Orgiazzi, T lymphocyte subsets at various stages of hyperthyroid Graves' disease : Effect of carbimazole treatment and relationship with thyroid -stimulating antibody levels or HLA status, J. Clin. Endocrinol. Metab. 62:117 (1986).
6. A.M. Madec, M.C. Laurent, Y. Lorcy, A.M. Le Guerrier, A. Stefanutti, J. Orgiazzi, and H. Allannic, Thyroid stimulating antibodies : an aid to the strategy of treatment of Graves' disease ? Clinical Endocrinology 21:247 (1984).
7. P. Kendall-Taylor, A.J.Knox, N.R. Steel, and S. Atkinson, Evidence that thyroid stimulating antibody is produced in the thyroid gland, Lancet, i:654 (1984).
8. A.A.R. Gossage, J.C.W. Crawley, S. Copping, D. Hinge, and R.C. Himsworth, Consistency and variability in the character of thyrotropin receptor antibodies in Graves'disease, Clinical Endocrinology 19:97 (1983).
9. D.C. Lowe, D.R. Hadden, D.A.D. Montgomery, and J.A. Weaver, Propranolol as the sole therapy for thyrotoxicosis : long term follow-up, in Thyroid Research, J. Robbins and L.E. Braverman ed., Excerpta Medica, American Elsevier, New York (1976).

TSH RECEPTOR AUTOANTIBODIES AFFECTING THYROID CELL FUNCTION

G.F. Fenzι, P. Vitti, C. Marcocci, L. Chiovato, and E. Macchia

Cattedra di Endocrinologia e Medicina Costituzionale

University of Pisa, Pisa, Italy

Introduction

Autoantibodies directed to different components of the thyroid cell are present in sera of patients with thyroid autoimmune disorders (1). Among the thyroid cell structures, the TSH receptor has been implicated as the putative antigen of autoantibodies having different biological effects. Autoantibodies able to mimic TSH in its ability to stimulate thyroid hormone production and cell growth have been found in sera of patients with Graves' disease and in minority of those with other thyroid autoimmune disorders (2). Furthermore it was observed that the IgG fraction from the same patients inhibited the binding of radiolabeled TSH to its receptor. More recently, autoantibodies able to inhibit some biological effects of TSH on the thyroid cell were found in sera of patients with idiopathic myxedema. These antibodies may be important in the pathogenesis of thyroid atrophy and hypothyroidism (3, 4). Thus, several data suggest that autoantibodies from patients with thyroid autoimmune diseases may either mimic or block the TSH action on the thyroid cell. In the present review we report the incidence and the biological effects of these antibodies detected by different assays using human thyroid cell membranes and FRTL-5 thyroid cells.

Thyroid adenylate cyclase stimulating antibodies (TSAb)

Historically, TSAb were detected by LATS bioassay, but a consistent number of Graves' patients were negative by this test even after concentration of the IgG fraction. This relatively low incidence of LATS positive responses has been attributed to the species-specificity of TSAb, so that only antibodies cross-reacting with the murine thyroid could be detected by LATS bioassay (1, 5). Results directly assessing thyroid stimulating activity in human thyroid plasma membranes or slices have been reported by several investigators. The average positivity obtained with Graves' IgG is about 80% in different laboratories. In a series of 49 Graves' patients with untreated Graves' disease studied in our laboratory using human thyroid membranes we found 71.4% positivity with the IgG fraction. No adenylate cyclase (AC) stimulatory activity was detectable in IgG preparations from 28 normal subjects and 12 patients with Hashimoto's thyroiditis or idiopathic myxedema (6). Cultured human thyroid cells have been also proved to be a sensitive system for assessing TSAb (7). More recently, a new sensitive method for the measurement of TSAb was developed using a continuous cell line of rat thyroid cells (FRTL-5 cells) (8). The ability of these cells to be growth under standard and highly reproducible conditions allowed easy optimization of the assay. Intracellular cAMP was measured by RIA after challenge of cells with the IgG specimens from 84 patients with hyperthyroid Graves' disease or from 42 normal subjects. In our series 90.5% (76/84) of IgG preparations from hyperthyroid Graves' patients exhibited AC stimulating activity, thus the sensitivity of this assay was similar to that reported when human thyroid cells or slices were used (9). Essentially similar results could be obtained with a different methodological approach.

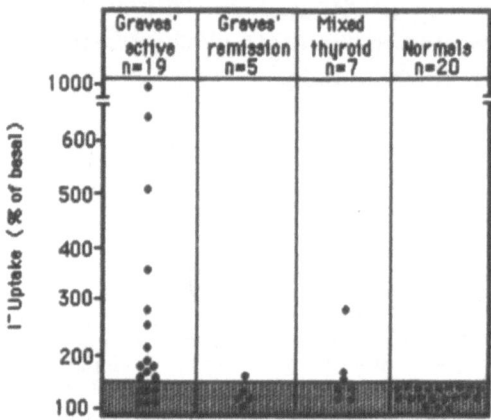

Fig. 1. Effect of IgG preparations from patients with Graves' disease and other thyroid disorders to stimulate the iodide uptake in FRTL-5 cells. Results obtained with IgGs from normal control subjects are also shown.

In a series of 24 patients with Graves' disease, all IgG which showed positive results in the cAMP assay using FRTL-5 cells, were also able to stimulate ^{125}iodide uptake in the same cells (Fig. 1) (10). Thus, the iodide uptake assay may be used as an alternative method for the measurement of TSAb, and appears to be simpler, less expensive and less time-consuming than assaying needing a cAMP radioimmunoassay.

Besides their ability to stimulate thyroid AC, we have attempted to study other effects of TSAb. In particular, we have investigated TSAb mimic TSH also in the induction of complex phenomena such as the desensitization of thyroid cells. Previous studies performed in several thyroid cell systems have shown that TSH preincubation induces refractoriness to further stimulation of cAMP accumulation by the hormone. The question of whether TSAb from Graves' patients have the same desensitizing effect as TSH was studied. Cells cultured in medium deprived of TSH for 4-5 days have an AC system exquisitively sensitive to TSH and TSAb. Refractoriness to TSH was induced in these cells by a 24 h preincubation with 250 μU/ml of the hormone. Four different TSAb preparation all induced refractoriness to acute TSAb as well as TSH-stimulated cAMP accumulation. TSAb-induced desensitization was dose-dependent and required prolonged exposure to TSAb. Furthermore, the desensitization induced by TSAb as well as that caused by TSH were significantly inhibited by cycloheximide, indicating the need for *de novo* protein synthesis (Fig. 2) (11). This gives further proof of the ability of TSAb to mimic the TSH action also in more complex physiologic events requiring several steps after AC stimulation.

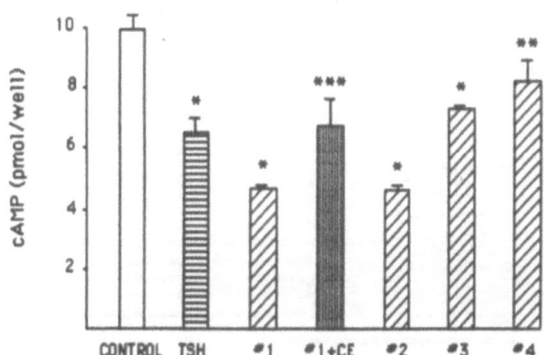

Fig. 2. Effect of different TSAb preparations on the desensitization of TSH-stimulated cAMP accumulation. Cells were preincubated for 24 hr with a pool for normal IgG (control); 250 µU/ml TSH (TSH) or TSAb preparations from four different patients with hyperthyroid Graves' disease (#1, #2, #3, #4) and TSAb #1 plus 10 µU cycloheximide (#1+CE).

Autoantibodies inhibiting the TSH stimulation of thyroid AC

Hypothyroidism is observed in patients with idiopathic myxedema and less frequently with Hashimoto's thyroiditis. In these two conditions autoantibodies to different thyroid cell components have been described (1). More recently, it was proposed that hypothyroidism may result from antibodies blcking the effect of TSH on the thyroid in the absence of cell damage (12, 13). Two cases of transient neonatal hypothyroidism in newborns of a mother with idiopathic myxedema were described in both cases it was possible to demonstrate the transplacental transfer of an antibody that was able to block TSH binding and TSH activated adenylate cyclase in human thyroid membranes. The occurrence of transient neonatal hypothyroidism due to TSH receptor blocking antibodies has been subsequently confirmed by other laboratories (14, 15). The observation that hypothyroidism was transient and that the time of recovery of thyroid function in newborns was strictly related to the disappearance from the circulation of maternal antibody, indicates that clinical hypothyroidism may be produced by antibodies reacting with the TSH receptor. Furthermore, a different thyroid autoantibody was described in a patient with idiopathic myxedema who gave birth to a neonate with transient hypothyroidism (14-16). This maternal antibody was able not only to inhibit TSH binding and TSH stimulated adenylate cyclase, but it also inhibited iodide uptake and organification at a post receptor level. However, the precise mechanism of this post receptor effect is still unclear and requires further investigation. Autoantibodies blocking the TSH stimulated adenylate cyclase (TBkAb) were also reported in several patients with adult idiopathic myxedema (3, 17). These antibodies were also shown to be able to inhibit the TSH binding to its receptor (18, 19). At variance with neonates with transient immunogenic hypothyroidism, it is still unclear whether these antibodies blocking TSH stimulation of thyroid function are the primary cause of hypothyroidism in adult patients with thyroid atrophy.

The incidence of TBkAb in autoimmune thyroid diseases has been studied in our laboratory by a sensitive technique that employes FRTL-5 cells. Twenty three out of 36 patients with idiopathic myxedema (Fig. 3) and 15 out of 38 patients with hypothyroid Hashimoto's thyroiditis had circulating autoantibodies able to

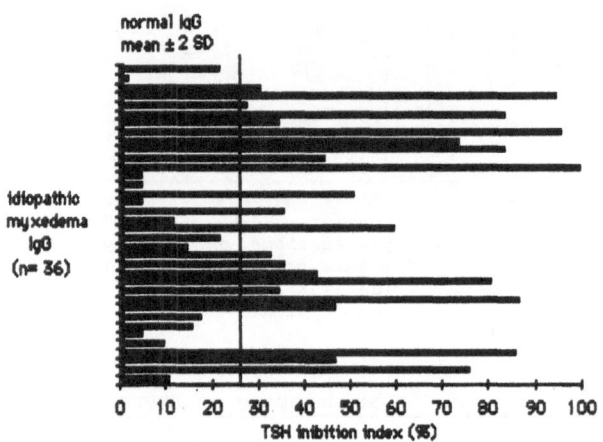

Fig. 3. Effect of IgG preparations from 36 patients with idiopathic myxedema on TSH stimulation of cAMP accumulation in FRTL-5 cells. The vertical dashed line represents the mean ± 2 SD of the effect produced by IgG from normal subjects. The amount of TSH used for the stimulation was 40 µU/ml.

significantly inhibit the TSH activation of adenylate cyclase in FRTL-5 cells. When the results obtained in this inhibition assay were compared with the titer of thyroid microsomal antibodies, as assessed by passive hemagglutination, no correlation was found, indicating that a different type of autoantibody was involved. Moreover, the inhibition of TSH-stimulated AC produced by these antibodies appeared to be competitive with respect to TSH, possibly indicating their interaction with the TSH receptor complex (Fig. 4).

These data suggest that autoantibodies blocking TSH stimulation of the AC may have a pathogenetic role in the development of hypothyroidism in some patients with thyroid autoimmune disorders. Preliminary data indicate that antibodies with the same blocking activity are also present in a minority of patients with Graves' disease.

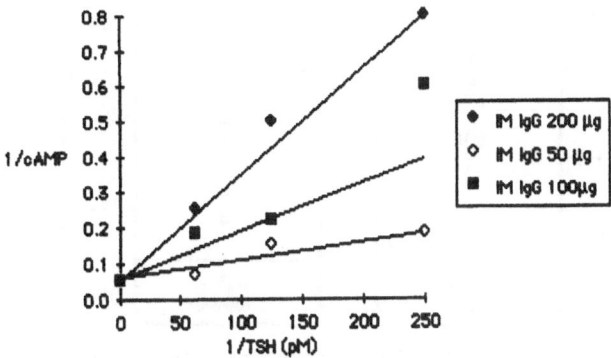

Fig. 4. Effect of different doses of idiopathic myxedema IgG on the inhibition of TSH-stimulated cAMP production in FRTL-5 cells.

Thyroid growth-stimulating antibodies (TSAb)

Recently, several reports have suggested that goiter may be linked to the presence of growth stimulating antibodies that may act through the TSH receptor but not necessarily involving the stimulation of the AC (2). FRTL-5 cells can be usefully employed for the measurement of TGSAb. Using this assay, we have found that IgGs from patients with active Graves' disease and Hashimoto's thyroiditis can increase thyroid cell growth as measured by cell number and ^{3}H-thymidine incorporation (20, 21). While several reports (21, 22) indicate that in sera of patients with Hashimoto's thyroiditis or nontoxic goiter TGSAb may be present in the absence of TSAb, it is still unclear whether these two thyroid stimulating activities may exist separately in Graves' disease. To investigate this problem we compared the results of TSAb and TGSAb assays using FRTL-5 in IgGs from 25 patients with Graves' disease. TSAb was measured by iodide uptake and AC stimulation of ^{3}H-thymidine incorporation was used to detect TGSAb. TGSAb were found in 15/25 IgGs; all of them were also able to stimulate cAMP accumulation and iodide uptake. Thus, in Graves' patients TGSAb activity could not be separated from TSAb activity. To further charify this point, peripheral lymphocytes from a goitrous patient with active Graves' disease were fused with mouse myeloma cells NS1. Eighteen out of 150 (12%) hybridoma supernatants showed a significant binding to solubilized human thyroid membranes. After appropriate subcloning and expansion, IgGs were prepared from spent media using DEAE-Sephadex. These monoclonal antibodies were tested for TSAb and TGSAb activities.A clear-cut increase of cAMP was produced by 9 out of 18 mAb. The same mAb were also able to stimulate ^{3}H-thymidine incorporation. Negative results in both assays were obtained with the remaining mAb (Fig. 5).

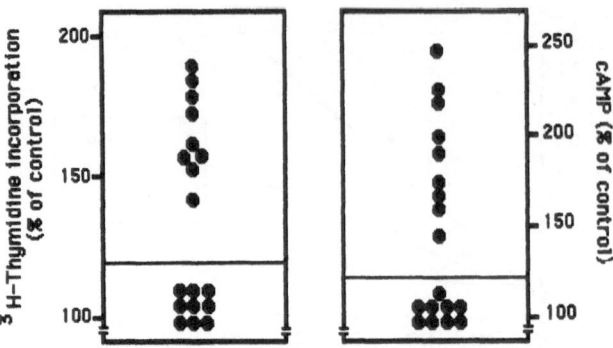

Fig. 5. Effect of monoclonal antibodies from a Graves' patient on ^{3}H-thymidine incorporation and cAMP accumulation in FRTL-5 cells.

These data indicate that, at least in Graves' disease, the TSAb and TGSAb activities coexist in the same IgG suggesting that the adenylate cyclase-cAMP system may be one of the pathways of the signal transmission resulting in the growth of thyroid cells (22). However, the existence of different mechanisms of thyroid growth not involving cAMP production is also suggested by the observation that TGSAb are present in sera from patients with no detectable TSAb activity (20, 21, 23) and by studies in which mAb to the TSH receptor were used (2, 13).

Conclusive remarks

TSH receptor related antibodies may possess multiple biological activities mimicking or interfering with the TSH function. Examples of the TSH-like effects of TSAb include their ability to stimulate thyroid AC and cell growth and to induce AC desensitization of thyroid cells. Autoantibodies blocking the TSH function but devoid of thyroid stimulating activity are present in sera of patients with autoimmune hypothyroidism. In Graves' IgGs thyroid adenylate cyclase and growth stimulating activities are correlated. Furthermore, mAb from a Graves' patient with goiter had simultaneously the ability to stimulate thyroid adenylate cyclase and growth, suggesting that cAMP may be one of the signals mediating thyroid growth. However, the results obtained with mAb from different patients showed that growth and adenylate cyclase stimulating activities could be separated (11). Further studies are needed to clarify this point.

REFERENCES

1. Pinchera A, Fenzi GF, Bartalena L, Chiovato L, Marcocci C, Baschieri L 1980 Antigen-antibody system involved in thyroid autoimmunity. In: A Pinchera, D Doniach, L Baschieri (Eds), Autoimmune Aspects of Endocrine Disorders, Academic Press, London, p 57.

2. Kohn LD, Aloj SM, Tombaccini D, Rotella CM, Toccafondi R, Marcocci C, Corda D, Grollman EF, 1985 The thyrotropin receptor. In: G Litwack (Ed), Biochemical Actions of Hormones, vol. XII, Academic Press, New York, p 457.

3. Konishi J, Iida Y, Endo K, Misaki T, Nohara Y, Matsuura N, Mori T, Torizuka K 1983 Inhibition of thyrotropin-induced adenosine-3',5' monophosphate increase by immunoglobulins from patients with

primary myxedema. J Clin Endocrinol Metab 57: 544.

4. Drexhage HA, Bottazzo GF, Bitensky L, Chayen J, Doniach D 1981 Thyroid growthblocking antibodies in primary myxedema. Nature 289: 594

5. McKenzie JM, Zakarija M, Sato A 1978 Humoral immunity in Graves' disease. Clin Endocrinol Metab 7: 31.

6. Macchia E, Fenzi GF, Monzani F, Lippi F, Giani C, Bartalena L, Baschieri L, Pinchera A 1981 Comparison between thyroid stimulating and TSH-binding inhibiting immunoglobulins of Graves' disease. Clin Endocrinol (Oxf) 17: 175.

7. Pinchera A, Fenzi GF, Bartalena L, Chiovato L, Marcocci C, Toccafondi R, Rotella C, Aterini S, Zonefrati R 1980 Thyroid cell surface antibodies in patients with thyroid autoimmune disorders. In: JR Stockigt, S Nagataki (Eds), Thyroid Research VIII, Australian Academy of Science, Canberra, p 707.

8. Vitti P, Valente WA, Ambesi-Impiombato FS, Fenzi GF, Pinchera A, Kohn LD 1982 Graves' IgG stimulation of continuously cultured rat thyroid cells: a potentially useful clinical assay. J Endocrinol Invest 5: 179.

9. Vitti P, Rotella CM, Valente WA, Cohen J, ALoj SM, Laccetti P, Ambesi-Impiombato FS, Grollman EF, Pinchera A, Toccafondi R, Kohn LD 1983 Characterization of the optimal stimulatory effects of Graves' monoclonal and serum immunoglobulin G on adenosine-3',5'-monophosphate production in FRTL-5 cell: a potential clinical assay. J Clin Endocrinol Metab 57: 782.

10. Marcocci C, Valente WA, Pinchera A, Aloj SM, Kohn LD, Grollman EF 1983 Graves' IgG stimulation of iodide uptake in FRTL-5 rat thyroid cells: A clinical assay complementing FRTL-5 assays measuring adenylate cyclase and growth-stimulating antibodies in autoimmune thyroid disease. J Endocrinol Invest 6: 463.

11. Vitti P, Chiovato L, Ceccarelli P, Lombardi A, Novaes M Jr, Fenzi GF, Pinchera A 1986 Thyroid-stimulating antibody mimics thyrotropin in its ability to desensitize the adenosine 3',5'-monophosphate response to acute stimulation in continuously cultured rat thyroid cells (FRT-L5). J Clin Endocrinol Metab 63: 454.

12. Pinchera A, Fenzi GF, Macchia E, Bartalena L, Mariotti S, Monzani F 1982 Thyroid-stimulating immunoglobulins. Hormone Res 16: 317.

13. Kohn LD, Rotella CM, Marcocci C, Toccafondi RS, Pinchera A, Tombaccini D, Valente WA, De Luca M, Grollman EF 1985 Monoclonal antibodies and autoimmune thyroid disease. In: A Pinchera, G Doria, F Dammacco, A Bargellesi (Eds) Monoclonal Antibodies '84: Biological and Clinical Applications, Editrice Kurtis, Milano, p 169.

14. Matsuura N, yamada Y, Nohara Y, Konishi J, Kasagi K, Endo K, Kojima H, Wataya K 1980 Familial neonatal transient hypothyroidism due to maternal TSH binding inhibiting immunoglobulins. N Engl J Med 303: 738.

15. Takasu N, Mori T, Koizumi Y, Takeuhi S, Yamada T 1984 Transient neonatal hypothyroidism due to maternal immunoglobulins that inhibit thyrotropin-binding and post-receptor processes. J Clin Endocrinol Metab 59: 142.

16. Iseki M, Shimizu M, Oikawa T, Hojo H, Arikawa K, Ichikawa Y, momotani N, Ito K 1983 Sequential serum measurements of thyrotropin binding inhibitor immunoglobulin G in transient familial neonatal hypothyroidism. J Clin Endocrinol Metab 57: 384.

17. Takasu N, Naka M, Mori T, Yamada T 1984 Two types of thyroid function-blocking antibodies in autoimmune atrophic thyroiditis and transient neonatal hypothyroidism due to maternal IgG. Clin Endocrinol 21: 345.

18. Arikawa K, Ichikawa Y, Yoshida T, Shinozawa T, Homma M, Momotani N, Ito K 1985 Blocking type anti thyrotropin receptor antibody in patients with non goitrous hypothyroidism: its incidence and characteristics of action. J Clin Endocrinol Metab 60: 953.

19. Konishi J, Iida Y, Kasagi K, Misaki T, Nakashima T, Endo K, Mori T, Shinpo S, Nohara Y, Matzuura N, Torizuka K 1985 Primary myxedema with thyrotropin-binding inhibiting immunoglobulins. Ann Int Med 103: 26.

20. Chiovato L, Hammond LJ, Hanafusa T, Pujol-Borrell R, Doanich D, Bottazzo GF 1983 Detection of thyroid growth immunoglobulins (TGI) by ^{3}H-thymidine incorporation in rat thyroid follicles. Clin Endocrinol (Oxf) 19: 581.

21. Valente WA, Vitti P, Rotella CM, Vaugham MM, Aloj SM, Grollman EF, Ambesi-Impiombato FS, Kohn LD 1983 Growth-promoting antibodies in autoimmune thyroid disease: a distinct population of thyroid-stimulating antibodies. N Engl J Med 309: 1028.

22. Marcocci C, Gianchecchi D, Masini I, Grollman EF 1986 TSH stimulation of thyroid cell proliferation; role of adenylate cyclase-cAMP system. Ann Endocrinol (Paris) 47: 50.

23. Drexhage HA, Bottazzo GF, Doniach D, Bitensky L, Chayen J 1980 Evidence for thyroid-growth-stimulating immunoglobulins in some goitrous thyroid diseases. Lancet 2: 287.

HETEROGENEITY OF TSH RECEPTOR-DIRECTED ANTIBODIES (TRAb)

AND THEIR SIGNIFICANCE

Margita Zakarija

Department of Medicine
University of Miami School of Medicine
Miami, FL

In reviewing TRAb in Graves' disease there is no longer need for debate about the role of TSAb itself. This antibody is generally accepted as causing hyperthyroidism through binding to a component of the TSH receptor and stimulation of adenylate cyclase. Formerly we used an assay based upon measurement of an increase in cAMP in human thyroid slices and found TSAb in over 90% of 102 patients (1). Now the procedure developed by Kasagi et al (2) and refined by Rapoport and his colleagues (3) has replaced the slice assay. This technique entails incubation of human thyroid cells in primary monolayer culture with patients' IgG in hypotonic medium and subsequent measurement of cAMP that has been released into the medium. With this assay we find 100% positive results with IgG from Graves' disease patients. This high sensitivity apparently is not associated with decreased specificity as judged by negative results with IgG from over 90 patients with thyroid disorders of non-autoimmune origin. A current alternate and more convenient procedure is the similar use of functioning rat thyroid (FRTL-5) cells in continuous culture (4), but not all IgG positive in the human thyroid cell assay give a response in this system.

Unlike antibodies that interact with the receptor for insulin (5) or acetylcholine (6), TSAb is active in the monovalent form, i.e., as the Fab fragment (7,8). An important additional characterization, recently confirmed by Knight et al (9), is that the antibody has restricted heterogeneity (10); the most telling piece of evidence in this regard is the finding that the TSAb-IgG from a given patient has only one type of L chain, i.e., either k or λ, and usually the latter. The full significance of such oligoclonality has yet to be established but undoubtedly its relevance will eventually be revealed at the level of DNA analysis. It should be emphasized that the data quoted above were obtained with unusually potent preparations of IgG (10). Typically such high levels are found in patients who have relapsed after one or more attempts to treat their hyperthyroidism by medical (antithyroid drug) or ablative therapy (1). Also, with a number of these patients, we have been able to show that their TSAb activity was of virtually unchanged potency over many years; the longest interval has been 16 years of such longitudinal collection of data. Furthermore, many of these patients, having been subjected to ablative therapy, sometimes in multiple episodes, were clinically hypothyroid, under treatment with thyroxine, and with no palpable thyroid tissue for much of the period of observation. These considerations are relevant to current debate regarding the importance of antigen modulation of antibody production and whether or not the thyroid is a major site of secretion of TSAb (11).

Much less is known about other antibodies that interact with the TSH receptor but their importance in some clinical situations is being increasingly reported. Most commonly observations in neonatal syndromes have led to recognition of these other TRAb. For instance, temporary hypothyroidism has been attributed to an antibody that, having passed across the placenta, blocks the action of TSH until the neonate metabolizes the maternal IgG (12). The incidence of such an inhibiting antibody is unknown but in Graves' disease it may be as frequent as 34%. This figure comes from our observations with IgG from 153 patients tested on human thyroid cells in hypotonic medium. By assaying IgG at 2 to 4 concentrations, over the range of 5–1500 ug per ml medium, 101 (66%) of the samples gave a straight line response, similar to that obtained with TSH. On the other hand, 52 (34%) gave a plateaued or biphasic response, i.e., an initial dose-related increment followed by a decrement in the concentration of cyclic AMP, with the maximum effect being less than that observed with TSH. Our interpretation of this pattern of response is that such IgG contains both TSAb and an inhibitor of TSAb, as we have described in detail with an especially potent example of the phenomenon (8). This IgG came from a woman who gave birth over 6 years to 3 children who suffered from intrauterine and delayed neonatal hyperthyroidism; this lasted from the 6th week post partum to approximately the 6th month of life (13,14). Our published data (8,13) indicated that the delayed onset reflected the preponderant effect of the TSAb-inhibitor in the initially high concentration of maternal IgG and subsequently yet another antibody acted as an enhancer of TSAb or stimulated the thyroid by itself. We have shown that unlike TSAb, the enhancer is active only as a divalent molecule, i.e. as IgG or $F(ab')_2$, but not as the Fab fragment (8).

Kohn and his colleagues have also studied antibodies from this patient, particularly as monoclonals secreted by heterohybridomas produced with her peripheral blood lymphocytes (15). Some of their data, obtained by assay of circulating IgG, were interpreted to indicate that the TSAb-inhibitor was an anti-idiotype to TSAb (15). That our observations (8,13) could not be explained by the action of an anti-idiotype was established by the following experiment. FRTL-5 cells were preincubated with the patient's IgG and then washed before incubation with either a laboratory standard TSAb-IgG or TSH; the effect of both stimulators was abolished. Obviously in these circumstances the inhibitory IgG was active directly on the TSH receptor. On the other hand, since the enhancing IgG is inactive as Fab, it is conceivable that it is an antibody to idiotopes on the inhibitory IgG molecule that are separate from the antigen-binding site. The divalent action of such an anti-idiotype might be to bridge adjacent Ab-receptor complexes and thus influence receptor kinetics. In this regard it is important to note that the enhancing effect is not obtained with solubilized preparations of the receptor (8,16) where clearly an aggregating effect would not be feasible. Enhancement of TSH binding to human thyroid, but not to FRTL-5 cells (8), may be explained by differing density of TSH receptor on the cell membranes. For example, if the spacing on human thyroid cells is such that an antibody molecule binds to the receptor only by one Fab, cross-linking by a putative anti-idiotype might explain the enhancing effect. Although cross-linking of the receptor is obviously not necessary for the action of TSAb or the inhibitory IgG [that is also effective as

Table 1. TSH—Receptor Antibodies (TRAb)

1. Thyroid—stimulating antibody (TSAb); IgG, effective as Fab
2. Inhibitor of TSH and TSAb (I); IgG, effective as Fab
3. Enhancer of TSH—binding (E);
   a) IgG, not effective as Fab
   b) Stimulator in its own right
4. Non—TSAb stimulator (S)
   a) IgG, effective as Fab
   b) Not blocked by inhibitor

All these TRAb are of restricted heterogeneity, i.e., the activities are associated with only k or λ light chains.

Fab (8)], these speculations regarding a possible anti—idiotype are currently being put to the test. It should be emphasized, however, that desipte all the polemics above, there is currently no clear cut evidence of the spontaneous (i.e., in man) regulation of TSAb by an idiotype—anti-idiotype network in Graves' disease.

The further confirmation of the existence and possible pathogenetic importance of an inhibitor of TSH (and in our experience of TSAb) action and binding comes from a survey of serum from patients with primary myxedema (17). Recently we have identified a patient (a volunteer "normal" control for another study) who appears to represent the early developmental phase of inhibitor production. This 47 year old female was found to have an increase in serum TSH over 1 year from 3.1 to 9.5 uU/ml (normal 0.5 - 4 uU/ml). She has no goiter but positive titers of antibody to thyroglobulin and microsomal antigen (1:640 and 1:25,600 respectively) and a family history of hypothyroidism. In the assay with human thyroid cells her IgG inhibited by 60% the response to 10 uU TSH per ml; in FRTL-5 cells there was a lesser but significant degree of inhibition of 100 uU TSH per ml. Regarding the syndromes of neonatal hypothyroidism we agree with the reports of others (12,18) that the mothers are generally hypothyroid requiring treatment with thyroxine. In our experience several children have been diagnosed as having athyrotic hypothyroidism. Subsequent studies, including confirmation of the maternal serum containing a potent inhibitor of TSH, led to the realization that neonatal evidence of thyroid agenesis, as judged by radioisotope scanning, no doubt reflected total inhibition of endogenous TSH.

A fourth TRAb has been identified by us, yet again through study of IgG from the mother of 3 children with transient neonatal hypothyroidism (19). In this instance the IgG is a thyroid—stimulator, effective as Fab, but distinct from "conventional" TSAb in that it is unaffected by the TSAb—inhibitor, that is also present in this woman's IgG. The stimulator is identified in the assays for TSAb only with high concentrations of IgG and we speculated that because of its low concentration or affinity for its antigen (that might be distinct from the TSH receptor) the effect of the inhibitor prevailed in the neonates. These observations thus lead to the categorization of 4 separate TRAb listed in Table I and illustrative data are given in Fig. 1. In this experiment, the inhibitory IgG (I) is shown to reduce the basal concentration of cAMP and to inhibit in a dose-dependent fashion the effects of enhancer (E) and TSAb. TSH was similarly inhibited (data not shown) and a detailed example of inhibition of TSH in the FRTL-5 system is given in Fig. 2. In addition, in Fig. 1, non-TSAb stimulator(S) is shown not to be inhibited by I. This is the only example

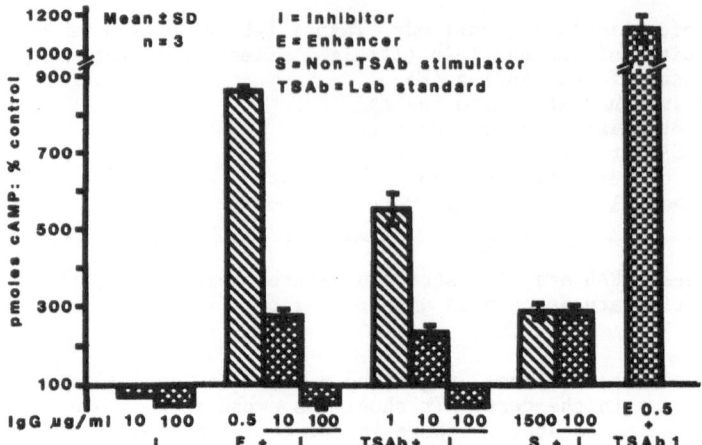

Fig.1. Interactions of TRAb. Assay was with human thyroid cells in
hypotonic medium. I,E, S and TSAb represent the activities
of different IgG obtained with 4 patients with autoimmune
thyroid disease. The E is shown to be effective at 0.5
ug/ml, i.e., stimulating by itself and additive with TSAb;
in a previous report (8) this IgG, that also contains
inhibitor, was shown to block TSAb action at 5 or more
ug/ml. The S, a weak stimulator, was not inhibited by I,
confirmed by similar data obtained with FRTL-5 cells. When
mixed with TSAb, E or TSH, S inhibited those effects and
retained the level of activity shown in this figure (19).

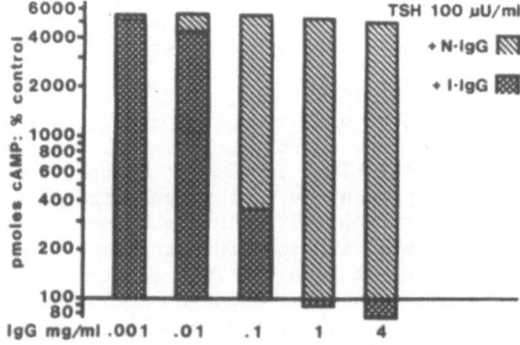

Fig.2. Effect of inhibitory IgG (I-IgG) on TSH stimulation of
FRTL-5 cells. Data are means of closely agreeing triplicate
observations. TSH was mixed with normal IgG (N-IgG) or I-
IgG as indicated and incubated with the cells for 2 hours.

94

in a series of 23 samples of TSAb tested in which stimulation was not prevented by I, thus leading to our suggestion that this represents a separate variety of stimulator, distinct from TSAb.

In summary, patients with autoimmune thyroid disease may present clinically as having Hashimoto's or Graves' disease. The thyroid status, that may be influenced by treatment, otherwise reflects the sum of effects of TRAb that may have stimulating or inhibiting effects on function. The clearest reflection of these actions may be seen in the neonatal syndromes and it is through the opportunity provided by such patients that the 4 TRAb listed in Table 1 have been defined.

As discussed in detail elsewhere in this symposium, evidence has been published purporting to establish a separate category of IgG that specifically stimulates the growth of thyroid cells and does not act through adenylate cyclase (20). This concept was given circumstantial support by the claim that the growth effect of TSH, as studied in FRTL-5 cells, was not cyclic AMP mediated (21). The initial studies were based upon the assessment of DNA in guinea pig thyroid as an index of cells being in the S phase of the growth cycle (22). By this index, the effect of TSH was shown to reach a plateau within 3 hours of its addition to the thyroid fragments (23). Since mammalian cells typically respond to a mitogen with a delay of 8-12 hours before entering the S phase and then exhibit an incremental response over 24 to 48 hours (24), as has indeed been confirmed with a canine thyroid preparation (25), it is difficult to interpret those initial studies (22). However, subsequently, there have been reports of stimulation of growth, as indexed by the incorporation of 3H-thymidine into DNA in FRTL-5 cells, with the IgG coming from patients with non-toxic sporadic goiter (26) or endemic iodine-deficiency goiter (26,27),i.e., conditions otherwise not considered to have an immunological pathogenesis.

Thus, to summarize these recent reports, TSH was viewed as stimulating growth through an action not dependent upon cyclic AMP (22) and a separate thyroid-growth promoting IgG (TGI), distinct from TSAb and also not acting through adenylate cyclase, was identified in sporadic (26) and endemic (27) goiter. There was, in addition, the speculation that TGI is active in Graves' disease, thus facilitating understanding of the acknowledged lack of correlation between goiter size and activity in that syndrome (20). We have attempted to confirm these various claims, but succeeded only in showing that TSH and TSAb effect on growth of FRTL-5 cells is in fact mediated by cAMP (28); similar experience has been reported by others (29,30,31). In addition, growth induced by these stimulators is suppressed or abolished by inhibitory IgG (data not shown) in proportion to the inhibition of cAMP as exemplified in Fig. 1 and 2. We also obtained data suggesting the identity of TSAb and TGI in that both activities in a given IgG preparation have the same isoelectric point and are retained in the Fab fragment (32).

In Graves' disease we have failed to find "TGI" in the absence of TSAb and the two activities have been of similar potency. It is important to realize that in our experience all patients with hyperthyroidism of Graves' disease have IgG that is positive for TSAb in the assay using human thyroid cells, but some are negative in the FRTL-5 system. These negative IgG are also without effect in the TGI assay. TSAb that are negative in the TGI assay might reflect different sensitivities of the two systems or the action of an inhibitory IgG. TSAb assay data relevant to this consideration are shown in Fig 3. This patient was subjected to a subtotal thyroidectomy for relapsing hyperthyroidism in June, 1984.

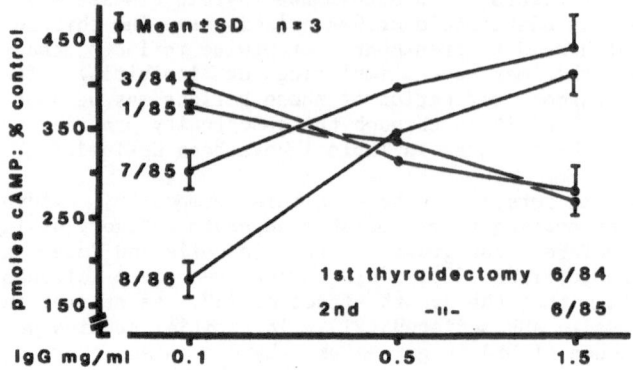

Fig.3. Assays of one patient's IgG with human thyroid cells in hypotonic medium. Dates refer to the time of collection of blood. The patient regrew the goiter and had recurrence of hyperthyroidism between 6/84 and 6/85.

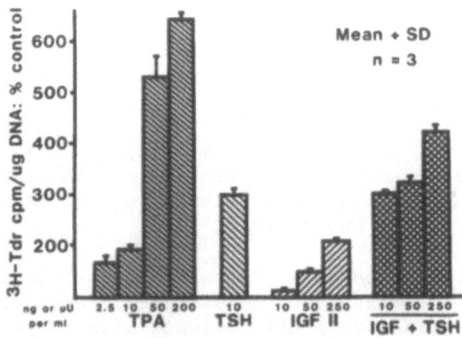

Fig.4. Growth assay with FRTL-5 cells. TPA = tetradodecanoyl phorbol acetate; IGFII = insulin-like growth factor II. Incubation was for 72 hours. TSH was combined with IGFII (IGF + TSH) at a concentration of 10 uU/ml.

Her TSAb at that time gave in human thyroid cells the negative dose response relationship typical of the presence of an inhibitory IgG (8). There was no response of FRTL-5 cells to her IgG, either in terms of an increase in the concentration of cAMP or in the incorporation of 3H-thymidine into DNA. Nonetheless, she rapidly regrew a goiter, and became hyperthyroid again, and so was subjected to a near-total thyroidectomy in June, 1985. One may only speculate that the in-vitro assay conditions facilitated inhibition in the TGI assay, although clearly in-vivo there was unequivocal thyroid growth. Samples from 1985 and 1986, showing only a positive dose-related response, probably reflect a reduced potency of both antibodies in her IgG. We have not yet tested those samples for effects in FRTL-5 cells.

To turn to TGI in non-immune goiter, our experience can be summarized as follows. We have assayed for TSAb and TGI preparations of IgG from 56 subjects with non-toxic goiter (32 sporadic goiter, most treated with thyroxine; 26 endemic goiter, before and after iodide therapy) and uniformly failed to detect either activity. We are at a loss to explain our failure to confirm the data published by others (26,27). One possibility we are currently exploring is that there may be other, non-IgG, growth factors involved in non-immune goiter. Insulin-like growth factor I (IGFI) and interleukin 1 (IL 1) have been shown to stimulate thyroid growth and to synergize with TSH in this regard (33). In view of this report we have tested two other factors and the initial experience is shown in Fig. 4. These data indicate that non-specific growth stimulators, TPA and IGFII, both enhance growth in FRTL-5 cells although the effect of IGFII was minor and only additive to that of TSH, unlike what was reported for IGFI (33). The actions of IGFI and II, TPA and IL1 are not cAMP mediated so it is clear that thyroid growth can indeed be stimulated by mechanisms not involving that nucleotide. The relevance of these considerations to "TGI" is unknown but because of the experiences summarized above the conclusions listed in Table 2 are presented as a synopsis of our understanding of thyroid growth control.

Table 2. Conclusions From Growth Assays With FRTL-5 Cells

---

1. TSH - cAMP mediated
2. TSAb- cAMP mediated
3. Growth factors - not cAMP mediated
4. TGI - to be confirmed

Acknowledgements

Original work carried out in the author's laboratory was supported by USPHS grant AM-31391. FRTL-5 cells were kindly provided by Drs. Valente and Kohn, NIH (Bethesda, MD). Highly purified NIH-bovine (b) TSH-10 (30 IU/mg) was a gift from NIADDK, NIH. I am grateful to Mrs. Gilda Manicourt for expert typing of this manuscript.

References

1. Zakarija M, McKenzie JM, Banovac K 1980. Ann Intern Med 93:28
2. Kasagi K, Konishi J, Iida Y, Ikekubo K, Mori T, Kuma K, Torizuka K 1982 J Clin Endocrinol Metab 54:108
3. Rapoport B, Greenspan FS, Filleti S, Pepitone M 1984 J Clin Endocrinol Metab 58:332
4. Vitti P, Rotella CM, Valente WA, Cohen J, Aloj SM, Laccetti P,

Ambesi-Impiombato FS, Grollman EF, Pinchera A, Toccafondi R, Kohn LD 1983 J Clin Endocrinol Metab 57:782

5. Kahn CR, Kasuga M, King GL, Grunfeld C 1982 In: Evered D, Whelan J (eds) Receptors, antibodies and disease. Ciba Foundation Symposium 90, Pitman, London, p 91

6. Drachman DB, Angus CV, Adams RN, Michelson JD, Hoffman GJ 1978 N Engl J Med 298:1116

7. Smith BR 1976 Immunol Commun 5:345

8. Zakarija M, Garcia A, McKenzie JM 1985 J Clin Invest 76:1885

9. Knight J, Laing P, Knight A, Adams D, Ling N 1986 J Clin Endocrinol Metab 62:342

10. Zakarija M 1983 J Clin Lab Immunol 10:77

11. Weetman AP, McGregor AM 1984 Endocrine Rev 5:309

12. Matsuura N, Yamada Y, Nohara Y, Konishi J, Kasagi K, Endo K, Kojima K, Wataya K 1980 N Engl J Med 303:738

13. Zakarija M, McKenzie JM, Munro DS 1983 J Clin Invest 72:1352

14. Zakarija M, McKenzie JM 1986 J Clin Endocrinol Metab 62:368

15. Kohn LD, Alvarez F, Marcocci C, Kohn AD, Corda D, Hoffman WE, Tombaccini D, Valente WA, de Luca M, Santisteban P, Grollman EF 1986 Ann NY Acad Sci 475:157

16. McKenzie JM, Zakarija M 1986 In: Ingbar SH, Braverman LE (eds) Werner's The Thyroid. Lippincott Co., Philadelphia, p 559

17. Konishi J, Iida Y, Kasagi K, Misaki T, Nakashima T, Endo K, Mori T, Shinto S, Nohara Y, Matsuura N, Torizuka K 1985 Ann Intern Med 103:26

18. Iseki M, Shimizu M, Oikawa T, Hojo H, Arikawa K, Ichikawa Y, Momotani N, Ito K 1983 J Clin Endocrinol Metab 57:384

19. Koizumi Y, Zakarija M, McKenzie JM In: Gaitan E, Medeiros-Neto G (eds) Frontiers in Thyroidology. Plenum Press, New York, in press

20. Valente WA, Vitti P, Rotella CM, Vaughan MM, Aloj SM, Grollman EF, Ambesi-Impiombato FS, Kohn LD 1983 N Engl J Med 309:1028

21. Valente WA, Vitti P, Kohn LD, Brandi ML, Rotella CM, Toccafondi R, Tramontano D, Aloj SM, Ambesi-Impiombato FS 1983 Endocrinol 112:71

22. Drexhage HA, Bottazzo GF, Doniach D, Bitensky L, Chayen J 1980 Lancet 2: 287

23. Drexhage HA, Bottazzo GF, Doniach D 1983 In: Chayen J, Bitensky L (eds) Cytochemical Bioassays. Marcel Dekker, New York, p 153

24. Mitchison JM 1971 The Biology of the Cell Cycle. Cambridge University Press, Cambridge, p 58

25. Roger PP, Dumont JE 1982 FEBS Lett 144:209

26. Kohn DL, Valente WA, Alvarez FV, Rotella CM, Marcocci C, Toccafondi R, Grollman EF 1985 In: Walfish PG, Wall JR, Volpe R (eds) Autoimmunity and the Thyroid. Academic Press, New York, p 217

27. Medeiros-Neto GA, Halpern A, Cozzi ZS, Lima N, Kohn LD 1986 J Clin Endocrinol Metab 63:644

28. Jin S, Hornicek FJ, Neylan D, Zakarija M, McKenzie JM 1986 Endocrinol 119:802

29. Dere WH, Rapoport B 1986 Molec Cell Endocrinol 44:195

30. Ealey PA, Emmerson JM, Bidey SP, Marshall NJ 1985 J Endocrinol 106:203

31. Tramontano D, Chin WW, Moses AC, Ingbar SH 1986 J Biol Chem 261:3919

32. Zakarija M, Jin S, McKenzie JM 1986 61st Annual Meeting of the American Thyroid Association, Phoenix, AZ, 1986, p T-17 (Abstract)

33. Tramontano D 1986 68th Annual Meeting of the Endocrine Society, Anaheim, CA, 1986, p 33 (Abstract)

HUMORAL FACTORS IN GRAVES' OPHTHALMOPATHY

Roberto Toccafondi, Carlo M. Rotella, Roberto Zonefrati, and Annalisa Tanini

Clinica Medica III
Universita' di Firenze
Firenze, Italy

The existence of specific receptors for thyrotropin (TSH) has been demonstrated in non-thyroidal cells such as fat cells of different animal species (1-5), as well as in retro-orbital tissue and lymphocytes (6), in fibroblasts, mouse L-cells, and neural membranes (7-10), in testicular and adrenal cells (11), and even in bacteria (12). It has been also demonstrated that TSH can exert a biological activity in fat cells (13-15) and this possibility lead many investigators to speculate whether Graves' ophthalmopathy could reflect an autoimmune reaction involving shared orbital and thyroid antigens (16-18).

The existence of shared orbital and thyroid antigens was first raised by studies of experimental ophthalmopathy. It is well known that pituitary extracts rich in TSH can induce exophthalmos in animals (19,20); besides, receptors in retrobulbar tissue capable of binding TSH or the so-called "exophthalmos-producing factor" have been described, this binding beeing enhanced by immunoglobulins of ophthalmic Graves' patients (21-24). The activity of this exophthalmogenic immunoglobulins, present in sera of ophthalmic Graves' patients, can be detected in the test for EPS in goldfish (25), but did not correlate with the presence in these sera of thyroid stimulating autoantibodies (TSAb), as determined by "in vivo" mouse bioassay (26). It was thus suggested that the shared antigens might involve determinants on the TSH receptor, but that the antibodies to these determinants would be a subpopulation of total anti-TSH receptor antibodies in the sera of patients with autoimmune thyroid disease.

The antigenic relevance of shared TSH receptor determinants to human ophthalmopathy has been questioned. In fact, it has been postulated that the disease may be initiated by the interaction between circulating antithyroglobulin autoantibodies and thyroid-derived thyroglobulin inserted in eye muscle membranes. Kriss and his collegues (27,28) have demonstrated that retro-orbital muscle has an affinity for both thyroglobulin and antithyroglobulin immunocomplexes. Mullin and co-workers (29) showed that thyroglobulin was a component of normal human eye muscle and that immunocomplexes bind to eye muscle membranes. Kriss and Medhi (30) confirmed these data by using artificial lipid vescicles containing eye muscle proteins. The importance of thyroglobulin as shared orbital and thyroid antigen has been also suggested using a monoclonal antibody approach (31). Despite these data, the involvement of a thyroglobulin determinant as common orbital and thyroid antigen has been questioned by Wall (32). In fact, the eye disease occurs occasionally in the absence of any thyroid disorder and there is no correlation between ophthalmopathy and: (i) the presence or levels of serum thyroglobulin (32), except in the study of Cupini and collegues (33); (ii) titres of antithyroglobulin antibodies; or (iii) levels of immunocomplexes (34). Furthermore, Kodama and co-workers (35) denied a role of thyroglobulin on eye muscle membranes with studies on the binding of monoclonal antibodies against human thyroglobulin to human eye muscles.

Independently from the nature of the shared orbital and thyroid antigens, in the past few years evidence has been accumulated that in the sera of ophthalmic Graves' patients immunoglobulins directed against retro-orbital eye muscle or connective tissue antigens exist. This has been demonstrated by radioimmunometric or enzyme-linked immunosorbent assays and using as substrate soluble antigens from eye muscle (36,37), or eye muscle plasma membranes (38,39), or orbital tissue plasma membranes (40,41), or fibroblast-like cells obtained from retro-orbital tissue (42,43). A soluble antigen has been characterized and partially purified from human eye muscle cytosol using a monoclonal antibody (36). However, recent studies from the same group (39) were unable to demonstrate convincing differences between patients with Graves' ophthalmopathy and normal subjects because of high background reactivity in the ELISA, due to non specific binding of serum proteins and enzyme-second antibody conjugates to plastic surface, and contaminations with other immunoglobulins. Finally, Mengistu and co-workers (44) have detected the presence of autoantibodies against an eye muscle soluble antigen in 33 out 44 patients with Graves' ophthalmopathy by immunofluorescence; however, this test was positive also in some patients affected by other thyroid autoimmune diseases. The titre of eye muscle autoantibodies appeared to be correlated to the degree of eye muscle involvement and the duration of the eye disease.

In reconsidering the problem of shared antigenic determinants between thyroid and retro-orbital tissues by a different methodological approach, evidence was presented that fibroblasts may be an important target for TSH receptor autoantibodies present in Graves' patients with ophthalmopathy (45). This was demonstrated by evaluating the effect of Graves' autoantibodies on fibroblast collagen biosynthesis. Using circulating IgG purified from Graves' sera or monoclonal antibodies to the TSH receptor, evidence was provided that shared thyroid and nonthyroid antigens exists, and that mainly consist of TSH receptor determinants on the thyroid and on nonthyroid tissues, and these are related to the connective tissue complications of Graves' disease (45,46).

For these purposes Graves' disease patients and other thyroid

disease patients attending the Florence University Clinic were selected
(45). Human skin fibroblasts were used as targets for biological
activities of immunoglobulins (45,46). Monoclonal anti-TSH receptor
antibodies were also used to demostrate the relationships between the
TSH receptor structures and the biological effects studied by us
(47,48). Collagen biosynthesis in human skin cultured fibroblasts was
evaluated by measuring the incorporation of tritiated proline into
pepsin-digested high salt-precipitable material (45). Glycosaminoglycan
production by human skin cultured fibroblasts was measured by
evaluating the incorporation of tritiated glucosamine into
pronase-digested cetylpiridinium low salt-precipitable material (46).

One of the more intriguing aspects of these studies was to
determine whether the collagen biosynthesis assay in human skin
fibroblasts was relevant to Graves' ophthalmopathy. IgGs obtained from
the sera of 82 patients with and without ophthalmopathy have been
studied. From results reported in Figure 1, it is clear that the
totality of Graves' patients with exophthalmos, were positive in this

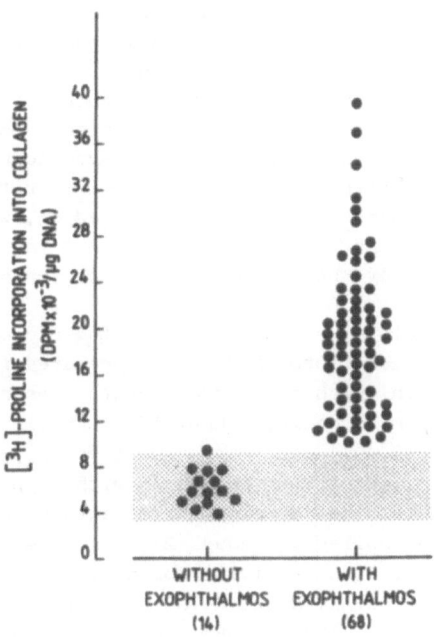

Figure 1. Collagen biosynthesis, evaluated as tritiated proline
incorporation into collagenous proteins synthetized by human skin
fibroblasts, induced by IgGs prepared from sera of Graves' patients
with or without ophthalmopathy. Shaded area corresponds to the mean ±
SD range of normal sujects.

assay, whereas 13/14 IgGs from Graves' patients without ophthalmopathy behaved like normal IgG. No activity was found in IgG from patients with nontoxic diffuse goiter, Hashimoto's thyroiditis or primary thyroid atrophy. The response of Graves' IgG in this assay was totally unrelated to that obtained in Thyroid Stimulating Antibody (TSAb), Thyrotropin Binding Inhibiting Antibody (TBIAb) and Thyroid Growth Promoting Antibody (TGPAb) assays.

To verify if the activity of these IgG could be related to anti-TSH receptor autoantibodies, the activity of a number of monoclonal antibodies (McAb) to the TSH receptor, produced by clones either obtained by fusing spleen cells of mice, immunized with solubilized thyroid membranes, with mouse mieloma cells, or heterohybridomas obtained by fusing circulating lymphocytes of Graves' patients with mouse mieloma cells, was tested in the collagen-fibroblast assay (45). McAb 307H6 was the more potent, among the heterohybridoma produced IgG, in stimulating collagen biosynthesis, while McAbs 129H8, 122G3, 208F7 were weak stimulators and a host of others were inactive. Several mouse IgG monoclonal autoantibodies (11E8, 22A6 and 13D11), were also potent stimulators of collagen synthesis by fibroblasts. Also in the case of monoclonal antibodies the activity in this assay is totally unrelated to that displayed in TSAb, TBIAb and TGPAb assays. More recently, using the heterohybridoma technique, clones from a patient with severe ophthalmopathy have been obtained (46,49). 142 clones of this fusion (the "800 series") were able to produce antibodies. Of these, 13 produced IgG that acted only as stimulators of collagen synthesis in fibroblasts. Thus far, only half of these antibodies fit criteria established for TSH receptor autoantibodies. These data suggest that distinct antibodies which are responsible for triggering the ophthalmopathy circulate in the sera of patients with Graves' disease and connective tissue complications. Considering that evidence for the involvement of thyroglobulin (31) and TSH receptor (45) as antigenic determinants in common between thyroid and retro-orbital tissue has been parallely carried on, we agree with the conclusion of Tao and collegues (31) that more than one antigen-antibody system may be involved in the pathogenesis of ophthalmopathy.

To further ascertain the specificity of the biological effect of Graves' autoantibodies on fibroblasts, IgGs prepared from patients with autoimmune diseases in which the thyroid system was not involved, for example, patients with myasthenia, reumatoid arthritis, or systemic lupus has been tested (46,49). All were inactive in the fibroblast collagen system, except IgGs from patients with type B insulin resistance, a form due to the development of autoantibodies to the insulin receptor. In the collagen assay 2/4 of the patient IgG preparations were positive. The activity of positive antibodies was more than additive with the 11E8 and 307H6 activities. It was noted that the positive antibodies (B7 and B8) were capable of interacting weakly with the insulin receptor, and more potently with the Insulin-like Growth Factor I (IGF-I) receptor; in contrast, the 2 negative antibodies reacted only with the insulin receptor. Neither insulin nor IGF-I alone could enhance collagen biosynthesis in the fibroblasts nor could they, alone, inhibit the activity of the B7 and

B8 antibodies or the 11E8 monoclonal to the TSH receptor, again raising the issue of multiple determinants.

Since modifications of glycosaminoglycan (GAG) synthesis have been also reported in connective tissue complications of Graves' disease (50), the possibility that IgGs from Graves' patients can increase GAG production of human fibroblasts has been investigated. IgGs from the same series of Graves' patients studied in Figure 1, either with or without pretibial myxedema, were not able to significantly affect GAG production of skin fibroblasts. Considering that lymphocytes which commonly infiltrate orbital tissues in ophthalmopathy induce GAG synthesis by fibroblasts derived from retro-orbital tissue of Graves' patients (51,52), our data prompt us to conclude that soluble factors circulating in ophthalmic Graves' patients are not involved in the GAG deposition in retro-orbital connective tissue.

After having defined the characteristics of the biological effects of Graves' IgG on human skin fibroblasts, we turned our attention to the problem of the possible differences between skin and orbital tissue fibroblasts. We have obtained fibroblasts in long-term culture from specimens of eye muscle of a patient undergoing surgery for an orbital injury, and we have compared the effects of IgG extracted from 9 patients with severe ophthalmopathy on eye muscle fibroblasts, with those elicited on skin fibroblasts obtained from the same patient. As reported in Figure 2, all IgG preparations induced an

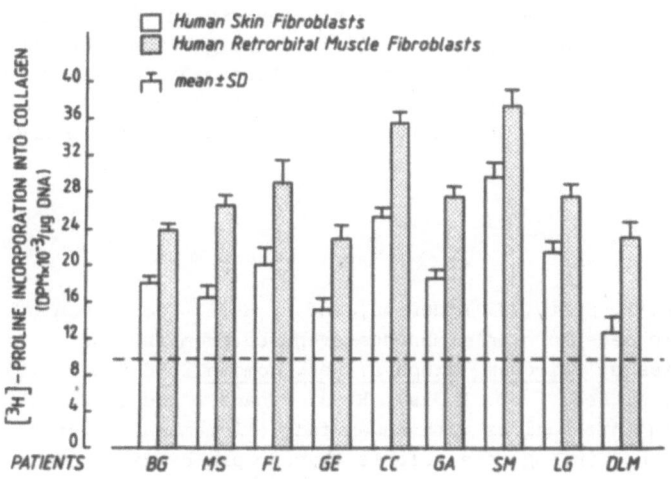

Figure 2. Collagen biosynthesis, evaluated as tritiated proline incorporation into collagenous proteins synthetized by human skin fibroblasts (white bars) or by human retro-orbital muscle fibroblasts (dotted bars), induced by IgGs prepared from the sera of 9 Graves' patients with severe ophthalmopathy. Broken line corresponds to the upper limit of normal range.

higher tritiated proline incorporation value in retro-orbital muscle fibroblasts with respect to skin fibroblasts. In order to evaluate the species-specificity of the biological effects exerted by IgG on retro-orbital muscle fibroblasts, we have compared the effect of IgG preparations of 9 patients studied in Figure 2 on collagen biosynthesis of porcine retro-orbital muscle fibroblasts. A good correlation between tritiated proline incorporation values obtained in porcine and human fibroblasts was found (r=0.91; p 0.001), but the collagen assay in porcine retro-orbital muscle fibroblasts was 5-6 times less sensitive than in human ones, thus far confirming that the latter model is the ideal to test the biological activity of ophthalmic Graves' patient IgG.

A final consideration can be addressed with respect to the effect of plasma exchange therapy in Graves' disease ophthalmopathy. Five of the nine patients reported in Figure 2 (CC, FL, LG, BG and DLM) were tested for the ability of their IgG to stimulate collagen biosynthesis in retro-orbital muscle fibroblasts also when their ophthalmopathy became dormient as a consequence of therapy with plasma exchange, which consisted of three cycles of a sequence of three sessions of plasma exchange at each of which 2 litres of plasma were removed and replaced by human serum albumin and saline; the interval between sessions was of 48 hours and between cycles of 4 weeks. In all patients, examined one month after the end of the last cycle of plasma exchange, the ophthalmopathy index decreased of 3 to 6 points, while the collagen-fibroblast assay became negative in 4 out 5 patients. In the patient in which the test was still positive (CC) the ophthalmopathy became again active after three months of quiescence.

In conclusion, (i) circulating factors (soluble antigens, autoantibodies) can directly or indirectly play a role in Graves' ophthalmopathy; (ii) shared thyroid and non-thyroid antigens exist and their nature may be heterogeneous; (iii) a significant portion of shared antigens consists of TSH receptor determinants on the thyroid and non-thyroid tissues; (iv) thus far, human retro-orbital muscle fibroblasts appear to be an useful tool in the study of the Graves' ophthalmopathy.

REFERENCES

1. C. S. Teng, B. R. Smith, J. Anderson, and R. Hall, Comparison of thyrotropin receptors in membranes prepared from fat and thyroid tissue, Biochem. Biophys. Res. Commun. 66:836 (1975).
2. B. R. Mullin, G. Lee, F. D. Ledley, R. J. Winand., and L. D. Kohn, Thyrotropin interactions with human fat cell membrane preparations and the finding of a soluble thyrotropin binding component, Biochem. Biophys. Res. Commun. 69:55 (1976).
3. D. L. Gill, N. J. Marshall, and R. P. Ekins, Characterization of thyrotropin binding to specific receptors in human fat tissue, Mol. Cell. Endocrinol. 12:41 (1978).
4. M. Kishinara, Y. Nakao, Y. Baba, S. Matsukura, K. Kuma, and T. Fujita, Interactions between thyroid stimulating immunoglobulins and thyrotropin receptors in fat cell

membranes, J. Clin. Endocrinol. Metab. 49:706 (1979).

5. K. Endo, S. M. Amir, and S. B. Ingbar, Development and evaluation of a method for the partial purification of immunoglobulins specific for Graves' disease, J. Clin. Endocrinol. Metab. 52: 1113 (1981).

6. T. F. Davies, C. S. Teng, S. M. Mc Lachlan, B. R. Smith, and R. Hall, Thyrotropin receptors in adipose tissue, retro-orbital tissue and lymphocytes, Mol. Cell. Endocrinol. 9:303 (1978).

7. R. M. Friedman, and L. D. Kohn, Cholera toxin inhibits interferon action, Biochem. Biophys. Res. Commun. 70:1078 (1976).

8. L. D. Kohn, R. M. Friedman, J. M. Holmes, and G. Lee, Use of thyrotropin and cholera toxin to probe the mechanism by which interferon initiates its antiviral activity, Proc. Natl. Acad. Sci. U.S.A. 73:3695 (1976).

9. G. Lee, E. F. Grollman, S. Dyer, F. Beguinot, L. D. Kohn, W. H. Habig, and M. C. Hardegree, Tetanus toxin and thyrotropin interactions with rat brain membrane preparations. J. Biol. Chem. 254:3826 (1979).

10. N. P. Morris, E. Consiglio, L. D. Kohn, W. H. Habig, M. C. Hardegree, and T. B. Helting, Interaction of fragments B and C of tetanus toxin with neural and thyroid membranes and with gangliosides, J. Biol. Chem. 255:6071 (1980).

11. K. M. Trokoudes, A. Sugenoya, E. Hazani, V. V. Row, and R. Volpe', Thyroid-stimulating hormone (TSH) binding to extra-thyroidal human tissues: TSH and Thyroid-stimulating immuno-globulin effects on adenosine 3',5'-monophosphate in testicular and adrenal tissues, J. Clin. Endocrinol. Metab. 48:919 (1979).

12. M. Weiss, S. H. Ingbar, S. Winblad, and D. L. Kasper, Demonstration of saturable binding site for thyrotropin in Yersinia Enterocolitica, Science 219:1331 (1983).

13. I. R. Hart, and J. M. McKenzie, Comparison of the effects of thyrotropin and long-acting thyroid stimulator on guinea pig adipose tissue, Endocrinology 88:26 (1971).

14. P. Kendall-Taylor, and D. S. Munro, The lipolytic activity of long-acting thyroid stimulator, Biochim. Biophys. Acta 231: 314 (1971).

15. D. Gospodarowicz, A comparative study of the lipolytic activity of thyroid-stimulating hormone and luteinizing hormone, J. Biol. Chem. 248:1314 (1973).

16. J. P. Kriss, V. Pleshakov, A. L. Rosenblum, M. Holderness, G. Sharp, and R. J. Utiger, Studies of the pathogenesis of the ophthalmopathy of Graves' disease, J. Clin. Endocrinol. Metab. 27:582 (1967).

17. D. Doniach, and A. Florin-Christensen, Autoimmunity in the pathogenesis of endocrine exophthalmos, Clin. Endocrinol. Metab. 4:341 (1975).

18. R. Day, Hyperthyroidism: clinical manifestations of eye changes. in: "The thyroid: a fundamental and clinical test", C. S. Werner, and S. H. Ingbar, eds., Harper-Row, New York, p.663 (1978).

19. J. Schokaert, Enlargement and hyperplasia of the thyroids in

young ducks from the injection of anterior pituitary extracts, Am. J. Anat. 49:379 (1932).

20. B. M. Dobyns, and S. L. Steelman, The thyroid stimulating hormone of the anterior pituitary as distinct from the exophthalmos producing substance, Endocrinology 52:705 (1953).

21. R. J. Winand, and L. D. Kohn, The binding of 3H-thyrotropin derived exophthalmogenic factor by plasma membranes of the Harderian gland, Proc. Natl. Acad. Sci. U.S.A. 69:1711 (1971).

22. L. D. Kohn, and R. J. Winand, Structure of an exophthalmos--producing factor derived from thyrotropin by partial pepsin digestion, J. Biol. Chem. 250:6503 (1975).

23. D. Bolonkin, R. L. Tate, J. H. Luper, L. D. Kohn, and R. J. Winand, Experimental exophthalmos. Binding of thyrotropin and an exophthalmogenic factor derived from thyrotropin to retro--orbital tissue plasma membranes. J. Biol. Chem. 250: 6516 (1975).

24. R. J. Winand, and L. D. Kohn, Stimulation of adenylate cyclase activity in retro-orbital tissue membranes by thyrotropin and an exophthalmogenic factor derived from thyrotropin. J. Biol. Chem. 250:6522 1975.

25. P. J. Der Kinderer, EPS, LATS, and exophthalmos, in: "Thyro-toxicosis", W. J. Irvine, Livingstone, Edinburgh, p.221 (1967)

26. J. M. Mc Kenzie, and E. P. Cullagh, Observation against a casual relationship between the long-acting thyroid stimulator and ophthalmopathy in Graves' disease, J. Clin. Endocrinol. Metab. 28:1177 (1968).

27. J. Konishi, M. Herman, and J. P. Kriss, Binding of thyroglobulin and thyroglobulin-antithyroglobulin immune complex to extraocular muscle membranes, Endocrinology 95:434 (1974).

28. J. P. Kriss, J. Konishi, and M. Herman, Studies on the patho-genesis of Graves' opthalmopathy (with some related observa-tions regarding therapy), Rec. Progress Horm. Res. 35:533, (1975)

29. B. R. Mullin, R. E. Levinson, A. Friedman, D. E. Henson, R. J. Winand, and L. D. Kohn, Delayed hypersensitivity in Graves' disease and exophthalmos. Identification of thyroglobulin in normal human orbital muscle, Endocrinology 100:351 (1977).

30. J. P. Kriss, and S. Q. Medhi, Cell-mediated lysis of lipid vesicles containing eye muscle protein: Implications regarding pathogenesis of Graves' ophthalmopathy, Proc. Natl. Acad. Sci. U.S.A. 76:2003 (1979).

31. T. W. Tao, P. J. Cheng, H. Pham, S. H. Leu, and J. P. Kriss, Monoclonal antithyroglobulin antibodies derived from immunizzation of mice with human eye muscle and thyroid membranes, J. Clin. Edocrinol. Metab. 63:577 (1986).

32. J. R. Wall, Autoimmunity and Graves' ophthalmopathy, in: "The eye and orbit in thyroid disease", C. A. Gorman, R. R. Waller, and J. A. Dyer, eds., Raven Press, New York, p.103 (1984).

33. C. Cupini, S. Mariotti, U. Del Ninno, A. Antonelli, and A. Pinchera, Humoral markers of Graves' ophthalmopathy, Ann.

Endocrinol. (Paris) 44:82A (1983).

34. D. Brohee, G. Delespesse, and M. Bonnyns, Circulating immune complexes in thyroid disease, _Ann._ _Endocrinol._ (Paris) 39:20A (1978).

35. K. Kodama, H. Sikorska, R. Baylyn, P. Bandy-Dafoe, and J. R. Wall, Use of monoclonal antibodies to investigate possible role of thyroglobulin in the pathogenesis of Graves' ophthalmopathy, _J._ _Clin._ _Endocrinol._ _Metab._ 59:67 (1984).

36. K. Kodama, H. Sikorka, P. Bandy-Dafoe, R. Bayly, and J. R. Wall, Demonstration of a circulating autoantibody against a soluble eye-muscle antigen in Graves' ophthalmopathy, _Lancet_ ii:1353 (1982).

37. S. Atkinson, M. Holcombe, and P. Kendall-Taylor, Ophthalmopathic immunoglobulin in patients with Graves' ophthalmopathy, _Lancet_ ii:374 (1984).

38. M. Faryna, J. Nauman, and A. Gardas, Measurement of autoantibodies against human eye muscle plasma membranes in Graves' ophthalmopathy, _Brit._ _Med._ _J._ 290:191 (1985).

39. M. Salvi, Y. Hiromatsu, L. Wasu, E. Lareya, J. How and J. R. Wall, Current status of autoantibodies against orbital antigens in the pathogenesis of Graves' ophthalmopaty, _in:_ "The thyroid and autoimmunity", H. A. Drexhage, and W. H. Wiersinga, eds, Excerpta Medica ICS 711, Amsterdam, p.255 (1986).

40. T. Kuroki, J. Ruf, L. Whelan, A. Miller, and J. R. Wall, Antithyroglobulin monoclonal and autoantibodies cross-react with an orbital connective tissue membrane antigen: a possible mechanism for the association of ophthalmopathy with autoimmune thyroid disorders, _Clin._ _exp._ _Immunol._ 62:361 (1985).

41. M. Salvi, J. S. How, and J. R. Wall, Detection of autoantibodies against affinity purified orbital membrane antigens in Graves' ophthalmopathy using a competitive binding ELISA, _in:_ "Proc. 61st Meeting of American Thyroid Association", Phoenix, Sept. 10-13, 1986 (Abstract).

42. R. S. Bahn, C. A. Gorman, C. J. Krco, L. W. De Santo, and C. M. Johnson, Binding of IgG to human retro-ocular cells in vitro, _in:_ "Proc. 68th Annual Meeting of Endocrine Society", Anaheim, June 25-27, 1986 (Abstract).

43. R. S. Bahn, C. A. Gorman, G. E. Woloschak, and C. M. Johnson, Serum IgG from patients with Graves' disease binds to a 23 KD protein from human retro-ocular connective tissue, _in:_ "Proc. 61st Meeting of American Thyroid Association", Phoenix, Sept. 10-13, 1986 (Abstract).

44. M. Mengistu, E. Laryea, A. Miller, and J. R. Wall, Clinical significance of a new autoantibody against a human eye muscle soluble antigen, detected by immunofluorescence, _Clin._ _exp._ _Immunol._ 65,19 (1986).

45. C. M. Rotella, R. Zonefrati, R. Toccafondi, W. A. Valente, and L. D. Kohn, Ability of monoclonal antibodies to the thyrotropin receptor to increase collagen synthesis in human fibroblasts: an assay which appears to measure exophthalmogenic immunoglobulins in Graves'sera. _J._ _Clin._ _Endocrinol._ _Metab._ 62:357 (1986).

46. C. M. Rotella, R. Toccafondi, L. D. Kohn, F. Alvarez, Monoclonal antibody studies in the connective tissue complications of Graves' disease: exophthalmos and pretibial mixedema, in: "Monoclonal antibodies: basic principles, experimental and clinical applications in endocrinology", G. Forti, M. B. Lipsett, and M. Serio, eds, Serono Symposia Pubblications for Raven Press, Vol. 30, New York, p. 253 (1986).

47. W. A. Valente, P. Vitti, Z. Yavin, E. Yavin, C. M. Rotella, E. F. Grollman, R. S. Toccafondi, and L. D. Kohn, Monoclonal antibodies to the thyrotropin receptor: stimulating and blocking antibodies derived from the lymphocytes of patients with Graves' disease, Proc. Natl. Acad. Sci. U.S.A. 79:6680 (1982).

48. L. D.Kohn, S.M. Aloj, D. Tombaccini, C. M. Rotella, R. Toccafondi, C. Marcocci, D. Corda, E. F. Grollman, The Thyrotropin Receptor, in : "Biochemical actions of hormones, Vol. XII", G. Litvak, ed., Marcel Dekker, New York, p.457 (1985).

49. C. M. Rotella, F. Alvarez, L. D. Kohn, and R. Toccafondi, Graves' autoantibodies to extrathyroidal TSH receptor: their role in ophthalmopathy and pretibial myxedema, Proceedings of "Advances in Thyroidology, Acta Endocrinologica (Kbh), (Suppl.), (1986) (in press)

50. J. F. O'Brien, Glycosaminoglycans and exophthalmos, in : "The eye and orbit in thyroid disease", C. A. Gorbman, R. R. Waller, and J. A. Dyer, eds., Raven Press, New York, p. 43, (1984).

51. J. C. Sisson, Stimulation of glucose utilization and glycosaminoglycan production by fibroblasts derived from retrobulbar tissue, Exp. Eye Res. 12:285 (1971).

52. J. C. Sisson, and J. A. Vanderburg, Lymphocyte–retrobulbar fibroblast interaction: mechanism by which stimulation occurs and inhibition of stimulation, Invest. Ophthalmol. 11:15 (1972).

IMMUNOREGULATORY ABNORMALITIES IN AUTOIMMUNE THYROID DISEASE

Robert Volpé and Vas V. Row

Endocrinology Research Laboratory, The Wellesley Hospital
University of Toronto, Toronto, Ontario, Canada
160 Wellesley Street, E.K. Jones Building Room 112D
Toronto, Ontario M4Y 1J3

This brief paper is divided into three elements:

1) Evidence for an organ-specific defect in suppressor T lymphocytes

2) The role of a generalized disturbance of suppressor T lymphocytes in active untreated Graves' disease

3) The nature of HLA-DR and antigen expression on thyrocytes in these disorders

ORGAN-SPECIFIC SUPPRESSOR T CELL DEFECT

In human autoimmune thyroid disease, much of the initial evidence with respect to an organ-specific suppressor T lymphocyte (Ts) defect initially came from studies of a modified migration inhibition factor (MIF) test using preparations of T lymphocytes [1-9]. This test reflects the production of a T lymphocyte lymphokine in response to antigen and thus can be considered as an index of (helper) T lymphocyte sensitization. Okita et al [1-4] have demonstrated that preparations of peripheral blood T lymphocytes from patients with Graves' disease (GD) or Hashimoto's thyroiditis (HT) will manifest MIF in response to thyroid antigen. If normal T lymphocytes are added to the sensitized T lymphocytes in ratios from 1:1 to 1:9 (normal : sensitized), then MIF production is abolished. If however, one adds populations of T lymphocytes from one patient with GD or HT to the T lymphocytes of another similar patient, MIF in response to thyroid antigen continues. Treatment of the normal T lymphocytes with irradiation, mitomycin C, or cimetidine (a histamine-2 receptor blocker), agents known to interfere with normal Ts activity, did indeed abolish that activity. On the other hand, T lymphocytes from patients with GD or HT were unable to ameliorate MIF production by lymphocytes from other similar patients, suggesting that there was a defect in Ts function in these disorders. There was no relationship to thyroid function, and indeed this apparent defect in specific Ts activity lasted in the majority of GD patients many years after ^{131}I [9]. Later Topliss et al [6] showed evidence that this Ts defect was disease specific. While Ludgate et al [10] were unable to reproduce these results, Vento et al [7,8] amply confirmed the findings in every detail. Indeed Vento et al [8] have recently provided evidence that the organ-specific defect in GD can be separated from that of HT. (Moreover, Corazza et al [28] have used the T lymphocyte direct MIF technique to demonstrate gluten-specific suppressor T cell dysfunction in coeliac disease).

Further evidence for an organ specific Ts defect in autoimmune thyroid disease has been reported by Noma et al [11], Mori et al [12] and Tao et al [13], all of whom utilized haemolytic plaque assays in their studies, which confirmed the above observations in relation to the regulation of anti-thyroglobulin production. In the study of Mori et al [12], the organ-specific Ts defect was in H2-receptor-bearing Ts cells, confirming the work of Okita et al [4]. Moreover, in the reports of Mori et al [12], the organ-specific Ts defect was clearly partial.

Balasz et al [14] have also studied antigen-specific Ts function (as well as non-specific Ts function) in a set of homozygous twins discordant for GD (one had active GD, one was healthy). Lymphocytes were first cultured with concanavalin A or thyroid membrane for 24 hours. These workers then added these lymphocytes to second groups of lymphocytes (lymphocyte indicator cells) that had been stimulated by concanavalin A for 72 hours, or thyroid membrane antigen for 96 hours, and measured the uptake of tritiated thymidine as an index of nonspecific or specific Ts function respectively. In the twin with active GD, there was a specific Ts defect accompanied by a much less severe nonspecific Ts defect, while in the healthy twin, no such abnormalities could be detected. In a study of intrathyroidal lymphocytes by Benveniste et al [15], a partial specific defect in Ts functions could be demonstrated in the thyroid gland of HT. Similar observations have recently been made by Ueki et al [16]. There thus appears to be a considerable body of evidence supporting the view that there is an organ-specific Ts defect in autoimmune thyroid disease.

GENERALIZED Ts FUNCTION IN AUTOIMMUNE THYROID DISEASE

Despite the above evidence, the magnitude of an organ-specific defect must be minimal; it would therefore not be expected that there would be any generalized Ts disorder in patients with these conditions. Such a generalized disturbance would be expected to result in multiple clinical disorders of immunoregulation. Nevertheless, a literature review [17], indicates that there does appear to be a reduction in the number and functions of generalized Ts in the hyperthyroid phase of GD; however, these tend to normalize as thyroid function itself improves. Although there are a few exceptions, most studies have not shown any subset abnormalities in euthyroid patients with HT. In a study of our own [18], in which an automated flow cytometer was employed, a reduction in the Leu 2a+15+ subset, ie., Ts numbers were clearly demonstrated in active untreated Graves' disease, most clearly evident when the hyperthyroidism was most severe. In one year following ^{131}I therapy, the abnormal values seen in untreated GD had returned to normal. Several patients still had very high titres of TSAb and other thyroid antibodies at that time and yet had returned to completely normal lymphocyte subsets: that is, their organ-specific abnormality (but not their non-specific Ts abnormality) was still manifest. It seemed evident that hyperthyroidism per se (or some factor related closely thereto) did have a deleterious effect on Ts numbers and that this might be additive to the antigen-specific Ts defect; it thus may be an important factor in causing self perpetuation of the disease (Figure 1). Our Ts and other lymphocyte subset values were normal in Hashimoto's thyroiditis and in non-toxic nodular goitre (unpublished data). Thus there is no evidence for an abnormality of lymphocyte subsets either in euthyroid autoimmune thyroid disease, or in non-toxic goitre, despite assertions to the contrary [27].

THE ROLE OF HLA-DR AND THYROID ANTIGEN EXPRESSION ON THE THYROID CELLS

Bottazzo et al [19] have claimed that local aberrant expression of HLA-DR by thyroid cells enables antigen on them to activate and stimulate T lymphocytes, and that these then activate effector cells to initiate autoantibody production. They suggested that interferon gamma

(IFNγ) produced by T lymphocytes secondary to local viral infections was a likely cause of the aberrant HLA-DR expression and was the initiating factor in precipitating autoimmune thyroid disease. (It is indeed clear that IFNγ is the only known inducer of thyrocyte HLA-DR antigen expression [20,21].)

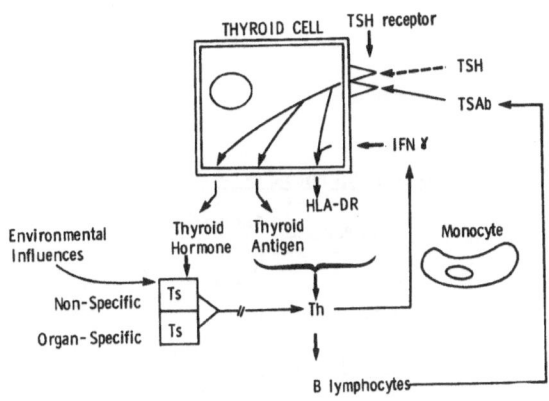

FIGURE 1

Hypothesis for the pathogenesis of Graves' disease (GD)

The basic factor necessary for the development of GD is considered to be an HLA-related genetically induced organ-specific defect in suppressor T lymphocyte (Ts) function. Precipitating factors from the environment (e.g., stress, infection) may cause a reduction in generalized Ts function and numbers which is additive (superimposed) on the organ-specific Ts defect. The resultant is to reduce suppression of a thyroid-directed helper T lymphocyte (Th) population. The specific Th will then (in the presence of monocytes and the specific antigen) produce interferon gamma (IFNγ) and will also stimulate specific B lymphocytes to produce thyroid stimulating antibody (TSAb). TSAb, like TSH, stimulates the TSH receptor and will result in antigen (e.g., microvillar antigen) expression. IFNγ causes HLA-DR expression on the thyroid cell surface and this effect is enhanced by TSAb (and TSH). Thus antigen presentation by the thyroid cell occurs directly (requiring the presence of the antigen and HLA-DR expression); this activates and stimulates the specific Th further and the cycle is repeated. Moreover, excess thyroid hormone acts on generalized Ts reducing their number and function, further stimulating Th and adding to the cycle and thus perpetuating the disease.

The sequence depicted in Figure 1 is interrupted by ATD acting on
thyroid cells directly. The primary action is to reduce thryroid hormone
production (1). This normalization of thyroid function increases the
inhibition of non-specific Ts and that function returns to normal (2); the
additive effect on the basic organ-specific Ts defect is thus lost.
Suppression of the specific Th population is brought about (3) in the subset
of patients who do not have a severe organ-specific defect in Ts. This

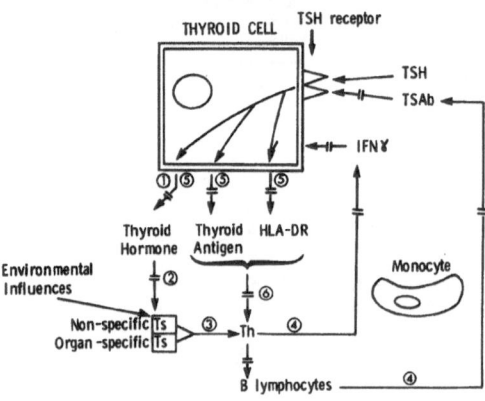

FIGURE 2

Induction of remissions in GD with antithyroid drugs (ATD)

results in a reduction of IFN ɣ production and reduced Th stimulation of
B lymphocytes to produce TSAb (4). The combined reduction of TSAb and
IFNɣ will reduce the thyroid antigen and HLA-DR expression, i.e., antigen
presentation by the thyroid cell; there will also be reduced thyroid
hormone production (5). The reduced hormone production will further
increase Ts inhibition, thus reducing Th activity, and similarly reduced
antigen presentation will have the same effect (6). This beneficial
cycle will then repeat itself, but will not occur in those patient with
a severe organ-specific Ts defect.

However, Iwatani et al [21], in our laboratory, have shown that the expression of HLA-DR antigen on thyrocytes in culture depends on the presence not only of T cells, but also of monocytes; moreover, there is nothing peculiar about GD thyroid cells that do express HLA-DR in vivo but lose this expression within a few days in tissue culture. Thereafter, their responses to mitogens (mediated only through the response of passenger lymphocytes in the cultures) is no different from that of normal thyroid cells. Indeed the thyroid cells from GD glands when xenoplanted into nude mice soon lose their HLA-DR expression. Moreover, they soon become perfectly normal in function as the lymphocytes disappear [22]. Thus unlike the situation in obese strain chickens[23], there is no evidence for an intrinsic thyroid cell abnormality prior to the onset of human auto-immune thyroid disease. Indeed, lymphocytes from patients with either active untreated GD or hypothyroid HT produce <u>less</u> IFNγ and thyrocyte HLA-DR expression following <u>non-specific</u> mitogenic stimulation than do normal lymphocytes. In contrast, lymphocytes from patients with GD or HT are capable of stimulating autologous thyroid cells (previously allowed to lose their DR expression) to again express aberrant DR expression; this occurs much more sharply and quickly than with normal lymphocytes. This is due to the fact that GD and HT lymphocytes are already sensitized to the thyroid antigen. The difference here is between non-specific (mitogenic) stimulation on the one hand, and specific (antigenic) stimulation on the other. Moreover, Davies [24] has shown that thyroid cells from normal individuals have the capacity to stimulate T lymphocytes after lectin-induced thyrocyte DR expression. From these data it seems evident that thyrocyte DR expression is a secondary phenomenon, ie, secondary to the immune assault itself. It is, however, possible that it might help to potentiate the T lymphocyte response once the immune process itself is initiated, but this will not continue once the underlying process abates. The latter point derives from the work of LeClère et al [25] in which they demonstrated HLA-DR expression on thyroid cells in the acute phase of subacute (deQuervain's) thyroiditis. We have confirmed this observation (unpublished data) and have shown that this thyrocyte HLA-DR expression disappears at the time of a second biopsy following recovery. It is important to emphasize, therefore, that HLA-DR expression on the thyroid cells does <u>not</u> establish a self-perpetuating, or "vicious" cycle on its own. If it <u>is</u> potentiating or amplifying, it can do so only as long as the underlying immunoregulatory abnormality or immune perturbation persists. The latter qualifying remark would also account for the focal immune disturbances (and thyrocyte HLA-DR expression) seen in thyroid carcinoma, non toxic goitre, etc.

It may also be emphasized that other environmental factors can influence generalized Ts function, including stress, infection, drugs and aging [17]. Such factors therefore may act as a precipitant in persons predisposed by virtue of a genetic disturbance in organ-specific Ts. Although space does not permit a discussion of an hypothesis as to how remissions could be brought about by drugs, a schema for this hypothesis is depicted in Figure 2 and legend [26].

REFERENCES

1. Okita N., Kidd A., Row V.V., Volpé R., (1980) Sensitization of T lymphocytes in Graves' and Hashimoto's diseases. J. Clin Endocrinol Metab 51: 316-320

2. Okita N., Row V.V., Volpé R., (1981) Suppressor T lymphocyte deficiency in Graves' disease and Hashimoto's thyroiditis. J. Clin Endocrinol Metab 52: 528-533

3. Okita N., Kidd A., Row V.V., Volpé R., (1981) T lymphocyte sensitization in Graves' and hashimoto's disease confirmed by an indirect migration inhibition factor test using normal T lymphocyte as indicator cells. J. Clin Endocrinol Metab 52: 523-527

4. Okita N., How J., Topliss D., Lewis M., Row V.V., Volpé R., (1981) Suppressor T Lymphocyte dysfunction in Graves' disease: role of the H-2 histamine recepto-bearing suppressor T lymphocytes. J. Clin Endocrinol Metab 53: 1002-1007

5. Topliss D.J., Okita N., Lewis M., Row V.V., Voplé R., (1981) Allosuppressor T lymphocytes abolish migration inhibition factor production in autoimmune thyroid disease: evidence from radio-sensitivity experiments. Clin Endocrinol 15: 335-341

6. Topliss D.J., How J., Lewis M., Row V.V., Volpé R., (1983) Evidence for cell-mediated immunity and specific suppressor T lymphocyte dysfunction in Graves' disease and diabetes mellitus. J. Clin Endocrinol Metab 57: 700-705

7. Vento S., Hegarty J.E., Bottazzo G.F., Macchia E., Williams R., Eddlestone A.L.W.F., (1984) Antigen-specific suppressor cell function in autoimmune chronic active hepatitia Lancet 1: 1200-1204

8. Vento S., O'Brien C.J., Cundy T., Williams R., Eddlestone A.L.W.F., (1985) T lymphocyte sensitization to discrete thyroid membrane antigens in patients with different autoimmune thyroid disorders. Proc. Seventh Europ. Immunol Meeting, Jerusalem, Israel, p. 205

9. How J., Topliss D.J., Strakosch C., Lewis M., Row V.V., Volpé R., (1983) T. lymphocyte sensitization and suppressor T. lymphocyte defect in patients long after treatment for Graves' disease Clin Endocrinol 18: 61-72

10. Ludgate M.E., Ratanachaiyavong S., Weetman A.P., Hall R., McGregor A.M., (1985) Failure to demonstrate cell-mediated immune responses to thyroid antigens in Graves' disease using in vitro assays of lymphokine mediating migration inhibition. J. Clin Endocrinol Metab. 60: 90-102

11. Noma T., Yata J., Shishiba Y., Inatsuki B., (1982) In vitro detection of antithyroglobulin antibody producing cells from the lymphcytes of chronic thyroiditis patients and analysis of the regulation. Clin Exper Immunol. 49: 565-571

12. Mori H., Hamada N., DeGroot L.J., (1985) Studies of thyroglobulin-specific suppressor T lymphocytes function in autoimmune thyroid disease J. Clin Endocrinol Metab 61: 306-312

13. Tao T.W., Gatenby P.A., Leu S.L., Pham H., Kriss J.P., (1985) Helper and suppressor activities of lymphocyte subsets on antithyroglobulin production in vitro. J. Clin Endocrinol Metab 61: 520-524

14. Balasz C.S., Stenszky V., Kosma L., Farid N.R., (1984) Specific suppressor T Cell function in a patient with Graves' disease and her healthy identical twin. Clin Endocrinol 20: 683-693

15. Benveniste P., Row V.V., Volpé R., (1985) Studies of the immunoregu-lation of thyroid autoantibody production in man. Clin Exper Immunol 61:274-282

16. Ueki Y., Fukuda T., Otsubo T., Kawabe Y., Shimomora Y., Matsunaga M., Tezuka H., Ishikawa N., Ito K., Eguchi K., (1986) The decrease of suppressor function of T cells in thyroid glands of Graves' disease. Ann d' Endocrinol 47: 53

17. Volpé R., (1986) Autoimmune thyroid disease-a perspective. Mol. Biol Med 3: 25-51

18. Gerstein H.C., Iwatani Y., Iitaka M., Row V.V., Volpé R., (1986) Enumeration of T lymphocytes subsets in Graves' disease: decreased suppressor cells in severe hyperthyroidism. Proc Ninth Internation. Thyroid Congress, Plenum Press (in press)

19. Bottazzo G.F. Pujol-Borrell R., Hanafusa T., Feldmann M., (1983) Role of aberrant HLA-DR expression and antigen presentation in induction of endocrine autoimmunity. Lancet 2: 1115-1119

20. Todd I., Pujol-Borrell R., Hammond L.J., Bottazzo G.F., Feldmann M., (1985) Interferonγ induces HLA-DR expression by thyroid epithelium Clin Exper Immunol 61: 265-273

21. Iwatani Y., Gerstein H., Iitaka M., Row V.V., Volpé R., (1986) Thyrocyte HLA-DR expression and interferon production in autoimmune thyroid disease. J. Clin Endocrinol Metab 63: 695-708

22. Leclère J., Béné M.C., Duprez A., Faure G., Thomas J.L., Vignaud J.M., Burlet C., (1984) Behaviour of human Graves thyroid disease in nude mouse. Proc 7th Internat. Congr. Endocrinol. July 1-7 Quebec City, Excerpt Medica, Internat. Congress Series 652, p. 1079 abstr. 1638

23. Bigazzi P.E., and Rose N.R., (1985) Autoimmune thyroid disease. In: The autoimmune diseases, ed. by Rose N.R., and MacKay I.R., Academic Press, New York pp. 161-199

24. Davies, T.F., (1985) Cocultures of human thyroid monolayer cells and autologeous T cells-impact of HLA Class II antigen expression. J. Clin Endocrinol Metab 61: 418-422

25. Leclère J., Faure G., Béné M.C., Thomas J.L., Paul J.L. Hartemann P., (1986) In situ immunological disorders in the De Quervain's thyroiditis. Proc Ninth Internat Thyroid Congress. Plenum Press (in press)

26. Volpé R., Karlsson A., Jansson R., Dahlberg P.A., (1986) Antithyroid drugs act through modulation of thyroid cell activity to induce remissions in Graves' disease. Clin Endocrinol 25: 453-462

27. Vander Gaag, R.D., VonBlomberg-van der Flier M., Van de Plassche-Boers, E., Kokje-Kleingeld M., and Drexhage H.A., (1986) T-suppressor cell defects in euthyroid nonendemic goitre. Acta Endocrinolagica 112: 38-86

28. Corazza, G.R., Sarchielli P., Londei M., Frisoni M., and Gasbarrini G., (1986) Gluten-specific suppressor T cell dysfunction in coeliac disease. Gut 27: 392-398.

INTRATHYROIDAL LYMPHOCYTES, THYROID AUTOANTIBODIES AND THYROID DESTRUCTION

S. M. McLachlan, C. A. S. Pegg, M. C. Atherton, S. Middleton,
P. Rooke, C. Thompson, S. Dahabra, E. T. Young, F. Clark,
and B. Rees Smith

Departments of Pathology and Medicine, University of
Newcastle upon Tyne and Department of Medicine, University
of Wales College of Medicine, Cardiff, UK

INTRODUCTION

Lymphocytes infiltrating thyroid tissue in Graves' and Hashimoto
patients may be found in aggregates or diffusely distributed between and
within thyroid follicles [1,2]. Using mechanical disaggregation and/or
enzyme digestion to isolate lymphoid cells from thyroid tissue, we have
obtained evidence which strongly suggests that thyroid autoantibodies
are secreted by lymphocytes in the diffusely distributed population [3,4].
The autoantibody secreting cells occur in close proximity to thyroid cells
and also to T cells bearing the cytotoxic/suppressor marker. These T
cells may be involved in regulation of autoantibody synthesis in vivo.
However, some recent studies suggest that the inhibition of thyroid autoantibody synthesis induced by Pokeweed mitogen in vitro is not mediated
by conventional suppressor T cells [5]. This population of cytotoxic/
suppressor T cells observed in thyroid sections may play a role in thyroid
cell damage and it is therefore of interest to note that a high proportion
of T cell clones from Hashimoto thyroid lymphoid suspension had non-specific
cytolytic activity [6]. Although cytotoxic T cells are likely to be important in thyroid destruction, studies in an animal model of Hashimoto's
disease, the Obese Strain chicken, indicate that thyroid autoantibodies
also play a role [7]. The mechanisms involved are not clear but they may
include complement fixation or an antibody dependent mechanism mediated
by killer or natural killer (K/NK) cells.

Autoantibodies to thyroid microsomal (Mic) antigen and thyroglobulin
(Tg) are predominantly of IgG class and they are usually restricted to
subclasses IgG1 and/or IgG4 [8,9]. Different forms of therapy for Graves'
disease are accompanied by characteristic changes in total serum autoantibody
levels. However, in a group of 21 Graves' patients treated with carbimazole,
131-iodine or surgery, the contribution made by each IgG subclass to Mic
and/or Tg antibodies remained relatively unchanged over a period of 8 -
24 months despite variations in total serum levels [10]. Similarly, in
7 Hashimoto patients taking thyroxine (all of whom had high titres of
Tg antibody), the % contribution of each IgG subclass to Tg antibody was
in general unaltered over 2 - 5 years [10]; nor was any major IgG subclass
change observed in 35 clinically euthyroid microsomal antibody positive
women studied during the postpartum rise in thyroid autoantibody levels [11].
Further, Mic antibodies may have a totally different subclass distribution

from Tg antibodies in the same patient [8]. Consequently, we have suggested that the IgG subclass distribution of Mic and/or Tg antibody may be regarded as a "fingerprint" of an individual's response to thyroid antigens [10].

Antibodies are bifunctional molecules, with the antigen binding site in the variable region and the biological activity residing in the constant region. We have therefore studied the potential role of thyroid auto-antibodies of different IgG subclasses in antibody mediated destruction using thyrocyte monolayers. In addition, we have investigated the auto-antibody IgG subclass distribution in sera from patients with autoimmune thyroid disease and their clinically unaffected relatives.

METHODS AND MATERIALS

Antibody dependent cell cytotoxicity (ADCC) was investigated in mono-layers of thyroid cells prepared by digestion of Graves' thyroid tissue and labelled with 51-Cr. The thyroid cells were exposed to immunoglobulins precipitated from Graves' or Hashimoto sera using ammonium sulphate; dilutions corresponding to serum concentrations of 1:100, 1:1000 and 1:10,000 were used. Peripheral blood lymphocytes (a source of K/NK cells) from normal donors were added at a ratio of 20 lymphoid cells : 1 thyroid cell. After an incubation period of 18 hours, aliquots of supernatant were col-lected and the extent of 51-Cr release (indicating thyroid cell death) was measured. The results are expressed as % Specific lysis defined as:

$$\frac{\text{Counts using lymphocytes + IgG - Counts using IgG only}}{\text{Total counts released using detergent}}$$

The method was based on that described by Creemers et al. [12] and Bognor et al. [13].

The levels of Mic or Tg antibodies (all IgG subclasses) were measured by ELISA in sera or IgG preparations at dilutions of 1:100 to 1:10,000 and the results have been expressed as an ELISA Index as previously defined [14,15]. The IgG subclass distribution of Mic and Tg antibodies was analysed by an ELISA technique using murine monoclonal antisera to human IgG sub-classes [8]. The results have been expressed as the optical density reading at 492 nm or as the % contribution made to Mic or Tg antibody by subclasses IgG1 to IgG4.

RESULTS

Using IgG preparations at concentrations equivalent to serum diluted 1:100, the extent of ADCC (measured as 51-Cr release) was higher when thyroid cells were incubated with K/NK cells and IgG from 8/9 patients with thyroid antibodies than with IgG from normal individuals (Table 1). ADCC was dependent on the dose of IgG used and although sera diluted 1:1000 still induced thyrocyte destruction, much lower values for ADCC were observed with serum diluted 1:10,000. The cytotoxic effect of sera showed no correlation with the levels of Tg antibody (Table 1) but the effect was significantly correlated with the levels of Mic antibody (Fig 1 A). When this was analysed in terms of IgG subclass, a significant association was observed between the extent of ADCC and the level of Mic antibody of subclass IgG1 (Fig 1 B) but not IgG4.

The IgG subclass distribution of Mic and/or Tg antibodies has been analysed in 42 thyroid autoantibody positive probands and relatives out of a total of 129 individuals from 11 families with autoimmune thyroid disease. An example of the results obtained for one family is shown

118

Table 1. Thyroid cell destruction measured as % specific 51-Cr release by Graves' thyroid cell monolayers incubated with peripheral blood lymphocytes and sera from patients with autoimmune thyroid disease or normal donors. Un: Undetectable.

| Donor | % Specific 51-Cr release with serum diluted. | | | ELISA Index | |
	1:100	1:1000	1:10,000	Mic Ab 1:1000	Tg Ab 1:1000
Sera from Patients with Autoimmune Thyroid Disease					
EB	29.7	36.1	12.6	1.46	1.70
KT	30.4	23.5	9.9	1.04	2.89
VW	22.5	19.6	10.9	1.15	2.62
CD	24.3	18.3	6.4	1.54	0.64
GH	17.3	16.9	11.3	1.30	0.13
JW	24.9	16.0	6.7	0.52	0.31
IP	12.3	10.3	6.9	1.54	2.54
PP	25.6	9.8	4.7	0.25	1.05
MF	5.7	3.5	3.6	0.29	0.98
Sera from Normal Donors					
PN	3.9	4.3	4.3	Un	Un
SM	6.7	-	-	Un	Un
MA	4.5	1.1	6.0	Un	Un

in Fig 2. Two individuals have Mic antibodies only, three have Mic and Tg antibodies and the ability to produce thyroid antibodies of different IgG subclasses varies from one individual to another. The IgG subclass pattern of Mic and Tg antibodies for the probands (individuals 3 and 4 who have Hashimoto's thyroiditis) are very similar. The older sister (12) of proband 3 also has a similar IgG subclass distribution pattern for serum Mic and Tg antibodies, although the levels (as indicated by the ELISA index values) are lower than the corresponding values for her mother and her sibling. Further, the maternally derived HLA antigens in individual 12 (A3, B7, DR2) are not the same as those inherited by individual 4 from her mother (A11, B44, DR7) and it is possible that this difference is associated with lack of expression (or perhaps delayed expression) of overt disease in individual 12.

DISCUSSION

Early studies of the destructive effects of thyroid autoantibodies in vitro showed that thyroid damage was associated with Mic antibodies and in particular with their ability to fix complement [16,17]. Recently we observed that the development of postpartum hypothyroidism tended to be associated with antibodies of subclass IgG1 rather than IgG4 [11].

119

This could have been due to the ability of antibodies of subclass IgG1 (but not IgG4) to fix complement [18]. However, an additional factor could be the greater efficiency of Mic antibodies of subclass IgG1 to mediate damage via K/NK cells and this possibility is supported by the results of our <u>in vitro</u> studies presented here.

Previous observations by others have shown that overt autoimmune thyroid disese is associated with the HLA markers and Gm allotypes of the

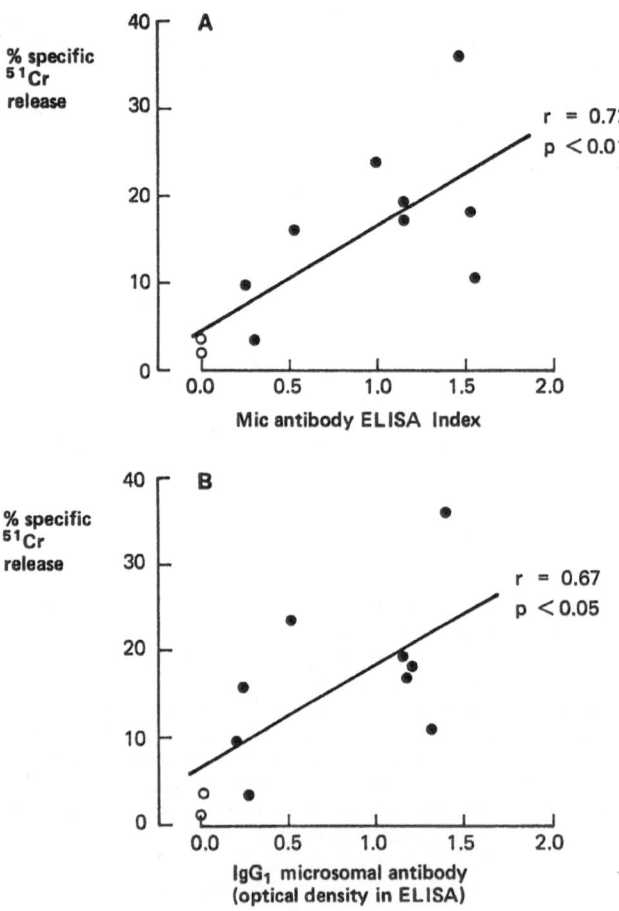

Fig. 1. Correlation between antibody dependent cell cytotoxicity in thyroid monolayers (measured as % specific 51-Cr release) and A, the level of Mic antibody (all IgG subclasses) present in serum or B the amount of Mic antibody of subclass IgG1 . Values for the ELISA Index or the optical density were obtained from sera diluted 1:1000. r = correlation coefficient. P; probability.

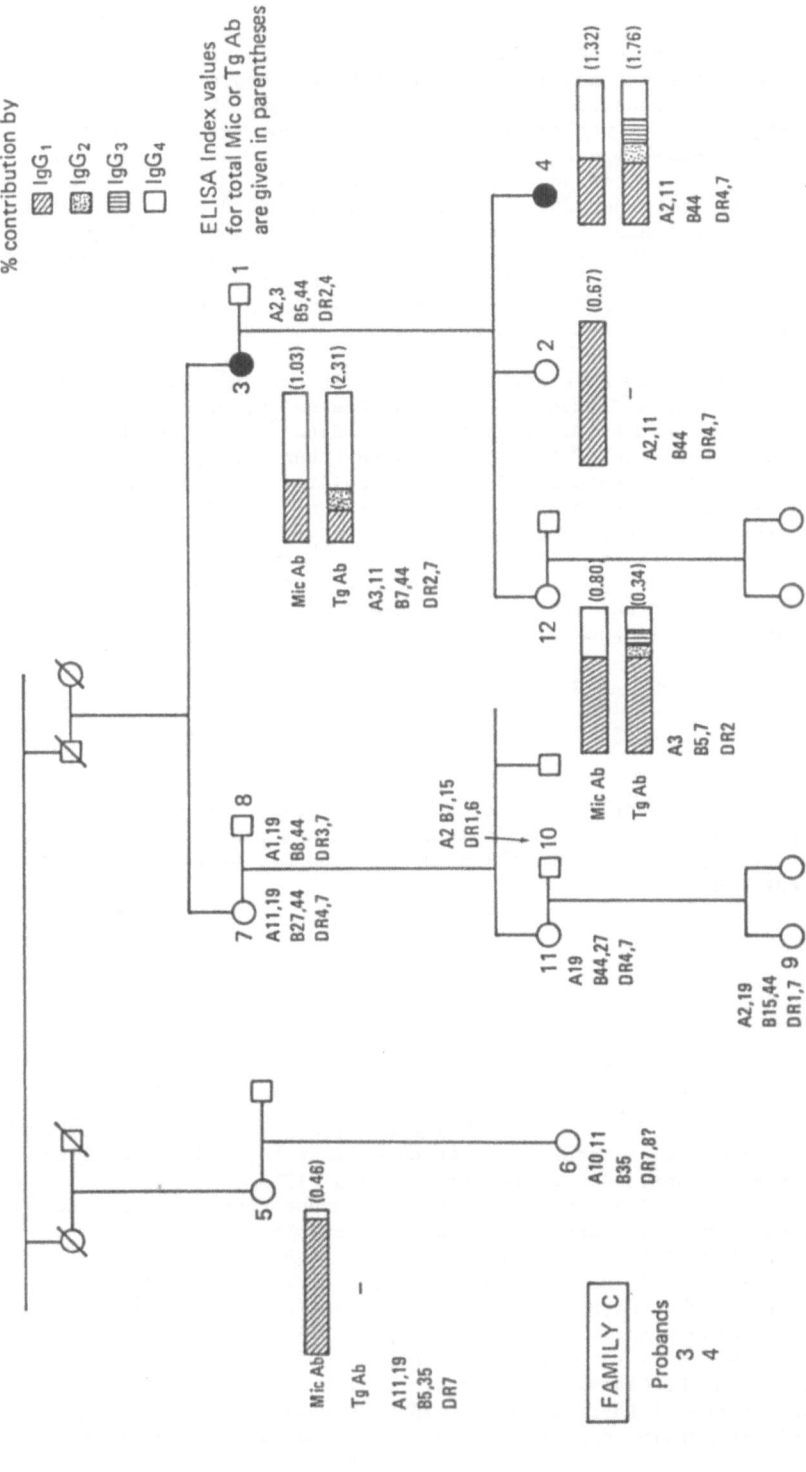

Fig. 2. Characterisation of Microsomal & Thyroglobulin Antibodies in Probands & Relatives in a Family Predisposed to Autoimmune Thyroid Disease

proband [19]. Such interactive effects between Gm allotypes and HLA markers have been described for the antibody response to the bacterial antigen, flagellin [20]. Since Gm allotypes are linked to IgG subclasses, it seems likely that the association between Gm and active autoimmune thyroid disease could arise because of the different biological capacities of autoantibodies of different subclasses in mediating thyroid destruction. An alternative (or additional) explanation could be that the subclass distribution might reflect the nature of the autoimmune response mounted by different individuals to different antigenic epitopes on thyroid auto-antigens. The ability to respond to one particular autoantigenic epitope rather than another could be associated both with the production of thyroid autoantibody of a particular subclass and with the development of thyroid specific cytotoxic T cells. If this hypothesis is correct, the IgG subclass distribution of microsomal and/or thyroglobulin autoantibodies, together with HLA markers, could reflect the potential capacity of the individual to destroy the thyroid by autoimmune mechanisms.

Many Graves' patients have high titres of Mic antibody and sometimes Tg antibody as well; in addition, therapy for Graves' hyperthyroidism may be followed by the development of hypothyroidism [21]. These observations as well as analyses of thyroid biopsies taken from patients at least 10 years after treatment for hyperthyroidism [22], suggest that in Graves' disease there is an underlying process of thyroid destruction which is overcome by the powerful stimulatory effects of TSH-receptor antibodies [23]. Consequently it is likely that on the basis of TSH-receptor antibody levels, IgG subclass distribution of Mic and/or Tg antibodies, Gm allotypes and HLA markers, in association with iodide availability and the well know effects of age and sex, it will ultimately be possible to predict the development of overt autoimmune hyperthyroidism in genetically predisposed individuals.

ACKNOWLEDGEMENTS

We would like to thank Miss Anne Stratton, Blood Transfusion Service, Newcastle General Hospital, for assistance with HLA-typing. These studies were supported by the Medical Research Council, Great Britain and the Newcastle Health Authority.

REFERENCES

1. J. B. Margolick, S. M. Hsu, D. J. Volkman, K. D. Burman and A. S. Fauci, Immuno-histochemical characterization of intrathyroid lymphocytes in Graves' disease, Am. J. Pathol., 41:425 (1984).
2. G. Aichinger, H. Fill and G. Wick, In situ immune complexes, lympho-cytic subpopulations and HLA-DR-positive epithelial cells in Hashimoto thyroiditis, Lab. Invest. 52:132 (1985).
3. S. M. McLachlan, C. A. S. Pegg, M. C. Atherton, S. L. Middleton, F. Clark and B. Rees Smith, TSH receptor antibody synthesis by thyroid lymphocytes, Clin. Endocrinol. 24:223 (1986).
4. S. M. McLachlan, C. A. S. Pegg, M. C. Atherton, S. L. Middleton, A. Dickinson, F. Clark, S. J. Proctor, G. Proud and B. Rees Smith, Subpopulations of thyroid autoantibody secreting lymphocytes in Graves' and Hashimoto glands, Clin. Exp. Immunol. 65:319 (1986).

5. S. M. McLachlan, C. A. S. Pegg, M. C. Atherton, S. L. Middleton, A. Dickinson, F. Clark and B. Rees Smith, The thyroid microenvironment in autoimmune thyroid disease: effects of TSH and lymphokines on thyroid lymphocytes and thyroid cells, Acta Endocrinol., In Press (1987).

6. G. F. Del Prete, E. Maggi, S. Mariotti, A. Tiri, D. Vercelli, D. Parronchi, D. Macchia, A. Pinchera, M. Ricci and S. Romagnani, Cytolytic T lymphocytes with natural killer activity in thyroid infiltrate of patients with Hashimoto's thyroiditis: analysis at clonal level, J. Clin. Endocrinol. Metab. 62:52 (1986).

7. E. Kromer, R. Sundick, K. Schauenstein, K. Hala and G. Wick, Analysis of lymphocytes infiltrating the thyroid gland of Obese Strain chickens, J. Immunol. 135; 2452 (1985).

8. A. B. Parkes, S. M. McLachlan, P. Bird and B. Rees Smith, The distribution of microsomal and thyroglobulin antibody activity among the IgG subclasses, Clin. Exp. Immunol. 57:239 (1984).

9. T. F. Davies, C. M. Weber, P. Wallack and M. Platzer, Restricted heterogeneity and T cell dependence of human thyroid autoantibody immunoglobulin G subclasses, J. Clin. Endocrinol. Metab. 62:945 (1986).

10. S. M. McLachlan, U. Feldt-Rasmussen, E. T. Young, S. L. Middleton, M. Blichert-Toft, K. Siersboek-Nielsen, J. Date, D. Carr, F. Clark and B. Rees Smith, IgG subclass distribution of thyroid autoantibodies : a 'fingerprint' of an individual's response to thyroglobulin and thyroid microsomal antigen. Clin. Endocrinol. In Press.

11. R. Jansson, P. M. Thompson, F. Clark and S. M. McLachlan, Association between thyroid microsomal antibodies of subclass IgG-1 and hypothyroidism in autoimmune postpartum thyroiditis, Clin. Exp. Immunol. 63:80 (1986).

12. P. Creemers, N. R. Rose and Y. C. Kong, Experimental autimmune thyroiditis : in vitro cytotoxic effects of T lymphocytes on thyroid monolayers, J. Exp. Med. 157:559 (1983).

13. U. Bognor, H. Schleusener and J. Wall, Antibody-dependent cell mediated cytotoxicity against human thyroid cells in Hashimoto's thyroiditis but not Graves' disease, J. Clin. Endocrinol. Metab. 59:734 (1984).

14. S. M. McLachlan, S. Clark, W. H. Stimson, F. Clark and B. Rees Smith, Studies of thyroglobulin autoantibody synthesis using a micro-ELISA assay, Immunol. Letters 4:27 (1982).

15. C. W. Schardt, S. M. McLachlan, J. Matheson and B. Rees Smith, An enzyme-linked immunoassay for thyroid microsomal antibodies, J. Immunol. Methods 55:155 (1982).

16. R. J. V. Pulvertaft, D. Doniach, I. M. Roitt and R. V. Hudson, Cytotoxic effects of Hashimoto serum on human thyroid cells in tissue culture, Lancet ii:214 (1959).

17. I. J. Forbes, I. M. Roitt, D. Doniach and I. L. Solomon, The thyroid cytotoxic autoantibody, J. Clin. Invest. 41:996 (1962).

18. H. L. Spiegelburg, Biological activities of immunoglobulins of different classes and subclasses, Adv. Immunol. 19:259 (1974).

19. H. Uno, T. Sasazuki, H. Tamai and H. Matsumoto, Two major genes linked to HLA and Gm control susceptibility to Graves' disease, Nature 292:768. (1981).

20. S. Whittingham, J. Mathews, M. Schanfield, J. Matthews, B. Tait, P. Morris and I. MacKay, Interactive effect of Gm allotypes and HLA-B locus antigens on the human antibody response to a bacterial antigen, Clin. Exp. Immunol. 40:8 (1980).

21. L. C. Wood and S. H. Ingbar, Hypothyroidism as a late sequela in patients with Graves' disease treated with antithyroid agents, J. Clin. Invest. 64:1429 (1979).

22. Y. Hirota, H. Tamai, Y. Hayashi, S. Matsubayashi, P. Matsuzuka, K. Kuma, L. F. Kumagai and S. Nagataki, Thyroid function and histology in forty-five patients with hyperthyroid Graves' disease in clinical remission more than ten years after thionamide drug treatment, J. Clin. Endocrinol. Metab. 62:165 (1986).
23. B. Rees Smith, Thyrotropin Receptor Antibodies in "Receptors and Recognition" Series B. (Receptor Regulation) Vol. 13, 217:244, Chapman & Hall. (1981).

CELLULAR MECHANISMS FOR AUTOIMMUNE DAMAGE IN THYROID-ASSOCIATED OPHTHALMOPATHY

J. How, Y. Hiromatsu, P. Wang, M. Salvi and J.R. Wall*

Thyroid Research Unit
The Montreal General Hospital Research Institute
1650 Cedar Avenue
Montreal, Quebec, Canada, H3G 1A4

INTRODUCTION

Idiopathic (thyroid-associated) ophthalmopathy is an autoimmune disorder of the extraocular muscles and orbital connective tissue (1-3). It is associated with Graves' hyperthyroidism in 80% of cases and Hashimoto's thyroiditis in 20%. Although a variety of antibodies against eye muscle (EM) and orbital connective tissue (OCT) antigens have been demonstrated (4-6) their role in the tissue damage of ophthalmopathy is unclear. We have recently identified antibodies which are cytotoxic to EM cells in antibody dependent cell-mediated cytotoxicity (ADCC), some of which cross-reacted with surface antigens on thyroid cells and orbital fibroblasts (7). The role of cellular immune mechanisms in the autoimmune reactions against eye muscle and OCT has not been extensively studied (reviewed in 8).

We now report preliminary results of studies of the nature and role of cell-mediated immunity and spontaneous (natural) cytotoxicity against EM and OCT cells and antigens in thyroid-associated ophthalmopathy.

CLINICAL SUBJECTS AND METHODS

We studied 50 patients, 8 men and 42 women, aged 14-82 (mean age 48 yr) with ophthalmopathy, all of whom had severe, active disease of less than 12 months duration. All had eye muscle involvement and generalized OCT inflammation. Forty-two had associated Graves' hyperthyroidism and 8 Hashimoto's thyroiditis. At the time of study 10 of the former group were hyperthyroid, while all the rest were euthyroid. Also studied were (i) 43 patients, 8 men and 35 women, aged 16-70 (mean age 42 yr) with Graves' hyperthyroidism without eye disease (ii) 10 patients, one man and 9 women, with Hashimoto's thyroiditis (iii) 10 patients with non autoimmune thyroid disorders (4 with subacute thyroiditis, 6 with non toxic goitre or nodules), all women, aged 30-80 (mean age 50 yr) (iv) 42 normal subjects, 10 men and 32 women, aged 18-62 (mean age 40 yr), as controls.

Antigen Preparation

Cytosol (soluble), membrane, and solubilized membrane fractions of eye muscle, other skeletal muscle, orbital connective tissue, liver, and thyroid were prepared as described previously (4,5). Human tissues were obtained at autopsy less than 4 h after death. The tissues were rinsed and minced, and homogenates centrifuged at 5400 x g to remove whole cells and debris. The supernatant was then separated into soluble and membrane fractions by centrifugation at 100,000 x g. Membrane proteins were solubilized by CHAPSO or SDS for 30 min, followed by centrifugation at 100,000 x g. Protein concentrations were determined and adjusted to 1 mg/ml, and the fractions stored at -75°C until use.

Affinity purified EM and OCT antigens were prepared from soluble and solubilized membrane fractions using human monoclonal antibodies (Ig) in affinity chromatography as described previously (8,9).

Natural Killer Cell-Mediated Cytotoxicity

Natural killer (NK) cell cytotoxicity was measured in ^{51}Cr release assays using human eye muscle and other (abdominal) skeletal muscle cells, orbital fibroblasts (OF), and thyroid cells as targets. Eye muscle was obtained at surgery from otherwise normal subjects undergoing strabismus repair. Abdominal muscle was obtained from patients undergoing cholecystectomy, and OCT at blepharoplasty carried out on normal subjects. Thyroid tissue was obtained at thyroidectomy undertaken for benign nodules. In some experiments target cells were pretreated with gamma interferon (γIFN) for 6 days. K562 cells, an NK cell-sensitive target, was also used. Unfractionated peripheral blood lymphocytes (PBL) or PBL depleted of adherent cells were used as effector cells. In a few experiments intrathyroidal lymphocytes were isolated from the thyroid cells using a PERCOLL gradient.

^{51}Cr-labelled target cells (5×10^3) in 100 μl were incubated in microtiter plates with 100 μl normal or patient PBL at various E:T cell ratios, at 37C in 5% CO_2 and 95% air. After 18 hr incubation, the plates were centrifuged, 100 μl aliquots of supernatant aspirated, and their radioactivity counted. Spontaneous release was determined by counting a 100 μl aliquot of medium, while total radioactivity was determined in a 100 μl aliquot of uncentrifuged incubation mixture. Cytotoxicity was expressed as percent specific lysis, calculated as: cpm released with test materials - cpm spontaneous release/cpm total - cpm spontaneous release x 100. Spontaneous release never exceeded 25% in 18 hr assays. Test samples were assayed in quadruplicate. PBL preparations from patients and age and sex-matched normal subjects were tested in equal numbers on the same assay plate.

Leukocyte Procoagulant Activity (LPCA) Assay

The LPCA assay was used as a test for cell-mediated immunity. This assay measures a lymphokine produced by sensitized helper T lymphocytes, which enhances clotting (10). Mononuclear cells were separated from citrated peripheral venous blood over Ficoll-Hypaque, washed twice in Hank's balanced salt solution (HBSS), and suspended in RPMI 1640. The cells (2×10^6 per culture) were then incubated with or without antigen, in Nunc "minisorb" tubes for 20 hr in a humid atmosphere of 5% CO_2 in air at 37°C, following which the cells were washed three times with cold HBSS and resuspended in RPMI 1640.

The ability of the cultured cells to enhance the clotting time of normal human plasma was determined using a one-stage recalcification time assay. To 0.2 ml of the cell suspension was added 0.1 of platelet-poor , pooled, normal human plasma and 0.1 ml of 0.025M $CaCl_2$. The clotting times were measured in triplicate in an automatic coagulometer and the results expressed as percentage reduction in recalcification time (RT) in seconds calculated as: RT without antigen - RT with antigen/RT without antigen x 100.

RESULTS

NK Cell Cytotoxicity:

NK cell-mediated cytotoxicity tests were carried out using PBL from patients with ophthalmopathy, autoimmune thyroid disorders without eye disease and normals, and various orbital and thyroidal cells and K562 cells as targets. Effector:target cell ratios were from 12.5:1 - 100:1. In the first experiments K562 cells were used as targets. There were no significant differences between patients with ophthalmopathy, GH (euthyroid) without eye disease, or patients with Hashimoto's thyroiditis without eye disease, and normal subjects at any E:T cell ratio. When PBL from hyperthyroid patients with Graves' disease (with or without ophthalmopathy) were tested against K562 cells a significant depression was, however, found at all E:T cell ratios tested (Table 1). When patients became euthyroid, following radioiodine or antithyroid drug treatment, K562 lysis returned to normal. In the 3 patients with subacute thyroiditis tested lysis was markedly increased, returning to normal during recovery (results not shown). Levels of NK cells, measured as leu 11b positive cells by immunofluorescence, were not increased in hyperthyroid patients (Table 1).

Natural cytotoxicity against orbital fibroblasts was low being <10% in all patients and normals tested, at all E:T cell ratios. The differences between patients with GO, Hashimoto's thyroiditis, GH (euthyroid) and normals were not significant at any E:T cell ratio (results not shown). There were no significant correlations between % specific lysis of OF and serum thyroxine levels for patients with GH or Hashimoto's thyroiditis. Studies were repeated using PBL depleted of adherent cells (as effectors) and K562, thyroid, and skeletal (SM) muscle cells as targets. In this experiment the target cells were pretreated with 𝛾IFN shown previously (11) to enhance susceptibility to lysis in ADCC. Although killing of K562 cells was decreased at all E:T ratios, the differences between the groups were not significant. Results were similar when adherent cell depleted effector populations were employed. In experiments with thyroid and SM cells as targets, although there was a tendency for increased killing of SM cells (but not thyroid cells) in patients with GO and HT, the difference, compared to normals, was not significant for either effector cell population.

TABLE I - NK cell activity against K562 target cells, and NK cell numbers, in patients with untreated Graves' hyperthyroidism.

| GROUPS | EFFECTOR:TARGET CELL RATIO | | | Leu 11b Positive Cells[•] |
	25:1	50:1	100:1	
Graves' Hyperthyroidism (n = 33)	8.5 ± 8.4*% P<0.01**	14.7 ± 11.5% P<0.001	24.5 ± 13.2% P<0.001	13.4 ± 4.1 NS#
Normals (n = 23)	19.1± 17.05	29.8 ± 19%	40.6 ± 15.6%	16 ± 6.0 (n = 20)

* mean (±SD) % specific lysis.
** Statistical analyses refer to differences compared to normals (student's 't' test).
• Determined on PBL using a mouse MCAB (anti-Leu 11b) and the immunofluorescence test expressed as mean (±SD) %.
Not significant.

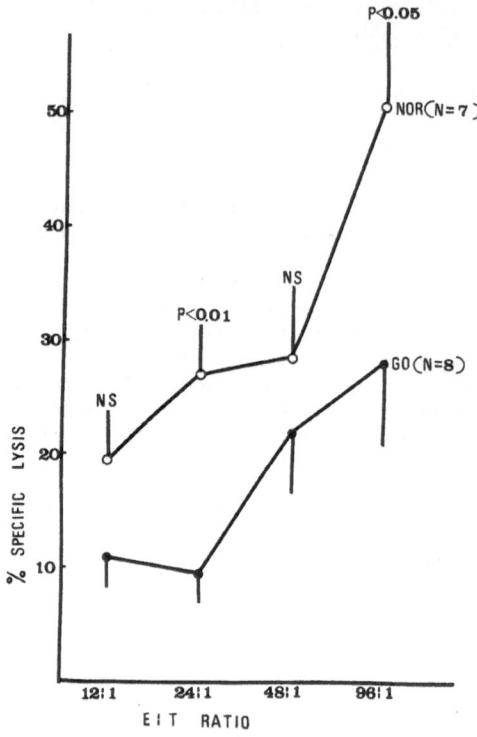

Figure 1.

NK cell cytotoxicity against human eye muscle cells using PBL from
patients with Graves' ophthalmopathy (●————●) and normal subjects
(o————o) at E:T cell ratios of 12:1-96:1 determined using a ^{51}Cr
release assay. Results are expressed as mean (±SE) % specific lysis.
Statistical analysis refers to differences compared to normals
(student's 't' test).

Next, tests were carried out using human EM cells as targets, and
PBL from patients with ophthalmopathy (with associated hyperthyroidism)
and normal subjects. Results are summarized in Fig. 1 which shows that
NK cell cytotoxicity or PBL from patients with ophthalmopathy against
human EM cells was less than that for normal subjects, the difference
being significant at E:T cell ratios of 24:1 { 8.3 ± 2.8% SE (n = 8) and
27 ± 3.6% (n = 8) P < 0.01 respectively}, and 96:1 {29.9 ± 8% (n = 8) and
51 ± 7% (n = 8) P < 0.01 respectively}. Intrathyroidal lymphocytes from
aspiration biopsy specimens gave levels of NK cell activity similar to
those of PBL in the three patients tested.

Finally, effects of γIFN treatment of K562 target cells and human
EM cells on their susceptibility to lysis in NK cell assays was tested.
As seen in Fig. 2, NK cell lysis of K562 cells was depressed in the two
patients tested compared to the normal, and further depressed when
target were treated with γIFN. NK lysis of EM cells was also low, in
the one normal subject tested, and further depressed when treated cells
were used as targets.

Effect of γIFN (200 ^{U}/ml) treatment of K562 target cells (a) and human eye muscle cells (b) on their susceptibility to lysis in natural killer (NK) cell assays. Unfractionated peripheral blood lymphocytes from patients with GO (-■- and -●-), and a normal subject (-▲-) were used as effector cells. K562 cells and human eye muscle cells were precultured with IFN for 5 days and then used as target cells. -------- = γIFN treated target cells. ————— = untreated target cells. Cytotoxicity was assessed as % specific lysis in a ^{51}Cr release assay.

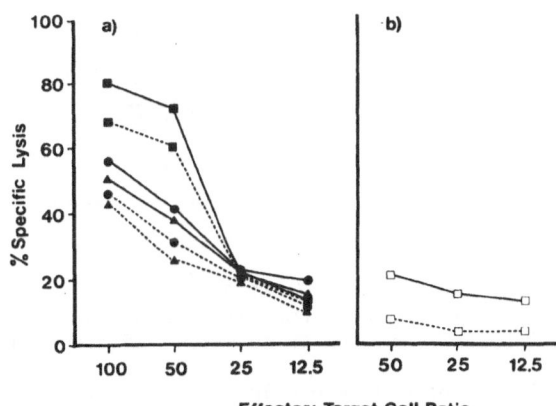

Figure 2.

CELL-MEDIATED IMMUNITY

The LPCA test was used to test for CMI against crude and affinity purified orbital antigens in patients with ophthalmopathy. As shown in Table 2, LPCA level was increased, compared to normals, for EM cytosol, OCT cytosol and OCT membranes, but not EM membranes. Taking a % recalcification time of mean +2SD for the normals as the upper limit of normal, tests were positive in 65% of patients to EM cytosol, 27% to OCT cytosol, 31% to OCT membranes but in only 7% (1 patient) to EM membranes. Tests were positive in less than 20% of patients with autoimmune thyroid disorders without eye disease, for all fractions.

LPCA tests have also been carried out using affinity purified orbital tissue antigens, prepared using human monoclonal antibodies as described previously (9). As shown in Table 3 there was a good correlation, for all patient groups, between reactivity in LPCA, and ELISA reactivity, suggesting a close correlation between B and T cell immuno-reactivity to EM and OCT soluble and membrane antigens.

TABLE 2. Leukocyte procoagulant activity against human orbital tissue antigens in patients with Graves' ophthalmopathy.

TISSUE FRACTION*	TEST GROUP		
	OPHTHALMOPATHY	NORMALS	
EM Cyt	20.7 ± 11.0%**	2.4 ± 12.2%	P<0.001***
EM Mem	5.7 ± 10.1%	1.2 ± 9.0%	N.S.
OCT Cyt	13.7 ± 15.0%	3.2 ± 8.4%	P <0.05
OCT Mem	15.1 ± 12.0%	0.7 ± 7.7%	P<0.001
	(n = 17)	(n = 17)	

*EM = eye muscle, OCT = orbital connective tissue, Cyt = cytosol, Mem = membranes.
**Results are expressed as % (±SD) recalcification time.
***Statistical analysis refer to the differences, assessed using Student's 't' tests, compared to normals. NS = not significant.

TABLE 3. Monoclonal antibody and helper T lymphocyte reactivity against MCAB affinity purified orbital tissue antigens in patients with ophthalmopathy and autoimmune thyroid disorders.

ANTIGEN NUMBER	ANTIGEN PREPARATIONS*	ELISA REACTIVITY	NUMBER OF TESTS	NUMBER+ LPCA**	PERCENTAGE+ LPCA
E2-2	OCT CYT	+	24	22	91.6
E12-1	EM SDS-SM	+	17	17	100
E12-2	EM SDS-SM	+	20	20	100
2E7-1	EM CHAP-SM	+	7	6	85.7
2E7-3	EM CHAP-SM	+	24	17	70.8
E7-2	EM CHAP-SM	+	8	7	87.5
2E9-2yt	EM CHAP-SM	+	6	5	83.3
	TOTAL	+	106	94	88.7
E4-2	EM CYT	–	17	3	17.6
E3-3B	EM CYT	–	15	0	0
E4-1	EM CYT	–	3	0	0
E3-3A	EM CYT	–	0	0	0
E1-2	EM CYT	–	9	3	33.3
2E9-4	EM CHAP-SM	–	2	1	50
E7-3	EM CHAP-SM	–	5	0	0
	TOTAL	–	58	7	12.1

*OCT = orbital connective tissue. EM = eye muscle. CYT = cytosol.
 SDS-SM = SDS-solubilized membranes.
 CHAP-SM = "CHAPSO"-solubilized membranes.
**All patient groups and normals.

DISCUSSION

We have shown CMI, measured as LPCA, against crude and affinity purified EM and OCT antigens in patients with endocrine ophthalmopathy. While a role of NK cell cytotoxicity against orbital targets was not demonstrated, decreased activity against EM cells was shown. This was not due to associated hyperthyroidism even though depressed NK cytotoxicity of K562 cells was found for hyperthyroid patients with or without ophthalmopathy. The mechanism for the decreased NK activity (which was not due to a decrease in blood NK cells) is unclear. Gamma interferon is known to enhance NK activity by an effect on the NK cells, but to depress target response (12). On the other hand we showed, earlier, that ɤ IFN markedly enhanced ADCC

On the other hand CMI and OCT antigens is likely to play a role in the autoimmune damage of ophthalmopathy. Our studies suggest that helper T cells are sensitized to a variety of orbital antigens and that there is a good correlation between antibody and lymphocyte reactivity to these antigens. We showed previously cytotoxic antibodies reactive in ADCC (7,19) and soluble and membrane antigen directed antibodies measured in ELISA (5), and by IF (6). The inter-relationship between the various parameters of immune damage to autoantigens is unclear. A role of cytotoxic T lymphocytes has not been tested although likely to be important.

Finally our studies shed some light on the identity of the orbital targets of idiopathic ophthalmopathy, and the mechanism for its association with autoimmune thyroid disease. Although the eye muscle is likely to be the main target LPCA tests were also positive with OCT fractions, and an OCT mem - thyroglobulin shared antigen and antibody reactivity against it, was previously found (4,13). On the other hand ADCC is only rarely positive to orbital fibroblasts (11). One can postulate that while the basic underlying reaction may be action of cytotoxic antibodies against eye muscle specific, and thyroid/eye muscle shared antigens, the observed T cell reactions against EM and OCT membrane and soluble antigens may be secondary, although playing a role in the inflammation and ensuing tissue damage.

SUMMARY

The role of natural killer (NK) cell-mediated cytotoxicity against human eye muscle (EM) cells and orbital fibroblasts and K562 cells, and of cell-mediated immunity (CMI), measured using the leukocyte procoagulant activity (LPCA) assay against crude and affinity purified orbital antigens, in thyroid-associated ophthalmopathy, were studied. NK cell cytotoxicity against K562 cells and orbital targets was normal in patients with autoimmune thyroid disorders with, or without ophthalmopathy, except for (i) depressed killing of K562 cells in hyperthyroid patients with Graves' disease which was unrelated to the eye disease and (ii) depressed killing of eye muscle cells in patients with ophthalmopathy which was independent of the thyroid status. LPCA tests were positive to crude EM cytosol and orbital connective tissue (OCT) membranes in over 60% of patients with ophthalmopathy, but in less than 20% of patients with Hashimoto's thyroiditis or Graves' disease without evident eye involvement. Tests were also positive, in most patients with ophthalmopathy, to a variety of affinity purified EM and OCT soluble and membrane antigens and there was a close correlation between humoral and T lymphocyte reactions to these antigens. Although endocrine ophthalmopathy is associated with many humoral and cellular immune reactions to eye muscle and, to a lesser extent, OCT antigens, including those shared with thyroid antigens tissue damage is likely to be caused by cytotoxic antibodies, in antibody-dependent cell-mediated cytotoxicity, and by lymphokines in CMI. The significance, and possible role, of depressed NK cell mediated cytotoxicity in hyperthyroidism and ophthalmopathy are unknown although likely to be secondary.

ACKNOWLEDGEMENTS

This work was supported by MRC (Canada) Grant #MT-698, an NIH Grant #EYO-5062-O1A1 of the NEI, and a St. Mary's Hospital Grant.

REFERENCES

1. D. Doniach, Autoimmune endocrine exophthalmos, Lancet ii:2878 (1982).
2. J.R. Wall, Immunological aspects of Graves' ophthalmopathy, in: "The eye and orbit in thyroid disease", C. Gorman, R. Waller and J. Dyer, eds., p 103, Raven Press, New York (1984).
3. J.R. Wall and T. Kuroki, Immunologic fators in thyroid disease, in: "Symposium on thyroid disorders", W.B. Saunders Co. Ltd., R. Larsen and M. Kaplan, eds., Med. Clin., N. Am. 69:913 (1985).
4. T. Kuroki, J. Ruf, A. Miller, L. Whelan and J.R. Wall, Anti-thyroglobulin monoclonal and autoantibodies cross-react with an orbital connective tissue membrane antigen - a possible mechanism for the association of ophthalmopathy with autoimmune thyroid disorders, Clin. exp. Immunol. 62:361 (1985).
5. K. Kodama, H. Sikorska, P. Bandy-Dafoe, R. Bayly and J.R. Wall, Demonstration of a circulating autoantibody against a soluble eye muscle antigen in Graves' ophthalmopathy, Lancet ii: 1353 (1982).
6. M. Mengistu, E. Laryea, A. Miller and J.R. Wall, Clinical significance of a new autoantibody against a human eye muscle soluble antigen detected by immunofluorescence, Clin. exp. Immunol. 65:19 (1986).
7. P.W. Wang, Y. Hiromatsu, E. Laryea, L. Wosu, J. How and J.R. Wall, Immunologically-mediated cytotoxicity against human eye muscle cells in Graves' ophthalmopathy, J. Clin. Endocrinol. Metab. 63:316. (1986).
8. J.R. Wall, J. How, M. Salvi and Y. Hiromatsu, Can endocrine exophthalmos now be viewed as separate from thyroid autoimmunity, in: "Clinics in allergy and immunology", D. Doniach and F. Bottazzo eds. W.B. Saunders Co. Ltd., (in press) (1986).
9. M. Salvi, Y. Hiromatsu, L. Wosu, E. Laryea, J. How and J.R. Wall, Current status of autoantibodies against orbital antigens in the pathogenesis of Graves' ophthalmopathy in: "Proceedings of an International Symposium on Thyroid and Autoimmunity", H. Drexhage and W. Wiersinga eds., p.255, Elsevier, Amsterdam, (1986).
10. J. How, A.W. Thomson, J.I. Milton, R. Scott, P. Bewshew, C.H.W. Horne, Thyroid antigen-induced leukocyte procoagulant activity: A novel approach to the study of cell-mediated immunity in Hashimoto's thyroidits, In: "Autoimmunity and the Thyroid", P.G. Walfish, J.R. Wall and R. Volpé eds.,p. 349, Academic Press (1985).
11. Y. Hiromatsu, P.W. Wang, L. Wosu, J. How and J.R. Wall, Mechanisms of tissue damage in Graves' ophthalmopathy. Hor. Res. (In press) (1986).
12. A. Trinchieri, D. Granato and B. Perussia, Interferon-induced resistance of fibroblasts to cytolysis mediated by natural killer cells: specificity and mechanism. J. Immunol. 126:335.

13. T. Kuroki, K. Kodama, P. Carayon, J. Ruf, A. Miller and J.R. Wall, Use of mouse and human monoclonal antibodies to investigate the immunologic basis of Graves' ophthalmopathy, <u>Mt. Sinai J. Med.</u> 53:60 (1986).

THYROID INFILTRATING T LYMPHOCYTES IN HASHIMOTO'S THYROIDITIS: PHENOTYPIC AND FUNCTIONAL ANALYSIS AT SINGLE CELL LEVEL

G.F. Del Prete, A. Tiri,*S. Mariotti,*A. Pinchera,
S.Romagnani, and M. Ricci
Allergology Clinical Immunology, University of Florence
and (*) Endocrinology, University of Pisa
Policlinico Careggi, 50134 Florence, Italy

In the last 30 years, studies of the thyroid-specific abnormal autoimmune response have mainly focused onto humoral rather than cellular mechanisms. Thus, both the initial events responsible for the breakdown in self-tolerance and the subsequent immunological mechanisms responsible for thyroid infiltration by lymphocytes and thyroid cell alterations are still poorly understood. The development of monoclonal antibodies (MoAbs) to lymphocyte membrane antigens made it possibile to analyze the phenotype of thyroid infiltrating lymphocytes by immunohistological staining techniques. Both B and T lymphocytes have been found in affected glands, the major cellular component being T cells. Some controversy, however, existed about the proportion of the $CD4^+$ and $CD8^+$ T cell subsets within autoimmune thyroid infiltrates. A reduction in intrathyroidal $CD8^+$ cells compared with peripheral blood (PB)[1] or a substantial identity between PB and thyroid infiltrates with regard to the proportions of CD4+ and CD8+ cells have been reported[2,3]. However, more recent studies agree that T cells with the CD8+ cytotoxic/suppressor phenotype are predominant in either Graves' disease (GD) or Hashimoto's thyroiditis (HT) infiltrates[4,5,6]. In any case, whatever the alteration of phenotypically defined T cell population may be, it is of uncertain significance. Since it is now clear that CD4 and CD8 antigens do not represent markers of specific functions, before any conclusion is drawn on the role of a given cell population, phenotypic analysis needs to be supported by functional studies. Unfortunately, functional assays performed on heterogeneous cell populations are difficult to interpret, because they do not provide information on the proportion of cells expressing a given function.

To overcome these difficulties, attempts have been recently made to grow long-term T cell lines and clones that represented the in vitro progenies of thyroid-infiltrating T lymphocytes[5,7,8,9]. We have recently used two protocols to raise clonal progenies of PB and thyroid infiltrating T lymphocytes in some patients with HT in order to analyze at clonal level their functional heterogeneity. To this purpose, T cells from patients and normal donors underwent two parallel cloning

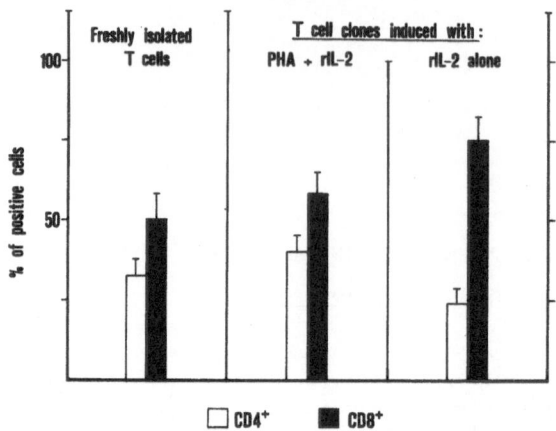

Fig.1. Phenotype distribution of freshly isolated T cells from
thyroid infiltrates of HT patients and of their clonal
progenies obtained with different cloning procedures.
Results represent the mean value ($\pm$ SE) of 5 experiments.

procedures. In one, T cells were seeded in limiting number in
microwells containing irradiated spleen feeder cells and
phytohaemagglutinin (PHA), followed by weekly addition of recombinant
IL-2 (rIL-2, Biogen, Geneva)[10] . In the other, rIL-2 alone, in the
presence of spleen feeder cells was used both at the beginning and
during the clonal expansion, in order to achieve exclusively the clonal
growth of T cells already activated in vivo[7] . Since, under the
microculture conditions used, high proportions of plated T cells
underwent clonal proliferation, the set of clones obtained could be
considered largely representative of the original T cell population.
Thus, following initial stimulation with either PHA or rIL-2 alone, high
proportions of CD8 T cell clones were established from thyroid HT
infiltrates showing an inverted CD4/CD8 ratio (Fig. 1). On the other
hand, since there was no abnormality in the percentages of CD4[+] and CD8[+]
cells in the PB of the same patients compared to those in normal
subjects, the phenotype distribution of patient PB-derived clones
substantially reflected that of clones established from control PB,
lymph nodes or spleens[5].

Cytolytic potential of thyroid-derived T cell clones.

All clones derived from HT patients and normal subjects were
assayed for cytolytic activity against the murine P815 cell line in the
presence of PHA (lectin-dependent cytotoxic assay - LDCC). The results
obtained in the LDCC assay, which allows the detection of cytolytic T
cell precursors (CTL-P) of any specificity,[11] are summarized in Fig.2.

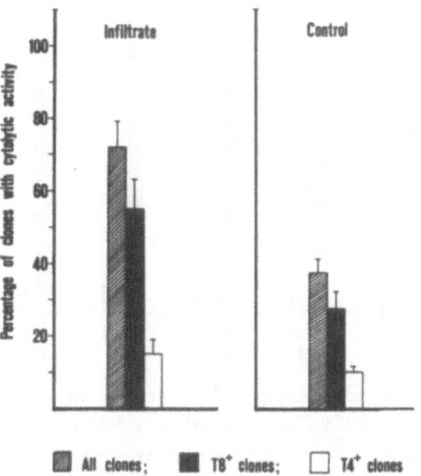

Fig.2. Cytolytic activity of single clones derived
        from 5 HT thyroid infiltrates or from normal
        lymphoid tissue (2 spleens and 3 lymph nodes)
        was assessed by lectin-dependent cytolytic assay
        using the murine P815 cell line as target at an
        E/T ratio of 4/1. Clones inducing ^{51}Cr release
        exceeding the mean spontaneous release by 5 SD
        were considered cytolytic.
        Results represent the mean percentage ($\pm$ SE)
        of clones with cytolytic activity.

The majority of PHA-induced clones and almost all (> 90%) rIL-2-elicited
clones from HT infiltrates were CTL-P with the CD8$^+$ phenotype. In
contrast, in the clonal progenies of normal PB, lymph node or spleen the
proportion of clones with cytolytic potential was consistently lower
than 45%.

Proliferative response of thyroid-derived T cell clones to autologous
thyrocytes.

The reason why HT infiltrates contain so high proportions of T
cells equipped with machinery for killing is unknown at the present
time. One possibility is that a number of these cells were thyroid
antigen-specific CTL able to exert a MHC-restricted cytolytic mechanism.
In order to investigate this possibility, thyroid infiltrating T cells

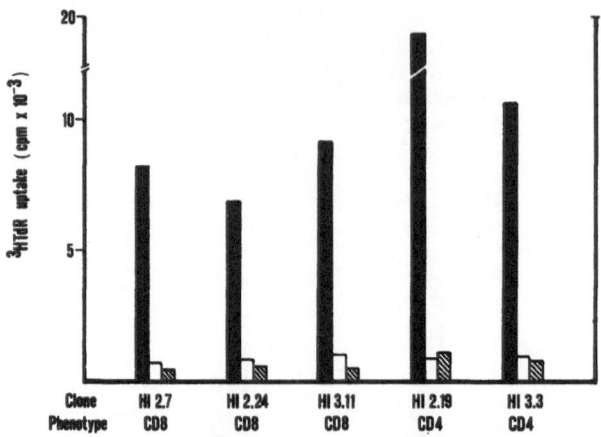

Fig.3. Proliferative response to autologous thyrocytes by thyroid-derived T cell clones of a patient with HT. 2×10^4 clonal T blasts were incubated for 3 days with 10^5 irradiated autologous non-T cells (▨) or with 10^4 autologous (■) or allogeneic (☐) thyrocytes in flatt-bottomed wells. Sixteen hr before harvesting, 0.5 µCi ^{3}HTdR were added to each culture. Results represent the mean value of ^{3}HTdR uptake of triplicate cultures.

from a patient with HT were cloned with rIL-2. Three CD8$^+$ and two CD4$^+$ out of 46 clones, all displaying cytolytic potential, showed significant proliferation when cultured for 3 days in the presence of cryopreserved autologous thyrocytes (Fig. 3). This observation is consistent with recent data obtained by other investigators who established thyroid antigen-specific T cell lines[9] or clones[8] from thyroid infiltrating lymphocytes of GD or HT patients by using different cloning procedures. It is of note, however, that none of the CD4$^+$ or CD8$^+$ clones derived from the thyroid infiltrate of our HT patient showed proliferative response in the presence of allogeneic thyrocytes or autologous PB non-T cells cultured in medium alone or with addition of a wide range of thyroglobulin (Tg) concentrations. These data indicate that a number of in vivo activated thyroid infiltrating T cells may show their cytolytic potential (CTL) and specific recognition of thyrocyte autoantigen(s) through a MHC-restricted mechanism made possible by the ectopic expression of class II MHC molecules on thyrocytes themselves[12-14]. Experiments are currently underway to establish whether T cell clones proliferating to thyrocyte antigen(s) are actually able to display specific killing in vitro of autologous autoantigen(s)-presenting thyrocytes.

Natural killer (NK) activity of thyroid-derived T cell clones.

In view of the possibility to investigate whether also MHC-nonrestricted cytolytic mechanisms play a role in thyroid cell damage, the clonal progenies of thyroid infiltrating T cells were tested for cytolytic activity of NK type. All clones established with PHA or rIL-2 were assayed for cytolytic activity against NK sensitive targets, such as K562 or MOLT-4 cells, as detailed elsewhere[5,7]. As shown in Table 1, high proportions of CD8+ clones established from thyroid infiltrates of HT patients displayed NK activity. A significant increase in the proportion of clones with NK activity was observed also in the clonal progenies of PHA-activated T cells from the PB of the same patients. This increase was due to CD4+ clones, since the proportion of patient PB-derived CD8+ clones with NK activity was similar to that observed in clones from normal PB or lymphoid tissues. Among thyroid-derived clones elicited with rIL-2, the proportion of CD8+ clones with NK activity was even greater than that found among clones derived from the same thyroid T cells by using PHA as initial stimulant. Thus, taken together, these findings support the concept that most of the CD8+ T cells activated in vivo within the affected HT gland have the potential to display NK-like cytolytic function[7]. The question of whether such a NK-like activity may represent an actual cytolytic effector mechansism in HT deserves further investigation.

Table 1. NK activity of T cell clones derived from thyroid infiltrates and PB of patients with HT

Source of T cells	Cloning procedure	% of clones showing NK activity	
		CD4+	CD8+
HT Infiltrate	PHA + rIL-2	20.2	55.5
	rIL-2	15.1	72.1
HT PB	PHA + rIL-2	25.1	21.2
	rIL-2	ND	ND
Normal Lymphoid tissue	PHA + rIL-2	7.0	26.5
	rIL-2	3.2	15.7
Normal PB	PHA + rIL-2	7.4	23.2
	rIL-2	ND	ND

NK activity was tested against the human K562 cell lines at an E/T ratio of 4/1. Clones inducing ^{51}Cr release exceeding the mean spontaneous release by > 5 SD were considered cytolytic. ND = Not done. Results represent the mean percent values obtained in 4 HT patients and 6 normal donors.

Interleukin production by thyroid-derived T cell clones

Since NK function may be induced or enhanced by interleukins, the ability to secrete interferon-γ (IFN-γ) and IL-2 of T cell clones derived from HT infiltrates and the corresponding PB was then investigated. Due to the obvious impossibility to use the appropriate antigen for every single T cell clone, a multivalent lectin was used in order to mimic the activation signals required for interleukin production by T cells. The choice of PHA was based on the recent observation that this lectin may mediate its mitogenic effect by binding to membrane activation molecules and particularly to a glycoprotein of the T3-Ti antigen-receptor associated complex on T cell surface[15]. As shown in Table 2, upon PHA stimulation, almost all CD8+ and CD4+ clones derived from HT thyroid infiltrating T cells were IFN-γ producers (IFN-P). In contrast, the proportion of the same clones able to produce IL-2 was comparable to that found in patient PB and normal PB or spleen, suggesting that this peculiar function had not been focused in the affected thyroid (data not shown). Besides the increased frequency of IFN-P T cell precursors, another feature of HT infiltrates was the capacity of several T cell clones (both CD8+ and CD4+) to produce considerable high amounts of IFN-γ. In contrast, in the clonal progeny of PB lymphocytes of the same HT patients only a proportion of CD4+ clones showed the ability to secrete high IFN-γ concentrations (Fig. 4).

Table 2. PHA-induced production of IFN-γ and IL-2 by T cell clones from thyroid infiltrates and PB from patients with HT

Source of T cells	Phenotype	No. of clones showing production of:	
		IFN-γ	IL-2
HT Infiltrate	CD4	61/ 69 (88%)	44/ 69 (64%)
	CD8	87/104 (84%)	55/104 (53%)
HT PB	CD4	104/170 (61%)	108/170 (64%)
	CD8	41/ 61 (67%)	36/ 61 (59%)
Normal Lymphoid tissue	CD4	32/ 53 (60%)	28/ 53 (53%)
	CD8	9/ 18 (50%)	10/ 18 (56%)
Normal PB	CD4	57/108 (53%)	73/108 (68%)
	CD8	26/ 40 (65%)	21/ 40 (52%)

T blasts from each clone (10^5) were washed and cultured in 0.2 ml medium containing PHA (1% vol/vol) for 40 h and supernatant removed and stored at -70° C ultil tested for its IFN-γ and IL-2 content. For the quantitative measurement of IFN-γ the IMRX Interferon-gamma RIA (Centocor Inc.) was used. IL-2 activity was assessed by ^{3}H-thymidine uptake by the murine CTLL cell line. Culture supernatants showing IFN-γ or IL-2 levels 5 SD over those of control supernatants derived from irradiated feeder cells alone were regarded as positive.

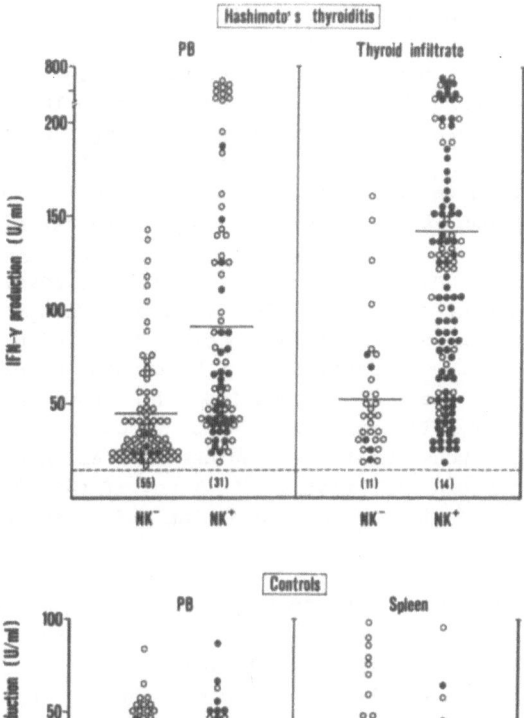

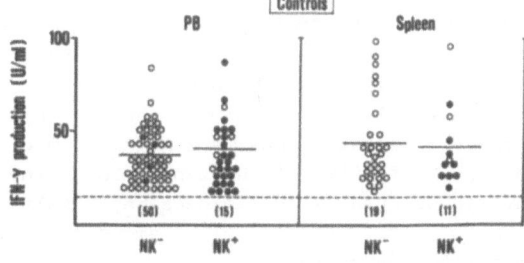

Fig.4. IFN-γ production by T cell clones derived from thyroid
infiltrates and PB of patients with HT and from control
PB or spleens. NK activity and PHA-induced IFN-γ
production were assessed in individual CD4+ (O) or
CD8+ (●) clones, as indicated previously. Values
in parentheses indicate the number of clones showing
IFN-γ production lower than 5 SD above the mean IFN-γ
level (---) found in culture supernatants of irradiated
feeder cells alone.

Whether such a circulating CD4+ T cell population derives from thyroid
infiltrates or it represents a disease-related abnormality of the PB T
cell compartment in HT, remains to be clarified.

A relationship existed between the capacitiy of secreting high
levels of IFN-γ and the potential to display NK activity shown by
thyroid-derived clones. In fact, as shown in Fig. 4, almost all clones
with NK activity (NK+) established from HT infiltrates could be
triggered to high IFN-γ production (mean ± SE: 139 ± 14 U/ml), while in
the few thyroid clones without NK activity (NK-) the mean IFN-γ
production (57 ± 9) was comparable to that obtained in either NK+ or NK-
clones derived from normal spleen (44 ± 4). On the other hand, in the
clonal progeny of patient PBL, only a number of CD4+ clones, all showing
NK activity, were potent IFN-γ producers.

Possible role of IFN-γ in thyroid autoimmunity.

Since IFN-γ is a pleiotropic lymphokine playing an important role during the immune response[16], the high potential to IFN-γ secretion shown by the clonal progenies of thyroid-infiltrating T cells might be responsible for some of the immunologic abnormalities found in patients with HT. IFN-γ has been recently shown to exert a B-cell growth factor (BCGF) activity on human B cells[17] and to act synergistically with other helper factors in the stimulation of B cell proliferation and differentiation into antibody-producing cells[18,19]. Thus, one may suggest that high concentrations of IFN-γ released within the affected thyroid may favour local activation and proliferation of B cells with consequent increase of the proportion of IL-2 receptor-bearing B cells recently shown in HT infiltrates. In addition, the promoting effect of IFN-γ on B cell differentiation might be of importance in the generation of cells spontaneously producing thyroid autoantibodies which have have been demonstrated in thyroid infiltrates[2,20]. Thus, if this is the case, IFN-γ might play an important role in maintaining and/or enhancing local autoantibody formation.

IFN-γ has also been found to play an important role in the generation of cytotoxic T lymphocytes[21-23]. Therefore, another possible suggestion is that the high potential to secrete IFN-γ by most thyroid infiltrating T cells may contribute to induce and/or maintain their cytolytic activity. Interestingly, T cell clones showing the ability to produce the highest IFN-γ concentrations were mainly found just among those displaying cytolytic activity of NK type. Thus, the cytolytic potential of most thyroid-derived T cell clones may result from their concomitant abnormal ability to secrete high amounts of IFN-γ in response to appropriate activation signals.

An additional property ascribed to IFN-γ is its ability to enhance MHC class I and to promote de novo expression of MHC class II antigens in a large number of cell types, including thyroid cells[12-14]. Thus, an additional effect of excessive intra-thyroidal IFN-γ secretion might be a persistent and diffused ectopic expression of MHC class II determinants on the membrane of thyroid cells. This phenomenon might result in recruitment of other T cells, including CTL, which contribute to maintain and expand the intrathyroid pathogenic process. In this respect, it has been demonstrated that autoimmune disease-exhibiting MRL-1pr/1pr mice show elevated IFN-γ synthesis by their T cells and lack suppressor cells capable of regulating its production[24]. Thus, the finding that T cell clones derived from thyroid infiltrates and PB of patients with HT show abnormal potential to IFN-γ secretion may have important implications for autoimmune diseases. Whether abnormal IFN-γ production is an inherent feature of a proportion of T cells from subjects who undergo autoimmune diseases or it is acquired by T cells generated in these patients, owing to particular (even though undefined) immune responses, remains to be established.

AKNOWLEDGEMENTS

This work was supported by grants from CNR (CT 85.00714.04) and from the Ministery of Education.

References

1. R. Jansson, T.H. Totterman, J. Sallstrom, and P.A. Dahlberg, Thyroid infiltrating T lymphocyte subsets in Hashimoto's thyroiditis, J Clin Endocrinol Metab 56:1164 (1983).

2. S.M. McLahlan, A.M. Dickinson, A. Malcom, J.R. Farndon, E. Young, S.J. Proctor, and B. Rees Smith, Thyroid autoantibody synthesis by cultures of thyroid and peripheral blood lympho cytes. I. Lymphocyte markers and response to pokeweed mitogen, Clin exp Immunol 52:45 (1983).

3. J.R. Wall, R. Baur, H. Schleusener, and P. Bandy-Dafoe, Pheripheral blood and intrathyroidal mononuclear cell populations in patients witn autoimmune thyroid disorders enumerated using monoclonal antibodies, J Clin Endocrinol Metab 56:164 (1983).

4. M.C. Bene, V. Derennes, G. Faure, J.L. Thomas, J. Duheille, and J. Leclere, Graves' disease: in situ localization of lymphoid T cell subpopulations, Clin exp Immunol 52:311 (1983).

5. G.F. Del Prete, E. Maggi, S. Mariotti, A. Tiri, D. Vercelli, P. Parronchi, D. Macchia, A. Pinchera, M. Ricci, S. Romagnani, Cytolytic T lymphocytes with natural killer activity in thyroid infiltrate of patients with Hashimoto's thyroiditis: analysis at clonal level, J Clin Endocrinol Metab 62:52 (1986).

6. J.B. Margolick, S.M. Hsu, D.J. Volkman, K.D. Burman, and A.S. Fauci, Immunohistochemical characterization of intrathyroid lymphocytes in Graves' disease, Am J Med 76:815 (1984).

7. G.F. Del Prete, D. Vercelli, A. Tiri, E. Maggi, S. Mariotti, A. Pinchera, M. Ricci, and S. Romagnani, In vivo activated cytotoxic T cells in the thyroid infliltrate of patients with Hashimoto's thyroiditis, Clin exp Immunol 64:140 (1986).

8. M. Londei, G.F. Bottazzo, and M. Feldmann, Human T-cell clones from autoimmune thyroid glands: specific recognition of autologous thyroid cells, Science 228:85 (1985).

9. A.P. Weetman, D.J. Volkman, K.D. Burman, J.B. Margolick, P. Petrick, B.D. Weintraub, and A.S. Fauci, The production and characterization of thyroid-derived T-cell lines in Graves' disease and Hashimoto's thyroiditis, Clin Immunol Immunopathol 39:139 (1986).

10. A. Moretta, G. Pantaleo, L. Moretta, J.C. Cerottini, and M.C. Mingari, Direct demonstration of the clonogenic potential of every human peripheral blood T cell. Clonal analysis of HLA-DR expression and cytolytic activity, J Exp Med 157:743 (1983).

11. A. Moretta, G. Pantaleo, L. Moretta, M.C. Mingari, and J.C. Cerottini, Quantitative assessment of the pool size and subset distribution of cytolytic T lymphocytes within human resting or alloactivated peripheral blood T cell populations, J Exp Med 158:571 (1983).

12. G.F. Bottazzo, R. Pujol-Borrell, and T. Hanafusa, Role of aberrant HLA-DR expression and antigen presentation in induction of endocrine autoimmunity, Lancet 2:1115 (1983).

13. T.F. Davies, Cocultures of human thyroid monolayer cells and autologous T cells: impact of HLA class II antigen expression, J Clin Endocrinol Metab 61:418 (1985).

14. Y. Iwatani, H.C. Gerstein, M. Iitaka, V.V. Row, and R. Volpe, Thyrocyte HLA-DR expression and interferon-γ production in autoimmune thyroid disease, J Clin Endocrinol Metab 63:695 (1986).

15. A. Valentine, C.D. Tsoukas, G. Rhodes, J.H. Vaughan, and D.A. Carson, Phytohemagglutinin binds to the 20-KD molecule of the T3 complex, Eur J Immunol 15:851 (1985).

16. G. Trinchieri, and B. Perussia, Immune interferon: a pleiotropic lymphokine with multiple effects, Immunol Today 6:131 (1985).

17. S. Romagnani, M.G. Giudizi, R. Biagiotti, F. Almerigogna, M.C. Mingari, E. Maggi, C.M. Liang, and L. Moretta, B cell growth factor activity of interferon-γ. Recombinant human interferon-γ promotes proliferation of anti-μ activated human B lymphocytes J Immunol 136:3513 (1986).

18. M. Brunswick, and P. Lake, Obligatory role of gamma interferon in T cell replacing factor-dependent, antigen-specific murine B cell responses, J Exp Med 161:953 (1985).

19. H.J. Leibson, M. Gefter, A. Zlotnik, P. Marrack, and J.W. Kappler, Role of γ-interferon in antibody producing responses, Nature 309:799 (1984).

20. G.F. Del Prete, S. Mariotti, A. Tiri, M. Ricci, A. Pinchera, and S. Romagnani, Characterization of thyroid infiltrating lymphocytes in Hashimoto's thyroiditis. Detection of B and T cells specific for thyroid antigens. Acta Endocrinol (in press).

21. W.L. Farrar, H.M. Johnson, and J.J. Farrar, Regulation of the production of immune interferon and cytotoxic T lymphocytes by interleukin-2. J Immunol 126:1120 (1981).

22. J.R. Klein, and M.J. Bevan, Secretion of immune interferon and generation of cytotoxic T cell activity in nude mice are dependent on interleukin 2: age-associated endogenous production of interleukin 2 in nude mice. J Immunol 130:1780 (1983).

23. A.G. Morris, Y.L. Lin, and B.A. Askonas, Immune interferon release when a cloned cytotoxic T-cell line meets its correct influenza-infected target cell, Nature 295:151 (1982).

24. Y.J. Rosenberg, A.D. Steinberg, and T.J. Santoro, The basis of autoimmunity in MRL-lpr/lpr mice: a role for self Ia-reactive T cells, Immunol Today 5:64 (1984).

AN IN VITRO MODEL FOR THYROID AUTOIMMUNITY

B.E. Wenzel, R. Gutekunst, S. Grammerstorf and
P.C. Scriba
Klinik für Innere Medizin, Med. Universität
zu Lübeck; D-2400 Lübeck, FR Germany

INTRODUCTION

Clinical observations have suggested an association between iodine intake and the occurance of autoimmune thyroiditis in man (1,2), while in areas with endemic goiter prevalence due to iodine deficiency a lower incident of Hashimoto's thyroditis was found (3). Others, however, have contested these claims (4,5). Experimentally, this association has been demonstrated with genetically susceptible chicken (6), rats (7) and dogs (8) on a high iodized diet. In the present study, we were interested in the effect iodine would have on the functional immune response of human T-lymphocytes in co-cultures with autologous thyroid epithilial cells (TECs). Classically, only immunocompetent cells, namely macrophages are able to present antigen together with the immunregulatory class-II surface antigen(9).These class-II antigens (in man HLA-D locii) can also be found in vivo (10) and induced by various agents in vitro(11) on TECs. With this background our in vitro model system was designed to i) modulate HLA-D expression on TECs and ii) to investigate,if a potential iodide induced autoantigen on TECs would be presented through HLA-D to autologous T-lymphocytes and thus initiate a proliferative cellular immunresponse. In order to modulate the hypothetical iodine induced autoantigen the influence of Methimazole (MMI) and perchlorate (PC) on the co-culture system was to be studied. MMI has been suspected to act immune suppressively during suppression therapy of Graves' disease (GD) in vivo and on antibody synthesis in vitro (12). Interestingly, when MMI therapy in GD hyperthyroidism was compared to PC treatment, which clearly is no immuno suppressive agent, both drugs had the same effect on the production of thyroid stimulating antibodies (TSab) (13).

METHODS

Subjects

Thyroid tissue was obtained from patients with GD or non toxic goiter (NTG). GD patients with the exception of two where in cpm = cpm (TEC + Ly) - cpm (TEC) - cpm (Ly)

Indirect immunoflorescence (IF) (11).

TEC$_3$ were plated and cultured on 8 chamber glass slides (20 x 10^3) cells (chamber) in the appropriate medium with or without inducing agents. After 4 days TECs were washed and incubated with specific monoclonal antibodies for HLA-D or M-antigen. Double stained slides were developed with a mouse IgG or a human IgG coupled to FITC or TRITC , respectively.

MATERIALS

Collagenase (Dispase II) was from Boehringer, Mannheim, FRG. Fetal calf serum (FCS), Isco ve (T) medium and all cell culture additives were from Biochrom, West Berlin. Mono-clonals, Tü-22/35/39 and interleukin 2 were from Biotest,Dreieich,FRG. FITC and TRITC conjugated second anti-bodies were from DAKOPATT, Hamburg, FRG. Interferonɣ, Methi-mazole and all hormone additives were from Sigma Chemie, Munich, FRG. Sodium iodide and Potassium perchlorate were from E. Merck, Darmstadt, FRG. Thyrotropin (Thyreostimulin) was from Organon, Munich, FRG. MicroLab slides (Miles) Phyto-hemagglutinin and sheep erythrocytes were from Flow, Mecken-heim, FRG. A Cell harvester,Multiwash 2000, Dynatech, Denken-dorf, FRG and a Flourescence-Photomicroscope, BH-2 from OLympus Europe, Hamburg, FRG were used.

RESULTS

We demonstrate simultaneous expression of HLA-D and M-antigen, when TECs are preincubated with bTSH in 5H (serum free) medium. In contrast, no M-antigen is re-expressed in TECs after incubation with PHA or IFNɣ (Table 1.). The HLA-D

Table 1. In vitro Expression[1] of HLA-D Polymorphism and Microsomal Antigen in Preincubated TEC Cultures.

	DR	DP/DR	DQ	M
PHA	+++	++	0	0
+NaI	++	+	0	0
TSH	++	+	0	+++
+NaI	+	+	0	++
IFNɣ	+++	++	+++	0
+NaI	++	+	++	0
NaI	(+)[2]	0	0	0
MMI	(+)	0	0	0
PC	0	0	0	0
Medium	(+)	(+)	0	(+)

[1]-assessed by IF   [2]-in some GD-TECs spontaneously

cases were iodine loaded for 10 days before surgery. They also had TSab and 6/7 had microsomal (M) antibodies. Patients with NTG were all void of thyroid antibodies.

Thyroid epithelial cells

Thyroid tissue was minced, washed and digested enzymatically with 4 mg/ml collagenase two times for 90 minutes at 37 C. Cells then were washed, separated from debris and erythrocytes by density centrigfugation, washed again and plated in Iscove medium containing insulin, hydrocortisone, somastatin, human transferrin and gly-his-lis tripeptide in 0,5% fetal calf serum (FCS) (5-hormone,(5H) medium).

Cell Cultures

TECs were allowed to adhere overnight in 250 ml/96 well flat bottom Microtiter plates ($20x10^3$ cells/well). After washing with medium, TECs were incubated for 4-5 days with Interferon γ (IFN γ) 10 U/ml, Phytohemagglutinin (PHA) 0.5 µg/ml, bovine thyrotropin (bTSH) 1-100 mU/ml together with or without sodium iodide (NaI), 0.1 mM, MMI, 1-100 µM and PC , 1-100 µM.

On day 5 after starting TEC cultures peripheral blood was drawn from the donor of the thyroid tissue. Lymphocytes were prepared by density centrifugation and T-cells were separated by rosetting with sheep red blood cells (SRBC).

When intra-thyroidal lymphocytes were prepared, the initial TEC suspension after collagenase digestion was divided up. One part was used for establishing TEC cultures, while the other part was allowed to adhere overnight, only that thereafter the non-adherend cells were purified by density centrifugation. All cells banding with lymphocytes were washed, frozen and stored in liquid nitrogen until use on the fifth day of autologous TEC cultures. The yield of intra thyroidal T-lymphocytes was very variable. Depending on the source of the thyroid tissue 1-30 million T-lymphocytes could be obtained.

Co-cultures

After the preincubation period for TECs $2-4x10^5$ T-lymphocytes were added to each Microtiter well ($1-2 x10^5$ cells /ml) using Iscove medium-T supplemented with 15% interleukin 2 (IL2). Co-cultures were incubated for another 6 days, whereafter the 24 hour tritiated thymidin (^{3}HTdR) uptake was measured.

^{3}HTdR uptake

To each Microtiter well 0.5 µCi/50µl ^{3}HTdR (2 Ci/mmol) were added. After 24 hours the non attached cells in co-cultures were resuspended, harvested with a cell-harvester on to cellulose acetate filter, precipitated with 10% tri-chloracetic acid (TCE) and washed with 96% cold ethanol. Filters were dried, punched out and disolved in scintillation cocktail. Samples were set up in quadruplicates and stimulation indices were calculated as:

cpm (+IL2) / cpm (- IL2) = SI + SD

Table 2. HLA-D Expression and Autologous T-Lymphocyte Response in Co-Cultures with TECs.

	HLA-D	SI ± SD
PHA	&+++	1.5 ±0.4 **
+NaI	++	5.6 ±1.1
+ " +MMI	+	1.1 ±0.6
+ " +PC	+	0.9 ±0.6
IFN γ	+++	1.6 ±0.2
+ NaI	++	5.1 ±0.6 *
+ "+MMI	++	1.8 ±0.5
+ "+PC	+	1.5 ±0.6
TSH	++	1.2 ±0.7
+NaI	+	4.1 ±0.8 *
+ "+MMI	+	0.9 ±0.4
+ "+PC	+	1.0 ±0.3
Medium	−	1.8 ±0.5

&-IF   *p < 0.05   **p < 0.01

inducing agents also differ, when HLA-D polymorphism was assessed. While IFM strongly induces HLA-DQ, PHA and TSH incubated TECs display only DR/DP and no -DQ (Table 1). Although NaI is reducing flourescence stain on induced TECs, there is no suppressing of HLA-D observed. The same applies for MMI and PC at concentration lower than 0.1 mM in cultures. In some TECs from GD-patients a spontaneous HLA-D expression occurs, which disappears after 3 days in culture.

As shown in Table 2.only those co-cultures,where HLA-D was induced together with NaI incubation, autologous T-lymphocytes responded with a significantly increased proliferation. This autologous MLR-likereaction was abolished by simultaneous incubation with MMI or PC. Both agents, however, did not suppress HLA-D expression under the same preincubation conditions.

Table 3. Proliferative Response in Co-Cultures of TECs with Autologous Intra-thyroidal T-lymphocytes from GD-Patients.

	IFN γ	IFN γ+NaI	Con A
Patient 1	§1.6 ±0.4	1.3 ±0.5	5.2 ±0.4
Patient 2	1.6 ±0.2	1.6 ±0.5	6.9 ±0.6

§ -SI ± SD

When intra-thyroidal T-lymphocytes were used under identical co-culture conditions, no proliferative response was observed on IFNɣ/NaI preincubated TECs (Table 3), although the ConA T-lymphocyte response was still intact and the T-suppressor T-helper ratio were not altered (visually checked by IF).

There appears to be a difference in T-lymphocyte responses according to iodine administration before surgery. Co-cultures of GD-patients which have not been loaded with iodine tend to have lower SI than those of patients "plummered" for 10 days (Table 4.). When co-cultures were set up with TECs from patients with NTG only 4/15 T-cell responses were observed (not shown).

Table 4.   The Influence of Iodine Load on the Autologous T-Lymphocyte response in Co-Cultures with TECs from GD-Patients.

	"Plummer"	SI ±SD
Patient 1	no	2.8 ±0.7
Patient 2	no	3.1 ±0.4
Patients, n=7	yes	5.8 ±0.6

" " Iodine loaded for 10 days pre-Op.

DISCUSSION

Our in vitro co-culture system appears to be a model for iodine induced autoimmunity(2).It is comparable to the animal models using obese chicken(6) or BB/W rats(7).Likewise in those models the autologous T-lymphocyte response in our in vitro system is genetically suszeptibility dependent,since 10/10 GD-donors with proliferative responses are contrasted by only 4/15 NTG-patients.Wether this could reflectalternatively the actual iodine deficiency in the goitrous thyroid is not yet understood.One hint in that direction could be the difference in magnitude of the response in iodine loaded and unloaded GD-patients.

In order to obtain a T-lymphocyte response two requirements have to be met: 1.An autoantigen has to be induced.In our model this is apparently iodine induced and dependent,since preventing the iodine uptake with PC abolishes the response. 2. The autoantigen has to be presented to immunocompetent lymphocytes.It appears that the thyrocyte is presenting its own autoantigen via HLA-D,since HLA-D expression of TECs is a condition for the response.This would confirm findings,where class-II antigen expressing epithelial cells were able to present viral proteins(14).MMI does not suppress class-II antigen,which reflects previous findings in recurrent hyperthyroidism od GD-patients(15).
Moreover,the similar behaviour of MMI and PC in our system recalls findings in GD therapy,where both agent had the same

effect on thyroid antibody titers during the course of the disease(13).

Our failure to produce a proliferatiye response with intra-thyroidal T-lymphocytes is puzzling and hard to interpret.Although the Ts/Th ratio and the mitogenic T-lymphocyte response are not altered,there might be a loss of T-helper cells during the preparation procedure.

Ongoing studies in our laboratory are designed to define the iodine dependent autoantigen.

SUMMARY

TSH,in contrast to PHA and IFNγ,induces in serum free medium both,class-II and microsomal antigen.The class-II polymorphism displays DR/DP locii rather than DQ,while IFN always strongly induces DQ.Iodine produces autoantigen in TECs which together with class-II expression gives rise to an autologous mixed lymphocyte reaction -like response.The iodine induced immune response in co-cultures prevails in TECs from GD-patients(10/10),while only 4/15 NTG-TECs gave response.Mehimazole as well as perchlorate abolish the re-sponse,although they do not suppress the class-II expression of TECS.Iodine could not induce a proliferative response with intra-thyroidal lymphocytes .The mitogenic T-cell response is not abolished.Responses in iodine loaded patients are higher than in the two GD-patients who were not " plummered" before operation.

ACKNOWLEDGEMENTS

The technical and organizationalhelp of Ms A. Bullasch is gratefully acknowledged.

This work was supported by "Deutsche Forschungsgemein-schaft", SFB 232/C4.

REFERENCES

1. Furszyfer J, Kurland LT, McConahey WM, Wooler BL, Elverback LR.Epidemiologic Aspects of Hashimoto's and Graves`Disease in Rochester,Minnesota(1935-1967) With Special Reference to Temporal Trends. Metabolism,21/3 : 197,(1972).

2. FradkinJE, Wolff J. Iodide-induced thyrotoxicosis. Medicine,62/1 : 1,(1983).

3. Asamer H, Riccabona G, Holthaus N, Gabel F. Immunhistologische Befunde bei Schilddrüsenerkrank-ungen in den endemischen Kropfgebiet. Archiv für Klinische Medizin 215 : 270,(1968).

4. Vollweider R, Stolkin I, Hedinger C. Fokale lympho-
    zytäre Thyreoditis und Jodsalzprophylaxe.
    Schweizer Med Wschr 112 : 482,(1982).

5. Harach HR, Escalante DA, Onativia A, Outes JL, Day
    ES, Williams ED. Thyroid carcinoma and thyroiditis
    an endemic goiter region before and after iodine
    prophylaxis. Acta Endocrinol(Kbh) 108 : 55,(1985).

6. Bagchi N, Brown TR, Urdanivia E, Sundick RS.
    Induction of autoimmune thyroiditis in chicken by
    dietary iodine. Science 230 : 325,(1985).

7. Allen EM, Appel MC, Braverman LE. The effect of
    iodide ingestion on the develpement of spontaneous
    lymphocytic thyrioditis in the diabetes-prone BB/W
    rat. Endocrinol 118 : 1977,(1986).

8. Evans TC, Beierwaltes WH, Nishiyama RH.
    Eperimental canine Hashimoto's thyrioditis.
    Endocrinology 84 : 641,(1969).

9. Balfour BM, Drexhage HA, Kamperdijk EWA, Hoefsmit
    ECM. Antigen-presenting cells,including Langerhans'
    cells,veiled cells and interdigitating cells; in
    microenvironments in haemopoietic and lymphoid dif-
    ferentiations. Ciba Symp 84 : 281,(1981):

10. Hafanusa T, Pujol-Borrell R, Chiovato L, Russel RCG,
    Doniach D, Bottazzo GF. Aberrant expression of HLA-
    DR antigen on thyrocytes in Graves' disease: rele-
    vance for auto-immunity. Lancet ii: 1111,(1983).

11. Wenzel BE, Gutekunst R, Mansky T, Schultek T,Scriba
    PC. Thyrotropin and IgG from patients with Graves'
    disease induce class-II antigen on human thyroid
    cells. in:The thyroid and autoimmunity,eds.H.A.
    Drexhage and W,M. Wiersinga;p. 141.,Elsevier,(1986).

12. McGregor AM, Petersen MM, McLachlan SM, Rocke P,
    Smith BR, Hall R. Carbimazole and the autoimmune
    response in Graves'disease. N Engl J Med 303 : 302,
    (1980).

13. Wenzel KW, Lente JR. Similar effects of thionamide
    drugs and perchlorate on thyroid-stimulating
    Immunoglobulins in Graves'disease: Evidence against
    an immunosuppressive action of thionamide drugs.
    J Clin Endocrinol Metab 58 : 62,(1984).

14. Londei M, Lamb JR, Bottazzo GF, Feldmann M.
     Epithelial cells expressing aberrant MHC class II
     determinants can present antigen to cloned human
     T-cell . Nature 312 : 639,(1984).

15. Carel JC, Remy JJ, Zuchman D, Salamero J, Charreire
     J. Role of Methimazole on DR antugen expression on
     human thyroid epithelial cell cultures. in: The thy-
     roid   and   autoimmunity;eds.   H.A.Drexhage   and
     W.M.Wiersinga .Elsevier,(1986).

GENETIC ASPECTS OF GRAVES' DISEASE

A. M. McGregor, S. Ratanachaiyavong, C. Gunn, K.W. Lee,
P.S. Barnett, C. Darke* and R. Hall
Department of Medicine, University of Wales College of Medicine,
Heath Park, Cardiff and *Tissue Typing Laboratory, Regional
Blood Transfusion Centre, Rhydlafar, Cardiff, Wales, U.K.

INTRODUCTION

The aetiology of Graves' disease is multifactorial (Table 1).
Environmental influences, immunological aberration and perhaps subtle target-
organ alterations (for which there is currently no evidence) all interacting
upon or as a result of a genetic predisposition and occurring particularly
in females are responsible for a disease in which hyperthyroidism results
from the generation of antibodies to the TSH receptor. The familial predisposition to such a course of events and the major histocompatibility
(HLA) association have until now been the most easily accessible means to
examining the genetic linkage of Graves' disease. The familial predisposition does not allow clear discrimination of the pattern of inheritance
(which in a disease upon which the environment has such an impact is not
surprising) and the HLA association is weak. There is no evidence for a
disease susceptibility gene nor does such a gene seem likely. Rather it
would make more sense if Graves' were to be a polygenic disease representing
the conjunction of several independent genetic traits. In this context a
greater understanding of the interactions between the immunologic and
genetic systems, coupled with the recent availability of reagents and new
technology offers the opportunity to examine further the impact which
genetic factors may have in Graves' disease.

In patients and families with Graves' disease living in South Wales
we have sought to define the genetic factors which are associated with the
disease. Using conventional techniques and restriction fragment length
polymorphism analysis based on Southern blotting we have examined the
contributions which family history, HLA class I, II and III antigen analysis,
Gm allotyping and immunoglobulin heavy chain switch region and T cell
receptor beta chain make to the development of the disease. The aim of
these studies, recognising the genetic predisposition to the development
of Graves disease, is to define genetic factors which will permit the
identification of individuals at risk of developing Graves' disease.

ENVIRONMENTAL AND CONSTITUTIONAL FACTORS

In considering environmental influences on the development of the
disease (Table 1) the importance of dietary iodine intake in influencing
the development of the disease is increasingly well recognised(1). The
variation in the incidence of the disease can be shown to correlate with

Table 1. Elements of a Multifactorial Disease

FACTORS		
GENETIC	CONSTITUTIONAL	ENVIRONMENTAL
GENES	AGE	TIME
-Specificity	SEX	GEOGRAPHY
-Dosage	DEVELOPMENTAL STAGE	CLIMATE
-Number	HOMEOSTATIC MECHANISMS	SOCIOECONOMIC STATUS
	-biochemical	OCCUPATION
	-immunological	EDUCATION
	-physiological	DIET
	MATERNAL FACTORS	OTHER
	COGNITIVE QUALITIES	-habits
	TEMPERAMENT	-diseases
	ETHNIC GROUP	INFECTIOUS AGENTS

iodine consumption (1,2). The seasonal variation in the disease in the U.K. may well reflect variation in iodine consumption which is related to marked seasonal changes in levels of iodine in dairy products (1).

Age certainly has an impact on disease development but is more difficult to evaluate though with increasing age detectable TSH receptor antibody activity is observed less frequently in patients presenting with hyperthyroid -ism (2). The influence of the sex of the patient on disease development is however more easily evaluated and it is clear that whilst the disease is more common in women, when it occurs in men it is more severe (Table 2). The impact of the developmental stage of an individual on Graves' disease and on any other autoimmune disease is best exemplified by the dramatic impact which pregnancy has on autoimmune thyroid disease (see Hall, R. et al in this volume). Immunological homeostatic mechanisms are clearly disturbed in Graves' disease and central to the development and maintenance of the disease (3). In this context a number of factors require consideration but in particular the role of the T cell regulatory process and of antibodies to the TSH receptor and these are considered in detail elsewhere in this monograph. Whilst stress has often been claimed to influence disease development it remains difficult to evaluate and the link is currently unsubstantiated. Ethnic origins clearly have an impact on the disease but whether they reflect only genetic differences rather than different environmental influences such as dietary iodine intake (which is certainly the case) is again uncertain.

Table 2. Graves' Disease - Influence of Sex of Patient on
Disease Activity in 172 Patients

	MALE	FEMALE
NUMBER WITH DISEASE	37(22%)	135(78%)
TSH RECEPTOR ANTIBODY POSITIVE	34(92%)	99(73%)
TSH RECEPTOR ANTIBODY ACTIVITY*	83.7	36.1
RELAPSE RATE (3years follow-up)	26(70%)	75(56%)

*Mean level in bioassay in bTSH equivalents (normal < 2)

GENETIC FACTORS

A. Familial aggregation

The familial occurrence of Graves' disease is undoubted and well established. Whilst increased concordance rates for the disease have been found in monozygotic as compared with dyzygotic twins, and support a genetic influence neither of these sets of observations allow firm conclusions on the genetic basis of the disease and its pattern of inheritance but point rather to an important influence of environmental and consitutional factors in genetically predisposed individuals. In considering situations in which the environment is constant/common, the elegant gene dosage effects on autoantibody development by Rose and his colleagues (4) further strengthen the likelihood of a genetic basis. Likewise combining factors in trying to assess the likelihood of developing autoimmune thyroid disease demonstrates an important influence of genetic elements in the process (Table 3).

Table 3. The Likelihood of Developing Post-Partum
Thyroid Dysfunction (PPTD) in 49 Women

PARAMETER	% DEVELOPING PPTD
FAMILY HISTORY (FH)	31.6%
AB TO TMA AT BOOKING (MAB)	50.0%
FH + MAB	68.8%
FH+MAB+HLA B8,DR3	83.3%

FUNG H.Y.M. et al (1986)

B. The Major Histocompatibility Complex (MHC)

The MHC, located on the short arm of chromosome 6 consists of at least 3 sets of antigen loci (class I, II, III);

GLO-·· DP DQ DR····C2 Bf C4B····21-OH····C4A ···21-OH··· B C A -

    II   III   III   I

Attempts to demonstrate statistically an association between Graves' disease and particular HLA phenotypes has resulted in considerable evidence, which whilst supporting such associations shows them to be incomplete (5). Improved reagents and techniques for serological tissue typing has not improved the situation. The relatively weak associations between Graves' disease and the various HLA alleles is open to a number of interpretations (Table 4).

1. Class II. The well recognised but incomplete association of DR3 with Graves' disease in our own population is associated with a relative risk of around 3. Whilst this may vary and be strengthened depending on the parameter defined (Table 5) nevertheless the weak influence of the association means that its impact on disease recognition and management is minimal. In attempting to extend and strengthen these observations we have made use of cDNA probes to the α and β chain genes of the D region (DRα, DRβ, DQα, DQβ) and restriction enzymes (BamH1, Pst1, EcoR1, Taq1, Bag12) to search for restriction fragment length polymorphisms (RFLP) by Southern blotting. Whilst associations between Graves' disease and various RFLP's have been observed when these have been analysed the associations have been weak or reflected an association between a particular fragment and a particular class II allele.

Table 4.   Possible Explanations For The Incomplete
Association Between Graves' Disease And HLA Alleles

DISEASE HETEROGENEITY
CONTRIBUTIONS OF
           -Other Genes
           -Environment
LINKAGE DISEQUILIBRIUM OF HLA WITH AS YET
     UNIDENTIFIED SUSCEPTIBILITY GENE
TECHNICAL INADEQUACY
POPULATION HETEROGENEITY
MIXTURE

Table 5. HLA And Thyroid Microsomal Autoantibody
(TMA) Status Association

AUTOANTIBODY TO TMA	HLA DQw3 FREQUENCY
Positive (n=108)	52.8%
Negative (n=113)	33.6%

Relative risk =2.2, x^2 =7.5, p = <0.01

Kologlu, M. et al (1986)

Whether use of different enzymes or probes will improve the situation
remains to be determined but seems unlikely.

2. Class III.   Three complement proteins are controlled by genes within
the MHC; factor B, C2 and C4. All 3 exhibit genetic polymorphism.   The
synthesis of C4 proteins is controlled by 2 loci, C4A and C4B.   The C4
loci have a number of alleles including a null or QO (quantity zero)
allele.   Whilst data on polymorphisms of C2 and Bf have been reported
in Graves' disease (6) little information is available on the C4 allele
distribution.   Our own data would suggest an association between the
C4AQO allele and Graves' disease (Table 6) but again the association
is weak but interestingly its presence is more strongly associated with
the likelihood of young healthy relatives of Graves' patients having
thyroid autoantibodies (Ratanachaiyavong S. et al unpublished).

Table 6. Graves' Disease And The C4AQO Complement Allele

	NORMALS	GRAVES' DISEASE
C4AQO+ve	30	57
C4AQO-ve	70	35
TOTAL	100	92

x^2 = 19.75, p= <0.001, RR = 3.8

3. Extended Haplotypes. Associations between class I, II and III antigens and Graves' disease may reflect linkage disequilibrium or differences in immune responsiveness in relation to different HLA antigens (1). Whereas little data is available in patients with Graves' disease. The use of extended haplotype/supratype data in patients and families with insulin-dependent diabetes mellitus (7) have demonstrated extended haplotypes covering class I (HLA-B), class II (DR) and class III (Bf, C2, C4A, C4B). Whilst conferring a significantly increased susceptibility to the disease these haplotypes only increase the relative risk to around 10.

4. Other Genes. Analysis of Gm allotypes of the IgG heavy chain constant region have provided conflicting data on the association between these markers and Graves' disease. Again preliminary data using cDNA probes to the immunoglobulin switch region have failed to show strong RFLP associations with Graves' disease, and this is also the case to date with RFLP analysis in Graves' disease using cDNA probes to the T cell receptor α and β chain. If associations are to be found with further restriction enzyme analysis, current data in other autoimmune diseases and in Graves' disease do not support the concept that these will be strong and therefore particularly significant.

CONCLUSIONS

We remain no clearer in our understanding of the genetics of Graves' disease. The long established recognition of the familial nature of the disease and the more recently recognised HLA associations provide inconclusive evidence. Newer techniques which permit both broadening of the analyses possible and also more sophisticated analysis of genes within, for example the HLA class II have failed to make a significant impact. Whether more intensive family studies with generation of extended haplotypes will clarify the problem remains to be seen. Increasingly however it appears more likely that whilst a genetic predisposition to Graves' disease is undoubted its influence is minor and in the absence of a "disease susceptibility gene", the roles of environmental and constitutional factors are much more relevant in this multifactorial disease.

REFERENCES

1. Chang, D.C.S., Barnett, P.S., Ratanachaiyavong, S. et al (1986) Graves' disease; factors associated with its development and subsequent course, in: The Thyroid and Autoimmunity H. A. Drexhage and W. M. Wiersinga Ed. Excerpta Medica, Amsterdam pp 37-49.
2. Phillips, D.I. W., Barker, D.J.P., Smith, B.R. et al (1985) The geographical distribution of thyrotoxicosis in England according to the presence or absence of TSH-receptor antibodies Clin. Endocrinol. 23: 283-287
3. Weetman, A.P., McGregor, A.M., (1984) Autoimmune Thyroid Disease; developments in our understanding. Endoc. Rev. 5: 309-355.
4. Burek, C.L., Hoffman, W.F., and Rose, N.R. (1982) The presence of thyroid autoantibodies in children and adolescents with autoimmune thyroid disease and in their siblings and parents. Clin. Immunol. Immunopathol. 25; 395-404
5. Farid, N.R., Stenszky, V., Balazs, C. and Bear, J.C. (1986) The MHC and autoimmune thyroid disease. Mt. Sinai J. Med. 53; 6-18.

6. Farid, N.R., and Bear, J.C. (1981) The human MHC and Endocrine
    disease. Endoc. Rev. 2: 50-86

7. Rich, S., O'Neill, G., Dalmasso, A.P. et al (1985) Complement and
    HLA. Further definition of high-risk haplotypes in insulin-
    dependent diabetes. Diabetes 34; 504-509.

THYROID AND RELATED AUTOIMMUNE DISORDERS:

CHALLENGING THE DOGMAS

Gian Franco Bottazzo, Ian Todd, Antonino Belfiore
Rita Mirakian, and Ricardo Pujol-Borrell

Department of Immunology
The Middlesex Hospital Medical School
London W1P 9PG, UK

INTRODUCTION

When, in 1973, one of us (GFB) joined Deborah Doniach and the Autoimmunity Group in the Department of Immunology at The Middlesex Hospital in London, the main area of research was the pathogenesis of autoimmune liver diseases. Indeed, it is of interest to recall that another young Italian research fellow in the team at that time was Mario Rizzetto who, a few years later, discovered the Delta particle, and thus made a fundamental advance in the understanding of viral hepatitis. No doubt he had the right training! But to return to the story of the young fellow from Venice, he knew that the Department was famous all over the world for the investigation of endocrine autoimmunity and he was hesitant to become involved in the 'diversion' of liver disorders. There is nothing wrong with this subject but, after all, Ivan Roitt and Deborah Doniach were the discoverers of human thyroid autoimmunity 17 years previously and had persued this line of novel investigation for several years. 'What about turning the emphasis again towards the first 'love' of endocrine autoimmunity?' he asked. Deborah Doniach enthusiastically agreed. It was in 1974 when he then tested a few sera of patients with Addison's disease on sections of human pancreas by the indirect immunofluorescence technique, that he observed the islets shining out against the dark background of the exocrine acini. With Alex Florin-Christensen, who actively collaborated in this new approach, the first dogma was thus challenged: a year previously during the first meeting on 'Immunology of Diabetes' held in Brussels, it was stated: 'We are afraid that islet cell antibodies do not exist'.

This was the opportunity Deborah was looking for, and all the endocrine autoimmunologists were excited to see her back in the area where she was much more at home. What then happened now belongs to history (doesn't time fly!). The field of autoimmunity and diabetes expanded tremendously, and a number of other conditions in the 'idiopathic limbo' were moved under the umbrella of autoimmune disorders. It was at this point that we had the temerity to ask: 'Shall we challenge other dogmas which have dominated the field for several years?'. All the progress which then followed was clearly made possibly by the collaboration and friendship of several colleagues who were attracted to the laboratory by the novel and exciting wind which was refreshing the subject and whose important contributions are gratefully acknowledged.

It would exceed the limits of this manuscript to summarize all the excitement of these years which derived primarily from working closely with Deborah Doniach, together with the constant support of Ivan Roitt. In keeping with the title assigned to us, we shall therefore concentrate on those themes which, we believe, most directly challenge some of the established dogmas.

DOGMA 1: INSULIN-DEPENDENT DIABETES IS NOT AN AUTOIMMUNE DISEASE

Following the first description of islet cell antibodies (ICA) in polyendocrine autoimmune diabetic patients (Bottazzo et al, 1974) and their subsequent identification in uncomplicated juvenile cases (Lendrum et al, 1975), speculation arose as to whether these serological markers merely represented a secondary phenomenon, with a specific attack by a common environmental agent(s) being responsible for the initial injury to the pancreatic beta cells. However, although Type I diabetes has an acute clinical onset, ICA were demonstrated in predisposed individuals years before the onset of the disease, and this lead to reconsideration of the 'common viral dogma' as the sole cause of diabetes. The new concept of a primary autoimmune attack emerged initially from studies of unaffected members of diabetic families and was subsequently confirmed in retrospective and prospective studies in identical twins discordant for the disease, in polyendocrine non-diabetic patients and even in single sporadic cases (reviewed by Bottazzo et al, 1986). A proportion of these individuals eventually became overtly diabetic.

More recently, full-blown immunological aggression has been uncovered around and inside islets in an acute diabetic patient who died of the disease close to the time at which symptoms became overt (Bottazzo et al, 1985). Most facets of an autoimmune attack were represented in the frozen pancreatic blocks, with abundant evidence of immune complex and complement deposition. $CD8^+$ (?cytotoxic) T cells were a predominant feature of the diseased tissue, with the lymphocytes expressing activation markers. No evidence of coxsackie, mumps or other common viruses was detected in the diabetic islets. We believe that because of this new evidence, previously advocated environmental agents should be considered to act more as precipitating rather than initiating factors of beta cell damage (Bottazzo, 1986). This strongly suggests that something more subtle and definitely more complicated is involved in the pathogenesis of this disease.

Regardless of the nature of the initial trigger, the major concern of most investigators and diabetologists is to try to efficiently hold the autoimmune attack against beta cells in check once it has been mounted. The initial pilot study with cyclosporin A (Stiller et al, 1984) and the more recent double blind trial in newly diagnosed diabetic patients (Feutren et al, 1986) is, in this context, the best indication that general opinion is coming round to the idea that autoimmunity plays a major role in the attack on the beta cells. However, it is important to point out that none of the presently available immunosuppressive drugs are sufficiently specific for those lymphocytes ultimately responsible for the destruction of beta cells. This conclusion is based on the fact that withdrawal of the drugs leads to recurrence of the disease and the need for re-introducton of conventional insulin therapy. Most importantly, they cause serious side effects which call for intensive management and monitoring by specialized units.

DOGMA 2: THE DIRECT PATHOGENIC ROLE OF THYROID MICROSOMAL ANTIBODIES 'IN VIVO'

Cytoplasmic antibodies remain an invaluable clinical tool for diagnostic and prognostic purposes, but the pathogenic role of any autoantibody must lie in its ability to bind autoantigens expressed on the cell surface. This is a prerequisite for activation of the complement cascade and of killer lymphocytes. Surface reactive antibodies have been demonstrated in several organ-specific systems but there are substantial differences in the nature of their reactivity patterns in the different diseases. In the thyroid, previous work has shown that passive transfer of thyroid microsomal antibodies to primates does not cause damage to the thyroids of these animals. In addition, mothers with Hashimoto's thyroiditis and high titres of thyroid antibodies give birth to perfectly normal children despite the fact that IgG autoreactive immunoglobulins cross the placenta. It is also well known that middle-aged women positive for these same antibodies do not necessarily become hypothyroid (reviewed by Belfiore & Bottazzo, 1987). Why this paradoxical ineffectiveness?

The work initially carried out by Emilio Khoury clearly demonstrated that virtually all sera containing thyroid microsomal antibodies (recently shown to react with the thyroid peroxidase complex (Czarnocka et al, 1985)) recognised surface antigens of viable thyroid cells in culture and in suspensions. Furthermore, the addition of complement lead to lysis of the thyrocytes (Khoury et al, 1981). These data, together with those almost simultaneously obtained by the Pisa Group (Reviewed by Pinchera et al, 1984) indicated that the cytoplasmic microsomal antigen was also expressed on the cell surface, suggesting perhaps rather prematurely, that these specific autoantibodies, contrary to expectation, could play a direct pathogenic role 'in vivo'. However, the situation was comlicated by the subsequent demonstration that the surface expression of this autoantigen was restricted to the microvillar apical border facing the colloid space on the interior of the thyroid follicles (Khoury et al, 1984). These results unexpectedly demonstrated the existence of a sequestered antigen which, like the eye and the sperm, is apparently inaccessible to the immune system. However, further work indicated that some thyroid follicles isolated from the glands of patients with autoimmune thyroid disease showed a spontaneous reversal of the cellular polarity with the microvillar border exposed at the vascular pole (Hanafusa et al, 1984). The precise stimuli which induce this phenomenon 'in vivo' in predisposed individuals is unknown, but it is interesting to note that a similar 'in-side-out' effect can be obtained 'in vitro' by culturing follicles in media with high protein content (Hanafusa et al, 1984), a phenomenon originally described with rat thyroid follicular cells (Nitsch & Wollman, 1980).

DOGMA 3: GOITRE FORMATION IS NOT MEDIATED BY AUTOIMMUNITY

Non-toxic simple and nodular goitres have been considered not to be autoimmune conditions. However, they are known to occur more frequently than expected, in families with autoimmune thyroid diseases and a proportion of these patients have low titres of autoantibodies to thyroid microsomal antigen and/or thyroglobulin. The discrepancy between toxicity and goitre size in Graves' disease and the flat TRH response in some cases of non-toxic goitre first lead Deborah Doniach to hypothesise that some forms of hyperplasia might be due to growth promoting antibodies (Doniach, 1976). The actual occurrence of thyroid growth-stimulating immunoglobulins (TGI) were first established by Hemmo

Drexhage when he joined forces with us in 1979 using a sensitive cytochemical bioassay devised by Jo Chayen and Lucille Bitensky at the Kennedy Institute in London (Drexhage et al, 1980). The autoantibodies are now known to be associated with goitre formation in Graves' disease, in two thirds of non-toxic goitre (Van der Gaag, 1985b; Smyth et al, in press) and in a proportion of Hashimoto goitres (Drexhage et al, 1980). The original method used for the detection of TGI is very labour intensive and is not suitable for extensive population studies. Advances in this connection have been made by measuring ^{3}H-thymidine incorporation into reconstituted rat thyroid follicles incubated with suitable patient sera, but at the expense of a much lower sensitivity of detection (Chiovato et al, 1983). The right balance between 'ease' in performing the assay and 'sensitivity' may be achieved by measuring TGI on the FRTL-5 cells. Effects of patients' immunoglobulins on the mitotic index in these cells may provide a better indication of the existence of growth-promoting antibodies (Ealey et al, 1985).

DOGMA 4: CONVENTIONAL AUTOANTIBODIES ARE SUFFICIENT TO EXPLAIN ATROPHIC ORGAN-SPECIFIC AUTOIMMUNITY?

Our contribution to this particular issue was again initially related to thyroid autoimmunity. By continuing his work on thyroid growth stimulating immunoglobulins, Hemmo Drexhage was also able to demonstrate the existence of receptor-associated 'blocking' antibodies primarily related to the pathogenesis of atrophy of the gland in primary myxoedema (Drexhage et al, 1981). Their presence may prevent re-growth of thyroid follicles despite increased pituitary output of TSH. The recent exciting news from the Amsterdam Group in collaboration with Jean Dussault in Canada indicates that, when transmitted through the placenta, these 'blockers' interfere with normal development of the foetal thyroid and are responsible for almost half the cases of athyreotic cretinism (Van der Gaag et al, 1985a).

As in atrophic thyroiditis, other similar organ-specific autoimmune disorders also seem to involve receptor blocking antibodies. The growing list in this particular field includes gastrin-receptor blocking antibodies in fundal gastritis (Loveridge et al, 1980) and, most recently, immunoglobulins with similar properties in Addison's disease (Wulffraat & Drexhage, 1986).

DOGMA 5: STIMULATORY AUTOIMMUNITY APPLIES ONLY TO THE THYROID GLAND

It is well established that destructive and stimulatory autoimmunity can affect the thyroid gland. By contrast, although destructive autoimmune processes are well documented in the atrophy of gastric parietal cells in the stomach, until recently no specific stimulatory immunoglobulins were identified at the level of the gastric cells. Clearly, duodenal ulcer represented another good challenge. In experiments performed in rats, Dobi and Lenkey (1982) originally showed that immunoglobulins from patients with acid hyper-secretory duodenal ulcer stimulated gastric secretion in the animal stomach and the number of gastric parietal cells increased. Interestingly, this parallels the experimental procedure originally adopted by Adams when also 30 years ago, he showed the existence of LATS (Adams, 1956). The findings of Dobi & Lenkey thus raised the possibility that both destructive and stimulating antibodies might also play an important role in gastric autoimmunity. This promoted Franca De Lazzari to examine whether a subgroup of patients with duodenal ulcer do indeed possess stimulating autoantibodies. She accordingly determined the ability of patients' IgGs to stimulate cyclic-AMP production by parietal cell suspensions prepared from the stomachs of young male guinea pigs (De Lazzari et al, 1986 and submitted). 13 out of 30 patients originally tested had immunoglobulins with stimulatory activity in this assay which suggested that they could act either on histamine receptors (H_2-R) of gastric parietal cells or on chief cells to stimulate pepsinogen production. In either case, their role in maintaining and perpetuating the gastric secretion could be of pathogenic importance. Furthermore, more than half our cases with stimulating antibodies did not respond to anti-H_2-R drugs. This may indicate 'in vivo' occupancy of the target receptor by antibodies and thus suggest the potential prognostic value of the test in predicting the responsiveness to specific treatment in these patients.

DOGMA 6: 'CONVENTIONAL ANTIGEN-PRESENTING CELLS MUST INITIATE AUTOIMMUNITY'

This story dates from around 1982 when we asked: could epithelial cells play an active role in stimulating autoimmunity? The initial experiments gave the first clue in that mitogens were able to trigger HLA Class II molecules on normal thyrocytes in culture (Pujol-Borrell et al, 1983). The next step was obvious: Toshi Hanafusa looked at sections of autoimmune thyroid glands and found that in Hashimoto's thyroiditis and, to a lesser extent, in Graves' disease, the specimens stained cytoplasmically for Class II molecules (Hanafusa et al, 1983). Interestingly, the phenomenon was also detected on the vascular pole of reconstituted follicles obtained from the same patients. These reports were soon confirmed (eg. Jansson et al, 1985; Aichinger et al, 1985; Davies, 1985) and extended to other tissues obtained from patients with a variety of autoimmune disorders (reviewed by Todd et al, 1986d) including beta cells in diabetic islets (Bottazzo et al, 1985; Foulis & Farquharson, 1986). These initial findings prompted us, in collaboration with Marc Feldmann, to put forward the hypothesis that the inappropriate expression of Class II molecules by epithelial cells might enable these cells to present their own surface molecules to autoreactive T cells, by-passing a requirement for 'conventional' antigen-presenting cells, like macrophages and dendritic cells (Bottazzo et al, 1983). Such a process could make an important contribution to the potentiation, and also possibly the initiation of the autoimmune process.

In order to test directly whether Class II⁺ thyrocyes can function as antigen-presenting cells, we furthered our collaboration with Marc Feldmann, and Marco Londei initially demonstrated that these cells were able to present a small peptide to HLA compatible human T cell clones known to respond to this antigen in other systems (Londei et al, 1984). However, these results did not necessarily indicate that thyroid cells could be autostimulatory, and for this reason more direct experiments were planned. Marco accordingly demonstrated that autoreactive cloned T cell lines, derived from the activated lymphocytes infiltrating Graves' disease thyroids, proliferated upon exposure to autologous thyrocytes, but were not stimulated by autologous peripheral blood mononuclear cells or allogeneic Class II⁺ thyrocytes (Londei et al, 1985). Furthermore, the interaction with autologous thyrocytes could be blocked with monoclonal anti-Class II antibodies. This experiment convincingly demonstrated that thyrocytes are capable of directly presenting their own autoantigens in an MHC Class II restricted, tissue-specific fashion to autoreactive T cells infiltrating the diseased gland.

Clearly, if HLA Class II expression by thyrocytes really does play an important role in pathogenesis, then the occurrence of this inappropriate expression would be expected to correlate with other features of the autoimmune pathology. In this regard, we have analysed a large series of glands from patients with a variety of thyroid diseases and found a significant correlation between HLA Class II expression by thyrocytes and the occurrence of circulating autoantibodies to thyroglobulin or thyroid microsomal antigen (Todd et al, 1986b; Lucas Martin et al, submitted). A more detailed analysis of a similar type was performed in Graves' disease patients in whom we examined expression of the HLA-D subregions DR, DQ and DP. The incidence and intensity of Class II subregion expression by thyrocytes was found to vary between patients, with DR being most expressed, followed by DP and DQ least expressed (Todd et al, 1986a). In this analysis, the most significant relationships were observed between high serum titres of thyroglobulin autoantibodies and thyrocyte expression of HLA-DQ, and between autoantibodies to microsomal antigen and HLA-DR. Although this type of analysis is indirect, these findings are consistent with different HLA-D subregion products expressed by thyrocytes being dominant in stimulating responses to different thyroid surface autoantigens (Todd et al, 1986b).

In view of these findings, an important question to be answered is: what are the mediators directly or indirectly responsible for the induction of Class II on the epithelial cells which are the targets for autoimmunity? Our findings indicate that human thyrocytes are relatively easily induced to express Class II whereas certain other cell types are much more resistant. This refers primarily to the effects of mediators produced by various immunocytes. Thus, interferon (IFN)-gamma (Todd et al, 1985) and IFN-gamma + TSH (Todd et al, 1986c) are potent inducers of Class II expression by thyrocytes. Conversely, we have also identified mediators which seem to down-regulate Class II products on the same cells. Epidermal growth factor, for example, significantly inhibits the induction exerted either by IFN-gamma alone or in combination with TSH (Todd et al, 1986c).

Turning to human pancreatic beta cells, the situation is much more complicated. A long list of mediators, including IFN-gamma, are unable to trigger Class II on beta cells in culture (Pujol-Borrell et al, 1986b). However, it is only recently that the combination of IFN-gamma + tumour necrosis factor or lymphotoxin have proved to be effective in this regard (Pujol-Borrell et al, 1986a and submitted). However, it is important to point out that this combination exerts similar effects on glucagon cells in the same cultures. This is different from the pathological situation in Type I diabetes, where only the beta cells inappropriately express Class II molecules and are targets of the destructive process. Thus, it appears that the 'in vitro' effects observed do not fully reproduce the situation in the diseased pancreas. This suggests that these immune mediators possibly play a role in potentiating the later stages of the pathogenesis, but may not be responsible for the initial inappropriate expression of Class II which is characteristically restricted to beta cells. Further evidence that immune mechanisms may not be involved in stimulating this expression are, firstly, that the majority of the islets containing Class II[+] beta cells in diabetic pancreases are devoid of lymphocytic infiltration (Foulis & Farquharson, 1986). Secondly, in other pathological conditions involving extensive infiltration of pancreatic exocrine tissue by lymphocytes, eg. chronic pancreatitis (Bovo et al, 1985) and cystic fibrosis (Foulis & Farquharson, 1986), the islets remain Class II[-]. The obvious question must then be, what else could be responsible for the disease-related Class II expression by beta cells.

One possibility is that certain viruses might directly induce Class II. This is supported by recent experiments in our laboratory in which epithelial cell lines were derived from thyroid monolayers by transfection with a plasmid containing the early region of SV-40 viral DNA: a proportion of the cells in these lines showed constitutive Class II expression (Belfiore et al, 1986). These lines have been cloned and maintained in culture for over a year. Although the transformed cells have lost some characteristic features (eg. full expression of microsomal antigen and significant sensitivity to TSH) they still fully maintain characteristics of epithelial cells and endocrine cells in general. Of most importance in the present context is the finding that a proportion of these cells (up to 50% in some of the clones) are constitutively Class II$^+$, and this is despite no Class II expression being detected in the parental cells. Although the level of Class II expression can be increased by stimulation of the clones with IFN-gamma, it is not dependent upon this lymphokine. This model system thus indicates the potential for direct Class II induction or stabilization in endocrine epithelia by viral infection/transformation without the need to invoke immune intervention. In view of the evidence just cited and the previous considerations, the possible relevance of this SV-40 model to the Class II expression by beta cells in Type I diabetes is clear; but the fact that immune mechanisms of induction are so effective on thyrocytes in no way precludes the model also being relevant to the pathogenesis of autoimmune thyroid disorders.

However, for the present a question mark remains over whether the inappropriate expression of Class II by thyrocytes is solely a secondary phenomenon associated with the established disease, or whether it could be involved in the initiation of the autoimmune attack. From the results discussed above, it appears very likely that immune mechanisms (particularly involving IFN-gamma) are responsible for the thyrocyte Class II expression associated with on-going autoimmunity, which is also the conclusion of others who have investigated this question (eg. Iwatani et al, 1986). It is therefore not surprising to find that thyrocytes from Graves' disease patients lose expression of Class II after a few days in culture (since such expression induced by IFN-gamma is not constitutive), and that this expression can be re-induced by IFN-gamma. Indeed, a parallel can be drawn with the loss of microsomal antigen in culture (Khoury et al, 1981), which is expressed again upon stimulation with TSH (eg. Chiovato et al, 1985). The observation that thyrocyte Class II expression and lymphocytic infiltration are often located together in autoimmune thyroid glands is also as one would expect. However, one cannot then assume that the mechanisms which propagate Class II expression in the infiltrated thyroid are identical to those responsible for its initial induction. Thus, examination of tissue from patients with advanced disease may give no clues as to the nature of the hypothetical initiating factors. It is possible that, even if the initial Class II expression by thyrocytes is not related to autoimmunity, it could result from activation of immune mechanisms, for example, in response to a local infection, as we originally proposed (Bottazzo et al, 1983). On the other hand, the fact that immune mechanisms are so effective at inducing Class II in thyrocytes does not preclude the possibility of similar effects being achieved by non-immune mechanisms. Indeed, the ease with which IFN-gamma induces Class II in thyocytes may almost be a disadvantge in experimental terms when it comes to building up a complete picture, since it tends to overshadow other potentially important possibilities.

FUTURE PROSPECTS: THE CHALLENGE OF THE DOGMAS CONTINUES

So much for the past and the present: what about the future? Clearly, it is important not to get into a rut, but to be constantly aware of the importance of critically evaluating scientific findings and analysing them in the right context. We found it extremely attractive to suggest an active role for the target epithelial cells, which no longer appear to be 'passive' as previously thought, but their role is now seen to be much more prominent following the demonstration that they can express HLA Class II molecules. It is also important to mention that these cells have an enhanced expression of Class I products and this finding correlates with an increased number of CD8[+] (?cytotoxic) T cells in the diseased tissue, as clearly shown in the diabetic pancreas (reviewed by Foulis & Bottazzo, 1987). Although the current debate is focused on the extent to which the autoimmune pathogenesis should be regarded as 'homicidal', ie. attack by common environmental factors and autoreactive immunocytes (either separately or in combination) on 'unsuspecting' target cells, we also consider this process to have a 'suicidal' element with the target making itself vulnerable by inappropriate expression of HLA Class II products (Bottazzo, 1986). The latter perspective certainly has a conceptual advantage in that both the afferent and efferent limbs of the autoimmune response then take place within the same organ, ie. at the surface of the target cells themselves. This may be contrasted with the conventional, but more complex models which require release of surface autoantigens from damaged target cells, their presentation by classical antigen-presenting cells in distant specialized lymphoid organs and the subsequent re-circulation of activated autoreactive lymphocytes to the target tissues. These steps clearly pose a number of logistical problems.

In order for Class II-positive target cells to effectively present their autoantigens, autoreactive T cells must come into close contact with them. Lymphocytic infiltration of the target tissues is clearly necessary for this to occur. An important part in permitting or promoting this infiltration could be played by the capillary endothelial cells, which physiologically constitute a discrete and selective barrier between the blood and the tissues. In organs affected by autoimmunity the capillaries are hypertrophic and strongly Class II-positive: this is apparent in the thyroids of ATD patients (Hanafusa et al, 1983), but is most marked in diabetic pancreases (Bottazzo et al, 1985; Foulis & Farquharson, in press). In the latter, these changes are observed in seemingly healthy endothelium around and inside islets (with or without infiltration), whereas the capillaries in the exocrine tissue are unaffected. The 'activated' endothelia could play a role in facilitating the 'homing' of lymphocytes, including those which are potentially autoreactive (Jalkanen et al, 1986) and/or could possibly be involved in the presentation of antigens cross-reactive with those expressed by the target endocrine cells (Nunez et al, 1983). However, regardless of the details, these observations, together with those of inappropriate Class II expression by the epithelial cells, highlight the major contribution of the target tissues to the stimulation of autoimmune pathogenesis.

We must also consider other areas which could ultimately help to elucidate important aspects of the pathogenesis of autoimmune disorders of the thyroid and other endocrine tissues. The possible existence of organ-specific suppressor T cells (Topliss et al, 1983; Vento et al, 1985) remains attractive although it is presently difficult to devise strategies for their isolation and unambiguous characterization. The possible involvement of anti-idiotypic responses in destructive autoimmunity has been proposed on several occasions (eg. Plotz, 1983) but it is hard to envisage how this particular type of mechanism can make a major contribution to this type of pathogenesis particularly since the lack of MHC restriction of such responses is difficult to reconcile with the observations of inappropriate HLA product expression by the target cells (reviewed by Bottazzo et al, 1984). On the other hand, the idiotype theory could explain the generation of antibodies to hormone receptors and it is possible that growth stimulating antibodies of this type could account for the regeneration of target tissues which is postulated to occur in the long latency period preceding the onset of clinical symptoms in many autoimmune diseases (Bottazzo, 1984).

The recent application of T cell cloning to autoimmunity (Hohlfeld et al, 1984; Londei et al, 1985; Del Prete et al, 1986) has greatly advanced the subject by facilitating the dissection of processes involved in the autoimmune attack (reviewed by Feldmann et al, 1985). With regard to Graves' disease, intrathyroidal lymphocytes from autoimmune glands proved to be the best source of starting material for the establishment of $CD4^+$ thyroid-specific, autoreactive cloned T cell lines (this followed several unsuccessful attempts over the years using peripheral blood lymphocyes from patients affected by the same disorders). Once again, epithelial HLA Class II expression proved to be a key factor, since autologous Class II^+ thyrocytes were successfully employed to stimulate expansion of the autoreactive T cells (Londei et al, 1985). Conversely, heavily infiltrated Hashimoto glands have proved to be the best source for cloning T lymphocytes with killer activity (Del Prete et al, 1986; Londei et al, 1986). Unfortunately, major problems still exist in applying T cell cloning technology to diabetes. Lack of sufficient numbers of insulin cells for 'in vitro' studies is one of the main limitations, but most important is the fact that the pancreas cannot be biopsied, so that the T cells most relevant to the diabetic process (ie. those present in the inflammatory infiltrate) are not available. As in Hashimoto's thyroiditis, the T cell clones which would most probably be derived from the diabetic pancreas are cytotoxic ones, since these appear to be the cells that dominate the infiltrate and finally destroy the beta cell. This concept is highlighted by the observation previously mentioned that the predominating lymphocytes in the diabetic pancreas at the time of diagnosis are of the CD8 phenotype (Bottazzo et al, 1985). Also relevant to the argument is the observation that in the pancreases transplanted from non-diabetic identical twins to the affected co-twins only the beta cells were destroyed. Only one of the four cases who underwent this particular surgical procedure showed the appearance of islet cell antibodies, but in all four pancreases $CD8^+$ T cells were the predominant features around the 'rejected' beta cells. As in the originally diabetic islets, glucagon and somatostatin cells were untouched (Sibley et al, 1985).

A more refined analysis of tissue-derived autoreactive lymphocytes should also permit investigations into the T cell receptors directed against specific autoantigens. Due to the organ-specific localization of the response, one would expect the frequency of the relevant T cells in the peripheral blood to be very low. Thus, T cell clones obtained from the lymphocytes invading the tissue would be the best material for the study. One could then accurately characterize the receptors at the genetic level, and also investigate whether viral integration might play a role in promoting the expansion of the self-reactive specificities.

Finally, there is an urgent need to produce appropriate epithelial cell lines to facilitate further 'in vitro' investigations. The usefulness of primary cultures of human epithelial cells is limited by their cellular heterogeneity and short life span. Furthermore, in diabetes research, for example, the lack of sufficient beta cells curtails experimentation. One approach to the development of human epithelial cell lines is exemplified by our experiments in transformation of thyroid cells with portions of the SV-40 genome (Belfiore et al, 1986). This has given insight into possible mechanisms of Class II induction, as discussed previously, but these lines no longer display all the features of the original cells. This implies that future efforts must be concentrated on devising new strategies which will allow cells to grow while retaining their original features.

In 1956, at the time of the discovery of thyroid autoimmunity, GFB and RM were ten years old, happily attending primary schools in Venice and Padua, respectively. RP-B, aged five, was caught between the Spanish and the Catalan languages in his native Barcelona and AB was three, thinking that, like Etna dominating Catania, all mountains should smoke. IT was only two, already showing signs of North European tallness in his Leeds upbringing. We were lucky: we first read of these findings in the text books and became fascinated with the subject; but, most importantly, we met, interracted, and worked with those mainly responsible for the discovery. They have taught us a great deal, and we are grateful to them.

ACKNOWLEDGEMENTS

We are also grateful to several Agencies and Institutions which so generously helped our work during the years and in particular: the British Diabetic Association, the Medical Research Council, The Wellcome Trust, The Juvenile Diabetes Foundation International (USA) and Novo Research Institute (Copenhagen). Miss Marian Pine patiently edited the manuscript.

REFERENCES

Adams, D.D., 1956, The clinical status of patients whose sera have given the abnormal response when assayed for thyrotropin, Proc. Univ. Otago. Med. Sch., 34:29-35.

Aichinger, G., Fill, H., & Wick. G., 1985, In situ immune complexes, lymphocyte subpopulations and HLA-DR positive epithelial cells in Hashimoto thyroiditis. Lab. Invest., 52:132-140.

Belfiore, A., Bottazzo, G.F., 1987, Epidemiology of autoallergic human thyroiditis. Monographs in Allergy, Karger, Basel (in press).

Belfiore, A., Pujol-Borrell, R., Mauerhoff, T., Mirakian, R. & Bottazzo, G.F., 1986, Effect of SV-40 transformaton on HLA expression by thyroid follicular cells: arise of a population of DR positive thyrocytes. Annales d'endocrinol, 47:17 (abstract).

Bottazzo, G.F., 1984, Beta cell damage in diabetic insulitis: are we approaching the solution?, Diabetologia, 26:241-249.

Bottazzo, G.F., 1986, Death of a Beta Cell: Homicide or Suicide? Diabetic Med., 3:119-130.

Bottazzo, G.F., Dean, B.M., McNally, J.M., MacKay, E.H., Swift, P.G.F. & Gamble, D.R., 1985, In situ characterization of autoimmune phenomena and expression of HLA molecules in the pancreas in diabetic insulitis, N. Engl. J. Med., 313:353-360.

Bottazzo, G.F., Florin-Christensen, A., Doniach, D., 1974, Islet cell antibodies in diabetes mellitus with autoimmune polyendocrine deficiencies, Lancet, ii:1279-1283.

Bottazzo, G.F., Pujol-Borrell, R., Gale, E., 1986, Autoimmunity and diabetes: progress, consolidation and controversy, The Diabetes Annual/2: K.G.M.M. Alberti & L.P. Krall Eds, Elsevier Science Pub., Amsterdam, pp13-29.

Bottazzo, G.F., Pujol-Borrell, R., Hanafusa, T. & Feldmann, M., 1983, Role of aberrant HLA-DR expression and antigen presentation in induction of endocrine autoimmunity, Lancet, ii:1115-1119.

Bottazzo, G.F., Todd, I., Pujol-Borrell, R., 1984, Hypothesis for the genetic contribution to the aetiology of diabetes mellitus. Immunol. Today, 5:230-231.

Bovo, P., Mirakian, R., Merigo, F., Angelini, G., Pujol-Borrell, R., Cavallini, G., Bottazzo, G.F. & Scuro, L.A., 1985, Chronic alcoholic pancreatitis: is autoimmunity involved?, Dig. Dis. Sci., 30:967 (Abstract).

Chiovato, L., Hammond, L.J., Hanafusa, T., Pujol-Borrell, R., Doniach, D., Bottazzo, G.F., 1983, Detection of thyroid growth immunoglobulins (TGI) by [^{3}H] thymidine incorporation in cultured rat thyroid follicles. Clin. Endocrinol., 19:581-590.

Chiovato, L., Vitti, P., Lombardi, A., Kohn, L.D. & Pinchera, A., 1985, Expression of the microsomal antigen on the surface of continuously cultured rat thyroid cells is modulated by thyrotropin, J. Clin. Endocrinol. Metab., 61:12-16.

Czarnocka, B., Ruf, J., Ferrand, M., Carayon, P., Lissitzky, S., 1985, Purification of the human thyroid peroxidase and its identification as the microsomal antigen involved in autoimmune thyroid diseases. FEBS Lett., 190:147-152.

Davies, T.F., 1985, Cocultures of human thyrid monolayer cells and autologous T cells: impact of HLA Class II antigen expression, J. Clin. Endocrinol. Metab., 61:418-422.

De Lazzari, F., Mirakian, R., Hammond, L., Venturi, C., Bartolami, M., Naccarato, R., Doniach, D., Bottazzo, G.F., 1986, Are there immunological forms of duodenal ulcer (DU) as a consequence of gastric parietal cell stimulating antibodies? Gut, 20:1116 (Abstract).

Del Prete, G.F., Maggi, E., Mariotti, S., Tiri, A., Vercelli, D., Parronchi, P., Macchia, D., Pinchera, A., Ricci, M., Romagnani, S., 1986, Cytotoxic T lymphocytes with natural killer activity in thyroid infiltrate of patients with Hashimoto's thyroiditis: analysis at clonal level, J. Clin. Endocrinol. Metab., 62:1-6.

Dobi, S., Lenkey, B., 1982, Role of secretagogue immunoglobulin in gastric acid secretion. Acta Physiol. Acad. Sci. Hung., 69:9-25.

Doniach, D., 1976, Clinical observations and hypotheses related to TSH receptors. in 'Biochemical Basis of stimulation and thyroid hormone action', A.V. Muhlen & M. Schleusener, eds. Georg Thieme, Stuttgard, pp24-36.

Drexhage, H.A., Bottazzo, G.F., Bitensky, L., Chayen, J., Doniach, D., 1981, Thyroid growth-blocking antibodies in primary myxedema, Nature, 289:594-596.

Drexhage, H.A., Bottazzo, G.F., Doniach, D., Bitensky, L., Chayen, J., 1980, Evidence for thyroid growth stimulating immunoglobulins in some goitrous thyroid diseases, Lancet, ii:287-292.

Ealey, P.A., Emmerson, J.M., Bidey, S.P., Marshall, N.J., 1985, Thyrotropin stimulation of the rat thyroid cell strain FRTL-5: a metaphas index assay for the detection of thyroid growth stimulators. J. Endocrinol., 106:203-210.

Feldmann, M., Doniach, D., Bottazzo, G.F., 1986, The heterogeneity of autoimmune response. in 'Immunology of Rheumatic Disease' S. Gupta & N. Talal, eds., Plenum Pub., New York, pp271-300.

Feutren, G., Assau, R., Karrenty, G., DuRostu, H., Sizumai, J., Papoz, L., Vialettes, B., Vexian, P., Rodier, M., Lallemand, A., Bach, J.F., 1986, Cyclosporin increases the rate and length of remissions in insulin-dependent diabetes of recent onset - results of a multicentre double-blind trail, Lancet, i:119-124.

Foulis, A.K., Bottazzo, G.F., 1987, Insulitis - 1986. in 'The Pathology of the Endocrine Pancreas in Diabetes'. P. Lefebvre & D. Pipeleers Eds. Springer-Verlag, Berlin (in press).

Foulis, A.K. & Farquharson, M.A., 1986, Aberrant expression of HLA-DR antigens by insulin containing beta cells in recent onset Type I (insulin-dependent) diabetes mellitus, Diabetes, (in press).

Hanafusa, T., Pujol-Borrell, R., Chiovato, L., Doniach, D., Bottazzo, G.F., 1984, In vitro and in vivo reversal of thyroid epithelial polarity: its relevance for autoimmune thyroid disease. Clin. exp. Immunol., 57:639-646.

Hanafusa, T., Pujol-Borrell, R., Chiovato, L., Russell, R.C.G., Doniach, D. & Bottazzo, G.F., 1983, Aberrant expression of HLA-DR antigen on thyrocytes in Graves' disease: relevance for autoimmunity, Lancet, ii:1111-1115.

Hohlfeld, R., Toyka, K.V., Heininger, K., Gross-Wilde, H., Kalies, I., 1984, Autoimmune human T lymphocytes specific for acetylcholine receptor, Nature, 310:244-246.

Iwatani, Y., Gerstein, H.C, Iitaka, M., Row, U.U. & Volpe, R., 1986, Thyrocyte HLA-DR expression and interferon-gamma in autoimmune thyroid disease, J. Clin. Endocrinol. Metab., 63:695-708.

Jansson, R., Karlsson, A. & Forsum, U., 1985, Intrathyroid HLA-DR expression and T lymphocyte phenotypes in Graves' thyrotoxicosis, Hashimoto's thyroiditis and nodular colloid goitre, Clin. exp. Immunol., 58:264-272.

Jalkanen, S., Steere, A.C., Fox, R.I. & Butcher, E.C., 1986, A distinct endothelial cell recognition system that controls lymphocyte traffic into inflamed synovium, Science, 233:556-558.

Khoury, E.L., Bottazzo, G.F., Roitt, I.M., 1984, The thyroid 'microsomal' antibody revisited: Its paradoxical binding in vivo to the apical surface of the follicular epithelium, J. Exp. Med., 159: 577-591.

Khoury, E.L., Hammond, L., Bottazzo, G.F., Doniach, D., 1981, Presence of organ-specific 'microsomal' autoantigen on the surface of human thyroid cells in culture: its involvement in complement-mediated cytotoxicity, Clin. exp. Immunol., 45:316-328.

Lendrum, R., Walker, S.G., Gamble, D.R., 1975, Islet cell antibodies in juvenile diabetes mellitus of recent onset, Lancet, 1:880-882.

Londei, M., Bottazzo, G.F. & Feldmann, M., 1985, Human T cell clones from autoimmune thyroid glands: specific recognition of autologous thyroid cells. Science, 228:85-89.

Londei, M., Lamb, J.R., Bottazzo, G.F. & Feldmann, M., 1984, Epithelial cells expressing aberrant MHC Class II determinants can present antigen to cloned human T cells, Nature, 312:639-641.

Loveridge, N., Bitensky, L., Chayen, J., Hausamer, T.U., Fischer, J.M., Taylor, K.B., Gardner, J.D., Bottazzo, G.F., Doniach, D., 1980, Inhibition of parietal cell function by human gamma-globulin containing gastric parietal cell antibodies, Clin. exp. Immunol., 41:264-270.

Lucas-Martin, A., Foz, M., Todd, I., Bottazzo, G.F., Pujol-Borrell, R., Inappropriate HLA Class II expression in a wide variety of thyroid diseases, (submitted for publication).

Nitsch, L. & Wollman, S.H., 1980, Ultrastructure of intermediate stages in polarity reversal of thyroid epithelium in follicles in suspension culture. J. Cell. Biol., 86:875-882.

Nunez, G., Ball, E.J. & Stastny, P., 1983, Accessory cell function of human endothelial cells. I. A subpopulation of Ia positive cells is required for antigen presentation. J. Immunol., 131:666-673.

Pinchera, A., Fenzi, G.F., Mariotti, S., Vitti, P., Macchia, E., Chiovato, L., Marcocci, C., Bartalena, L., 1984, Membrane antigens in thyroid autoimmune diseases. in 'Endocrinology' F. Labri & L. Proulx, eds., Excerpta Medica, Amsterdam, pp 469-472.

Plotz, P.H., 1983, Autoantibodies are anti-idiotype antibodies to antiviral antibodies, Lancet, ii:824-826.

Pujol-Borrell, R., Hanafusa, T., Chiovato, L. & Bottazzo, G.F., 1983, Lectin-induced expression of DR antigen on human cultured follicular thyroid cells. Nature, 303:71-73.

Pujol-Borrell, R., Todd, I., Adolf, G.R., Feldmann, M. & Bottazzo, G.F., 1986a, In vivo and in vitro demonstration of HLA Class II products on human islet beta cells. in 'Proceedings of Symposium on Immunology of Diabetes, Edmonton, Canada, June 1986' G.D. Molnan & M.A. Jaworski, eds. (in press). Elsevier Science Publishers, Amsterdam.

Pujol-Borrell, R., Todd, I., Doshi, M., Gray, D., Feldmann, M. & Bottazzo, G.F., 1986b, Differential expression and regulation of MHC products in the endocrine and exocrine cells of the human pancreas, Clin. exp. Immunol., 65:128-139.

Sibley, D.K., Sutherland, D.F.R., Goetz, F.C., Michael, A.F. (1985). Recurrent diabetes mellitus in the pancreas iso and allograft : a light and electron microscopic and immuno-histochemical analysis. Lab. Invest., 53:132-145.

Smyth, P.P.A., McMullan, N.M., Grubeck-Loebenstein, B., O'Donovan, D., 1986, Thyroid growth-stimulating immunoglobulins in goitrous disease, Acta Endocrinol., in press.

Stiller, C.R., Dupre, J., Gent, M., Venmer, M.R, Keown, P.A., Laupacis, A., Martell, R., Rodger, N.W., Groffenied, B.V., Wolfe, B.J.J., 1984, Effect of cyclosporine immunosuppression in insulin-dependent diabetes mellitus of recent onset. Science, 223:1363-1367.

Todd, I., Abdul-Karim, B.A.S., Pujol-Borrell, R., Feldmann, M. & Bottazzo, G.F., 1986a, Dissection and characterization of the spontaneous and induced expression of HLA-D/DR by thyroid epithelium, in 'Frontiers in Thyroidology', Plenum Press, New York, pp. 1587-1592.

Todd, I., Lucas Martin, A., Abdul-Karim, B.A.S., Hammond, L.J. & Bottazzo, G.F., 1986b, HLA-D subregion expression by thyrocytes is associated with the occurrence of circulating thyroid autoantibodies, Ann d'Endocrinol, 47:20 (Abstract).

Todd, I., McNally, J.M., Hammond, L.J. & Pujol-Borrell, R., 1986c, TSH enhances expression by thyrocytes of interferon-gamma induced HLA-D/DR, in 'Frontiers in Thyroidology', Plenum Press, New York, pp. 1551-1554.

Todd, I., Pujol-Borrell, R., Hammond, L.J., Bottazzo, G.F., Feldmann, M., 1985. Interferon-gamma induces HLA-DR expression by thyroid epithelium. Clin. exp. Immunol., 61:265-273.

Todd, I., Pujol-Borrell, R., Londei, M., Feldmann, M., Bottazzo, G.F., 1986c, Inappropriate HLA Class II expression on epithelial cells: consolidation and progress. in 'The Thyroid and Autoimmunity', H.A. Drexhage and W.M. Wiersinga, eds. International Congress Series, 711. Excerpta Medica, Amsterdam, pp 112-138.

Van der Gaag, R.D., Drexhage, H.A., Dussault, J.H., 1985a, Role of maternal immunoglobulin blocking TSH-induced thyroid growth in sporadic forms of congenital hypothyroidism, Lancet, 1:246-250.

Van der Gaag, H.A., Drexhage, H.A., Wiersinga, W.M., Brown, R.S., Docter, R., Bottazzo, G.F., Doniach, D., 1985b, Further studies on thyroid growth-stimulating immunoglobulins in euthyroid nonendemic goiter, J. Clin. Endocrinol. Metab, 60:972-979.

Wulffraat, N.M. & Drexhage, H.A., 1986, Immunoglobulins stimulating and blocking adrenal growth, in: Proceedings of First International Conference on Hormones and Immunity, Toronto, July 1986, (Abstract).

Correspondence to:

G F Bottazzo
Department of Immunology
Arthur Stanley House
The Middlesex Hospital Medical School
40-50 Tottenham Street
London W1P 9PG, UK

MOLECULAR AND FUNCTIONAL CHARACTERIZATION OF GENES ENCODING ANTI-THYRO-

GLOBULIN AND ANTI-TSH RECEPTOR ANTIBODIES

Marc Monestier and Constantin A. Bona

Mount Sinai Medical Center
One Gustave Levy Place
New York, New York 10029

Autoimmune thyroiditis covers a wide spectrum of diseases ranging from hyperthyroid forms, like Graves' disease to hypothyroidism forms like Hashimoto's disease.

The major characteristic of these diseases is the presence of organ-specific autoantibodies specific for thyroid antigens. The presence of anti-thyroid antibodies is not associated with hyperglobulinemia as in SLE or with defects in the number or functions of T and B cells. While the autoantibodies found in Graves' disease stimulate the thyrocytes since they bind to TSH receptor (1) probably because they are anti-Id antibodies carrying the internal image of the receptor for thyrotrophine (2), the auto-antithyroglobulin antibodies have a distinctive effect (3) leading to thyroid atrophy like in atrophic autoimmune or Hashimoto thyroiditis or goiter formation like in goitrous autoimmune thyroiditis (4).

Distinctive effect of autoanti-TG antibodies was also demonstrated in experimental models. Thus, in mice, injection of thyroid extract or thyroglobulin in FCA results in the occurrence of autoanti-TG antibodies followed by lymphocyte infiltration which leads to lymphocyte thyroiditis (5). The production of autoanti-TG antibodies requires T cells and is under Ir gene control. Whereas mice of H-2^q,^{s},or^k haplotype are high responders, mice of H-2^d or ^{b} haplotypes are low responders (6). However, the "forbidden" TG-reactive clones can be activated in BALB/c mice by B cell polyclonal activators such as LPS.

Because of the prominent role of antithyroid antibodies in autoimmune thyroiditis, we have studied functional and molecular characteristics of murine anti-TG and anti-TSH receptor antibodies.

I. ORIGIN OF ANTI-THYROID ANTIBODIES

Our studies have been conducted on a panel of 19 monoclonal antithyroid antibodies from various origins (Table 1). Four thyroglobulin-specific antibodies have been obtained from BALB/c mice immunized with TG and six from CBA/J mice immunized with the same antigen. Five monoclonal antibodies have been obtained from 1-month-old "motheaten" mice and three from BALB/c and NZB splenic lymphocytes following in vitro stimulation with LPS.

Table 1. **Origin, specificity and isotypes of monoclonal antibodies**

Origin	Specificity	Designation and Isotypes	Reference
BALB/c immunized with TSH	TSH receptor	LE-4(γ1k)	(7)
BALB/c immunized with TG	TG	1-15(γ1k),62Id(γ1k) B10H$_2$A$_2$(γ1k),APDB6(γ1k)	(8)
CBA/J immunized with TG	TG	10.VA2(μk),10.IA1(γ1k)8.4A3 (μk),8.ID2(γ2bk),8.IB1(μk), 8.4D1(μk)	(9)
Motheaten "spontaneous"	TG	UN59-9(μk),UN37-5(μk),UN40-3(μk) UN40-6(μk),UN40-9(μk)	(10)
LPS stimulated BALB/c lymphocytes	TG	B93(μk)	(11)
LPS stimulated NZB lymphocytes	TG	Z113(μk),Z51(μk)	(11)

The data presented in Table 2 show the binding activity of the panel of anti-TG antibodies and the inhibition of this binding by 150ng of TG. The binding of this antibody to microtiter plates coated with TG was considerably higher than the background binding to BSA. Furthermore, various degrees of inhibition were obtained by preincubation of 500ng of antibody with 150ng of thyroglobulin. A single antibody obtained from LPS-stimulated BALB/c lymphocyte was not antigen-inhibitable.

Table 2. **Antigen inhibition of binding of monoclonal antibodies by thyroglobulin**

Antibody	Plates coated with BSA	TG	% inhibition with 150ng
Z51	550±61	2,754±587	24
Z113	681±43	5,242±717	15
B93	365±39	1,276±56	0
UN37-5	1,115±120	6,587±38	15
UN59-9	618±62	2,610±2	80
UN40-3	910±59	7,567±1134	50
UN40-6	1,181±54	16,741±267	40
UN40-9	1,330±24	9,933±184	70
8.I.B1	116±8	6,537±696	76

II. BINDING PROPERTIES OF ANTI-THYROID ANTIBODIES TO OTHER AUTOANTIGENS

There are numerous data indicating that monoclonal antibodies produced by B cells from young animals (12,13) exhibit binding to various autoantigens. It was therefore interesting to investigate whether or not our TG binding monoclonal antibodies exhibited binding to other autoantigens. In this experiment, we use a large panel of auto-Ag known to be involved in human or experimental auto-immune diseases such as DNA, (cardiolipin), Sm, Fc fragment of IgG, Collagen, Intrinsic factor, acetylcholine receptor transferrin, thymocytes, red blood cells, etc. Interestingly, we found that 7 MAb exhibited multispecific binding. Furthermore, in reciprocal competitive inhibition, we found that their binding is inhibited by auto-

antigens. A summary of these experiments is illustrated in Table 3.
Our data clearly show that antibodies obtained from "motheaten" mice or
from LPS stimulated lymphocytes obtained from "normal" strains (BALB/c)
or auto-immune prone strains (NZB) exhibit multispecific binding properties for various self-antigens including TG.

Table 3. Binding properties of TG specific antibodies to
          various auto-antigens

Monoclonal antibody	Binding specificity	Inhibition of binding (>50%)	
		to	by
UN59-9	MBP,TG	MBP	MBP,TG
		TG	TG
UN37-5	TG,AcR Fc	TG	TG,G2a
		AcR	AcR,G2a,TG
		IgG2a	G2a
B93	TG,Card	TG	none
		Card	none
Z113	TG,Card,Fc	TG	none
		Card	none
		IgG2a	none
UN40-3	IF,TG,AcR,Fc	IF	IF,TG
		TG	G2a,TG
		AcR	G2a,TG
		IgG2a	G2a,TG
UN40-6	TG,Sm,TF	TG	TG,MBP,G2a,Sm
	MBP,Fc	Sm	Sm,MBP,G2a
		TR	MBP,G2a
		MBP	MBP,TG,G2a,Sm
UN40-9	IF,TG,Fc	IF	IF,TG,G2a,Br-MRBC
	Br-MRBC	TG	TG,G2a,Br-MRBC
		Br-MRBC	TG,G2a,Br-MRBC
		IgG2a	IF,G2a,Br-MRBC

MBP-myelin basic protein, IF-intrinsic factor, TG-thyroglobulin,
ACR-acetylcholine receptor, TR-transferrin, Br-RBC-bromalin treated MRBC,
Card-cardiolipin.

III. BINDING OF TG-SPECIFIC AUTOANTIBODIES TO FOREIGN ANTIGENS

A major question related to auto-immune processes is whether or not
self-reactive clones can be expanded by autoantigens or by foreign antigens. We addressed this question by studying the binding of a panel of
auto-Ab encoded by V_H J558 genes to a large panel of foreign antigens known
to be bound by antibodies encoded by genes from the same family, J558. Surprisingly, we found two TG-specific antibodies deriving from CBA/J mice
immunized with TG which bound to two synthetic polypeptides (Table 6). This
81.B1 bound to GT (co-polymer of L-glutamic acid[50] and L-Tyrosine[50]) and
8.4A3 binds to GT and GLØ (co-polymer of L-glutamic acid[35], L-lysine[56]
and L-phenylalanine[9]).

The data presented in Table 4 show that the binding of these Ab to TG
was inhibited by auto-Ag as well as by synthetic peptides. Conversely, the
binding to synthetic peptides was inhibited by TG and by homologous synthetic peptides. This suggests strongly that this multiple binding is paratope-
inhibitable and not related to a non-specific protein-protein interaction.

Table 4. Inhibition of binding of V_H J558 TG-specific antibodies by foreign antigens

Monoclonal antibody (10µg/ml)	Binding to plates coated with	% of inhibition of binding with 15ng antigen/well		
		TG		GT
8.I.B1	TG 6,537±696*	76.3%		84.8%
	GT 5,070±347	74.4%		88.2%
		TG	GT	GLø
	TG 2,203±640	62.3%	80.3%	80.6%
	GT 2,905±654	52.5%		81.3%
	GLø 4,908±307	66.7%	31.4%	

*
cpm-average of triplicate ± SD
Microtiter plates coated with 10 µg/ml antigen, incubated with 10 µg/ml chromatographically purified antibody and then with ^{125}I-monoclonal rat anti-murine kappa antibody.

Since we found the unexpected reactivity of TG-specific autoantibodies with foreign antigens, we studied the presence of shared idiotypes of mono-clonal autoantibodies or antibodies specific for foreign antigens. The data presented in Table 5 show that five anti-TG antibodies share idiotopes of rheumatoid factors (LPS10-1), one Ab share idiotypes of anti-Sm anti-bodies (Y2) two with anti-DNA antibodies (H130), one express the J558 cross-reactive idiotype which dominate the anti-α1-3 dextran response, one shares an idiotype with Py211 specific for the influenza virus hemag-glutinin and another shares the cross-reactive idiotype of anti-arsonate Ab. These results clearly demonstrate that TG-specific autoantibodies share idiotopes of auto-Ab of other specificities and even with Ab specific for foreign antigens.

Table 5. Idiotypic cross-reactivity of thyroid-specific antibodies with various autoantibodies and antibodies specific for foreign antigens

Idiotypic systems	Specificity of idiotype	Antibodies exhibiting 50% inhibit-ion with 500ng chromatographically purified antibody
Y19-anti-LPS10	Fc fragment of IgG	10VA2,8.4A1,8.4A3,8.IB1,LE4
Y2-anti-Y2	Sm	Z113
H130-anti-H130	DNA	10VA2,8.I B1
J558-CD3-2	α1-3 dextran	8I B1
PY211-63.4	HA of PR8 influenza virus	8I D2
36-65-AD8	Arsonate	10VA3

V. V_H GENES USED BY ANTIBODIES SPECIFIC FOR THYROGLOBULIN AND TSH RECEPTOR

The RNA extracted from all hybridomas used in this study has been hybridized in Northern-blotting technique with 8 V_H probes, each one a prototype for a V_H gene family (14,15). The data presented in Table 6 show that 11 use genes for V_H7183, one from QPC52, 5 for J558 and one for J606. It appears that among our small panel of anti-TG antibodies, there is a high usage of the 3' V_H gene families.

Table 6. VH genes used by antibodies exhibiting specificity for thyroglobulin and TSH receptor

VH gene family

J606	UN37-5
J558	10VA2,8.4A3,8IB1,8ID2,UN59-9
QPC52	8.4D1
7183	10IA1, 1-15,62-Id,B10H$_2$A$_2$,UN40-9,UN40-6
	UN40-3,B93,Z113,Z51,B93,LE4

VI. DISCUSSION

Injection of mice with crude mouse thyroid extract or purified thyroblogulin results in lymphocytic thyroiditis associated with the production of anti-TG antibodies. The production of these autoantibodies is under Ir gene control; various strains of mice are low or high responders. BALB/c mice (H-2^b) are low responders to TG.

Nevertheless, we obtained TG specific monoclonal antibodies from spleen cells of BALB/c mice stimulated with LPS. This fact clearly proves that TG specific precursors are present in the repertoire of mice which do not develop autoimmune thyroiditis and are low responders. The LPS, a strong polyclonal activator, is able to break tolerance and to expand clones which are silent under physiological conditions.

We have also obtained TG specific MAbs from motheaten mice that undergo a persistent in vivo activation of B cells stimulated by the secretion of activating factors (16).

It is important to note that the majority of TG binding MAbs from LPS stimulated BALB/c lymphocytes or motheaten mice bound to other self-antigens. One of TG specific MAbs also binds to intrinsic factor. This kind of autoantibody could provide a clue for the concomitant appearance of pernicious anemia and autoimmune thyroiditis in some patients (17) and even for the existence of autoimmune processes affecting several organs such as polyendocrine syndrome.

In contrast, the study of binding of MAbs obtained from animals immunized with TG in FCA, to a large panel of foreign antigens showed that two of them bound to synthetic antigens GT and GLφ. This observation clearly suggests that TG reactive clones can be activated by foreign antigens. In addition, TG specific MAbs share idiotopes with either autoantibodies with various specificities or antibodies specific for foreign antibodies. Zanetti et al. (18) described in BALB/c and rat anti-TG antibodies, a shared regulatory idiotope. Murine and rat TG reactive clones expressing this idiotope can be expanded by the administoration of rabbit anti-Id antibodies.

These results indicate that TG-reactive clones can be activated either by foreign antigens or alternatively by anti-Id antibodies produced subsequent to stimulation by autoantibodies or antibodies specific for foreign antigens which share cross-reactive idiotopes with anti-TG antibodies.

In conclusion, our results suggest that the silent or forbidden TG reactive clones can be expanded by a multitude of factors including: polyclonal activators, either of microbial origin such as B cell mitogens or of endogenous origin such as the lymphokines, by the immunization with thyroglobulin, with foreign antigens or anti-idiotypic antibodies specific for cross-reactive idiotopes shared by TG specific antibodies and autoantibodies with different specificities or specific for foreign antigens. This latter idiotype determined cross-regulation phenomenon which we described in the case of antibody responses against foreign antigens (19) could play an important role in the activation of autoreactive clones and therefore could contribute to the onset of certain auto-immune diseases.

AKNOWLEDGEMENTS

This study was supported by grant AG/A 10271601 from the National Institute of Aging, United States Public Service.

REFERENCES

1. D.D. Adams and H.D. Purves, Proc. Univ. Otago Med. Sch. 34,11 (1956).
2. N.R. Farid and T.C.Y. Log, Endocrine Rev. 6,1-23 (1985).
3. I.M. Roitt, D. Doniach, and P.N. Campbell, Lancet 2,830 (1956).
4. T.F. Davies, and E. deBernardo, Auto-Immune Endocrine Diseases, J. Wiley & Sons, New York pp127-139, (1983).
5. N.R. Rose, F.J. Twarog, and A.J. Crowle, J. Immunol. 106,698 (1971).
6. K.W. Beisel and N.R. Rose, Auto-Immune Endocrine Diseases, J. Wiley & Sons, New York pp41-58 (1983).
7. W.L. Cleveland, N.H. Wasserman, P. Sarangurajan, A.S. Penn, and B.F. Erlanger, Nature (Lond) 305-56-57 (1983).
8. M. Zanetti, M. De Baets, and J. Rogers, J. Immunol. 131:2342-2457, (1983).
9. N.R. Rose, M.A. Accavitti, and M.A. Leon, In Antibodies: Protective, Destructive and Regulatory Role. F. Milgrom, C.J. Abeyounis, and B. Albini, editors, Karger, Basel, Switzerland 171-178 (1985).
10. C. Painter, M. Monestier, B. Bonin, and C.A. Bona, Immunol. Rev. 94:75-98, (1986).
11. B. Bellon, A. Manheimer-Lory, M. Monestier, T. Moran, A. Dimitriu-Bona, and C. Bona. (In press).
12. D. Holmberg, G. Wennerstrom, L. Andrade and A. Coutinho, Eur. J. Immunol 16:82-87 (1986).
13. P. Lymberi, G. Dighiero, T. Ternynck, and S. Avrameas, Eur. J. Immunol. 15:702-707 (1985).
14. P. Brodeur, and R. Riblet, Eur.J. Immunol. 14:922-930 (1984).
15. R. Dildrope, Immunology Today, 5,85 (1984).
16. C.L. Sidman, L.D. Schultz, and R. Evans, J. Immunol. 135,870-872, (1985).
17. D. Doniach and I.M. Roitt, in P.G.H. Gell, R.R.A. Coombs, and P.J. Lackmann, Eds. Clinical Aspects of Immunology, Blackwell Scientific Publications, Philadelphia p.1355, (1975).
18. M. Zanetti, Crit. Rev. Immunol, 6,151 (1986).
19. C. Kobrin - Victor, F.A. Bonilla, B. Bellon, and C.A. Bona, J.Exp.Med. 162-647, (1985).

AUTOANTIGENICITY OF MURINE THYROGLOBULIN

B. Champion, P. Hutchings, D. Rayner, K. Page, P. Byfield*,
J. Chan*, I. Roitt, and A. Cooke

Immunology Department, Moddlesex Hospital Medical School,
London, W1P 9PG, and *Endocrinology Department, Clinical
Research Centre, Harrow, Middx, U.K.

PRESENTATION OF THYROGLOBULIN BY PRIMED B-CELLS

It is only comparatively recently that convincing evidence has
emerged for the involvement of B-cells in antigen presentation[1,2,3,4].
Because of the unique binding property of the Ig receptor, the antigen
concentration for effective presentation may be many times lower than
that needed by a non-specific antigen presenting cell (APC)[3,5]. In
autoimmunity where antigen concentration may be limiting, presentation
by B-cells could play an important part in the development of disease,
particularly as it has been shown that such autoantigen-specific B-cells
do exist in the repertoire of normal individuals[6]. To test this
hypothesis, we have employed as a source of APC, normal murine B-cells
which have been primed in vivo to the autoantigen thyroglobulin (Tg).
B-cells obtained in this way were treated for their efficiency at
presenting Tg to CH9, an Lyl^+2^-, $L3T4^+$, $I-A^k$ restricted T-cell hybridoma
specific for Tg[7].

When Tg primed spleen cells were cultured with CH9, a concentration
of 0.1 to 1.0 μg/ml Tg was sufficient to activate the hybridoma cells.
Activation was measured by increased production of IL-2 which was
assayed using an IL-2-dependent CTL line as an indicator cell. In
contrast, when non-primed spleen cells were used as APC, comparable
activation was only seen at an antigen concentration of 50 μg/ml. High
efficiency antigen presentation by primed cells at 1 μg/ml was
unaffected by the removal of T-cells (anti-Thy 1.2 treatment), whereas
B-cell removal (treatment with the B-cell specific monoclonal antibody
LR-1; a gift from S. Marshall-Clarke, University of Liverpool)
completely abrogated presentation at 1 μg/ml while leaving presentation
at 50 μg/ml intact (Fig.1). This indicates the presence of at least two
distinct antigen presenting populations in primed spleen cells which
vary both in their sensitivity to LR-1 treatment and in the range of
antigen concentrations over which they are active. In non-primed spleen
cells, only the low efficiency component was detectable (at 50 μg/ml)
and this was resistant to both anti-Thy 1.2 and LR-1 treatment.

Because LR-1 is known also to affect dendritic cells (S. Knight,
personal communication), B-enriched rat Tg primed spleen cells were
further treated with 33D1 and rabbit complement to remove dendritic

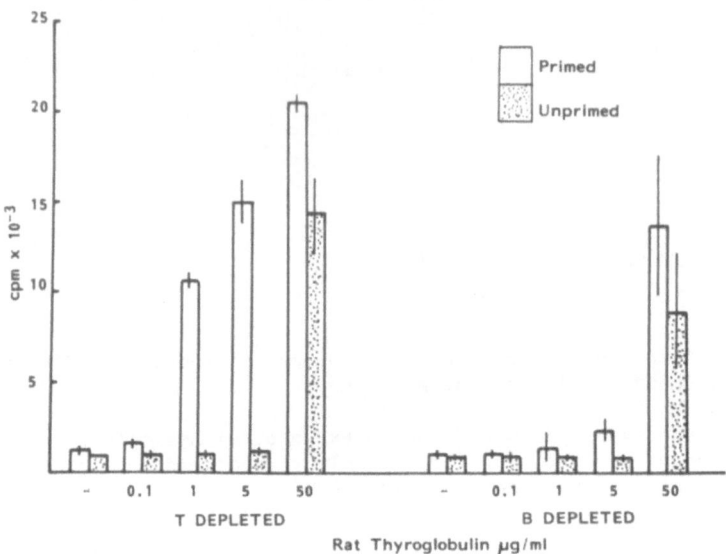

Fig. 1. EFFECT OF T- OR B- LYMPHOCYTE DEPLETION ON PRESENTATION OF Tg TO
CH9 BY PRIMED SPLEEN CELLS. Primed or non-primed spleen cells
were depleted of T- or B-cells as described in the text, irradiated
(2000R) and used to present rat Tg to the Tg-specific T-cell
hybridoma, CH9. Results are expressed as ^{125}I-deoxyuridine
incorporation by the IL-2-dependent CTLL cells cultured in supernatants (50%) from CH9 cultures (mean of triplicates + S.E.).

cells from the presenting population (33D1 is a monoclonal antibody
specific for dendritic cells, kindly provided by Dr. R. Steinman,
Rockefeller University, New York). Primed cells treated in this manner
presented rat Tg over a dose range of 1-50 µg/ml as efficiently as
primed cells treated with rabbit complement only. When mice were primed
with ovalbumin or rat Tg, presentation of rat Tg to CH9 at 1 µg/ml only
occurred with Tg primed cells, although all populations, regardless of
priming specificity, could present Tg at 50 µg/ml.

We next examined the role of the surface Ig receptor in the
efficient presentation by B-cells. Rat Tg primed B-cells were pulsed
overnight with rat Tg (1-10 µg/ml), washed twice and used to present to
CH9 without further addition of Tg. Such pulsed cells were efficient
presenters but if the primed B-cells were preincubated with sheep anti-
mouse F(ab')$_2$ (SaM) (50 µg/ml) for 30 minutes before the pulse,
presentation of antigen to CH9 was blocked (Fig.2). Preincubation with
purified normal sheep immunoglobulin however, had no effect on
presentation to CH9. In other experiments, preincubation with LR-1
(1/250), which is known to bind to a marker other than the surface Ig
receptor, also had no effect. Presentation was similarly blocked by
adding SaM directly to mixtures of B-cells, CH9 and Tg in culture.
These data indicate that B-cell surface immunoglobulin receptors are
involved in antigen specific presentation. There appears to be a

reciprocal interaction between CH9 and primed B-cells, since when CH9 is cultured with a T-cell depleted, primed spleen cell population and low concentrations of antigen, it can induce the primed B-cells to produce Tg antibody. This antibody was detected both in an Elispot assay which enumerates the specific antibody forming cells[8] and in a radioimmunoassay which measures the amount of antibody produced (Fig.3). Therefore, in this system, the primed B-cells not only present antigen

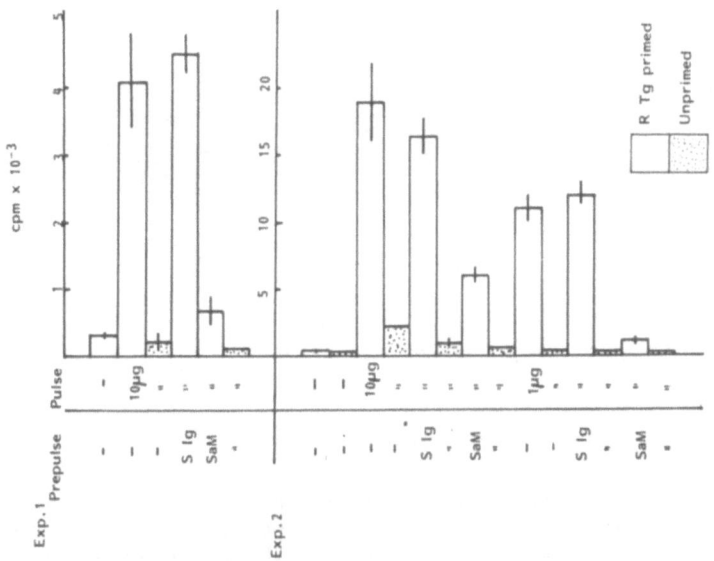

Fig. 2. BLOCKING OF PRESENTATION BY PRIMED B-CELLS WITH SHEEP ANTI-MOUSE F(ab')$_2$. Tg-primed B-cells were pulsed overnight with rat Tg and, where indicated, were prepulsed with sheep anti-mouse F(ab')$_2$ (SaM) or sheep immunoglobulin (SIg). Next day, the B-cells were washed and used to present rat Tg to CH9 as in Fig.1. No further antigen was added to the culture.

to the T-cells but the T-cells then provide help for the B-cells to produce specific antibody. In the system described here, it appears that B-cells primed to the autoantigen Tg, are capable of presenting that antigen to a T-cell hybridoma CH9, in a highly efficient and antigen-specific manner. It seems probable from the experiment using SaM to block the surface Ig receptors, that antigen binding to specific immunoglobulin on the B-cell is obligatory for presentation at low antigen concentrations. This supports observations by several other workers using foreign antigens[3,4,5].

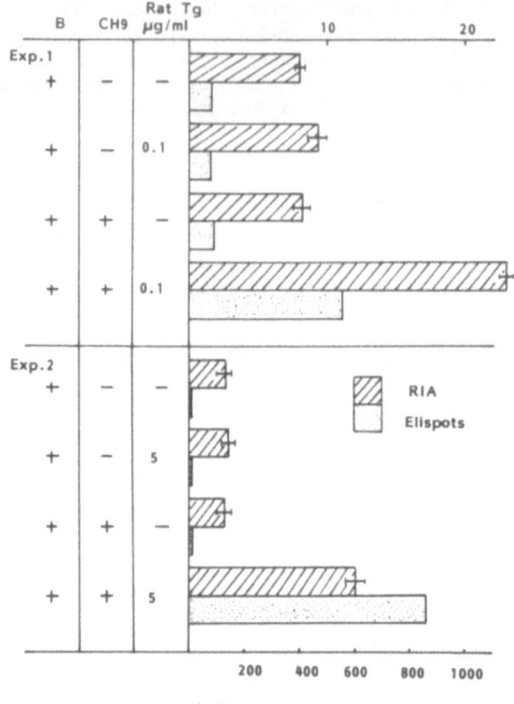

Fig. 3. RESPONSE OF PRIMED B-CELLS TO HELP PROVIDED BY STIMULATED CH9.
Rat Tg was presented to CH9 (irradiated, 1500R, to prevent over-
growth in cultures) by rat Tg primed B-cells. The ability of
such stimulated CH9 to help B-cell antibody production was
measured by an Elispot assay after 5 days of coculture. Secreted
anti-Tg antibody from these washed B-cells was also assessed by
RIA after a further 7 days in culture.

Removal of dendritic cells by treatment with 33D1 did not affect
presentation at low antigen concentrations. However, this does not
preclude dendritic cells from being involved in presenting Tg at higher
antigen concentrations; the role of dendritic cells in primary
responses to a variety of antigens is well documented[9,10]. It is
unlikely that there are enough antigen specific B-cells in non-primed
animals to contribute significantly to presentation of antigen during a
primary response.

We show here that not only do Tg-primed B-cells present antigen to
CH9 at low concentrations, but that they can subsequently be induced by
stimulated CH9 to secrete anti-Tg antibodies. B-cell presentation may
represent a means by which an initial triggering event, priming both B-
and T-cells, may allow maintenance of autoreactive responses in vivo in
the presence of low concentrations of circulating antigen.

THE ROLE OF IODINATION IN AUTOANTIGENICITY

A number of studies have suggested a link between the level of dietary iodine and the incidence of thyroid autoimmunity both in man[11,12] and experimental animals[13,14]. Since the thyroid gland incorporates iodine into Tg for the synthesis of the thyroid hormones thyroxine (T_4) and tri-iodothyronine (T_3), it seems reasonable to suggest that iodination influences the immunogenicity of Tg. Sundick and colleagues[15] have shown recently that highly iodinated chicken Tg is more autoimmunogenic than poorly iodinated Tg. Although the immunologic basis for this observation is not yet clear, one possibility is that T-cells will only recognise Tg when it is sufficiently iodinated. We have analyzed our mouse autoreactive T-cell lines and hybridomas specific for murine Tg[7,16] for their ability to recognise Tg iodinated to different degrees. For simplicity, the results with one T-cell clone (MTg9B3) will be presented although a second, independently-derived cloned T-cell population gave similar results.

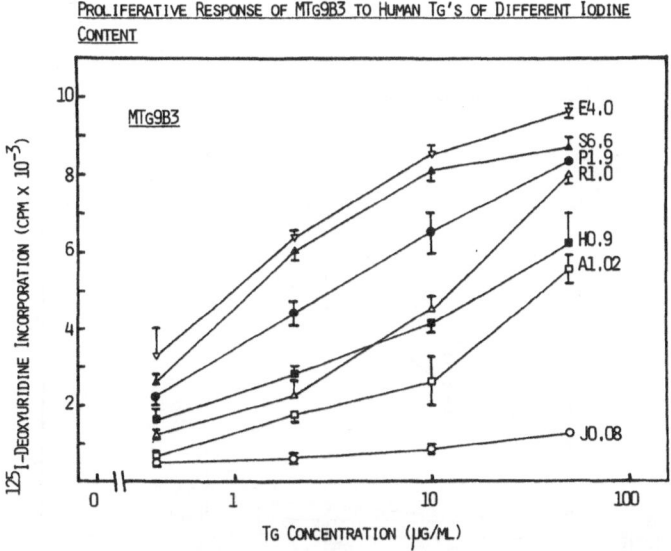

PROLIFERATIVE RESPONSE OF MTg9B3 TO HUMAN Tg'S OF DIFFERENT IODINE CONTENT

Fig. 4. EFFECT OF IODINATION ON ANTIGENICITY OF HUMAN Tg. The Tg-specific T-cell clone (MTg9B3) was tested in a 3-day proliferation assay, using syngeneic irradiated spleen cells to present antigen, for its ability to respond to a panel of human Tg's differing in their degree of iodination(prepared from post-mortem thyroid tissue). The different preparations are labelled with their code-letter and degree of iodination represented by their T_4 content (T_4 residues per mole Tg). Proliferative responses were assessed by the incorporation of ^{125}I-deoxyuridine.

The mouse autoreactive Tg-specific clones have been shown to recognise an epitope which is also present on human Tg[7],[17]. We tested MTg9B3 for its ability to respond to a panel of human Tg's, which differed in their degree of iodination (as measured by their content of T_4 and T_3). As shown in Fig.4, the level of response was dependent upon the degree of Tg iodination. Thyroglobulins with very low iodine content (J0.08 in Fig.4 and others not shown) failed to stimulate the T-cells. The level of response did not show a strict rank-order correlation with iodine content, but this is not surprising since a number of tyrosine residues can be iodinated and it is not yet known which region of the Tg molecule is recognised by the T-cell clone.

To substantiate these observations, we prepared normal (iodinated) and non-iodinated mouse Tg from matched groups of mice. Non-iodinated Tg was produced by supplementing the diet with the peroxidase-blocking drug, aminotriazole (ATA), for 3-6 weeks prior to collecting the thyroids. This procedure induced large goitrous thyroids, the Tg from which was shown to have undetectable levels of T_4 (compared with approximately 3 T_4 residues per mole for normal Tg). These Tg preparations were then examined for their ability to trigger MTg9B3. As shown in Fig.5, two separate preparations of non-iodinated Tg (ATA Tg) were unable to stimulate the T-cell clone, whilst the normally-iodinated Tg preparations triggered the cells perfectly well. This confirms the observation made with human Tg preparations, that this T-cell clone will only recognise Tg if it is sufficiently iodinated. As stated previously, this conclusion is also true for another independently-derived Tg-specific T-cell clone.

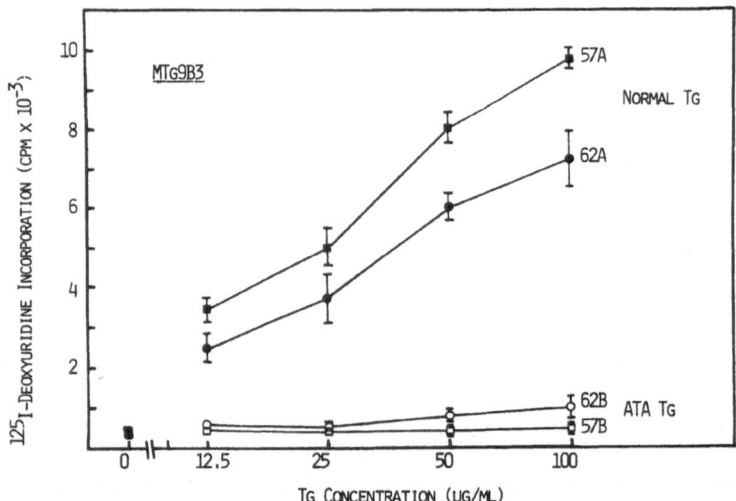

Fig. 5. EFFECT OF IODINATION ON ANTIGENICITY OF MOUSE Tg. MTg9B3 T-cells were tested in a proliferation assay (as described in Fig.4) for their ability to respond to normal and non-iodinated (ATA) Tg preparations. Two separate preparations (57 and 62) of each Tg were made from groups of sibling mice. Normally iodinated Tg (57A and 62A) was prepared from mice on a conventional diet where-as non-iodinated Tg was prepared from mice which had their diet supplemented with the peroxidase-blocking drug aminotriazole (ATA) for three (57B) or six (62B) weeks.

This observation in the mouse appears to be specific for T-cells since, unlike data from chickens[15], Tg autoantibodies (both polyclonal and monoclonal) fail to discriminate between normal and non-iodinated autologous Tg preparations (data not shown). Preliminary observations also indicate that non-iodinated mouse Tg may be unable to induce thyroiditis when injected with an appropriate adjuvant. If confirmed, this implies that iodination of Tg is a requirement for recognition by T-cells involved in pathogenesis but not for all T-helper cells important in antibody production.

The mechanistic basis for the involvement of Tg iodination in antigen recognition by these T-cells is still open to speculation. An iodinated tyrosine residue (mono- or di-iodotyrosine) or thyroid hormone (T_3 or T_4) may form part of the epitope recognised by the T-cell or may be important for the appropriate association of correctly processed Tg with the MHC class II molecule (I-A^k in this case). Alternatively, iodination may be important for the correct processing of Tg by the antigen presenting cell. A further possibility is the involvement of dehydroalanine residues created in the molecule at the site of donor tyrosine residues used to form T_4 and T_3. We are currently attempting to determine which of these (or other) possibilities are correct by further characterization of the epitope(s) using Tg fragments.

It is tempting to speculate that the influence of dietary iodine on human thyroid autoimmunity might be due to a similar mechanism to that described here, although there is as yet no data available to support this. Since the thyroid is very efficient at producing T_3 and T_4 residues even under conditions of low iodine content, it may be that the important regions of Tg are those tyrosine residues not involved in hormonogenesis.

REFERENCES

1. R. Chesnut and H. Grey, _J. Immunol._ 126:1075 (1981).
2. R. Shimonkevitz, J. Kappler, P. Marrack and H. Grey, _J. Exp. Med._ 158:303 (1983).
3. K.L. Rock, B. Benacerraf and A.K. Abbas, _J. Exp. Med._ 160:1102 (1984).
4. A. Lanzavecchia, _Nature_ 314:537 (1985).
5. A.K. Abbas, S. Haber and K.L. Rock, _J. Immunol._ 135:1661 (1985).
6. A.D. Bankhurst, G. Torrigiani and A.C. Allison, _Lancet_ i:226 (1973).
7. D.C. Rayner, P.J. Delves, D. Warren, I.M. Roitt and B.R. Champion, _Immunology_ (in press).
8. J.D. Sedgwick and P.G. Holt, _J. Immunol. Meth._ 57:301 (1983).
9. K. Inaba, M.D. Witmer and R.M. Steinman, _J. Exp. Med._ 160:858 (1984).
10. G.H. Sunshine, D.R. Katz and M. Feldmann, _J. Exp. Med._ 152:1817 (1980)
11. D.K. Weaver, R.H. Nishiyama, W.D. Burton and J.G. Batsakis, _Arch. Surg._ 92:796 (1966).
12. W.H. Beierwaltes, _Bull. All. India Med. Sci._ 3:145 (1969).
13. N. Bagchi, T.R. Brown, E. Urdanivia and R.S. Sundick, _Science_ 230:325 (1985).
14. E.M. Allan, M.C. Appel and L.E. Braverman, _Endocrinology_ 118:1977 (1986).
15. R.S. Sundick, D.M. Herdegen, T.R. Brown and N. Bagchi, _J. Exp. Med._ (in press).
16. B.R. Champion, P. Hutchings, S. Davies, S. Marshall-Clarke, A. Cooke and I.M. Roitt, _Immunology_ 58:51 (1986).
17. B.R. Champion, A-M. Varey, D. Katz, A. Cooke and I.M. Roitt, _Immunology_ 54:513 (1985).

IgG SUBCLASS DISTRIBUTION OF ANTI-Tg ANTIBODIES AMONG THYROID DISEASE

PATIENTS AND THEIR RELATIVES AND IN HIGH AND LOW RESPONDER MOUSE STRAINS[*]

N.R. Rose, I.M. Outschoorn[**], C.L. Burek, and R.C. Kuppers

Department of Immunology and Infectious Diseases
The Johns Hopkins University
Baltimore, Maryland 21205, U.S.A.

INTRODUCTION

A large body of clinical and experimental evidence points to a genetic predisposition toward the development of autoimmune thyroid disease.
During the past several years, work in our laboratory[1] as well as by
others[2] has resulted in significant progress in sorting out the several
genetic factors that influence thyroid autoimmunity in human populations.
In these investigations, we have derived considerable benefit from our
earlier analyses of the genetic determinants of autoimmune thyroiditis in
the Obese strain (OS) chicken.[3] This strain of birds develops a spontaneous form of thyroiditis that closely resembles human Hashimoto's disease.
It is marked by extensive mononuclear infiltration of the thyroid gland
and production of thyroid-specific autoantibodies, especially to thyroglobulin (Tg). In our studies of the OS chicken, the key finding was that
the occurrence of disease is not the result of any single gene, but rather
a conglomeration of several unrelated genetic lesions.[4,5] We found no
evidence for "disease susceptibility" genes as such. Rather, our findings
suggested that genes widely distributed among chickens derived from the
original Cornell colony have a number of consequences that, in the aggregate, favor the spontaneous development of autoimmune thyroid disease.
We recognize that this view differs substantially from that of many other
investigators, who suggest that etiology of autoimmune disease is based on
an abnormal gene in the major histocompatibility complex (MHC).[6]

---

[*] This study was supported by grants from the National Institutes of
Health, #AG04362, #AI21088, #AM31632, and #AR35383.
[**]Present address: Centro Nacional de Microbiologia, Majadahonda, Madrid,
Spain.

Our conclusions derive largely from investigations by our own group and those of Wick and his colleagues,[7] which have delineated at least three broad categories of genes that seem to favor the development of thyroid autoimmunity. The first set of genetic traits is associated with the MHC of the chicken, the B-locus.[8] Based on parallel studies in the mouse, it seems likely that this gene, or set of genes, regulates the immune response to thyroglobulin.

We later found evidence for a second, independent genetic abnormality in some members of the OS.[9] The major impact of this lesion is on the developmental sequence of T-cell subpopulations in the thymus, so that thymic cells that are mainly suppressive in their function emigrate from the gland somewhat later than T cells with a helper-inducer function. Evidence for a thymic lesion is based both on indirect functional studies as well as on direct investigations of the thymic cells.[10]

Finally, there is an increasing body of evidence pointing to an intrinsic defect in the thyroid gland of OS and related strains of chickens. The probable effect of this lesion is to alter the incorporation of iodide into thyroglobulin, an abnormality that seems to increase the immunogenicity of this molecule. These important studies, carried out primarily by Sundick and his colleagues,[11,12] emphasize the importance of a physiological lesion in the target tissue for the development of the pathological manifestations of thyroiditis.

It is useful to compare the interplay of these three types of lesions with respect to the development of an organ-localized disease, such as thyroiditis. The defects in the immunoregulatory system associated with the MHC give rise to a more vigorous response to one, or a small number of, epitopes on the thyroglobulin molecule and, therefore, can be considered antigen-specific. The abnormality in thymus function, on the other hand, pertains to a number of immunological responses and perhaps is the explanation for the production by OS chickens of several autoantibodies in addition to the antibodies to thyroglobulin. It should be noted that these additional autoantibodies do not usually result in disease. Finally, the genetic lesions of the thyroid gland suggest that there may be thyroid abnormalities in the OS, which may or may not pertain to an autoimmune response. The juxtaposition of these three apparently unrelated lesions, however, produces the thyroid specificity of the autoimmune process.

GENETICS OF EXPERIMENTAL AUTOIMMUNE THYROIDITIS IN THE MOUSE

Experimental autoimmune thyroiditis (EAT) can be induced in mice by injection of mouse thyroglobulin (MTg) with an adjuvant, such as complete Freund's adjuvant (CFA). Some mouse strains are highly susceptible to EAT,

producing elevated titers of antibodies to thyroglobulin and severe
lesions; other strains are relatively resistant, as evidenced by lower
antibody titers and minimal or no lesions in their thyroids. The availability of inbred mouse strains allowed us to map the major gene predisposing to EAT to the MHC, a finding that was directly confirmed using
congenic strains. Strains of the H-2 k, s or q haplotypes were designated high responders, whereas strains with the b, d, g, i or v haplotypes
were low responders [13] The susceptibility to EAT is inherited as an autosomal dominant, since F_1 animals between high- and low-responder parents
are generally good responders. In the F_2 generation, high response segre-
gates with the high-responder H-2 haplotype.

Detailed studies, using intra-H-2 recombinant mouse strains, permitted
further localization of the major MHC gene controlling the EAT to the I-A
locus.[14] This gene has been referred to as Ir-Tg. The basic pattern of
H-2-regulated response to MTg has been shown to hold, regardless of the
particular procedure or adjuvant used for inducing disease; for example,
Okayasu[15] has found similar genetic control of thyroiditis induced by thyroid transplantation to the renal capsule together with injections of
lipopolysaccharide. Thus, it is safe to conclude that the immune responsiveness relates to recognition of the thyroglobulin rather than to the
action of an auxiliary factor, such as adjuvant.

Cell transfers were carried out in order to determine the cellular
basis of genetic control of the immune response. Mice reconstituted with
T lymphocytes from good responder strains developed high responses to
thyroglobulin, whereas animals reconstituted with T cells from poor responder strains developed only low responses. Therefore, the site of genetic
regulation is the T-cell population rather than other immunologically
active cells or the thyroid gland itself.[16] The responsible population of
T cells was identified as the helper-inducer subset of Lyt 1+ cells by
means of lymphocyte proliferation assays.[17] In adoptive transfer experiments with EAT, lymphocytes were primed in vivo with MTg and adjuvant and
then restimulated in vitro with MTg. Only activated lymphocytes from good
responder strains of mice were able to transfer disease.[18] A similar pattern of I-A-determined responsiveness was found by Salamero and
Charreire[19] by in vitro induction of thyroid autoimmunity.

Initial studies by Tomazic et al.[20] suggested that additional genetic
controls of the response to thyroiditis are encoded to the right of I-A in
the H-2 region. Using intra-H-2 recombinant mice, a second locus of genetic control was traced to the D end of H-2.[21] This locus dealt primarily
with the severity of thyroid lesions rather than the titers of antibodies
to thyroglobulin. The K end of H-2 also seems to affect the development of

thyroid lesions.[22] These findings suggest that the Class I gene products, H-2D and H-2K, are restricting elements for the cytotoxic effector cells of autoimmune thyroiditis, whereas Class II gene products, such as Ia, are involved in recognition of thyroglobulin and initiation of the immune response.

MHC genes are the major elements determining the autoimmune response to MTg. In addition, genes outside of the MHC affect the disease process. A clear indication of the influence of non-MHC genes can be seen when strains of mice matched at the H-2 region but varying in background genes are compared. Significant differences in antibody titers and incidence of disease can be shown to depend upon non-H-2 background genes. We have been exploring these non-H-2 genes, using recombinant-inbred and congenic strains of mice. It has been possible to localize one gene influencing the autoantibody titer to MTg to chromosome 12. The gene appears to map close to the 5'-end of the Igh-V complex. The results suggested that the IgG subclass distribution of the anti-MTg antibody response may be controlled by gene(s) linked to or within the Igh locus.

To investigate the role of Igh-V genes in regulating the distribution of antibody subtypes, we have examined the influence of the Igh haplotype on isotype expression of MTg antibodies in a large number of strains of inbred mice. The relative IgG subclass distribution was measured using an ELISA assay. Animals were immunized with MTg in CFA and bled periodically to trace their relative IgG subclass distribution. The IgG-1 subclass was dominant in the anti-MTg response. The IgG-3 subclass was present only in very small amounts and often not detectable. IgG-2b antibody was found in all strains and IgG-2a in most strains tested. However, C57BL/6 mice failed to produce a significant IgG-2a antibody response to MTg. This subclass restriction did not apply to unrelated antigens given to the same strain of mice.

To determine directly whether the diminished IgG-2a response of C57BL/6 mice to MTg was due to the Igh^b gene, we tested the congenic CBA and CBA-Igh^b strains. Since both of these strains are H-2^k, they are high responders to MTg and differ only around the Igh locus. The Igh^b-bearing strain failed to produce a significant IgG-2a response to MTg. Nevertheless, the overall response of CBA-Igh^b mice to MTg was as high or higher than that of the comparable CBA mice, indicating that the anti-MTg response in other subclasses was raised.

To confirm the location of the gene regulating the IgG-2a response to MTg, BXH recombinant-inbred mice were tested. These strains represent genetic mixtures of C3H and C57BL/6 parental lines. These experiments also mapped regulation of the IgG-2a response to the IgH region.

These findings make it clear that one of the non-H-2 genes regulating the immune response of mice to MTg is closely associated with the IgH locus. The cellular basis of this regulation has not yet been determined, but we suggest that it is based on a T-cell restriction in the subclass switching of the MTg response. Further experiments are necessary to ascertain what effect, if any, this subclass restriction has on the pathological changes in the thyroid gland.

ISOTYPE DISTRIBUTION OF HUMAN ANTI-THYROGLOBULIN IgG ANTIBODIES

In most respects, the principal genetic traits influencing thyroid autoimmunity in mice have found their counterparts in humans. The major genetic risk factor in autoimmune thyroid disease is the human MHC, HLA. A second level of genetic control is associated with the Gm allotype, suggesting the IgG heavy chain may also be involved.[23] We decided, therefore, to investigate the isotype distribution of thyroid autoantibodies to see if we could find evidence of IgG subclass restriction.

Among patients with autoimmune thyroid disease, the distribution of antibodies to human thyroglobulin (HTg) among Ig classes and subclasses has remained controversial for more than twenty years. Early reports showed that HTg antibodies can occur in IgM, IgA and IgG isotypes and in all four IgG subclasses.[24,25,26] More recent reports have pointed to a possible subclass restriction, mainly to the IgG-4 subclass.[27,28,29] Since the question may be important in deciding on the origin of autoantibodies to thyroglobulin, we reinvestigated isotype distribution using a unique collection of serum samples from juvenile patients with chronic lymphocytic thyroiditis or thyrotoxicosis, from their parents and siblings, and from healthy, age-matched controls.[30,31] In some instances, two or three serum samples were available at two- to four-year intervals over an eight-year period, enabling a long-term study to be undertaken. An occasional sibling developed thyroiditis or thyrotoxicosis during the eight-year study period. Several sets of identical twins were also included. Subclass distribution was determined with an ELISA, using monoclonal antibodies of defined specificity.

In comparing juvenile patients with thyrotoxicosis with those having chronic lymphocytic thyroiditis, it was evident that subclass restriction was marked in some thyrotoxicosis patients. Black patients with thyrotoxicosis were especially striking in subclass restriction; for instance, of 7 black patients examined, only 1 had anti-HTg in all four subclasses, while 2 had IgG-1 antibodies exclusively and the remainder had antibody in the IgG-1 and IgG-3 subclasses. Among white children with thyrotoxicosis, most had Tg antibodies in all four subclasses, but 2 of 9 patients had antibodies only in the IgG-1 subclass. Where it was possible to follow the patients, these subclass restrictions diminished over the eight-year observation period.

Among parents of the thyrotoxicosis patients, 19 of 32 showed antibody to HTg. Of these, 6 of 12 were restricted to the IgG-1 subclass and 1 to the IgG-3 subclass. It was also possible to compare the patients with their unaffected siblings. In this population, antibodies to HTg were relatively prevalent. Among the unaffected brothers and sisters of the juvenile thyrotoxicosis patients, titers were generally low and, in many cases, found only in the IgG-1 subclass.

Of 12 juvenile patients with chronic lymphocytic thyroiditis, 6 had antibody in all four IgG subclasses; 3 in IgG-1, IgG-2, and IgG-3; 1 each in IgG-1 and IgG-3 or IgG-1 and IgG-2; and 2 in IgG-1. Thus, no particular pattern of isotype restriction was characteristic of the disease, nor were there any pronounced differences in the distribution of subclasses comparing patients with their unaffected siblings. However, 5 of 23 parents of the juvenile thyroiditis patients showed antibody restricted to IgG-1.

In studies of humans with autoimmune thyroid disease and their relatives, therefore, 50% of thyrotoxicosis patients and their asymptomatic family members showed HTg antibodies mainly or exclusively in the IgG-1 subclass. Antibodies seemed to appear first in this subclass, followed over time by IgG-3 or IgG-4, with IgG-2 appearing last. This sequential appearance of subclass-specific anti-HTg, as seen best in thyrotoxicosis patients and their asymptomatic relatives, was not so readily appreciable in cases of chronic lymphocytic thyroiditis.

To summarize, in thyroiditis families all possible subclass combinations occurred. The relatively minor contribution of the IgG-2 subclass is analogous to the very minor contribution of mouse IgG-3 subclass to the anti-MTg response. Serum samples obtained at two- to four-year intervals from thyrotoxicosis or thyroiditis patients showed significantly more patients than unaffected siblings had anti-HTg antibody in all four IgG subclasses.

DISCUSSION

The antibody response to thyroglobulin is controlled by a number of different genes. The MHC, in particular the I-A subregion, has been shown to be the major locus in regulating the recognition of MTg in mice. This H-2 influence on the anti-MTg response is at the level of T cells and probably determined by the magnitude of T-cell proliferation to MTg during initiation of the immune response. This MHC regulation itself may be complex, since the control of induction of the immune response and production of autoantibodies differs from regulation of the cellular functions responsible for thyroid lesions. Even the inductive phase of the immune response itself depends on the balance of two T-cell populations with differing genetic controls, one favoring the development of the immune response, a T_H subpopulation, and the second depressing antibody production, development of lesions and T-cell proliferation, a T_S subpopulation.[15] Control of the helper response is based mainly at the I-A locus, whereas the putative suppressor cell population is regulated by a gene, or genes, to the right of I-A, perhaps at I-E. On the other hand, the cytotoxic effects of the immune response to thyroglobulin are regulated by genes at the D end and the K end of the H-2 complex.

We have now found that the Igh region on chromosome 12 plays an important role in regulating the antibody response to MTg. The responsible genes reside within the boundaries of the Igh locus or are closely linked to that locus. Although Igh-associated genes affect the antibody response, their influence seems to be less in magnitude than the MHC-associated genes.

Igh-linked variable-region structural genes have been shown to influence the antibody response to several antigens through changes in fine specificity, affinity or idiotypic expression. One explanation for these findings is that there is a favored selection of V_H used in the MTg response according with the IgG-2a heavy chain allele. It is also possible that isotype selection depends upon isotype-specific helper T cells, such cells may not be stimulated in the presence of Igh^b-bearing B cells specific for MTg. In any case, it is clear that a gene associated with the Igh locus regulates the subclass distribution of antibodies to MTg.

In humans, subclass restriction is much more problematical. It does appear, however, that in selected populations of juvenile patients with thyrotoxicosis there is relative restriction of IgG subclass during the earliest immune response. Later, there is a broadening in subclass distribution, so that in most patients with fully developed thyrotoxicosis or lymphocytic thyroiditis HTg autoantibodies are found in all IgG subclasses.

SUMMARY

The genetic influence on subclass distribution was studied in the mouse experimental autoimmune thyroiditis (EAT) model and in human serum samples from patients and their first-degree relatives taken over an eight-year period. An IgG subclass-specific ELISA assay for thyroglobulin-specific antibody was developed, which was sensitive enough to detect subclass differences even in low-titer sera. The murine EAT model clearly demonstrates that genetic control of anti-Tg antibody responses is regulated by the MHC (H-2) region. In the mouse, the studies show a linkage of the control of subclass distribution to the IgG heavy chain locus. It could be mapped using several strains, including mice congenic around the Igh locus and in recombinant-inbred strains. Mouse strains bearing the IgH^b haplotype only produced minor amounts of IgG-2a antibodies. Data from both the congenic strains CBA versus CBA-Igh^b and from the BXH recombinant-inbred mouse strains map this restriction in response to the Igh locus. In the human studies, sera from families of juvenile patients suffering from chronic lymphocytic thyroiditis or thyrotoxicosis were examined. In 50% of thyrotoxicosis patients and in asymptomatic family members, Tg antibodies seemed to appear first in the IgG-1 subclass followed over time by IgG-3 or IgG-4, with IgG-2 appearing last. The sequential appearance of subclass-specific anti-Tg antibodies as seen in the thyrotoxicosis families was not so readily appreciable in the case of the patients with chronic lymphocytic thyroiditis and their relatives. Combinations of IgG-1 together with IgG-2, IgG-3 and IgG-4 were occasionally found in thyrotoxicosis families, while in families with chronic lymphocytic thyroiditis all possible subclass combinations could occur. The relatively minor contribution of the IgG-2, at least among the thyrotoxicosis patients, is analogous to the very minor contribution of the mouse IgG-3 subclass to the anti-Tg responses. Serum samples obtained at two- to four-year intervals from seven thyrotoxicosis families and eight families with chronic lymphocytic thyroiditis showed significantly more patients than unaffected siblings had anti-Tg antibody in all four IgG subclasses.

REFERENCES

1. N. R. Rose and C. L. Burek, The genetics of thyroiditis as a prototype of human autoimmune disease, Ann. Allergy 54:261 (1985).
2. N. R. Farid and J. C. Bear, Autoimmune endocrine disorders and the major histocompatibility complex, in: "Autoimmune Endocrine Disease," T. F. Davies, ed., John Wiley & Sons, New York (1983).
3. N. R. Rose, Y. M. Kong, I. Okayasu, A. A. Giraldo, K. Beisel, and R. S. Sundick, T-cell regulation in autoimmune thyroiditis, Immunol. Rev. 55:299 (1981).
4. N. R. Rose, L. D. Bacon, R. S. Sundick, and Y. M. Kong, The role of genetic factors in autoimmunity, in: "The Menarini Series on Immuno-pathology - First Symposium on Organ Specific Autoimmunity," P. A. Miescher, L. Bolis, S. Gorini, T. A. Lambo, G. J. V. Nossal, and G. Torrigiani, eds., Schwabe and Co., Ltd., Basel (1978).
5. N. R. Rose, Y. M. Kong, and R. S. Sundick, The genetic lesions of auto-immunity, Clin. Exp. Immunol. 39:545 (1980).
6. G. T. Nepom, HLA Class II variants: Structural studies and disease associations, in: "Autoimmunity: Experimental and Clinical Aspects," B. Boland, J. Cullinan, and S. Malmoli, eds., The New York Academy of Sciences, New York (1986).
7. G. Wick, R. Boyd, K. Hála, L. de Carvalho, P.-U. Müller, and R. K. Cole, The Obese strain (OS) of chickens with spontaneous autoimmune

thyroiditis: Review of recent data, Curr. Top. Microbiol. Immunol. 91:109 (1981).

8. L. D. Bacon, J. H. Kite, Jr., and N. R. Rose, Relation between the major histocompatibility (B) locus and autoimmune thyroiditis in obese chickens, Science 186:274 (1974).

9. M. Jakobisiak, R. S. Sundick, L. D. Bacon, and N. R. Rose, Abnormal response to minor histocompatibility antigens in Obese strain chickens, Proc. Natl. Acad. Sci. 73:2877 (1976).

10. M. D. Livezey, R. S. Sundick, and N. R. Rose, Spontaneous autoimmune thyroiditis in chickens. II. Evidence for autoresponsive thymo-cytes, J. Immunol. 127:1469 (1981).

11. R. S. Sundick and G. Wick, Increased iodine uptake by Obese strain thyroid glands transplanted to normal chick embryos, J. Immunol. 116:1319 (1976).

12. M. D. Livezey and R. S. Sundick, Intrinsic thyroid hyperreactivity in avian strains susceptible to autoimmune thyroiditis, Gen. Comp. Endocrinol. 41:243 (1980).

13. K. W. Beisel and N. R. Rose, Genetics of the autoimmune endocrino-pathies: Animal models, in: "Autoimmune Endocrine Disease," T. Davies, ed., John Wiley & Sons, New York (1983).

14. K. W. Beisel, C. S. David, A. A. Giraldo, Y. M. Kong, and N. R. Rose, Regulation of experimental autoimmune thyroiditis: Mapping of sus-ceptibility to the I-A subregion of the mouse H-2, Immunogenetics 15:427 (1982).

15. I. Okayasu and S. Hatakeyama, A combination of necrosis of autologous thyroid gland and injection of lipopolysaccharide induces auto-immune thyroiditis, Clin. Immunol. Immunopathol. 31:344 (1984).

16. A. O. Vladutiu and N. R. Rose, Cellular basis of the genetic control of immune responsiveness to murine thyroglobulin in mice, Cell Immunol. 17:106 (1975).

17. I. Okayasu, Y. M. Kong, C. S. David, and N. R. Rose, In vitro T-lymphocyte proliferative response to mouse thyroglobulin in experi-mental autoimmune thyroiditis, Cell Immunol. 61:32 (1981).

18. Y. M. Kong, L. L. Simon, P. Creemers, and N. R. Rose, In vitro T cell proliferation and cytotoxicity in murine autoimmune thyroiditis, Mt. Sinai J. Med. 53:46 (1986).

19. J. Salamero and J. Charreire, Syngeneic sensitization of mouse lympho-cytes on monolayers of thyroid epithelial cells. V. The primary syngeneic sensitization is under I-A subregion control, Eur. J. Immunol. 13:948 (1983).

20. V. Tomazic, N. R. Rose, and D. C. Shreffler, Autoimmune murine thyroi-ditis. IV. Localization of genetic control of the immune response, J. Immunol. 112:965 (1974).

21. Y. M. Kong, C. S. David, A. A. Giraldo, M. ElRehewy, and N. R. Rose, Regulation of autoimmune response to mouse thyroglobulin: Influ-ence of H-2D-end genes, J. Immunol. 123:15 (1979).

22. N. R. Rose, Y. M. Kong, P. S. Esquivel, M. ElRehewy, A. A. Giraldo, and C. S. David, Genetic regulation of autoimmune thyroiditis in the mouse, in: "Immunopathology - 6th International Convocation on Immunology," F. Milgrom and B. Albini, eds., S. Karger, Basel (1979).

23. N. R. Rose and I. R. Mackay, Genetic predisposition to autoimmune dis-eases," in: "The Autoimmune Diseases," N. R. Rose and I. R. Mackay, eds., Academic Press, Inc., Orlando (1985).

24. W. D. Terry and J. L. Fahey, Standards of human γ2 globulin based on differences in the heavy polypeptide chains, Science 146:400 (1964).

25. E. A. Lichter, Thyroglobulin antibody activity in the γ-globulins γ-A, γ-B and γ-C of human serum, Proc. Soc. Exp. Biol. Med. 116:555 (1964).

26. F. C. Hay and G. Torrigiani, The distribution of anti-Tg antibodies in the immunoglobulin G subclasses, Clin. Exp. Immunol. 16:517 (1974).

27. A. B. Parkes, S. M. McLachlan, P. Bird, and B. Rees Smith, The distribution of microsomal and thyroglobulin antibody activity among the IgG subclasses, Clin. Exp. Immunol. 57:239 (1984).
28. T. F. Davies, C. M. Weber, P. Wallack, and M. Platzer, Restricted heterogeneity and T cell dependence of human thyroid autoantibody immunoglobulin G subclasses, J. Clin. Endocrinol. Metab. 62:945 (1986).
29. A. P. Weetman and S. Cohen, The IgG subclass distribution of thyroid autoantibodies, Immunol. Letters 13:335 (1986).
30. C. L. Burek, W. H. Hoffman, and N. R. Rose, The presence of thyroid autoantibodies in children and adolescents with autoimmune thyroid disease and in their siblings and parents, Clin. Immunol. Immunopathol. 25:395 (1982).
31. C. L. Burek, N. R. Rose, G. M. Najar, W. H. Hoffman, A. Gimelfarb, C. M. Zmijewski, H. F. Polesky, and W. M. Hoffman, Autoimmune thyroid disease, in: "Immunogenetics," G. S. Panayi and C. S. David, eds., Butterworths, London (1984).

GENETIC BASIS OF SPONTANEOUS AUTOIMMUNE THYROIDITIS

Georg Wick, Guido Krömer, Hermann Dietrich, Konrad Schauenstein and Karel Hála

Institute for General and Experimental Pathology, University
of Innsbruck, Medical School
Fritz-Pregl-Strasse 3, A-6020 Innsbruck, Austria

INTRODUCTION

Autoimmune diseases, both organ-specific and systemic, have a multi-factorial basis with a definite genetic component. Most investigations on the theoretically and practically important problem of autoimmunity have focussed on the genetic basis of the aberrant immunological reactivity in experimental animals and man afflicted with autoimmune disease (for Review see 1,2). Much less emphasis has been given to the role of hormones as facultative factors modulating the development and severity of autoimmune diseases, reflected, e.g., by the preponderance of most - but not all - of these conditions in females[3,4]. Our own group has advocated a role for genetically determined primary alterations of the target organ as an obligatory prerequisite for the emergence of sponta-neous autoimmune thyroiditis (SAT) based on studies on the Obese strain (OS) of chickens. This new concept is schematically depicted in Figure 1 and has been presented in several recent reviews[5,6]. As can be seen in Figure 1 both obligatory and facultative factors, the latter having a modulatory role only, contribute to the final outcome of a given auto-immune disease. The OS chickens, which spontaneously develop an autoimmune thyroiditis early in life that closely parallels human Hashimoto thyroi-ditis, are especially suited as an animal model for the study of the relative contributions of the different factors outlined in Figure 1. Chickens have several advantages over mammalian species for this kind of investigation: (a) the extramaternal development of the embryo, (b) large numbers of offspring can be obtained from each pair of parents, (c) the expression of major histocompatibility complex (MHC = B locus in the chicken) antigens on the surface of the nucleated erythrocytes which allows easy and efficient tissue typing, (d) the characteristic morphological dichotomy of the avian immune system, and (e) the availabi-lity of inbred and even congenic normal strains of chickens for cross-breeding and backcross experiments.

The present discussion will be based on the results of classical immunogenetic breeding experiments performed in our laboratory during the past few years, but will also take into account data from ourselves and others during the earlier stages of the development of this strain.

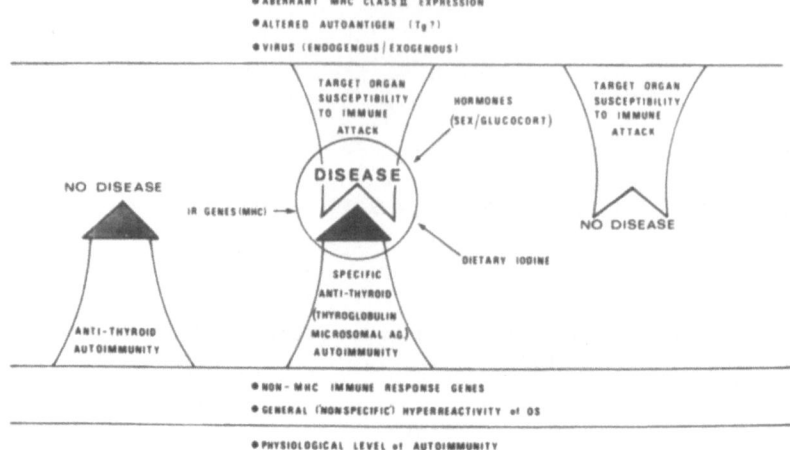

Figure 1. Schematical representation of the multigenic basis for SAT.

DEVELOPMENT OF THE OS

The OS was originally developed by Dr. R.K. Cole, now Professor emeritus, at Cornell Veterinary College, Ithaca, New York, by selective breeding of a few female animals of the Cornell C strain (CS) showing phenotypic symptoms of hypothyroidism, such as small body size and relatively high body weight due to subcutaneous and abdominal fat deposits, long silky feathers, small combs, cold sensitivity, low reproduction rate, etc.[7,8]. Although at first only 1% females of the closed colony (for 35 years) of CS chickens showed the hypothyroid trait, selective breeding from 1956 - 1958 increased the frequency to 10% and at the end of this period the first males were also found with lymphoid infiltration of the thyroid gland underlying the phenotypic symptoms of the disease. In the late sixties both females and males were afflicted to the same degree underlining the statement made above that sex hormones have a modulatory role but are not an absolute prerequisite for the development of spontaneous autoimmune thyroiditis (SAT)[5].

SAT is characterized by severe lymphoid infiltration of the thyroid glands and the occurrence of autoantibodies against thyroglobulin[9] and thyroid microsomal antigens[10], but also against a variety of non-thyroid autoantigens[10,11]. The degree of infiltration is arbitrarily graded from + to ++++, where + corresponds to mononuclear cell infiltration involving up to 25% of the histological thyroid cross-section and ++++, 75% to total infiltration. Thyroid infiltration can be seen as early as 2-5 weeks after hatching and efficient breeding of the OS can only be achieved with animals receiving thyroid hormone supplementation[12].

The genetic basis of Hashimoto thyroiditis is still an enigma and formal genetic studies aimed at the elucidation of possible correlations of the susceptibility for this disease and the presence of certain HLA haplotypes have so far been inconclusive[3]. An association of goitrous thyroiditis with HAL-DR 5 has been reported[13,14,15]. In contrast atrophic thyroiditis has been found to be associated with a high frequency of HLA-DR 3 and HLA-DR 8 and a low frequency of HLA-DR 5[14] possibly pointing to a different nature of atrophic and Hashimoto thyroiditis.

In the OS initial immunogenetic investigations by Bacon et al.[16] raised the possibility that the B-locus plays an important role in the development of SAT. Before discussing this point it should be mentioned that the nomenclature of the chicken MHC was unified and standardized by the participants of a workshop held in Innsbruck, Austria, in 1980 and the designation of haplotypes in the present context will adhere to the now generally accepted nomenclature[17]. The studies of Bacon et al.[16,18] showed that in the original OS colony kept by R.K. Cole at Cornell birds homozygous for B^{13} appeared as high responders with respect to the degree of SAT and the frequency and titer of thyroglobulin autoantibodies (TgAAb), OS B^5B^5 were low responders, and $B^{13}B^5$ heterozygotes intermediate. Studies in our own colony which at that time had been separated from the original flock for more than 10 years and was kept under similar selective breeding conditions leading to 100% SAT in both sexes showed that both B^{13} and B^5 homozygotes were high responders while a third haplotype, B^{15}, was associated with low responsiveness. Taking advantage of the rather wide variations in the degree of thyroid infiltration and TgAAb titers we selectively propagated high and low responders, respectively, of our OS B^{15} line and after 3 generations obtained an OS B^{15} high responder and an OS B^{15} low responder subline. We interpreted these and the previous data of Bacon et al.[17] as proof that a given MHC haplotype only has a modulatory role but is not instrumental in determining the degree of SAT. At that time we first put forward our "three-locus model" theory[19] which postulated the existance of 3, then still hypothetical, loci influencing the final outcome of SAT, viz. (a) the B-locus, (b) non-MHC associated genes with a pivotal role for the altered immune reactivity, and (c) genes responsible for a primary susceptibility of the target organ for the autoimmune attack.

IDENTIFICATION OF NON-MHC GENES INFLUENCING THE AUTOIMMUNE RESPONSE

Table 1 summarizes data from cross-breeding and backcross experiments using OS B^{15} and CB B^{12} chickens. The CB is a highly inbred strain[20] that is unrelated to the OS and thus provides a constant genetic background for the crosses. The F_1 birds were tested for the degree of SAT, the titer of TgAAb and various other parameters, such as the hyperresponsiveness of peripheral blood and spleen lymphocytes to Con A and the hyperproduction of Interleukin 2 (IL-2)[21,22] which are characteristic of the OS. The F_1 birds exhibited high titers of TgAAb, and elevated spontaneous and Con A-induced proliferation of lymphoid cells resembling that found in the OS (Table 1) but revealed a complete lack or only very mild degree of SAT[23]. Furthermore, if SAT occurred at all, it was found late in life (at the age of 20-23 weeks) in contrast to the usual early appearance of the disease in OS chicks.
Two conclusions were drawn from these data:
(i) We were for the first time able to produce animals that showed pathological parameters for autoimmunity, but did not develop SAT, thus speaking for our success in attempting to segregate those genes responsible for an aberration of the immune system and those

coding for susceptibility of the target organ.

(ii) Assuming a Mendelian pattern of inheritance the previously described general hyperreactivity of the immune system is a dominant trait.

Table 1

T-Cell Hyperreactivity

Strain (Cross)	n[b]	Spontaneous[a] ^{125}IUdR uptake of spleen cells ($\bar{x} \pm$ SEM, cpm)	n[c]	Con A (2.5 µg/ml) stimulation of PBL ^{3}H-thymidine incorporation ($\bar{x} \pm$ SD, cpm)
CB	10	587 ± 183	22	22,987 ± 5,558
OS	18	4,785 ± 3,544	14	55,188 ± 6,403
F_1(♀ OS x ♂ CB)		n.d.	7	52,109 ± 2,256
♀ F_1(OSxCB)x ♂ CB		n.d.	37	high responders: (n = 10) 41,489 ± 1,821
				low responders: (n = 27) 22,035 ± 790

[a]10^6 spleen cells or peripheral blood lymphocytes (PBL) were incubated without or with Con A, respectively for 48 hr in medium RPMI 1640 supplemented with 50 mM L-glutamine, 100 U/ml penicillin and 100 µg/ml streptomycin. The cells were cultured at 40°C in a humified atmosphere containing 5% CO_2.

[b]1 day old, n = number/group

[c]12-16 weeks old

Data partly from ref. 22.

IDENTIFICATION OF GENES CODING FOR A PRIMARY ABNORMALITY OF THE TARGET ORGAN

Human patients with various organ-specific autoimmune diseases often show antibodies to a variety of organ-specific autoantigens but nevertheless generally develop overt autoimmune disease only in a single organ, e.g. the pancreas, the adrenal or the thyroid gland.

Also in the OS model a broad variety of organ-specific and non-organ-specific AAb can be found[10,11] but careful histopathological and clinical analysis of these birds reveal thyroiditis as the only manifested autoimmune process. In the above mentioned original "three-locus model" we thus suggested that there must be genetic factors responsible for a primary alteration of the target organ which makes it susceptible to autoimmune damage.

We first concentrated our efforts on the elucidation of the genetic basis for a previously described phenomenon, i.e. the unexpected finding that thyroid glands of OS chicks analyzed <u>before</u> mononuclear cell infiltration (e.g. in the embryo or the first days after hatching) reveal an increased ^{131}I-uptake as compared to age-matched normal white Leghorn (NWL) controls. Cross-breeding experiments showed that this functional alteration is encoded by a single gene, inherited in a dominant fashion, and was proven to be independent of the MHC and the susceptibility to SAT[24].

As far as a genetic susceptibility of the thyroid gland for the development of SAT is concerned it was shown previously that the disease cannot be transferred by lymphoid cells and/or serum into histocompatible normal animals, but only from older OS into histocompatible newborn OS (resulting in accelerated very early development of the disease) and from OS B[13] into CS B[13], which normally only develop very mild, if any, SAT[25].

Passive transfer of TgAAb into (OS x CB) F[1] recipients did not result in SAT[24].

In order to identify the number of genes that might possibly be responsible for the susceptibility of the OS thyroid glands for the autoimmune attack we used (OS x CB) F[1] x OS backcrosses for the passive transfer experiments which are exemplified in <u>Table 2</u>. Assuming a Mendelian pattern of inheritance the frequency of about 10% backcrosses susceptible to passive transfer and developing severe SAT points to the existence of at least 3 genes that are responsible for this susceptibility[24], at least one of which is recessive.

In summary, we conclude that the non-MHC encoded alterations of the immunological reactivity in OS chickens is a dominant trait whereas the primary target organ abnormalities are recessive traits[6]. Furthermore, the original "three-locus model" has to be extended but the total number of genes, the role of which is absolutely essential for the development of SAT, is still rather small. In order to develop severe SAT an OS bird has to possess all of the necessary non-MHC genes (at least 2) influencing the immune system and all of the genes conveying target organ susceptibility (at least 3). Additional known (MHC, sex) and unknown factors have a modulatory function.

Space does not permit discussion of our ideas on the actual manifestations of the different genetic factors outlined above. These have already been the subject of two recent reviews[5,6]. As far as the immune system is concerned the general T-cell hyperreactivity and the characteristic hyperproduction of IL-2 have already been mentioned. For the latter a defect of a small molecular weight antagonist of IL-2 activity has been identified in the OS[21]. Furthermore, OS chickens show an interesting deficiency of thymic nurse cells, the possible role of which for altered T-cell differentiation is now under investigation[26,27]. In respect to the target organ abnormality changes in the ultracentrifuge sedimentation behaviour of thyroglobulin but no altered immunological reactivity of this antigen have been found[6]. In addition, OS thyroid epithelial cells aberrantly express MHC class II (B-L) antigen in the vicinity of infiltrating activated T-cells[5]. Finally, a new endogenous virus has been found by Southern blot analysis of the DNA of OS chickens, but is absent in all normal strains investigated so far[5,6]. Further studies of these interesting issues should provide insight not only into the immunogenetic basis of SAT in the OS, but also the human counterpart of this model, Hashimoto thyroiditis.

Table 2

Susceptibility of the Target Organ
Passive Transfer Experiments

Line (Cross)	No. of animals	Treatment[a]	No. of animals with/without thyroiditis[b]	Degree of thyroiditis[c]
OS	5	A	5/0	3.4 ± 0.9
	4	B	3/1	1.5 ± 1.0
	6	C	4/2	1.5 ± 0.6
CB	7	A	0/7	0
	12	B	0/12	0.1 ± 0.3[d]
	11	C	0/11	0.1 ± 0.3
F_1 (♀ CB x ♂ OS)	10	A	0/10	0.2 ± 0.4
	12	B	0/12	0
	12	C	0/12	0
F_1 (♀ OS x ♂ CB)	11	A	0/11	0.3 ± 0.5
	9	B	0/9	0.1 ± 0.3
	12	C	0/12	0.4 ± 0.5
Backcross	39	A	4/35	2.5 ± 0.6
(F_1 x OS)	33	C	0/33	0

[a]Treatment: A - injection of OS serum containing TgAAb
B - Injection with Tg-absorbed OS serum
C - untreated controls

[b]greater than 1+ infiltration

[c]estimated from the degree of infiltration of histological cross-sections.

[d]Minor well secluded lymphoid foci not infiltrating between thyroid follicles can occasionally be found in normal birds.

Data partly from ref. 23.

ACKNOWLEDGEMENTS

This work was supported by the Austrian Research Council (G.W., project S-41/05) and the Austrian Cancer Research Fund (K.H.). The competent secretarial help of Miss Anita Fuchs is gratefully acknowledged. Dr.Karine Keen-Traill kindly corrected our English.

REFERENCES

1. N.R.Rose, and I.R.Mackay (eds.) The Autoimmune Diseases. Academic Press, Inc., New York - London - Sydney, 1985
2. H.R.Smith, and A.D.Steinby, Autoimmunity - A Perspective. Ann.Dev. Immunol. 1:175 (1983)

3. R.Volpé, Monographs in Endocrinology. Autoimmunity of the Endocrine System. Springer Verlag, Berlin - Heidelberg - New York, 1981.
4. J.R.Roubinian, N.Talal, J.S.Greenspan, J.R.Goodman, and P.K.Siiteri, Effect of castration and sex hormone treatment on survival, artinucleic acid antibodies, and glomerulonephritis in NZB/NZW F_1 mice. J.Exp.Med. 147:1568 (1977)
5. G.Wick, J.Möst, K.Schauenstein, G.Krömer, H.Dietrich, A.Ziemiecki, R.Fässler, N.Neu, and K.Hála, Spontaneous autoimmune thyroiditis - a birds eye view. Immunol.Today 6:359.
6. G.Wick, K.Hála, H.Wolf, A.Ziemiecki, R.S.Sundick, M.Meilicke-Stöffler, and M.DeBaets, The role of genetically determined primary alterations of the target organ in the development of spontaneous autoimmune thyroiditis in Obese strain (OS) chickens. in: Immunological Reviews Vol. 94, G.Möller, ed., Munksgaard Int.Publ. (in press)
7. R.K.Cole, Hereditary hypothyroidism in the domestic fowl. Genetics 53:1021 (1966)
8. A.van Tienhoven, and R.K.Cole, Endocrine disturbance in Obese chickens. Anat.Rec. 142:111 (1962)
9. R.K.Cole, J.H.Kite, Jr., and E.Witebsky, Hereditary autoimmune thyroiditis in the fowl. Science 160:1357.
10. E.L.Khoury, G.F.Bottazzo, L.C.Pontes de Carvalho, G.Wick, and I.M.Roitt, Predisposition to organ-specific autoimmunity in Obese strain (OS) chickens: reactivity to thyroid, gastric, adrenal and pancreatic cytoplasmic antigens. Clin.exp.Immunol. 49:273 (1982)
11. G.Aichinger, H.Kofler, O.Diaz-Merida, and G.Wick, Nonthyroid autoantibodies in Obese strain (OS) chickens. Clin.Immunol.Immunopathol. 32:57 (1984)
12. R.K.Cole, J.H.Kite, Jr., G.Wick, and E.Witebsky, Inherited autoimmune thyroiditis in the fowl. Poultry Sci. 49:840 (1970)
13. M.Weissel, R.Höfer, H.Zasmeta, and W.R.Mayr, HLA-DR and Hashimoto thyroiditis. Tissue Antigens 16:256 (1980)
14. N.R.Farid, L.Sampson, H.Moens, and J.M.Barnard, The association of goitrous autoimmune thyroiditis with HLA-DR5. Tissue Antigens 17:265 (1981)
15. H.Tamai, H.Uno, Y.Hirota, S.Matsubayashi, K.Kuma, H.Matsumoto, L.F.Kumagai, T.Sasazuki, and S.Nagataki, Immunogenetics of Hashimoto's and Graves' disease. J.Clin.Endocrinol.Metab. 60:62 (1985)
16. L.D.Bacon, J.H.Kite, Jr., and N.R.Rose, Relation between the major histocompatibility (B) locus and autoimmune thyroiditis in Obese chickens. Science 186:274 (1974)
17. W.E.Briles, N.Bumstead, D.L.Ewert, D.G.Gilmour, J.Gogusev, K.Hála, C.Koch, B.M.Longenecker, A.W.Nordskog, J.R.L.Pink, L.W.Schierman, M.Simonsen, A.Toivanen, P.Toivanen, O.Vainio, and G.Wick, Nomenclature for chicken major histocompatibility (B) complex. Immunogenetics 15:441 (1982)
18. L.D.Bacon, and N.R.Rose, Influence of the major histocompatibility haplotype in autoimmune disease varies in different inbred families of chickens. Proc.Natl.Acad.Sci. 76:1435 (1979)
19. G.Wick, R.Gundolf, an K.Hála, Genetic factors in spontaneous autoimmune thyroiditis in OS chickens. J.Immunogenetics 6:177 (1979)
20. K.Hála, The major histocompatibility system of the chicken. in: The Histocompatibility System in Man and Animals, D.Götze, ed., Springer-Verlag, Berlin - Heidelberg - New York, pp. 291-312, 1977
21. G.Krömer, K.Schauenstein, N.Neu, K.Stricker, and G.Wick, In vitro T cell hyperreactivity in Obese strain (OS) chickens is due to a defect in nonspecific suppressor mechanism(s). J.Immunol. 135:2458 (1985)
22. K.Schauenstein, G.Krömer, R.S.Sundick, and G.Wick. Enhanced response to Con A and production of TCGF by lymphocytes of Obese strain

(OS) chickens with spontaneous autoimmune thyroiditis. J.Immunol. 134:872 (1985)

23. N.Neu, K.Hála, H.Dietrich, and G.Wick, Genetic background of spontaneous autoimmune thyroiditis in the Obese strain of chickens studied in hybrids with an inbred line. Int.Archs.Allergy appl.Immun. 80:168 (1986)

24. N.Neu, K.Hála, H.Dietrich, and G.Wick, Spontaneous autoimmune thyroiditis in Obese strain chickens: A genetic analysis of target organ abnormalities. Clin.Immunol.Immunopathol. 37:397 (1985)

25. I.Jaroszewski, R.S.Sundick, and N.R.Rose, Effects of antiserum containing thyroglobulin antibody on the chicken thyroid gland. Clin.Immunol.Immunopathol. 10:95 (1978)

26. R.L.Boyd, G.Oberhuber, K.Hála, and G.Wick, Obese strain (OS) chickens with spontaneous autoimmune thyroiditis have a deficiency in thymic nurse cells. J.Immunol. 132:718 (1984)

27. G.Wick, and G.Oberhuber, Thymic nurse cells: a school for alloreactive and autoreactive cortical thymocytes? Eur.J.Immunol. 135:855 (1986)

HETERO-TRANSPLANTATION OF AUTOIMMUNE HUMAN THYROID TO NUDE MICE AS A TOOL FOR IN VIVO AUTOIMMUNE RESEARCH

K. H. Usadel, R. Paschke, J. Teuber, and U. Schwedes

II. Medical Department, Klinikum Mannheim
University of Heidelberg, Theodor-Kutzer-Ufer
6800 Mannheim, FRG

INTRODUCTION

Various experimental transplantation models have been used in order to investigate the physiology, pathophysiology, and treatment of grafted tissues under in vivo conditions(1). Since in homologous and especially in heterologous transplantation models severe immunological problems exist, the description of thymus aplastic nude(nu/nu)mice(2)and nude(rnu/rnu)rats(3)has stimulated experimental transplantation research. The genes governing thymic agenesis and hairlessness proved to be linked and inherited as autosomal traits. This effect is linked with loss of immunocompetend T-lymphocytes, resulting in a lack of immune resistance. If nude mice or rats are used as recipients, hetero(xeno-)transplantation can be achieved without immunosuppressive therapy. Beside malignant and also various benign human tissue were successfully transplanted to nude mice.

Recently our interest centered on the behaviour of hetero-transplanted human thyroid tissue of patients with Graves' disease, toxic adenoma, and thyroidal carcinoma in the nude mouse.

MATERIAL AND METHODS

Human thyroid tissues were obtained from surgery of patients with Graves' disease, toxic adenoma, and thyroidal carcinoma. Small fragments(size 4x3x2 mm)of these thyroid tissues were transplanted s.c. adjacent to mammary glands of athymic nude mice immediately after surgery of the patient. For details of the method see reference 1 . Nude mice of an outbred strain(NMRI, initial body weight of approximately 28-30 gr., 5-6 weeks old)served as recipient animals and were maintained as described ealier(1).

RESULTS AND DISCUSSION

In summary of a variety of experiments the following results could be obtained:

Significance of the nude mouse bioassay for the biologic activity of thyroidal receptor antibodies.

We previously could demonstrate(4)that thyroid tissue of
patients with Graves' disease and toxic adenoma can succsess-
fully be transplanted to nude mice without rejection, and
that the grafts show typical function in the recipients.

Histological studies, determination of nuclear volume,
and 131 J-uptake, and scintiscanning of the grafts indicates
that thyroid tissues of toxic adenomas still show all signs
of a hyperfunctional state even 8 weeks after transplantation.
These findings contrast with those in tissues from Graves'
disease which lacks the patients TSI after transplantation
and presumably therefore then looses its stimulated hyperfunctional state. These results clearly show that thyroid
tissues of thyroidal autonomy are based on an intrinsic activity. Grafts from Graves' disease, however, depend upon the
activity of extrinsic applicated thyroid immunoglobulins
(TSI, TBIAb, TRAb).

The screening of hormone derivatives by in vitro assays
with subsequent testing in bio assays could demonstrate the
limited value of in vitro assays for the determination of
hormones biologic action and the need to cast a wide net of
parameters to determine a hormones biologic profile. Regarding TRAb the discrepancies of in vitro assay results on the
basis of different views concerning the TRAb receptor, TRAb's
messenger and different pathophysiological qualities of TRAb
further ilustrate this problem.

The nude mouse bio assay(4)permits the simultaneous determination of several parameters, 131 I incorporation by
gamma-counter and/or gamma-camera, thyroglobuline secretion
of transplants, histoautoradiographic ^{3}H thymidine incorporation and 131 I incorporation and histologic characterization of transplant viability after stimulation of transplanted human thyroid tissue with TRAb positive serum or IgG. Behaviour parameters after stimulation with 0.5 ml serum, TRAb
506 mU/ml(radioligand assay)$^{\pm}$ SEM compared to normal serum
is as follows: nuclear volume:88.7($^{\pm}$ 17.1)/68.8($^{\pm}$ 14.3)epi-
thelial hight: 9.0($^{\pm}$ 1.0)/7.5($^{\pm}$ 0.9)stimulation index determined by colloid resorption:72.9/59.3 stimulation index determined by colloid content: 71.3/57.3. Thyroglobulin secretion determined by radioimmuno-assay: 322 cpm/195 cpm, 131 I
incorporation (gamma-counter) 100.400 cpm/mg/47.000 cpm/mg.
By gamma-camera some of the histologically intact transplants
did only show small amounts of 131 I incorporation 30 min
and 2 h p.i. Parallel determination of nuclear volume (μm^3)
and ^{3}H thymidine incorporation (% of labeled cells) for TRAb
positive sera compared to normal serum showed the following
results: TRAb 279 mU/ml, 67μm^3/10.3%, TRAb 700 mU/ml, 86μm^3/
16.7%, controls: 39μm^3/9.4%. Scar tissue formation in some
transplants results in a proportional decrease of biologic
parameters. The mouse thyroids do show a parallel but less
obvious behaviour of biologic parameters.

Conclusions: 1)Biologic parameters are not proportional to TRAb values determined by radioligand assay.2)The
parallel stimulation of all biologic parameters by all the
investigated sera do not permit the characterization of a selective stimulation profile(as it could be shown by mixing
experiments). 3)TRAb does show in some transplants relative
species specifity. 4)Scar tissue formation influences the
bio assays sensitivity. 5)Determination of 131 I incorporation by gamma-counter is more reliable than the gamma-camera.

Using this model further studies might become possible in
order to differentiate various thyrotropin receptor antibo-
dies(5).

Experimental in vivo model for examination of iodine-indu-
ced hyperthyroidism

The effect of different doses of continuous iodine infusion on xenotransplanted human thyroid tissue or toxic adenoma and Graves' disease was examined using 131 I-scintigraphy
in athymic nude mice(6). The data obtained clearly demonstrated, for the first time under in vivo conditions, that high
iodine doses accelerate iodine turnover rate and presumably
the hyperfunction of human thyroid of toxic adenoma dose de-
pendently. Transplanted tissue of autoimmune thyroid disease
responds to high iodine dosis like normal nontoxic thyroid
tissue due to loss of extrinsic stimulators, but becomes hyperfunctional again by Graves' disease serum or TSH.

These results demonstrate again that exposure to iodine is
dangerous for patients with autonomously functioning thyroid
as well as with active Graves' disease.

Antiidiotypic antibodies involved in human autoimmune
thyroid diesease

Idiotype-antiidiotypic regulation of autoimmunity is discussed as pathophysiological mechanism of several autoimmune
diseases. Recently antiidiotypic antibodies could be demonstrated in sera of Graves' disease patients(7). Using different sera from patients with Graves' disease(active state
and remission)the stimulating effect of human follicle cells
was tested in the xenotransplantation nude mouse model. As
expected serum from active Graves' disease(with high TRAb)
serum stimulated in the usual way and serum from the same
patient for more than 1 year later and being in remission(no
detectable or low TRAb titers) of the disease did not stimulate the heterotransplanted grafts.

1:1 mixtures(active Graves' disease)of the sera from each
patient resulted in a blocking of the stimulation by sera
with high TRAb-titers. The observed blocking effect is probably caused by antiidiotypic antibodies in the low TRAb
sera neutralising stimulating antibodies in high TRAb serum.
These results demonstrated the first time in vivo that sera
from patients with Graves' disease who had developed low titers of TRAb(remission)can potentially block stimulating activity of sera with high TRAb titers. Further studies will
use chemically more defined fractions of gammaglobulins.

Evidence for DR-AG-expression by RHS-cells and not by thyroid epithelial cells

Several investigators described DR-AG-expression of thyroid epithelial cells in various thyroid disorders. DR-AG-expression was subsequently discussed as a relevant factor in the pathogenesis of autoimmune thyroid diseases. In contrast to these theories we could demonstrate that DR-AG-expression is likely to be an epiphenomenon in autoimmune diseases. Therefore we asked whether thyroid epithelial cell lines express DR-AG. For more details see Teuber et al.(this issue).

In conclusion one can say that by the use of xenotransplanted human endocrine tissues to nude mice investigations are available for the study of the physiology, the pathophysiology and therapy of various diseases especially the thyroid. It is wortwhile to point out that capillaries of surviving grafts are mainly of hosts's origine, and that grafted white blood cells and lymphocytes of the donor do not survive in the transplant.

REFERENCES

1. Bastert G, Eichholz H, Althoff PH, Steinau U, Klempa I, Fortmeyer HP, Schwedes U, Usadel KH (1981) Xenografts of benign and malignant endocrine tissues in thymus-aplastic nude mice and rats: Development and function. In: Bastert G et al. (eds): Thymusaplastic nude mice and rats in clinical oncology. Gustav Fischer Verlag, Stuttgart, New York, p 383.

2. Pantelouris EM (1968) Absence of thymus in a mouse mutant. Nature (London) 217: 370.

3. Festing MFW, Lovell D, Sparrow S (1978) The rowett athymic rat. Symposium: The laboratory rat and biological variation. Cambridge.

4. Usadel KH, Schumm PM, Wenisch HJC, Maul FD, Schwedes U, (1984) Transplantation of thyroid tissue nude mice: A method for demonstrating extrinsic stimulators, and a new bioassay for thyroid stimulating antibodies (TSI). In: Doniach D, Schleusener H, Weinheimer B (eds) Current topics in thyroid autoimmunity. G. Thieme, Stuttgart, New York, p 187.

5. Smith BR, Creagh FM, Hashim FA, Howells RD, Davies Jones E, Kajita Y, Buckland PR, Petersen VB (1985) Thyrotropin receptor antibodies. Drug res. 35 (II): 1943.

6. Schumm-Draeger PM, Senekowitsch R, Maul FD, Wenisch HJC, Pickardt CR, Usadel KH (1987) Evidence of in vivo iodine-induced hyperthyroidism in hyperfunctional autoimmune and autonomous human thyroid tissue xenotransplanted to nude mice. Klin. Wochenschr. in press.

7. Raines Kb, Baker JR, Lukes YG, Wartoffsky L, Burman KD (1985) Antithyrotropin antibodies in the sera of Graves disease patients. J. c. Endocr. Metab. 61: 217.

POST-PARTUM THYROID DYSFUNCTION

R. Hall[1], H. Fung[1], M. Kologlu[1], K. Collison[1], J. Marco[1], AB.
Parkes[1], B.B. Harris[2], C. Darke[4], R. John[3], C.J. Richards[5], and
A.M. McGregor[1]

Departments of Medicine[1], Psychiatry[2] and Medical Biochemistry[3]
University of Wales College of Medicine, Heath Park, Cardiff.,
Regional Tissue Typing Laboratory[4], Rhydlafar and Department
of Obstetrics[5], Caerphilly District Miners Hospital, Caerphilly
S. Wales

I INTRODUCTION

   Normal pregnancy is associated with two major series of alterations in
the endocrine system.   On the one hand hormonal changes necessary for the
maintenance of pregnancy must occur and on the other pregnancy itself may
influence the function of endocrine glands, such as the thyroid, which are
not themselves directly involved in the maintenance of the pregnancy.   In
pregnancy therefore, and as a result of these normal physiological regulatory mechanisms, thyroid function must be interpreted with caution (Table
1).   The situation is further complicated in those women with known (or
previously unrecognised) thyroid disease, particularly if the aetiological
basis of their disease is autoimmune (Table 1).   In these women pregnancy
may have a profound impact on their disease with amelioration during the
pregnancy itself but with exacerbation in the post-partum period.   In
addition and as a result of their thyroid disease, alterations in the
function of the foetal and neonatal thyroid may occur.   Considerable
interest has been focussed recently on alterations in thyroid function in
pregnancy and the post-partum period in both normal women and women with
known autoimmune thyroid disease and has been extensively reviewed (1-3).
In the present study we have sought to examine prospectively the thyroid
function of a group of normal women with no known history of thyroid
disease, through pregnancy and the post-partum period.   Our aim was to define
the true prevalence of post-partum thyroid dysfunction (PPTD) in such women,
to characterise the syndromes of PPTD developing and to determine the
factors associated with their development.

II STUDY GROUP

   Nine hundred and one consecutive women attending the ante-natal booking
clinic at the Caerphilly District Miners Hospital in South Wales between
April 1983 and January 1985 were studied.   At booking all were screened for
the presence of autoantibodies to thyroglobulin (TG) and the thyroid microsomal antigen (TMA) by ELISA (4).   All the booking samples were assayed
within the same assay and on the basis of data from 98 normal non-pregnant
subjects also assayed in the same assay, 117 (12.98%) of the pregnant women

Table 1. ALTERATIONS IN THYROID FUNCTION IN PREGNANCY

I   NORMAL WOMEN

A.   OESTROGEN-INDUCED SYNTHESIS OF THYROID-HORMONE
     BINDING PROTEINS

B.   ALTERED THYROID FUNCTION WITHIN THE NORMAL RANGE
     (see Table 2)

II   WOMEN WITH "AUTOIMMUNE" THYROID DISEASE

A.   OESTROGEN-INDUCED SYNTHESIS OF THYROID-HORMONE
     BINDING PROTEINS

B.   INFLUENCE OF PREGNANCY ON MATERNAL DISEASE
         - DURING PREGNANCY
         - POST-PARTUM

C.   INFLUENCE OF MATERNAL DISEASE ON FOETUS/NEONATE

---

were considered to be antibody positive. An age-matched antibody negative
group (AB-) and the antibody positive group (AB+) formed the basis of the
subsequent prospective study. With patients being lost to follow-up the
final study group (n=232) consisted of 100 women who were AB+ (43%) and 132
who were AB- (57%). The women in the two groups did not differ significantly for age, primigravid or multigravid status or mean gestational age at
delivery.

The study group were seen at booking thence at 6 weekly intervals
through the pregnancy and during the first 12 months post-partum. Normal
thyroid function through pregnancy was established using data obtained from
analysis of the serial samples of 120 of the 132 AB- women using
commercially available assay kits (Amersham International plc). The
remaining 12 conceived again before completing their years of follow-up
post-partum. On the basis of this information (Table 2) it is clear that
during pregnancy a significant fall in free T3 and free T4 as pregnancy
progresses is accompanied by a significant and compensatory rise in serum
TSH. All three parameters had normalised (compared with the levels at 12

Table 2. ALTERATIONS IN SERUM FREE T4, FREE T3 and TSH
          IN 120 NORMAL WOMEN THROUGH PREGNANCY

PARAMETER	TIME (weeks)					
	8-16	17-25	26-34	35-43	DELIVERY	49-56
fT4 (pmol/L)	15.7±4.5	14.0±3.9 **	12.9±3.4 **	12.5±3.8 **	12.8±4.9 **	16.3±5.1
fT3 (pmol/L)	5.9±1.6 **	5.1±1.4 **	4.8±1.4 **	4.6±1.3 **	4.3±1.7 **	6.4±1.8
TSH (mU/L)	2.0±1.5 **	1.8±1.3 *	1.9±2.0 *	2.1±1.8 **	2.3±2.2 **	1.5±1.7

* p = < 0.05, ** p = <0.001 as compared with the value at 49-56
weeks post-partum.

Results expressed as mean ± 2SD.

months post-partum) by 9 to 16 post-partum. Levels of hormone at a
particular time point which were greater than 2SD outside the normal range
for that time point were considered abnormal. When two or more consecutive
abnormal results were detected in a woman post-partum she was defined as
having post-partum thyroid dysfunction (PPTD).

II   POST-PARTUM THYROID DYSFUNCTION

a.   SYNDROME

Of the study group of 232 women, 49 (21.1%) developed PPTD. They could
be divided into 4 groups;

  A.   Hyperthyroidism followed by hypothyroidism (n=9).
  B.   Hyperthyroidism alone (n=21).
  C.   Hypothyroidism followed by hyperthyroidism (n=2).
  D.   Hypothyroidism alone (n=17).

The time of onset of PPTD (in weeks mean $\pm$ SEM) was 13 ± 2.3 for hyperthyroidism and 20 ± 2.5 for hypothyroidism in group A, 18.4 ± 2.8 for group B
and 21.3 ± 3.2 for group D. The episode of PPTD resolved spontaneously in all
the women but for one in group D who developed persistent hypothyroidism.
Clinical symptoms or signs did not provide any reliable guide to the
development of PPTD.

b.   AUTOANTIBODY STATUS

Of the 49 women who developed PPTD 37 (76%) were thyroid autoantibody
positive during the study but only 30 (61%) were AB+ve at booking and of
these 27 (55.1% of the total) had detectable antibodies to the TMA. Of the
7 women who became AB+ve later in pregnancy or in the post-partum 5 were TMA
AB+ve so that in total 32 of the 49 women developing PPTD (65.3%) were TMA
AB+ve at some time during their pregnancy. Assay of all 174 samples from
the 21 women in group B (hyperthyroidism alone) in the same human thyroid
cell bioassay (5) failed to reveal any evidence of Graves' autoantibodies to
the TSH receptor. In 7 of these women who were not breast feeding, a
thyroid ^{123}I uptake scan at the time of their episode of hyperthyroidism,
revealed suppressed uptakes at 4 and 48hr post 10mBq ^{123}I orally.

Assessment of changes in the level of the TMA AB in relation to the
development of PPTD revealed that although i) the level of TMA rose
significantly post-partum in all the women with PPTD and ii) the mean time
of onset for the particular PPTD syndromes might differ, nevertheless the
peak level of TMA activity tended to coincide with the mean time of onset of
the particular PPTD syndrome (Fig. 1).

c.   ASSOCIATED CLINICAL FACTORS

There was no difference in the age of the women developing PPTD
(24.8 ± 4.9 mean $\pm$ SD) from that of the women who did not develop PPTD, nor in
the number who were either primigravid (n=19, 38.8%) or multigravid (n=30,
67.1%) in the PPTD group as compared with the non-PPTD group. The presence
of a family history of thyroid disease though more common (n=12, 25.5%) in
the PPTD group was not significantly different from the numbers found in the
non-PPTD group (n=26, 15.3%). On the basis of the smoking habits of the
women during the post-partum period, though 60.6% (n=220) of the women were
non-smokers, when women smoking more than 20 cigarettes a day were considered, they were significantly more commonly found in the PPTD group
(n=7, 15.2%) than in the non-PPTD group (n=7, 4.2%; $p = < 0.01$). The
frequency and duration of breast feeding was no different in the PPTD and
non-PPTD groups. No significant difference existed in the mean birth

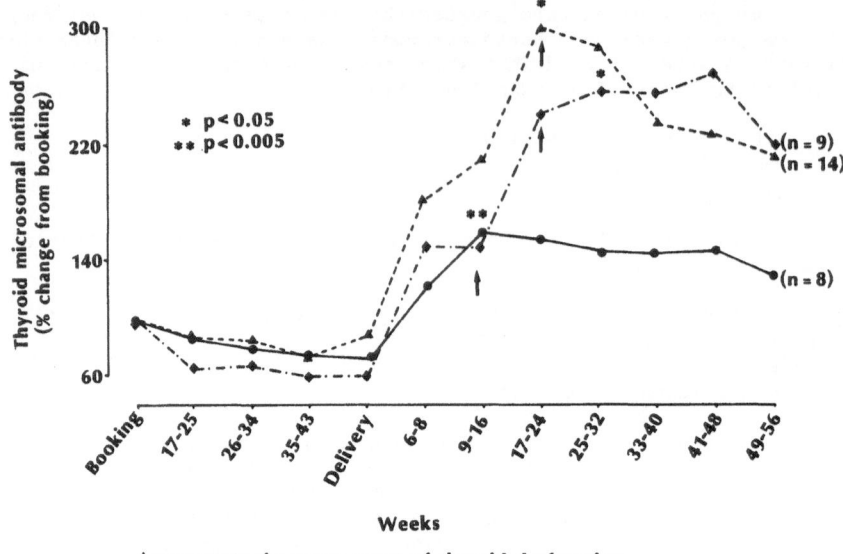

Fig. 1. Alterations in thyroid microsomal antibody activity in relation to the onset of thyroid dysfunction in 31 women with post-partum thyroid dysfunction.

weights of the infants born to the mothers in the two groups. Whilst the ratio of female to male infants was 0.75:1.0 in the PPTD group as compared with 1.28:1.0 in the non-PPTD group the difference was not significant. Grading of thyroid gland size (1 to 5) allowed serial assessment of thyroid alteration through pregnancy. Thyroid gland size at booking was 2.0±1.7 (mean ± 2SD, n=49) in the PPTD group and 1.98±1.6 (n=160) in the non-PPTD group and this was not significantly different.

d. THYROID FUNCTION

Besides assessment of free T3, free T4 and TSH through pregnancy (Table 2) and the post-partum, thyroid gland size and serum thyroglobulin (TG) were assessed serially.

i. Thyroid gland size. Thyroid gland size at 52 weeks post-partum was considered to reflect the norm and the serial size of the gland in the preceding pregnancy and post-partum period were compared with it. There was a significant increase in thyroid gland size (Figure 2). which paralleled the alteration in serum TSH through pregnancy. Though the gland size in the PPTD group continued to increase post-partum and remained significantly different at 24 weeks from the size at 52 post-partum (Fig. 2) the size at each point post-partum was not significantly different when compared with the non-PPTD group. The gland size however was significantly larger in the AB+ve women (n=100) as compared with the AB-ve women (n=132) at booking (p = < 0.05).

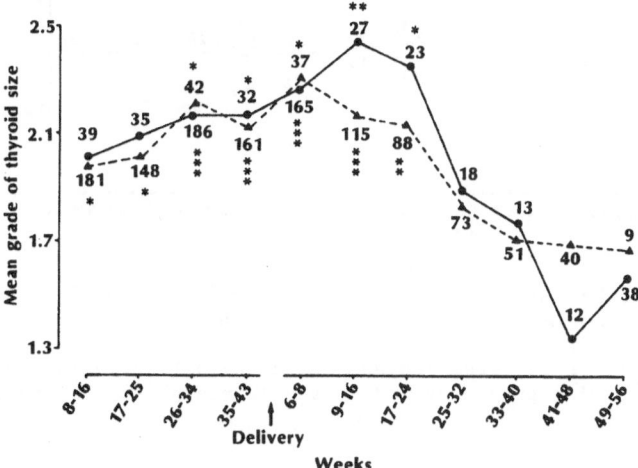

Alterations in thyroid gland size in 220 women throughout pregnancy and in the 12 months post-partum

*p< 0.05 **p <0.01 ***p<0.001 as compared with the value at 52 weeks post-partum

▲ Total (Syndrome + ve and Syndrome -ve) ● Syndrome + ve

Fig. 2. Alterations in thyroid gland size in 220 women through pregnancy and in the 12 months post-partum.

ii. Serum thyroglobulin. Establishment of a normal range for serum TG was performed using an ELISA on (6) serial samples from 107 syndrome negative, autoantibody negative women. The skewed distribution was normalised after logarithmic transformation. Alterations in serum TG through pregnancy and in the post-partum followed the changes in serum TSH (Fig. 3) and gland size (Fig. 2). In the 17 women developing PPTD in whom no TG antibody activity was ever detected, serial alterations in their TG level increased markedly post-partum and by non-parametric analysis using the Mann-Whitney U test could be shown to be significantly different from that of 107 normal, TG antibody negative women in the post-partum period (p =< 0.005).

ᴀ. IMMUNE STATUS

i. Total serum immunoglobulin levels. It has remained uncertain whether the significant fall in autoantibody activity frequently reported in a variety of diseases reflects the result of immunosuppression occurring in pregnancy or is the result of the normal physiological haemodilution associated with the condition. To examine this we studied serial changes in total IgG, IgM and albumin. Since autoantibodies to the TMA are primarily of the IgG class only the IgG data is considered here. IgG levels fell significantly during pregnancy and this was paralleled by the fall in albumin so that when the ratio of IgG to albumin was plotted the level was normalised, though in the AB+ve group a small but significant fall in the ratio persisted. When 42 women who were TMA autoantibody positive throughout pregnancy and the post-partum had their TMA activity against albumin ratio examined the small but significant fall in the ratio during pregnancy was followed by a marked and significant rebound post-partum which was maximal 25-32 weeks post-partum (Fig. 4) suggesting that the alterations in

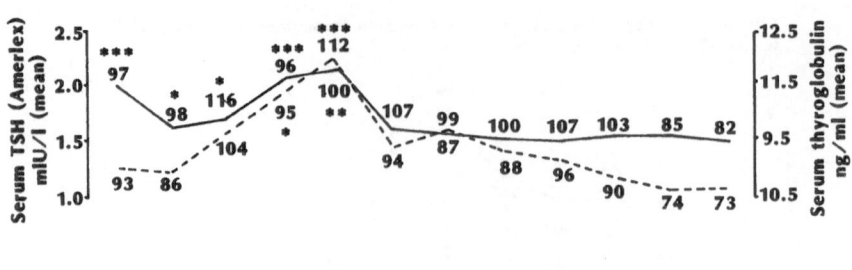

Fig. 3. Alterations in serum TSH and serum thyroglobulin in 120 normal
women during pregnancy and in the 12 months post-partum.

disease state in pregnancy could not be explained purely on the basis of
haemodilution.

.ii. <u>IgG sub-class of the thyroid microsomal antibody.</u> Using serial
samples from 84 women with antibodies to the TMA of whom 32 developed PPTD,
the IgG sub-classes of their TMA AB were examined by ELISA (7). The aim was
to assess the possibility that alterations in TMA IgG subclass activity with
the resulting implications for their ability to bind complement could have an
impact on whether the development of PPTD was determined by the IgG subclass of the TMA antibody. The analyses were performed so information was
obtainable on the subclass alterations with time through pregnancy and the
post-partum but also allowed comparisons between the sub-classes at each
time point.

IgG$_2$ (data not shown) and IgG$_3$ (Fig.5) levels increased significantly
in the post-partum period in the sub-group of women developing hyper-
followed by hypothyroidism with the IgG$_3$ level peak coinciding with the mean
time of onset of the episode of hyperthyroidism.

f. HLA STATUS

Two hundred and twenty-one women were HLA typed of whom 108 (49%) were
AB+ve and 113 (51%) were AB-ve, of these women 45 developed PPTD. A total
of 12 A, 18 B, 8 DR and 2 DQ HLA antigens were typed for and the data on
the pregnant women was compared with that of 600 non-pregnant Caucasians for
the A and B antigens and 382 of this population for HLA-DR antigens. When
all the women developing PPTD (n=45) irrespective of their autoantibody
status were considered, there was an increase in the frequency of HLA A1,

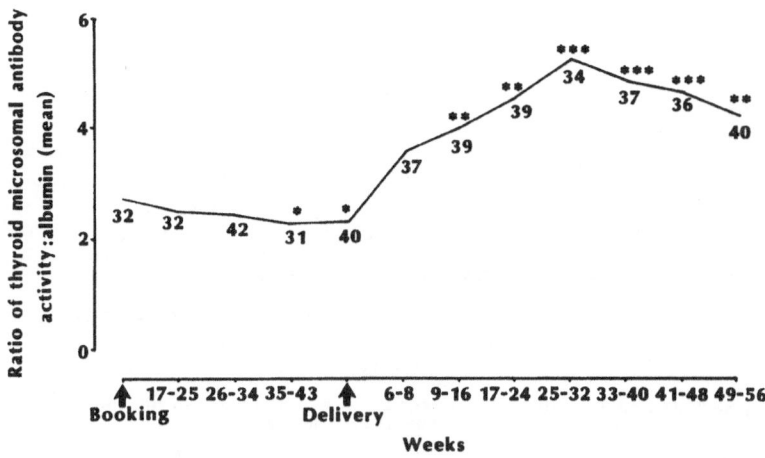

Fig. 4. Ratio of thyroid microsomal antibody activity to total serum albumin in 42 women during pregnancy and in the 12 months post-partum.

B8 and DR3 as compared with the controls which were not significant after correction. In contrast analysis of the combinations B8, DR3 and A1, B8, DR3 showed an increased frequency in the PPTD group which remained significant after correction. No association of HLA DR4 was observed with either the presence of thyroid autoantibodies or the development of PPTD. There was however a significant association in 108 AB+ve women with HLA-DQw3 when compared with 113 AB-ve women so that 52.8% of the AB+ve and only 33.6% of the AB-ve group were DQw3 positive (relative risk 2.2, $X^2 = 7.5$, p = <0.01). This remained significant using multiplex analysis.

g. POST-NATAL DEPRESSION

The possibility that the development of PPTD might be associated with the well recognised changes in mood that are recognised as occurring in the post-partum was examined. One hundred and forty-seven women of the study group (n=232) were assessed at 6 to 8 weeks post-partum by a psychiatrist with the use of 3 questionnaires (Edinburgh post-natal depression scale, Montgomery-Asberg depression rating scale and the Raskin depression scale). On the basis of these criteria 22 women were diagnosed as having post-natal depression (15%) and 21 as having borderline depression (14.3%). Of the women with PPTD (n=24) 4 (16.7%) met the criteria for post-natal depression and 2 (8.3%) for borderline depression. The frequency of depression was no different from that in the PPTD -ve group (n=123). Likewise no relationship existed between thyroid antibody status and presence or absence of depression.

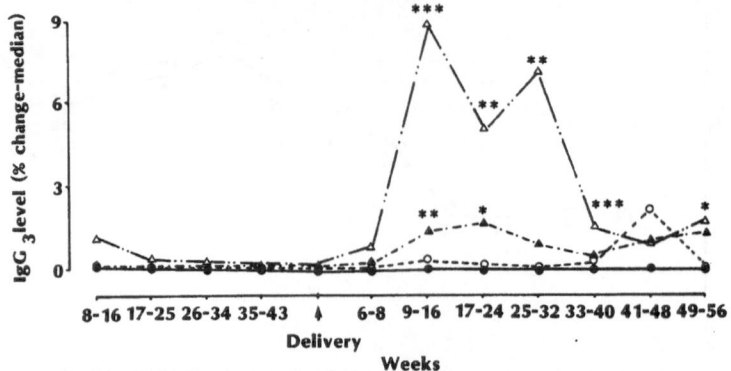

*p < 0.05 **p < 0.01 ***p < 0.001 as compared with the value of the control group at each time-point

△ Hyper/Hypo (n = 8)   ○ Hyper (n = 9)   ▲ Hypo (n = 14)   ● Control (n = 49)

Fig. 5.   Alteration in IgG_3 thyroid microsomal activity in 31 women with post-partum thyroid dysfunction (PPTD) in comparison with 45 women with normal thyroid function.

IV   CONCLUSIONS

Of 901 pregnant women with no previous history of thyroid disease, 12.98% were shown to have detectable antithyroid antibodies at the time of booking. In subsequent follow-up through the post-partum period of an antibody positive group (n=100) and an antibody negative group (n=132), 49 of the women (21.1%) were shown to develop PPTD. In highlighting the frequency of significant alterations in thyroid function in the post-partum period this study has defined the kinds of dysfunction observed and indicated a number of parameters which may help in defining the population at risk as well as in clarifying the underlying events leading to PPTD.

REFERENCES

1.   Amino, N. and Miyai, K., 1983, Post-partum autoimmune endocrine syndromes, in: Autoimmune Endocrine Disease T.F. Davies ed., J. Wiley and sons, New York., pp247-272.

2.   Davies, T.F. and Cobin, R., 1985, Thyroid disease in pregnancy and the post-partum period. Mount Sinai J. Med., 52:59-77.

3.   Jansson, R. and Karlsson, A., 1986, Autoimmune thyroid disease in pregnancy and the post-partum period, in: Immunology of Endocrine Diseases pp181-196, A.M. McGregor, ed., M.T.P. Press Ltd, Lancaster.

4.   Weetman, A.P., Rennie, D.P., Hassman, R., Hall, R. and McGregor, A.M., 1983, Enzyme-linked immunosorbent assay of monoclonal and serum microsomal autoantibodies, Clin. Chim. Acta., 138:237-244.

5. Weetman, A.P., Ratanachaiyavong, S., Middleton, G.W. et al. 1986, Prediction of outcome in Graves' disease after carbimazole treatment, Quart. J. Med. (New Series), 59:409-419.

6. Kilduff, P., Black, E.G., Hall, R. and McGregor, A.M., 1985, An enzyme-linked immunosorbent assay for the measurement of thyroglobulin in human serum using mouse monoclonal antibodies. J. Endocrinol., 107:383-387.

7. Parkes, A.B., McLachlan, S.M., Bird, P. and Rees Smith, B., 1984, The distribution of microsomal and thyroglobulin antibody activity among the IgG subclasses, Clin. Expt. Immunol., 57:239-243.

AUTOIMMUNE AND AUTONOMOUS TOXIC GOITER: DIFFERENTATION
AND CLINICAL OUTCOME AFTER DRUG TREATMENT

H. Schleusener, G. Holl, J. Schwander, K. Badenhoop, J.
Hensen, R. Finke, G. Schernthaner[+], W.R. Mayr[++], and
P. Kotulla, R. Holle[**]

Endocr. Dept., Medical Clinic, Klinikum Steglitz, Freie
Universität Berlin, Berlin, West-Germany
[*]IInd Medical Clinic[+] and Institute of Blood Group
Serology[++], University of Vienna, Vienna, Austria
[**]Center for Methodical Guidance of Therapeutic Studies
University of Heidelberg, Heidelberg, West Germany

Our own data presented in this paper are taken from investigations of
a multicenter prospective study[*], in which the following colleagues
participate:
Althoff (Frankfurt), Badenhoop (Mannheim), Benker (Essen), Beyer
(Mainz), Börner (Würzburg), Bogner (Berlin), Bretzel (Gießen), Fiek (Berlin), Finke (Berlin), Gräf (Berlin), Grebe (Gießen), Hengst (Münster),
Hensen (Berlin), Holl (Berlin), Hopf (Berlin), Hüfner (Heidelberg), Joseph
(Marburg), Jungmann (Frankfurt), Kahaly (Mainz), Kotulla (Berlin), Koppenhagen (Berlin), Müller-Eckardt (Gießen), Pickardt (München), Raue (Heidelberg), Reiners (Würzburg), Reinwein (Essen), Schatz (Gießen), Schleusener
(Berlin), Schöffling (Frankfurt), Schumm (Frankfurt), Schwander (Berlin),
Schwedes (Mannheim), Seif (Tübingen), Usadel (Mannheim), Witte (München),
Ziegler (Heidelberg)

SUMMARY

Graves' disease and autonomous goiter are the main reasons for the development of hyperthyroidism. In about 90% of untreated patients, the differentiation is possible either by clinical findings, i.e., concomitant
Graves' ophthalmopathy, or by laboratory data, i.e., measuring of TSH-receptor-antibodies. Very recently it has become evident that in patients
with longstanding Graves' disease autonomous cell clones may also proliferate, thus leading to a mixed histological pattern.

In patients with Graves' disease, the relapse rate is in the range of
50% to 70% one year after an antithyroid drug therapy. The data of some
publications suggest that a higher maintenance dose or a longer duration
of treatment can reduce this high rate. Many groups have investigated on
whether clinical signs, i.e., size of goiter and presence of ophthalmopathy, or laboratory investigations such as HLA-typing, measurement of TSH-

---

[*]This study was supported by the Bundesminister für Forschung und
Technologie (FRG)

receptor-antibodies or suppression tests will give reliable information about the risk of relapse. These data are very conflicting. In a multicenter prospective study, we obtained strong evidence that none of these parameters are of clinical importance.

DIFFERENTIATION

The two main causes of hyperthyroidism are Graves' disease (GD) and Plummer's disease (PD).

The pathogenetic factor in Graves' disease is the presence of autoantibodies directed against the TSH-receptor. They act like TSH itself (McKenzie, 1980; Burman et al., 1985).

In contrast, hyperthyroidism in Plummer's disease is caused by replication of autonomous cell clones because of an "inborn growth advantage" (Studer et al., 1985a). The individual cells vary in hormone production from nearly none to excessive. The combination of the "inborn growth advantage" and exogenous factors (e.g. iodine, goitrogens) leads to a heterogeneity of goiter ranging from simple goiter, on the one hand, to nodular goiter, toxic nodular goiter, or toxic adenoma, on the other hand (Studer et al., 1985b) (fig. 1).

There are also morphological differences between Graves's disease and

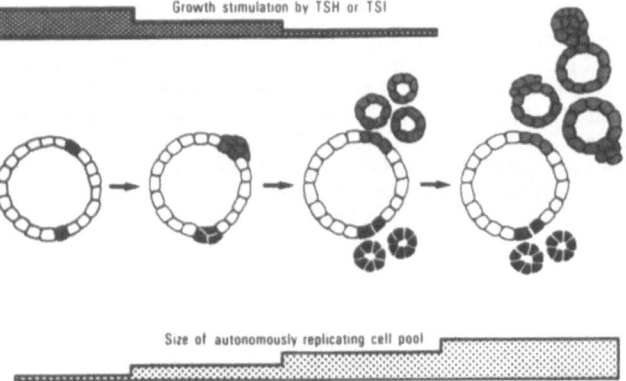

Fig. 1: Pathogenesis of autonomous goiter growth. Diagrammatic representation of the sequence of TSH (or TSI) depending and autonomous goiter growth. The follicle is assumed to contain two clones of epithelial cells with high intrinsic growth potential (shaded cells). The clone shown in the upper part of the follicle is assumed to possess inborn growth potential high enough to maintain cell replication and, hence, follicle neogeneration, even in the absence of exogenous stimuli, while the cell clone in the lower segment of the follicle multiplies only in response to exogenous growth factors. Any goitrogen will enhance growth of both cell clones and gradually lead to an increase of the total cell mass. Upon cessation of the goitrogenic stimulus, the clone with the highest spontaneous replication rate will multiply at the initial rate but, since its total size has increased, considerable autonomous goiter growth is now apparent (Studer et al., 1985b). (Reproduction with kind permission of H. Studer.)

Plummer's disease. In experiments in which tissue from autonomous goiters was transplanted into nude mice, Peter and co-workers (1985) could show that the follicles kept their original histologic structure and function, although autonomous growth and autonomous function are two different characteristics not always present in the same follicle at the same time.

In contrast, tissue from GD-thyroids also transplanted into nude mice (Dralle et al., 1985, Leclère et al., 1984) lost the hyperplasia of cells in the original tissue due to the absence of stimulating autoantibodies. In a personal communication, Dralle recently reported us about a few cases in which this loss of hyperplasia could not be seen in some follicles and thus represents a mixed histological pattern of GD and PD (fig. 2). This is in accordance with the theory of Studer (1985c) that, in GD thyroids, there are also autonomous cell clones which replicate and may mask the autoimmune process. At least they may contribute to a relapse of hyperthyroidism in an autoimmune thyroid.

Patients with newly arising hyperthyroidism can mostly be subdivided into GD- and PD-patients based on the existence of an endocrine ophthalmopathy and/or measurement of TSH-receptor-antibodies (TBIAb); in 80-90% TBIAb can be detected at the beginning of a drug treatment (Schicha et al., 1985; Schleusener et al., 1986). Thyroids of GD patients appear in ultrasound as tissue with diffuse, low echogenicity; autonome areas are indicated by demarcated foci with varying low echogenicity (Pfannenstiel 1983). In patients with a longstanding history of GD, ultrasound can reveal some focal alterations which are typical for autonomous areas (Müller-Gärtner et al., 1986). These show higher echogenicity similar to healthy thyroid tissue inside the low echogenic ultrasound appearance of a GD thyroid gland. "Histology of these areas revealed adenomas with a normal or macrofollicular structure" (Müller-Gärtner et al., 1986).

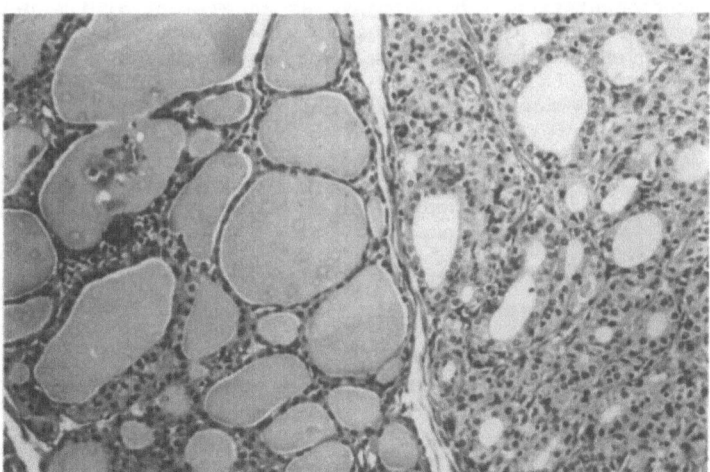

Fig. 2. Thyroid tissue of a Graves' disease patient transplanted to a nude mouse. The left side shows the typical histology of GD tissue after transplantation. After loss of stimulation the epithelium becomes flat and the structure macrofollicular. The right side represents the high epithelium of adenoma-tissue which remains high after transplantation. Both tissues are from the thyroid of a single patient.
(Reproduction with kind permission of H. Dralle.)

In accordance with these findings, we have some GD patients with nodular goiters in our own clinic (Hensen et al., 1984).

CLINICAL OUTCOME

General Comments

Since the introduction of thiouracil to the antithyroid therapy by Astwood in 1944, it has been widely used as the first choice for patients with GD, at least in Europe.

Methimazole (MMI) acts by blocking the peroxidase system, which is responsible for the building-in of iodine into thyroglobulin and the condensation of tyrosine to thyronine. In-vivo and in-vitro investigations suggest that methimazole also has an immunosuppressive effect, but this is still under discussion (McGregor et al., 1980; Jansson et al., 1983; Weetman et al., 1984; Wenzel et al., 1984). Patients with PD have been treated with surgery or radioiodine more often than with antithyroid drugs, based on the idea that the autonomous process cannot be cured otherwise.

In Europe, there has recently also been a tendency towards a more definite therapy for GD as has long been common practice in the USA (Hennemann et al., 1986).

The reason for this change of mind is the fact that the frequency of relapses after antithyroid drug therapy ranges between 50% and 70% (Wartofsky, 1973; Greer et al., 1977). Although studies on the clinical course after an antithyroid drug treatment are difficult to compare – because of different length of the therapy, different therapy schemes or different follow-up time – the relapse rate seemed to increase with time (Wartofsky, 1973). In the USA, one of the reasons might be the introduction of iodine supplementation. In Germany, as an area of iodine deficiency, iodine contamination plays the major role. Excessive doses of iodine have been proven to not only cause hyperthyroidism in PD (Herrmann et al., 1984), but to also destabilize the immune system in GD patients (McGregor et al., 1985). Some authors even discuss iodine as an inducer of the autoimmune process. Boukis and co-workers (1985) reported that, after application of iodinized oil, primarily microsomal-antibody-negative patients became positive. In a review of the recent literature, McGregor et al. (1985) demonstrated an increased rate of GD hyperthyroidism after the introduction of iodine supplementation.

Choice of Therapy for Hyperthyroidism

A number of groups investigated on whether clinical or laboratory parameters can point out which therapy is the best for an individual patient with hyperthyroidism.

Meng and co-workers (1982) reported about a prospective study (n=288) in which the influence of Graves' ophthalmopathy and size of the goiter was investigated. They found a higher risk of relapse after drug treatment in cases of large goiter, nodules within a goiter, and severe states of ophthalmopathy. The persons investigated were GD and PD patients. Another group (Laurberg et al., 1986) compared GD patients with and without goiter to patients with toxic nodular goiter (n=124). The patients with toxic nodular goiter quickly relapsed after cessation of drug therapy, as expected. A 5-year remission rate was attained by 83% of the GD patients without goiter but by only 37% of those with it. However, calculating sensitivity and specificity from the figures of the mentioned studies as an indicator of the validity of these parameters, these statistically clear results show no values which make these parameters important for clinical decisions.

Since 1982, there has been a prospective multicenter study in Germany to clarify the value of clinical and laboratory parameters for the managing of hyperthyroid patients. GD patients were treated mainly with thiamazole, beginning with 40 mg MMI. After the patients had become euthyroid, the dose was reduced to 5–10 mg MMI and 50 μg thyroxine were added. This treatment lasted for about 1 year. After the end of therapy, regular checks of the hormone levels and antibody titers were carried out for at least one further year. Our preliminary results – the study will end in December 1986 – show that 188 of 319 patients (59%) had relapsed one year after the end of an antithyroid drug therapy. One quarter of the patients with normal thyroid hormone levels showed no TSH response to TRH application ("latent hyperthyroidism"). Neither goiter size nor ophthalmopathy have any influence in predicting the success of an antithyroid drug treatment (tables 1, 2).

Tab. 1

Clinical Status of 274 Patients One Year after an Antithyroid Drug Treatment According to the Size of Goiter.

	goiter size		
	WHO 0-Ib	WHO II-III	
no relapse	67	47	114
relapse	67	93	160

sensitivity　0.58　　　　　　　　　　　　　　　　n=274
specificity　0.59

(preliminary results of the multicenter study)

Tab. 2

Clinical Status of Graves' Disease Patients One Year after an Antithyroid Drug Treatment According to the Degree of Ophthalmopathy at the Beginning of Therapy.

	WHO 0 - II	WHO III-VI	
no relapse	82	25	107
relapse	88	53	141

sensitivity　0.38　　　　　　　　　　　　　　　　n=248
specificity　0.77

(preliminary results of the multicenter study)

One could assume that GD patients who have high titers of microsomal (cytotoxic) antibodies (mab) might have a better chance to remain euthyroid after drug treatment, although the presence of mab does not necessarily lead to a destruction of thyroid cells (Lazarus et al., 1984; Wick et al., 1985). A Japanese group recently reported 22 patients who were tested for microsomal antibodies at the end of a one-year antithyroid drug therapy and who were still euthyroid 10 years later (Hirota et al., 1986). In these patients, both an increase in mab-frequency and a marked increase in mab-titers were found; no data about the mab-status of patients who relapsed were given. Hirota and coworkers (1986) concluded that GD may evolve in chronic thyroiditis in some patients who stay in remission.

Preliminary results of our study mentioned above indicate that neither microsomal antibody titers at the beginning of a drug treatment nor their course during treatment give any help in planning an optimal treatment. As far as one can judge this question by the short follow-up time of one year, the mab-titers at the end of therapy do not have any influence on the clinical course thereafter (n=197, sensitivity 0.39, specificity 0.59).

A number of groups have investigated on whether HLA-typing can predict the clinical outcome and came to conflicting results (for review see Schleusener et al., 1986). In our prospective study, we found no clinically relevant difference in the recurrence rate of DR3-positive and -negative patients (n=187, sensitivity 0.38, specificity 0.67, see Schleusener et al., 1986).

Dose and Duration of Therapy

In Europe, the dose of MMI is about 20-40 mg initially and 5-10 mg after euthyroidism has been achieved. Romaldini et al. (1983) advocate a high dose therapy because they saw a remission rate of about 75% after a one-year treatment with 60 mg MMI in 65 patients compared to 42% in 48 patients who were treated with a maintenance dose of about 15 mg MMI. A European multicenter study (Benker et al., 1986) will provide more information on this topic.

There is also no general agreement as to how long hyperthyroidism should be treated. The duration of therapy depends so far on the experience of each clinic and varies from 4 months to 4 years. Nearly all these studies were evaluated retrospectively and sometimes involved small numbers of patients. Greer et al. (1977), for example, show that the relapse rate does not differ among 31 patients treated for 5 months and 9 patients, who got a one-year treatment after their first relapse. In contrast to this, Slingerland et al. (1979) found that, in a total of 80 patients, the relapse rate was significantly different (p=0.001) among those patients who were treated for 1 year and those with a 4-year therapy. In the investigations by Tamai and coworkers (1980), the relapse rate depended on the duration of treatment: 6, 12, 18 and 24 months of therapy showed relapse rates of 69% (n=13), 56% (n=9), 25% (n=12) and 18% (n=11), respectively. In contrast Meng (1982) found in 288 patients a similar relapse rates after 1,2,3 and >3 years treatment.
Because of these differing results, several investigators looked for parameters which would indicate remission and help to predict the further course of the disease after an antithyroid drug therapy.

Criteria of Remission

Several parameters have been tested, especially the measurement of TSH-receptor-antibodies at the end of therapy with the radioligand receptor assay, and very controversial results were published (for review see Schleusener et al., 1986). In our study, we found a high statistical significance (p=0.0008) in relapse characteristics of the patients who were positive or negative for this parameter (n=269), the value for sensitivity (0.49) and specificity (0.72), however, show that this is not of any clinical importance (Schleusener et al., 1986).

A number of groups investigated whether a suppression test at the end of the therapy can predict the outcome and came to different conclusions (table 3). In our study, we could not show that a normal suppression at the end of an antithyroid drug treatment can predict the future course of an individual patient (table 4), although the result is of statistical significance (p=0.0001).

Investigations as to whether the TRH test at the end of therapy is an indicator for remission yielded encouraging results. In a study of Meng et al. (n=52), only 21% of the patients with a normal TSH response to TRH application relapsed. In patients with lacking TSH response, the relapse rate was 89% (Meng et al., 1983). Dahlberg and coworkers (1986) recently published similar results. In our study, we found for this parameter a sensitivity and specificity of 0.49 and 0.80, respectively, which shows the insignificance of this parameter for the prediction of outcome.

CONCLUSION

We feel that all these methods mentioned can only reflect the thyroid status at the time they were performed, but cannot predict the further clinical course. The reason for this thinking lies in the multifactorially caused genesis of autoimmune thyroid disease (Wick et al., 1985; Schleusener et al., 1986). Additional doubts base on the theory developed by Studer et al. saying that GD goiters could also contain autonomous cell clones. Further prospective studies in a sufficient number of patients should answer the question as to whether a high maintenance dose (e.g. 20 mg MMI/day) or a treatment for more than 2 years can yield satisfactory results. In view of the high relapse rate and the difficulties in finding parameters which can predict a future course of GD, it should be discussed whether surgery or radioiodine should be chosen at earlier times.

Tab. 3

Suppression of Radioiodine-Uptake at the End of an Antithyroid Drug Treatment and Future Clinical Course.

	n	normal n	Suppression relapses	no Suppression n	relapses
Cassidy 1970	184	48	21%	136	87%
Alexander et.al. 1970	93	51	31%	42	76%
Hackenberg et al. 1973	80	41	23%	39	61%
Meng et al. 1983	97	49	29%	48	69%
Yamamoto et.al. 1983	193	120	4%	-	-
Yamada et.al 1984	115	65	10%	-	-

Tab. 4

Suppressiontest at the End of an Antithyroid Drug Therapy and Clinical Status One Year Later.

	normal Suppression	no Suppression	
no relapse	56	22	78
relapse	36	59	95

sensitivity   0.62   n=173
specificity   0.72

(preliminary results of the multicenter study)

REFERENCES

Alexander, W.D., McLarty, D.G., Robertson, J., Shimmins, J., Brownlie, B.E.W., Harden, R.M., and Patel, A.R., 1970, Prediction of the long-term results of antithyroid drug therapy for thyrotoxicosis, J. Clin. Endocr., 30: 540.

Benker, G., Reinwein, D., Grobe, R., Creutzig, H., and Hirche, H., 1986, Effects of high and low dose of methimazole in patients with Graves' thyrotoxicosis, International Symposium "Advances in Thyroidology, Lübeck 1986, Acta Endocrinol, in press.

Boukis, M.A., Koutras, D.A., Souvatzoglu, A., Evangelopoulou, A., Vrontakis, M., Karaiskos, K.S., Piperingos, G.D., Kitsopanidis J., and Moulopoulos, S.D., 1985, Iodine-induced autoimmunity, in: "Thyroid Disorders Associated With Iodine Deficiency And Excess", Serono Symposium, R. Hall, J. Köbberling, eds., Raven Press, New York, p. 217.

Burman, K.D., Baker, and J.R., Jr., 1985, Immune mechanisms in Graves' disease, Endocr. Rev., 6: 183.

Cassidy, C.E., 1970, Thyroid suppression test as index of outcome of hyperthyroidism treated with antithyroid drugs, Metab., 19: 745.

Dahlberg, P.A., Karlsson, F.A., Jansson, R., and Wide L., 1985, Thyrotropin-releasing hormone testing during antithyroid drug treatment of Graves' disease as an inidcator of remission, J. Clin. Endocr. Metab., 61: 1100.

Dralle, H., Böcker, W, Döhler, K.D., Schröder, S., Haindl, H., Geerlings, H., Schwarzrock, R., and Pichlmayr, R., 1985, Growth and function of thirty-four human benign and malignant thyroid xenografts in untreated nude mice, J. Clin. Endocrinol. Metab., 59: 175.

Greer, M.A., Kammer, H., and Bouma, D.J., 1977, Short-term antithyroid drug therapy for the thyrotoxicosis of Graves' disease, New Engl. J. Med., 297: 173.

Hackenberg, K., Reinwein, D., Schemmel, K., 1973, Rezidivhäufigkeit methimazolbehandelter Hyperthyreosen und Suppressibilität der Schilddrüse, Münch. med. Wschr., 115: 2216.

Hennemann, G., Krenning, E.P., and Sankaranarayanan, K., 1986, Place of radioactive iodine in treatment of thyrotoxicosis, Lancet I, 1369.

Hensen, J., Kotulla, P., Finke, R., Badenhoop, K., Koppenhagen, K., Meinhold, H., and Schleusener, H., 1984, 10 years experience with consecutive measurement of thyrotropin binding inhibiting antibodies (TBIAB), J. Endocrinol. Inves., 7: 215.

Herrmann, J., Emrich, D., Kemper, F., Köbberling, J., Pickardt, R.C., and Stubbe, P., 1984, Jodexzeß und seine Auswirkung, Dtsch. Med. Wschr., 109: 1077.

Hirota, Y., Tamai, H., Hayashi, Y., Matsubayashi, S., Matsuzuka, F., Kuma, K., Kumagai, L.F., and Nagataki, S., 1986, Thyroid function and histology in fourty-five patients with hyperthyroid Graves' disease in clinical remission more than ten years after thionamide drug treatment, J. Clin. Endocrinol. Metab., 62: 165.

Jansson, R., Dahlberg, P.A., Johansson, H., and Lindström, B., 1983, Intrathyroidal concentrations of methimazol in patients with Graves' disease, J. Clin. Endocrinol. Metabol., 57: 129.

Laurberg, P., Hansen, P.E.B., Iversen, E., Jensen, S.E., and Weeke, J., 1986, Goitre size and outcome of medical treatment of Graves' disease, Acta Endocrinol., 111: 39.

Lazarus, J.H., Burr, M.L., McGregor, A.M., Weetman, A.P., Ludgate, M., Woodhead, J.S., and Hall, R., 1984, The prevalence and progression of autoimmune thyroid disease in elderly, Acta Endocrinol., 106: 199-202.

Leclère, J., Bene, M.C., Duprez, A., Fuare, G., Thomas, J.L., Vignaud, J.M., and Burlet, C., 1984, Behaviour of thyroid tissue from patients with Graves' disease in nude mice, J. Clin. Endocrinol. Metab., 59: 175.

McGregor, A.M., Petersen, M.M., McLachlan, S.M., Rooke, P., Smith, B.R., and Hall, R., 1980, Carbimazole and the autoimmune response in Graves' disease, New Engl. J. Med., 303: 302.

McGregor, A.M., Weetman, A.P., Ratanachaiyavong, S., Owen, G.M., Ibbertson, H.K., and Hall, R., 1985, Iodine: an influence on the development of autoimmune thyroid disease?, in: "Thyroid Disorders Associated With Iodine Deficiency And Excess", Serono Symposium, R., Hall, J. Köbberling, eds., Raven Press, New York, p. 209.

McKenzie, J.M., 1980, Thyroid-stimulating antibody in Graves' disease, in: "Thyroid Today," J.H. Oppenheimer, ed., 3 (5), 1.

Müller-Gärtner, H-W., Schneider, C., and Schröder, S., 1986, Autoimmune-resistance in Graves' disease tissues: indication of a structural and functional heterogenicity, Acta Endocrinol., 113: 233.

Meng, W., Meng, S., Stöwhas, H., Männchen, E., Ventz, M., and Hampel, R., 1982, Ergebnisse der thyreostatischen Langzeittherapie der Hyperthyreose – Einfluß der Struma, der Orbitopathie und der Behandlungsdauer, Dt. Gesundh.-Wesen, 37: 1956.

Meng, W., Stöwhas, H., Männchen, E., Weber, A., Ventz, M., Hampel, R., Meng, S., and Jäger, B., 1983, Prospektive Studie zur Frage der Erkennung einer Remission und zur Einschätzung der Prognose bei thyreostatisch behandelter Hyperthyreose. Dt. Gesund-Wesen, 38: 365.

Peter, H.J., Gerber, H., Studer, H., and Smeds, S., 1985, Pathogenesis of heterogeneity in human multinodular goiter, J. Clin. Invest., 76: 1982.

Pfannenstiel, P., 1983, Heutiger Stellenwert und Indikationen der Sono-graphie der Schilddrüse, Akt. Endokr. Stoffw., 4: 142-150.

Romaldini, J.H., Bromberg, N., Werner, R.S., Tanaka, L.M., Rodrigues, H.F., Werner, M.C., Farah, C.S., and Reis, L.C.F., 1983, Comparison of effects of high and low dosage regimens of antithyroid drugs in the management of Graves' hyperthyroidism, J. Clin. Endocrinol. Metab., 57: 563.

Schicha, H., Emrich, D., Schreivogel, I., 1985, Hyperthyroidism due to Graves' disease and due to autonomous goiter, J. Endocrinol. Invest., 8: 399-407.

Schleusener, H., Schwander, J., Holl, G., Badenhoop, K., Hensen, J., Finke, R., Schernthaner, G., Mayr, W.R., and Kotulla, P., 1986, Do HLA-DR-typing and measurement of TSH-receptor antibodies help in the prediction of the clinical course of Graves' thyrotoxicosis after antithyroid drug treatment?, International Symposium "Advances in Thyroidology, Lübeck 1986, Acta Endocrinol., in press.

Slingerland, D.W., Burrows, B.A., 1979, Long-term antithyroid treatment in hyperthyroidism, JAMA, 242: 2408.

Studer, H., Peter, H.J., and Gerber, H., 1985a, Toxic nodular goiter, Clinics Endocrinol. Metabol., 14: 351.

Studer, H., Peter, H.J., and Gerber, H., 1985b, Morphologic and functional changes in developing goiters, in: "Thyroid Disorders Associated With Iodine Deficiency And Excess," R. Hall, J. Köbberlin, eds., Raven Press, New York, p. 227.

Studer, H., 1985c, Growth control and follicular cell neoplasia, in: "New Frontiers In Thyroidology," G.A. Medeiros-Neto, E. Gaitan, eds., Proceedings of the 9th International, Thyroid Congress Sao Paulo, Brazil, Plenum Press, New York.

Tamai, H., Nakagawa, T., Fukino, O., Ohsako, N., Shinzato, R., Suematsu, H, Kuma, K., Matsuzuka, F., and Nagataki, S., 1980, Thionamide therapy in Graves' disease: Relation of relapse rate to duration of therapy, Ann. Int. Med., 92: 488.

Wartofsky, L., 1973, Low remission after therapy for Graves' disease, JAMA, 226: 1083.

Weetman, A.P., McGregor, A.M., and Hall, R., 1984, Evidence for an effect of antithyroid drugs on the natural history of Graves' disease, Clin. Endocrinol., 21: 163.

Wenzel, K.W., and Lente, J.R., 1984, Similar effects of thionamide drugs and perchlorate on thyroid-stimulating immunoglobulins in Graves' disease: Evidence against an immunosuppressive action of thionamide drugs, J. Clin. Endocrinol. Metab., 58: 62.

Wick, G., Möst, J., Schauenstein, K., Krömer, G., Dietrich, H., Ziermiecki, A., Fässler, R., Schwarz, S., Neu, N., and Hala, K., 1985, Spontaneous autoimmune thyroiditis - a bird's eye view, Immunology Today, 6: 359-364.

Yamada, T., Koizumi, Y., Sato, A., Hashizume, K., Aizawa, T., Takasu, N., and Nagata, H., 1984, Reappraisal of the 3,5,3'-triiodothyronine-suppression test in the prediction of long term outcome of antithyroid drug therapy in patients with hyperthyroid Graves' disease, J. Clin. Endocrinol. Metab., 58: 676.

Yamamoto, M., Totsuka, Y., Kojima, J., Yamashita, N, Togawa, K., Sawaki, N., and Ogata, E., 1983, Outcome of patients with Graves' disease after long-term medical treatment guided by triiodothyronine (T3) suppression test, Clin. Endocr., 19: 467.

Addendum

24 out of our 319 patients were treated for > 18 months and 42 patients had a maintenance of > 20 mg thiamazol daily. Both subgroups had not a higher remission rate than the total group.

POSTPARTUM ONSET OF GRAVES' DISEASE

Nobuyuki Amino, Haruo Tamaki, Mieko Aozasa, Yoshinori Iwatani
Junko Tachi, Kiyoshi Miyai, Masao Mori and Osamu Tanizawa

Department of Laboratory Medicine and Obstetrics and
Gynecology, Osaka University Medical School
1-1-50 Fukushima, Fukushima-ku Osaka 553, Japan

1. INTRODUCTION

Pregnancy markedly influences the clinical course of autoimmune thyroid diseases (1, 2). Graves' disease is aggravated in early pregnancy but ameliorated in the later half of pregnancy (3). Hashimoto's disease is also ameliorated during pregnancy and slightly increased levels of serum TSH are often returned into normal range in association with the progress of pregnancy (4). Contrary to amelioration of disease during pregnancy, both Graves' disease and Hashimoto's disease are aggravated after delivery and various types of thyroid dysfunction, as shown in Figure 1, are frequently observed (3~5).

Subclinical autoimmune thyroiditis (6, 7) is also aggravated after delivery and thyroid dysfunction was found in 5.5~7.1 per cent of postpartum women in general population (8-10). Fortunately more than 90 per cent of these postpartum thyroid dysfunction are transient but persistent Graves' thyrotoxicosis also developes after delivery (9, 10). In the present report we deal with postpartum onset of Graves' disease.

2. HISTORICAL REMARKS

Graves' disease was first described by Caleb H. Parry. In 1825, 3 years after Parry's death, a collection of his hitherto unpublished medical writings was assembled and published by his son. The first case of his 6 patients seen in 1786 had experienced palpitation, neck swelling and protrusion of eyes after delivery (11). Thus the first patients with Graves' (Parry's) disease described in the medical literature was the case of postpartum onset. In 1840, Karl A. von Basedow reported 4 cases of Graves' (Basedow's) disease (12). Interestingly one of his patients was also the case of postpartum onset. Reviewing these old reports, it is easily supposed that postpartum onset of Graves' disease may be frequently observed in general population. However, as far as we know, no systematic study was done on the postpartum onset of Graves' disease (postpartum Graves' disease).

3. PREVALENCE OF POSTPARTUM GRAVES' DISEASE

Considering the reports described above, we first examined the prevalence of postpartum onset of Graves' disease.

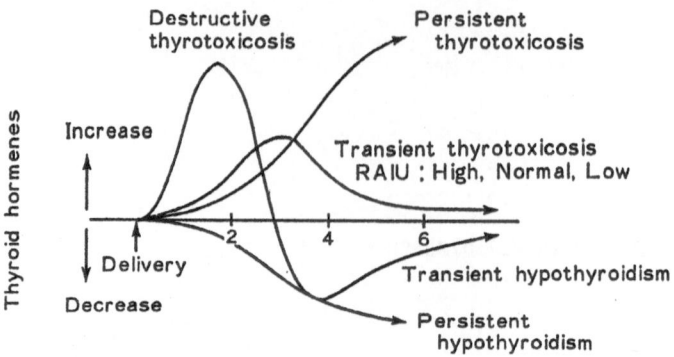

Figure 1. Changes of free thyroxine index in various types of postpartum thyroid dysfunction. Numbers indecate months postpartum.

Table 1 Screening of thyroid dysfunction
at 3 months postpartum among 680 subjects

Type of Thyroid Abnormality	Patients No. (%)	Number of cases Goiter	TGHA	MCHA
Transient thyrotoxicosis	13 (1.91)	6	5	11
Transient thyrotoxicosis followed by transient hypothyroidism	7 (1.03)	4	3	6
Persistent thyrotoxicosis	1 (0.15)	1	0	0
Transient hypothyroidism	8 (1.18)	7	3	7
Persistent hypothyroidism	1 (0.15)	1	1	1
Total	30 (4.41)	19	12	25

Table 2 Screening of thyroid dysfunction
at 7 months postpartum among 507 subjects

Type of thyroid abnormality	No. of patients (%)	Number of cases Goiter	MCHA
Transient thyrotoxicosis alone	1 (0.20)	0	0
Transient thyrotoxicosis followed by transient hypothyroidism	1 (0)	0	0
Persistent thyrotoxicosis Postpartum onset	1 (0.20)	0	0
Prediagnosed Graves' disease	1 (0.20)	1	1
Transient hypothyroidism alone	10 (1.97)	4	6
Persistent hypothyroidism	1 (0.20)	0	1
Total	13 (2.56)	5	8

A.SCREENING STUDY AT 3 MONTHS POSTPARTUM

Postpartum thyroid dysfunction was examined in 680 monthers at 3 months postpartum. The neck was palpated by one of us (N.A.) and serum T4, T3, TSH, anti-thyroglobulin antibody (TGHA), anti-thyroid microsomal hemagglutination antibody (MCHA), complete blood counts, and 25 biochemical constituents were measured in all subjects. Any subjects in whom the transverse width of the thyroid gland was more than 4.0cm was considered to have a goiter. When the subjects had abnormal thyroid function, enlarged thyroid gland and/or positive reaction for MCHA, they were followed longer. In subjects with high or low serum levels of thyroid hormones, free T4 and TBG were also measured.

Finally one patient with persistent Graves' disease was found (Table 1). At 7 months postpartum her serum T4 was 19.0 μg/dl, T3 593 ng/dl and radioactive iodine uptake (RAIU) was 69.4% (24hours) and anti-thyroid drug was started. She had slightly enlarged goiter (transverse width 4.7cm) but no anti-thyroid antibodies. Thirty of 680 subjects (4.41%) were found to have various types of thyroid dysfunction and 28 patients were transient type

B. SCREENING STUDY AT 7 MONTHS POSTPARTUM

A similar screening study was performed at 7 months postpartum, instead of 3 months postpartum, in order to detect more effectively the persistent types of thyroid dysfunction. In all 507 subjects the neck was palpated and thyroid dysfunction was evaluated by measuring serum free T4 and TSH, using new analog free T4 radioimmunoassay and highly sensitive immunoradio-radiometric assay, respectively. Anti-thyroid antibodies, complete blood counts and blood biochemical constituents were also measured.

Compared with the study at 3 months postpartum, incidence of transient thyrotoxicosis was markedly reduced as expected, but transient hypothyroidism was still observed frequently (Table 2). In this study persistent thyrotoxicosis was found in two subjects but one of them was revealed to be a prediagnosed active Graves' disease. Thyrotoxicosis in the patient with postpartum Graves' disease was mild, and her serum T4 was 14.3 μg/dl, T3 228 ng/dl and RAIU 37.5% at 10 months postpartum. This patient had no goiter or anti-thyroid antibodies. Anti-thyroid drug therapy was started at 16 months postpartum.

C. FOLLOW UP STUDY OF SUBCLINICAL AUTOIMMUNE THYROIDITIS

Postpartum thyroid dysfunction was thought to be induced by the aggravation of subclinical autoimmune thyroiditis. Therefore, the patients with subclinical autoimmune thyroiditis was screened by measurement of anti-thyroid microsomal antibody (MCHA) in early pregnancy.

One hundred and ninety-seven (15.3%) of 1285 subjects who were seen in our maternity clinic had positive reaction for MCHA: of these, 62 had prediagnosed Graves' disease and 17 had prediagnosed Hashimoto's disease and the remaining118subjects(9.2%)was newly diagnosed as having a subclinical autoimmune thyroiditis (Table 3). Thirty-four cases of these patients could be followed monthly during pregnancy and after delivery until 6 months postpartum. Finally Graves' disease occured after delivery in two patients (Table 4). Serial changes of thyroid function and anti-thyroid antibodies is described later.

D. PREVALENCE OF POSTPARTUM ONSET

We combined the 3 studies described above and calculated the overall incidence of postpartum onset of Graves' disease. As shown in Table 5, four patients with Graves' disease were newly found after delivery in 2472 mothers examined and thus the incidence was 0.16 per cent.

Table 3 Screening of anti-thyroid microsomal antibodies
in early pregnancy

MCHA Positive	197 (15.3%)
Prediagnosed Graves' disease	62 (4.8%)
Prediagnosed Hashimoto's disease	17 (1.3%)
Subclinical autoimmune thyroiditis	118 (9.2%)
MCHA Negative	1088 (84.7%)
Total	1285

Table 4 Postpartum development of thyroid dysfunction
in patients with subclinical autoimmune thyroiditis

Postpartum thyroid function	Case No.	%
Euthyroid	14	41.2
Destructive thyrotoxicosis alone	2	5.9
Destructive thyrotoxicosis followed by transient hypothyroidism	9	26.5
Transient hypothyroidism alone	7	20.6
Graves' disease	2	5.9
Total	34	100

Table 5 Prevalence of postpartum onset of Graves' disease

	No. of postpartum Graves' disease	(%)	Total subjects examined
Postpartum screening study			
3 months	1	(0.15)	680
7 months	1	(0.20)	507
Follow up study	2	(0.16)	1285
Total	4	(0.16)	2472

4. PREDICTION OF POSTPARTUM GRAVES' DISEASE

Postpartum occurrence of thyroid dysfunction could partially be
prevented by the short-term steroid therapy (13). Therefore it is very
important to predict exactly the postpartum onset of Graves' disease.
We could predict the relapse of Graves disease by the increase of free T4
at both 10-15 and 30-32 weeks of pregnancy (14). However this parameter
was not useful for the patients with subclinical autoimmune thyroiditis.
We analyzed various parameters in early pregnancy and the relation to the
postpartum onset of Graves' disease was examined in the patients with
subclinical autoimmune thyroiditis. In the follow-up study as described

above, anti-thyroid microsomal antibody (MCHA) was measured at first, and then TSH-binding inhibitory immunoglobulin (TBII) and peripheral lympho-cyte subsets were measured only in the subjects with positive MCHA.

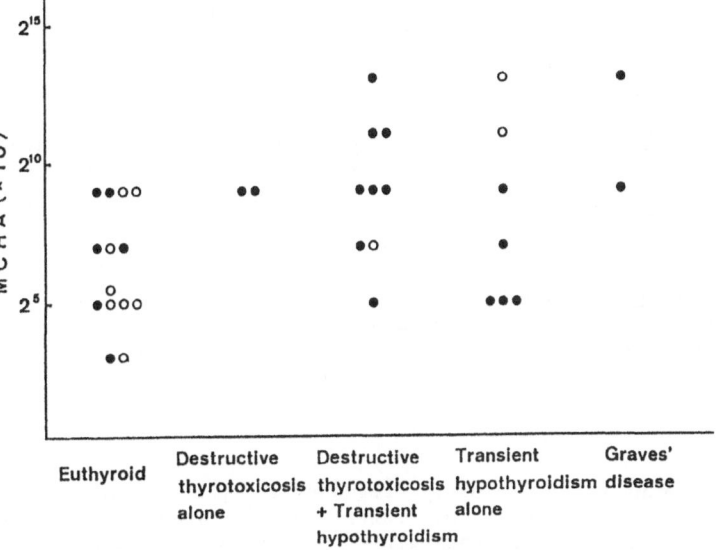

Figure 2. Relation of anti-thyroid microsomal antibodies (MCHA) in early pregnancy and postpartum changes of thyroid function in the patients with subclinical autoimmune thyroiditis. Closed and open circles indecate female and male babies, respectively.

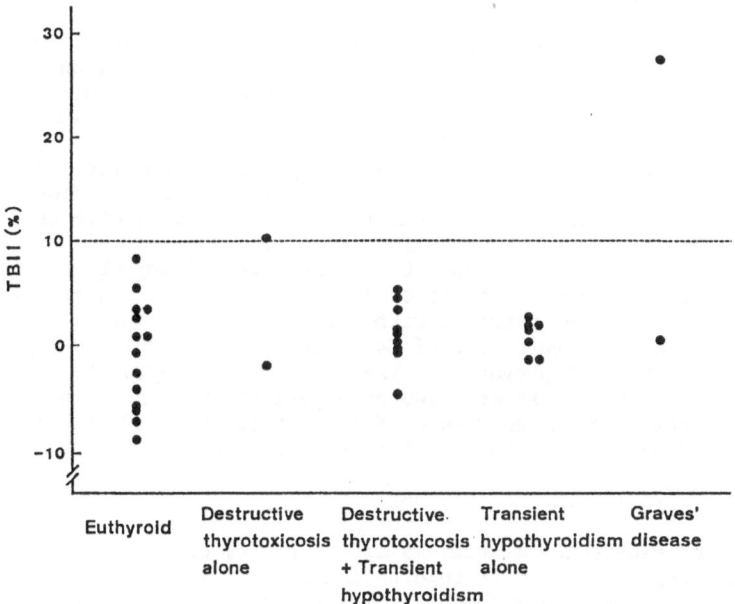

Figure 3. Relation of TSH-binding inhibitory immunoglobulin (TBII) in early pregnancy and postpartum changes of thyroid function in the patients with subclinical autoimmune thyroiditis.

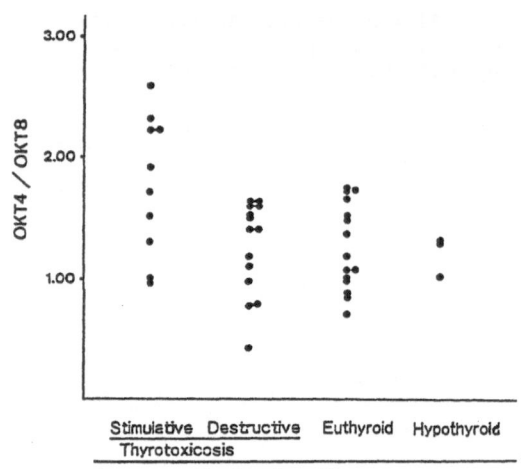

Figure 4.

Relation of OKT4/OKT8 lymphocyte ratio in early pregnancy and postpartum changes of thyroid function in Graves' disease in remission.

Relation of MCHA titers in early pregnancy and postpartum thyroid dysfunction in the patients with subclinical autoimmune thyroiditis is shown in Figure 2. All six patients with MCHA titers more than 2^{10}x10 developed thyroid dysfunction, but MCHA titers overlapped between the patients with postpartum Graves' disease and those of destructive thyrotoxicosis and hypothyroidism. In the whole group of postpartum thyroid dysfunction, 17 of 20 patients (85%) delivered a female baby,whereas 6 of 14 patients (43%) who did not develop postpartum thyroid dysfunction (Euthyroid group in Figure 2) delivered a female baby.The difference between the two was significant (p<0.05).

The relation of serum levels of TBII in early pregnancy and postpartum thyroid dysfunction was observed in the patients with subclinical autoimmune thyroiditis (Figure 3). Very interesting,one of two patients with postpartum Graves' disease had positive TBII. The other patients showed negative or borderline activity of TBII.

In order to evaluate the measurement of peripheral lymphocyte subsets, pilot study was done in the patients with Graves' disease in remission. All six patients with Graves' disease, who had lower levels of OKT8 cells less than 22%, relapsed Graves' thyrotoxicosis after delivery. All patients with   OKT4/OKT8 ratio more than 2.0 relapsed Graves' thyrotoxicosis (Figure 4). Usefullness of measurement of lymphocyte subsets was applied to the follow-up study of the patients with subclinical autoimmune thyroiditis. As shown in Figure 5, 3 of 34 patients showed lower OKT8 cells less than 20% in early pregnancy. Two of these developed the postpartum onset of Graves' disease. Two of 4 patients with subclinical autoimmune thyroiditis who showed OKT4/OKT8 ratio more than 2.0 in early pregnancy developed postpartum Graves' disease (Figure 6).

5. MECHANISM OF POSTPARTUM GRAVES' DISEASE

In order to elucidate the mechanisms of postpartum onset of Graves' disease, serial changes of serum thyroid hormones, anti-thyroid antibodies and lymphocyte subsets were examined in prospectively observed above two patients with postpartum Graves' disease (Figures 7-10). In both patients MCHA titers decreased during pregnancy and increased after delivery, as in the other cases of autoimmune thyroid diseases (15). However,increases of activities of TBII and thyroid stimulating antibody

(TSAb), which was detected by sensitive cAMP production assay using FRTL-5 cells, were delayed after increase of thyroid hormones (Figures 7, 9).

As for lymphocyte subsets, the percentages of OKT3 cells decreased

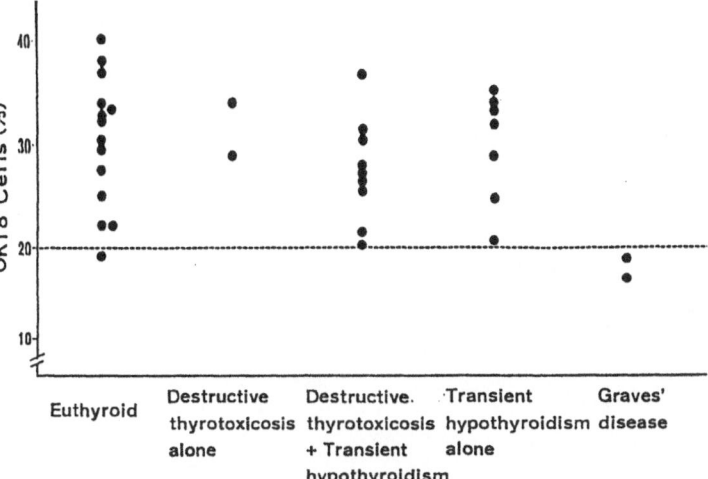

Figure 5. Relation of peripheral OKT8 lymphocytes in early pregnancy and postpartum changes of thyroid function in patients with subclinical autoimmune thyroiditis.

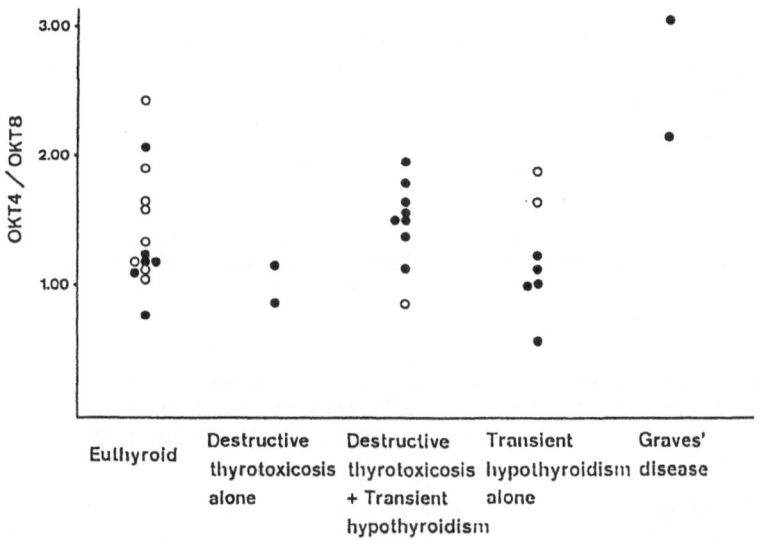

Figure 6. Relation of OKT4/OKT8 lymphocyte ratio in early pregnancy and postpartum changes of thyroid function in patients with subclinical autoimmune thyroiditis. Closed and open circles indicate female and male babies, respectively.

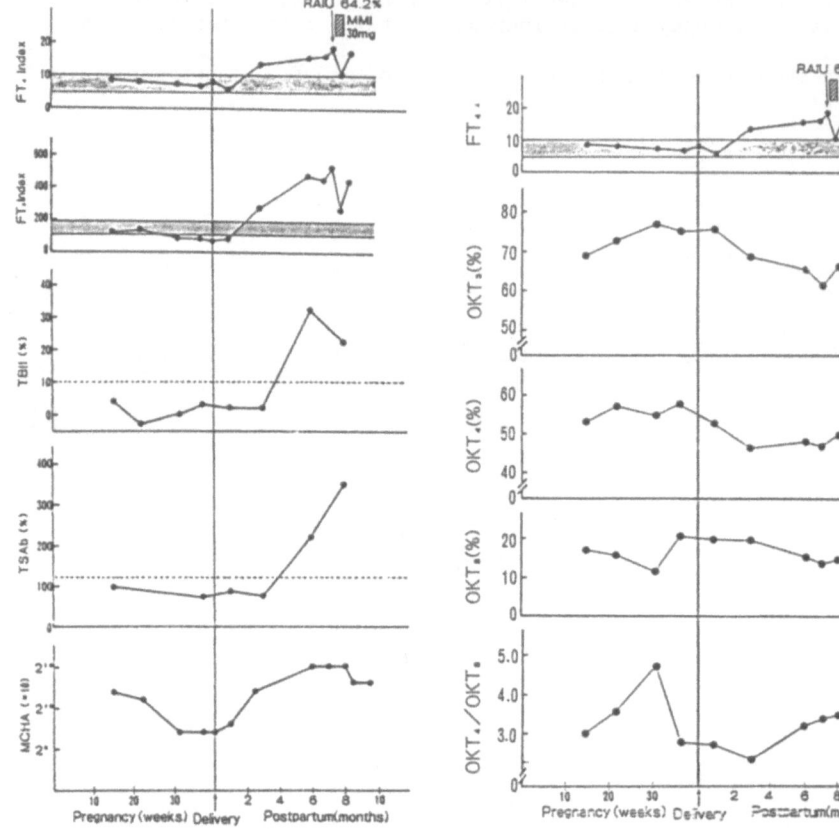

Figure 7. Serial changes of serum free T4 index, free T3 index, TBII, TSAb and MCHA in the patient who developed postpartum Graves' disease.

Figure 8. Serial changes of free T4 index, percentages of OKT3, OKT4 and OKT8 lymphocytes and OKT4/OKT8 lymphocyte ratio in the patient who developed postpartum Graves' disease.

(same patient in Figure 7).

after occurrence of Graves' thyrotoxicosis (Figures 8, 10) but no consistent changes were observed in other subsets to predict the postpartum onset of Graves' disease.

6. SUMMARY

Prevalence of postpartum onset of Graves' disease was 0.16% in general population. Measurement of MCHA, TBII and OKT4/OKT8 lymphocyte ratio in early pregnancy was partially useful for prediction of postpartum Graves' disease.

An increase of serum thyroid-stimulating antibody was associated with postpartum Graves' thyrotoxicosis, but delayed for 1-3 months after the increase of thyroid hormones.

In association with thyrotoxicosis percentage of OKT3 lymphocytes decreased, but no consistent changes were observed in other lymphocyte subsets to predict postpartum Graves' disease.

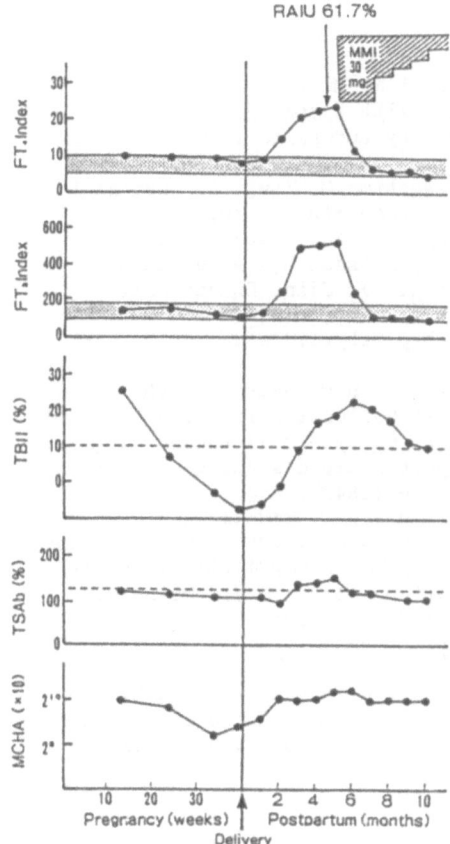

Figure 9.
Serial changes of serum free T4 index, free T3 index, TBII, TSAb and MCHA in the patient who developed postpartum Graves' disease.

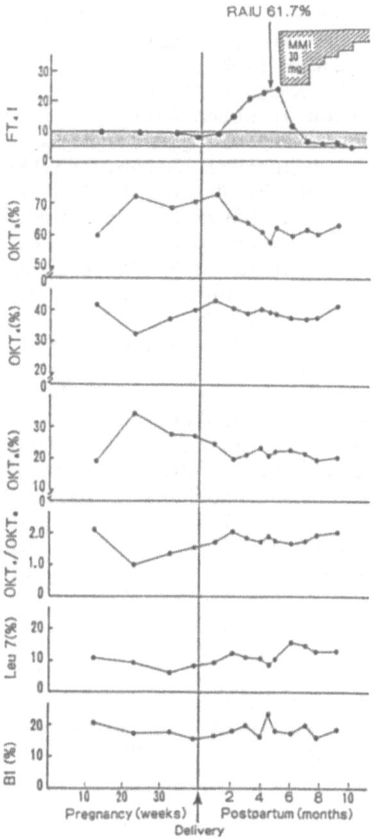

Figure 10.
Serial changes of free T4 index, percentages of various lymphocyte subsets and OKT4/OKT8 ratio in the patient who developed postpartum Graves' disease.

(same patient in Figure 9).

REFERENCES

1. Amino N, Miyai K, Onishi T, Hashimoto T, Arai K, Ishibashi K and Kumahara Y, Transient hypothyroidism after delivery in autoimmune thyroiditis. J. Clin. Endocrinol. Metab. 42:296 (1976).
2. Amino N, Miyai K, Yamamoto Y, Kuro R, Tanaka F, Tanizawa O and Kumahara Y, Transient recurrence of hyperthyroidism after delivery in Graves' disease. J. Clin. Endocrinol. Metab. 44:130 (1977).
3. Amino N, Tanizawa O, Mori H, Iwatani Y, Yamada T, Kurachi K, Kumahara Y and Miyai K, Aggravation of thyrotoxicosis in early pregnancy and after delivery in Graves' disease. J. Clin. Endocrinol. Metab. 55:108 (1982).
4. Amino N and Miyai K, Postpartum autoimmune endocrine syndromes. In Davies TF (ed) Autoimmune Endocrine Disease, pp.247-272, John Wiley & Sons, New York (1983).
5. Amino N, Miyai K, Kuro R, Tanizawa O, Azukizawa M, Takai S, Tanaka S, Nishi K, Kawashima M and Kumahara Y, Transient postpartum hypothyroidism: fourteen cases with autoimmune thyroiditis.

Ann. Intern. Med. 87:155 (1977).

6. Amino N, Miyai K, Autoimmune thyroiditis and Hashimoto's disease.
Lancet 2:585 (1978).

7. Yoshida H, Amino N, Yagawa K, Uemura K, Satoh M, Miyai K and Kumahara Y,
Association of serum antithyroid antibodies with lymphocytec infiltra-
tion of the thyroid gland: studies of seventy autopsied cases.
J. Clin. Endocrinol. Metab. 46:859 (1978).

8. Amino N, Mori H, Iwatani Y, Tanizawa O, Kawashima M, Tsuge I, Ibaragi K
Kumahara Y and Miyai K, High prevalence of transient postpartum
thyrotoxicosis and hypothyroidism. New Eng. J. Med. 306:849 (1982).

9. Jansson R, Bernander S, Karlsson A, Zevin K, Nilsson G, Autoimmune
thyroid dysfunction in the postpartum period. J. Clin. Endocrinol.
Metab. 58:681 (1984).

10. Walfish, P.G., Chan, J.Y.C., Post-partum hyperthyroidism.
Clin. Endocrinol. Metab. 14:417 (1985).

11. Parry, C.H., Enlargement of the thyroid gland in connection with
enlargement of palpitation of the heart. In Collection from the
Unpublished Papers of the late Caleb Hilliel Parry 2:111 London (1825).

12. von. Basedow K.A., Exophthalmos durch Hypertrophie des Zellgewebes in
der Augenhöhle. Wochenschr Heilk 6:197, 220 (1840).

13. Amino N, Iwatani Y and Tamaki H, Mori H, Miyai K and Tanizawa O,
Mechanism of postpartum thyroid disease. In Endocrinology. Labrie, F. and
Proulx, L. eds. Elsevier Science Publishers, New York, pp.461-464(1984).

14. Amino N, Iwatani Y, Tamaki H, Tamaki H, Mori H, Aozasa M and Miyai K,
Postpartum autoimmune thyroid syndromes. In Autoimmunity and The
Thyroid. Walfish, P.G., Wall, J.R., Volpe, R. eds. Academic Press,
Orland, Florida, pp.289-314 (1985).

15. Amino N, Kuro R, Tanizawa O, Tanaka F, Hayashi C, Kotani K, Kawashima M,
Miyai K and Kumahara Y, Changes of serum anti-thyroid antibodies during
and after pregnancy in autoimmune thyroid diseases. Clin. Exp. Immunol.
31:30 (1978).

THYROTROPIN-BINDING INHIBITOR IMMUNOGLOBULINS IN PRIMARY HYPOTHYROIDISM

Junji Konishi, Kanji Kasagi, Yasuhiro Iida, and Kanji Torizuka

Department of Nuclear Medicine
Kyoto University School of Medicine
Kyoto, Japan

INTRODUCTION

It is now widely accepted that immunoglobulins which inhibit the binding of 125-I-labeled thyrotropin to its receptor (TBII) are present not only in most patients with Graves' disease, but also in some sera from patients with primary hypothyroidism. In contrast to the thyroid-stimulating nature of IgG from patients with Graves' disease, TBII-positive IgG from hypothyroid patients has been found to be inhibitory against thyroid-stimulation induced by TSH. Thus, they are now considered to be blocking antibodies against thyrotropin receptors. In this paper, we will review the cases of TBII-positive hypothyroid patients so far reported in the literature to define characteristic features of the patients and the nature of TBII in these patients, and would like to discuss the pathogenetic role of the TBII in primary hypothyroidism.

INCIDENCE OF TBII IN HYPOTHYROID PATIENTS

The first case of a patient with primary myxedema who had potent TBII was reported in 1978 from our laboratory (1). Since then increasing number of TBII-positive hypothyroid patients have been found in Japan and recently in other countries (2-18). In a Japanese survey performed in 1984, 51 patients were reported from 9 institutions (14). Among them, 39 patients were nongoitrous. The incidence of TBII in nongoitrous and goitrous hypothyroid patients were 30.4% and 7.8%, respectively. In our screening of 43 each of nongoitrous and goitrous patients with hypothyroidism, TBII were positive in 9 (21%) and 7 (16%) patients, respectively (10). In another series of 20 nongoitrous patients, Arikawa et al.(9) reported that 8 (40%) patients were positive for TBII. Thus, the incidence of TBII in patients with primary nongoitrous hypothyroidism ranged from 21 to 40% in Japan. In other countries, Cho et al.(15) reported 2 cases in Korea, and Karlsson et al.(16) described a similar case in Sweden in 1984. Recently, 3 patients were reported by Clavel et al.(17) in France and one by Macchia et al.(18) in Italy. Although the number of cases are still limited in western countries, these findings clearly indicate that the condition is universal.

Table 1. Clinical and Laboratory Findings in Hypothyroid Patients Who Have TBII Activity Higher Than 50 %

No	Sex	Age at Onset	Goiter	Thyroglobulin Antibodies	Microsomal Antibodies	TBII (%)	Neonatal Hypothyroidism in Offspring	Author (Reference)
1	F	15	(-)	160	2,560	88	(-) 2	Endo (1)
2	F	15	(-)	25,600	25,600	97	(+) 2	Matsuura (2)
3	F	24	(-)	100	1,600	90	(+) 3	Iseki (3)
4	F	24	(-)	(-)	400	98	---	Konishi (4)
5	F	44	(-)	1,600	6,400	76	---	Konishi (4)
6	F	22	(-)	160	>40,960	90	(+) 1	Ninomiya (5)
7	F	15	(-)	100	25,600	89	(+) 1	Takasu (6)
8	F	21	(-)	(-)	640	72	---	Takasu (7)
9	F	36	(-)	(-)	160	92	---	Takasu (7)
10	F	32	(-)	(-)	(-)	104	---	Takasu (7)
11	F	32	(-)	(-)	(-)	51(x50)	latent(+) 1	Tamaki (8)
12	F	26	(-)	80	80	68(x50)	(+) 1	Tamaki (8)
13	F	27	(-)	(-)	100	79	(-) 1	Arikawa (9)
14	M	49	(-)	100	25,600	86	---	Arikawa (9)
15	F	29	(-)	6,400	100,000	89	---	Arikawa (9)
16	F	16	(-)	(-)	1,600	88	(-) 2	Arikawa (9)
17	F	32	(-)	400	(-)	89	---	Arikawa (9)
18	F	58	(-)	(-)	409,600	90	---	Arikawa (9)
19	M	51	(-)	(-)	1,600	81	---	Arikawa (9)
20	F	34	(-)	6,400	25,600	80	---	Konishi (10)
21	F	22	(-)	(-)	(-)	63	(-) 1	Konishi (10)
22	F	49	(-)	(-)	320	56	---	Konishi (10)
23	F	39	(-)	(-)	100	89	---	Konishi (10)
24	F	28	(-)	100	1,600	83	(+) 1	Konishi (10)
25	M	23	(-)	(-)	102,400	73	---	Konishi (10)
26	F	19	(-)	100	102,400	93	(+) 1	Yokota (11)
27	F	30	(-)	(-)	100	98	(+) 1	Inomata (12)
28	F	17	small	25,600	102,400	83	(-) 1	Inomata (12)
29	F	54	(-)	(-)	(-)	58	---	Mori (13)

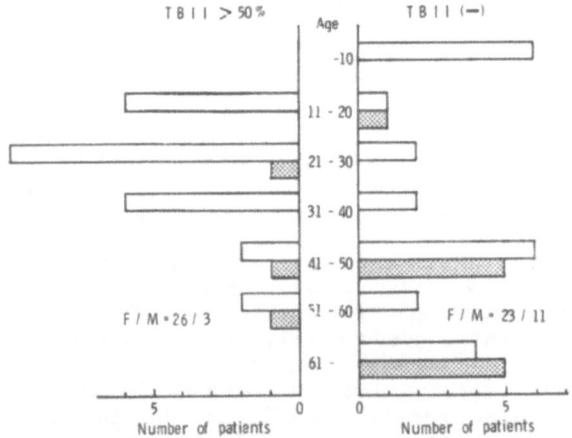

Fig. 1. Comparison of age and sex distributions of patients with primary myxedema who have TBII activity higher than 50% and those who have no detectable TBII.

CLINICAL AND LABORATORY FINDINGS IN TBII-POSITIVE HYPOTYROID PATIENTS

Twenty-nine cases of hypothyroid patients having potent TBII (>50% inhibition of 125-I-TSH binding) have so far been published (Table 1). They are composed of 26 females and 3 males. They rapidly developed hypothyroidism at ages ranging from 15 to 58, mean age 30.4 + 12.3 (S.D.), the highest incidence being in the third decade (Fig.1). Among them, only one female patient had a small goiter.

No significant difference was observed in serum TSH levels between TBII-positive and negative patients with primary myxedema. However, thyroid uptake in the former was signicantly lower than that in the latter (10). Antithyroid antibodies, especially antimicrosomal antibodies, were often positive in these patients (Table 1).

A characteristic feature was the ocurrence of transient hypothyroidism in newborn babies from these patients (2). Among 26 female patients, fourteen gave birth to 19 babies after the onset of the disease. Transient hypothyroidism was observed in 12 babies born in 9 (64%) families (Table 1). It is clinically important to note that TBII in hypothyroid mothers do not change substantially in their titer after replacement therapy and once a patient gave birth to a transiently hypothyroid baby, all the subsequent babies born in the same family suffered from this complication. In a recent survey of neonatal transient hypothyroidism performed in Japan by Matsuura et al. (19), 21 babies born in 15 families including cases described above, were reported. All of their mothers had potent TBII. TBII were also detected in all 14 babies studied, and became negative 2 to 10 months after delivery, being accompanied with the recovery from hypothyroidism. All babies except three who were only mildly hypothyroid, received thyroid replacement. However, in 3 babies whose mothers were hypothyroid during the pregnancy, retardation in mental and physical development was noted. Although mothers of hypothyroid infants had potent TBII without exception and the severity of hypothyroidism in infants appeared to be in accordance with the titer of TBII (10), there has been a report of discordant cases (20), and the complication did not occur in some instances of high maternal TBII activity like Case 1 in our series (Table 1). The fact suggests that some other factors which might influence the susceptibility of the thyroid cells are also involved in the development of this complication. Similar findings have been known as to the development of neonatal Graves' disease in infants from mothers with high titer of thyroid-stimulating antibody (21).

The characteristic clinical features of patients with primary hypothyroidism having TBII may be summarized as follows: They have female preponderance similar to Hashimoto's disaease, but their age distribution appears similar to that of Graves' disease; goiter is not palpable or small if any; they are mostly positive for antimicrosomal antibodies; they have a markedly diminished thyroid uptake; and transient hypothyroidism is often seen in their offspring.

BIOLOGICAL ACTIVITY OF TBII IN HYPOTHYROID PATIENTS

Immunoglobulin G from these patients showed no thyroid-stimulating activity both in vitro (cAMP) and in McKenzie bioassay. It inhibited human thyroid adenylate cyclase stimulation by TSH or Graves' IgG (1), and caused a significant inhibition of 131-I release induced by TSH or Graves' IgG in the bioassay (22). Titers of TSH-binding inhibitory activity in these IgGs were significantly correlated with their thyroid-stimulation blocking activity (Fig. 2)(10). The mode of the inhibition, when analyzed using Lineweaver-Burk plots, was mostly competitive (23), but non-competitive or mixed inhibition was also reported using few preparations (9). Papain digestion of an IgG preparation resulted in the complete preservation of both TSH-binding inhibitory and thyroid-stimulation inhibitory activities in Fab fragment (23).

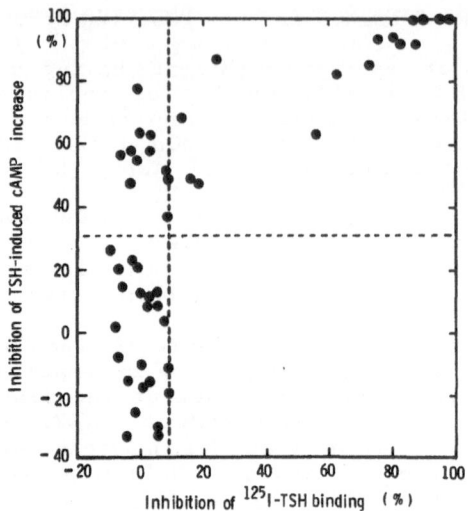

Fig. 2. Relation between TBII activity and thyroid-stimulation
blocking activity of IgG from patients with primary myxedema.

IgG preparations from these patients were also inhibitory against TSH-induced 3-H-thymidine incorporation into FRTL-5 cells (24). The growth-blocking activity was significantly correlated with their TSH-binding inhibitory activity.

The direct binding of the TBII to human thyroid membranes was observed after purification of the 125-I-labeled IgG by receptor adsorption using guinea pig fat membranes (22). The binding was significantly inhibited by TSH as well as the unlabeled TBII.

These data indicate that TBII in these patients are blocking antibodies directed against TSH receptors.

RELATION BETWEEN THYROID-STIMULATING ANTIBODY AND BLOCKING ANTIBODY

In order to analyze the difference between antigenic sites of the blocking antibodies and those of thyroid-stimulating antibodies (TSAb), we studied the influence of the blocking antibodies on various TSAb from Graves' patients. Blocking antibodies from a patient with primary myxedema inhibited TSAb activity of all immunoglobulin preparations from 21 patients with Graves' disease (Fig. 3)(25). The grade of inhibition was inversely correlated with TSAb or TBII activity of the Graves' immunoglobulins. Thus, TSAb without detectable TBII was most markedly inhibited by the blocking antibodies. Blocking activity against cAMP increase induced by TSAb of 11 immunoglobulin preparations from hypothyroid patients, was significantly correlated with both their TSH-binding inhibitory activity and blocking activity against TSH-induced cAMP increase (25). Thus, all of the blockig antibodies we tested inhibited both TSH and TSAb-induced cAMP increase in a similar manner. Being discordant with the results obtained by Valente et al. using monoclonal antibodies (26), these findings support the concept tha most of the thyroid-stimulating and blocking antibodies in patients with autoimmune thyroid diseases recognize the same or very closely located antigens in the TSH receptors.

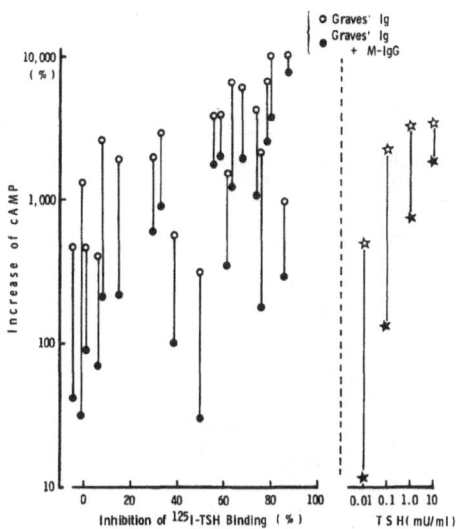

Fig.3. Left: Relation between TSH—binding inhibitory activity and
thyroid—stimulating activity of Graves' immunoglobulins, and
change of the thyroid—stimulating activity by the addition of
an IgG preparation from a patient with primary myxedema
(M—IgG).
Right: Effect of the addition of M—IgG on the dose—response
relationship of bovine TSH. Open and closed symbols
(connected by solid lines) indicate the responses in the
absence and the presence of M—IgG, respectively.

THYROID—STIMULATION BLOCKING ANTIBODY WITHOUT TBII ACTIVITY

In patients with primary myxedema, thyroid—stimulation blocking
antibodies which do not inhibit the binding of 125—I—TSH to its receptors
have also been reported . They have been detected by the inhibition of
adenylate cyclase activation (Fig. 2)(10), T3 release (27), 131—I uptake (6)
or thyroid growth (28) induced by TSH or other stimulators. The mechanism of
the action of these antibodies and their etiological role await further
clarification.

THYROTROPIN—RECEPTOR BLOCKING ANTIBODY IN GRAVES' DISEASE

The blocking nature of the TBII in hypothyroid patients is in marked
contrast to the thyroid—stimulating activity of TBII usually observed in
Graves' disease. However, heterogeneity in TSH—receptor antibodies in this
disease has been suggested by several previous studies (29—31). In 1982, Bech
et al. (32) reported the presence of blocking antibodies in 2 patients with
Graves' disease after radioiodine treatment. Creagh et al.(33) also described
TSH antagonist activity in IgG preparations from 2 patients. Recently, we
found a change of the biological activity of IgG from stimulating to blocking
one in a patient with Graves' disease concomitant with the development of
hypothyoidism after 3 years of antithyroid drug treatment (34). Since then,
we have confirmed the appearance of blocking antibodies in 4 other cases who
developed hypothyroidism after antithyroid drug treatment (35,36).
In connection with these findings, it is of special interest that
primary myxedema and Graves' disease are associated with the same HLA

ROLE OF TSH-RECEPTOR ANTIBODIES IN AUTOIMMUNE THYROID DISEASES

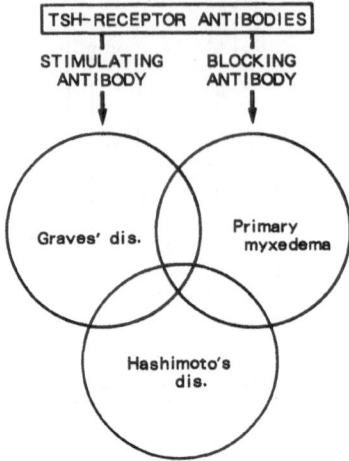

Fig. 4. Role of TSH-receptor antibodies in autoimmune thyroid diseases.

antigen, HLA-DR3, in white populations (37-39).

ROLE OF THYROTROPIN-RECEPTOR ANTIBODY IN HYPOTHYROIDISM

Both the biological nature of TBII and the close clinical association of the antibody with thyroid dysfunction emphasize the importance of this type of antibodies as a cause of hypothyroidism. As shown in Fig. 4, Graves' and Hashimoto's disease are known to be closely related, both clinically and in familial incidence. The presence of thyroid-stimulating antibody differentiates the former from the latter. On the other hand, primary myxedema has been considered to be an atrophic variant of Hashimoto's thyroiditis. However, at least a part of them is now disclosed to be a disease closely associated with thyrotropin-receptor blocking antibody. Furthermore, it was recognized that alteration in the population of receptor antibodies could lead a patient with Graves' disease to hypothyroidism. These findings support the concept that some type of primary myxedema and Graves' disease are at the opposite ends of a spectrum of autoimmune thyroid diseases caused by thyrotropin-receptor antibodies.

ACKNOWLEDGMENTS

The studies of the authors were supported in part by a Reseach Grant for the Intractable Diseases from the Ministry of Health and Welfare , and a Grant-in-Aid for Scientific Research from the Ministry of Education, Science and Culture, Japan.

REFERENCES

1. Endo K, Kasagi K, Konishi J, Ikekubo K, Okuno T, Takeda Y, Mori T, Torizuka K, J Clin Endocrinol Metab 46:734 (1978)
2. Matsuura N, Yamada Y, Nohara Y, Konishi J, Kasagi K, Endo K, Kojima K, Wataya K, N Engl J Med 303:738 (1980)
3. Iseki M, Shimizu M, Oikawa T, Hojo H, Arikawa K, Ichikawa Y, Momotani N, Itoh K, J Clin Endocrinol Metab 57:384 (1983)
4. Konishi J, Iida Y, Endo K, Misaki T, Nohara Y, Matsuura N, Mori T, Torizuka K, J Clin Endocrinol Metab 57:544 (1983)
5. Ninomiya M, Goji K, Takahashi T, Morishita Y, Kodama S, Iida Y, Kasagi K, Konishi J, Acta Paediatr Jpn 87:939 (Jpn) (1983)
6. Takasu N, Mori T, Koizumi Y, Takeuchi S, Yamada T, J Clin Endocrinol Metab 59:142 (1984)
7. Takasu N, Naka M, Mori T, Yamada T, Clin Endocrinol (Oxf) 21:345 (1984)
8. Tamaki H, Amino N, Iwatani Y, Watanabe Y, Mori H, Aozasa M, Harada T, Kaneya S, Maki I, Nose S, Mori M, Tanizawa O, Kumahara Y, Miyai K, Clin Endocrinol (Tokyo) 32:1089 (Jpn) (1984)
9. Arikawa K, Ichikawa Y. Yoshida T, Shinozawa T, Homma M, Momotani N, Itoh K, J Clin Endocrinol Metab 60:953 (1985)
10. Konishi J, Iida Y, Kasagi K, Misaki T, Nakashima T, Endo K, Mori T, Shinpo S, Nohara Y, Matsuura N, Torizuka K, Ann Intern Med 103:26 (1985)
11. Yokota Y, Oyama N, Otsuka K, Koshimizu T, Clin Endocrinol (Tokyo) 33:601 (Jpn) (1985)
12. Inomata H, Sasaki N, Tamaru K, Ushiku H, Niimi M, Nakajima H, Clin Endocrinol (Tokyo) 34:Supplement p.142 (Jpn) (1986)
13. Mori T, Ishii H, Akamizu N, Yokota T, Nakamura H, Kasagi K, Imura H, Clin Endocrinol (Tokyo) 34:Supplement p.130 (Jpn) (1986)
14. Nagataki S, in "Report of Research Committee on HormoneReceptor Anormality", Ogata E, ed., Ministry of Health and Welfare,Japan, p.29 (Jpn) (1985)
15. Cho BY, Koh CS, Lee M, in "Current Problems in Thyroid Disease", Lee M, Koh CS, Cho BY, eds., Korean Thyroid Society, Seoul, p.169 (1985)
16. Karlsson FA, Dahlberg PA, Ritzen EM, Acta Med Scand 215:461 (1984)
17. Clavel S, Madec AM, Stefanutti A, Orgiazzi J, Ann Endocrinol 47:p.87 (Abs) (1986)
18. Macchia E, Concetti R, Borgoni F, Carone G, Gasperini L, Fenzi GF, Ann Endocrinol 47:p.88 (Abs) (1986)
19. Matsuura N, Konishi J, Momotani N, Arikawa K, Nohara Y, Fujieda K, Kasagi K, Nakajima H, Inomata H, Mori T, Ishihara T, Suwa S, Tachibana K, Shimizu T, Igarashi H, Kaise K, Yamaguchi S, Koda N, Oyama N, Kurashige H, Ninomiya M, Ono S, Yamada Y, Clin Endocrinol (Tokyo) 34:809 (Jpn) (1986)
20. Amino N, Iwatani Y, Tamaki H, Mori H, Aozasa M, Miyai K, Mori M, Tanizawa O, in "Autoimmunity and the Thyroid", Walfish PG, Volpe R, eds., Academic Press, Orlando, Florida, p.289 (1985)
21. Rapoport B, Greenspan FS, Filetti S, Pepitone M, J Clin Endocrinol Metab 58:332 (1984)
22. Endo K, Konishi J, Misaki T, Iida Y, Nohara Y, Yamada Y, Matsuura N, Ingbar SH, Torizuka K, in "Current Problems in Thyroid Research", Ui N, Torizuka K, Nagataki S, Miyai K, eds., Excerpta Medica, Amsterdam, p.473 (1983)
23. Konishi J, Iida Y, Kasagi K, Endo K, Misaki T, Torizuka K, in "Endocrinology", Labrie F, Proulx L, eds., Excerpta Medica, Amsterdam, p.559 (1984)
24. Iida Y, Konishi J, Kasagi K, Misaki T, Arai K, Tokuda Y, Torizuka K, J Clin Endocrinol Metab in press
25. Konishi J, Kasagi K, Iida Y, Misaki T, Arai K, Nakashima T, Endo K, Nohara Y, Matsuura N, Torizuka K, in "Frontiers in Thyroidology", Plenum Publishing Co., N.Y., p.1505 (1986)

26. Valente WA, Vitti P, Yavin Z, Rotella CM, Grollman EF, Toccafondi RS, Kohn LD, Proc Natl Acad Sci USA 79:6680 (1982)
27. Steel NR, Weightman DR, Taylor JJ, Kendall-Taylor P, Brit Med J 288:1559 (1984)
28. Drexhage HA, Bottazzo GF, Bitensky L, Chayen J, Doniach D, Nature 289:594 (1981)
29. Orgiazzi J, Williams DE, Chopra IJ, Solomon DH, J Clin Endocrinol Metab 42:341 (1976)
30. Carayon P, Adler G, Roulier R, Lissitzky S, J Clin Endocrinol Metab 56:1202 (1983)
31. Zakarija M, McKenzie JM, J Clin Invest 72:1352 (1983)
32. Bech K, Bliddal H, Siersbaek-Nielsen K, Friis T, Clin Endocrinol (Oxf) 17:395 (1982)
33. Creagh FM, Howells RD, Williams S, Didcote S, Hashim FA, Petersen VB, Rees Smith B, Clin Endocrinol (Oxf) 24:79 (1986)
34. Kasagi K, Iida Y, Konishi J, Misaki T, Arai K, Endo K, Torizuka K, Kuma K, Acta Endocrinol 111:474 (1986)
35. Tamai H, Hirota Y, Kasagi K, Matsubayashi S, Kuma K, Iida Y, Konishi J, Okimura MC, Walter RM, Kumagai L, Nagataki S, J Clin Endocrinol Metab submitted for publication
36. Miki K, Takamatsu J, Kasagi K, Konishi, unpublished data
37. Farid NR, Sampson L, Noel EP, Barnard JM, Mandeville R, Larsen B, Marshall WH, J Clin Invest 63:108 (1979)
38. Weissel M, Hofer R, Zasmeta H, Mayer WR, Tissue Antigens 16:256 (1980)
39. Farid NR, Sampson L, Moens H, Barnard JM, Tissue Antigens 17:265 (1981)

THYROID FUNCTION MODULATES THYMIC ENDOCRINE ACTIVITY

Aldo Pinchera, Stefano Mariotti, Furio Pacini, Nicola Fabris* and Eugenio Mocchegiani*

Cattedra di Endocrinologia, Università di Pisa and (*) Dipartimento Ricerche Gerontologiche, I.N.R.C.A., Pisa and Ancona, Italy

INTRODUCTION

Several evidences have been accumulated indicating that thyroid function influences the immune system[1], but the precise mechanism(s) involved remain to be elucidated. Some of the more common thyroid disorders such as Hashimoto's thyroiditis, idiopathic myxedema and Graves' disease are typical organ-specific autoimmune disorders[2,3]. These conditions have a common basic immunologic disturbance, but differ in the abnormality of thyroid function, which ranges from hypothyroidism to hyperthyroidism. Whether and to what extent the altered thyroid function observed in thyroid autoimmune diseases may affect the immune system in general and/or thyroid immune surveillance is still unclear.

As reviewed in detail elsewhere[1], in spite of some inconsistencies, the immunological abnormalities observed in animals with experimental hypothyroidism appear to be mediated by impaired thymic function. In keeping with this notion, several recent data obtained in our and other laboratories provided evidence that thyroid function modulates the endocrine activity of the thymus[4-7]

In the present paper, attention will be focused on the studies showing that thyroid status affects in humans the plasma concentration of the thymic hormone called thymulin. Before reporting these results, we shall briefly review present knowledge on the relationship between the thyroid gland and the thymus.

THYROID FUNCTION AND THYMUS

Both experimental and clinical data suggest that thymic function is not completely autonomous, but appears to be regulated by the neuroendocrine system[4] and, in particular, by thyroid status[8-10] There is indirect evidence that the outflow of T cells from the thymus is altered by thyroid dysfunction, as judged from the distribution of T cell subsets[11,12] and from their functional capacity in peripheral lymphoid organs[13,14]. In both animals[15] and in man[16] hyperthyroidism and hypothyroidism are associated with hyper-and hypoplasia of the thymus, respectively.

Thymic function may also be evaluated by measuring plasma concentrations of thymic hormones. It is in fact presently recognized that the thymus produces hormone-like substances, some of which have been chemically characterized, such as thymosin-alpha[17], thymopoietin[18] and the factor called "Facteur Thymique Serique" (FTS)[19], more recently called thymulin in its zinc-bound biologically active form (Zn-FTS)[20]. No biochemical similarity exists among these different factors, although they are all produced by the epithelial cells of the thymus[21] and circulating plasma levels of such factors reflect the functional state of the thymus[22]. In particular, plasma concentrations of these factors decline progressively with advancing age, and this decline parallels the age-dependent involution of the thymus[22-24]. Since these factors are required to sustain the proliferation and the differentiation of thymocytes to mature T-cells[17-19], which are responsible for cell-mediated immunity, the major cause of the age-associated decline in immune capacity might be due to the progressive failure of thymic hormonal production[25].

As stated before, previous studies provided evidence that in experimental animals the secretion of thymic factors is modulated by thyroid hormones. In rodents thyroidectomy[4,5] and propylthiouracil treatment[6] cause reduction of circulating thymulin. Furthermore, the lack of detectable thymulin levels in old mice is reversed by administration of thyroxine (T4), and this reversal is followed by an increased immune efficiency at peripheral level[10,26].

In contrast to experimental animal models, until recently no information was available on the relationship between thyroid function and the circulating thymic hormones in humans. To study this problem, we measured thymulin by a rosette inhibition assay in a variety of conditions associated with abnormal thyroid function, as detailed below.

PLASMA THYMULIN LEVELS IN HYPERTHYROID AND HYPOTHYROID PATIENTS

The purpose of this section of the study[7] was to measure circulating thymulin concentrations in a series of hypothyroid or hyperthyroid patients before and after correction of the metabolic disturbance by appropriate treatment.

Patients

A total of 64 patients was studied. The hypothyroid group included 28 patients (6 men and 22 women aging 16-76 years) with untreated hypothyroidism due to total thyroidectomy for thyroid carcinoma (n=22), previous radioiodine therapy for toxic diffuse goiter (n=3), or idiopathic myxedema (n=3). The hyperthyroid group included 36 patients (16 men and 20 women, aging 26-28 years) with untreated hyperthyroidism due to toxic diffuse goiter (n=18), toxic multinodular goiter (n=12), or toxic adenoma (n=8). Eight hypothyroid (2 men and 6 women) and 9 hyperthyroid (3 men and 6 women) patients were studied after L-T4 or antithyroid drug treatments, respectively. The control group included 88 normal subjects (47 men and 41 women, aging 1 month - 90 years).

In all cases measurementes of serum T4 and triiodothyronine (T3) concentrations was done by radioimmunoassay using commercial kits (T4-RIA and T3-RIA, ARIA II, Becton Dickinson S.p.A., Milan, Italy). Anti-thyroglobulin and anti-thyroid microsomal antibodies were determined by passive hemagglutination and immunoradiometric assays[27,28].

Thymulin determination

Thymulin activity was measured in plasma samples by the method of Dardenne and Bach[29] with minor modifications. Briefly, plasma was filtered through a Centriflo Amicon Membrane with a cut-off of 50,000 daltons (Amicon Corp., Lexington, Ma, U.S.A.). Duplicate 50 μl of filtrate or serial dilutions of it made with Hank's solution were mixed with 200 μl of spleen cell suspension from thyroidectomized mice (final suspension 7.5×10^6/ml) and incubated at 37 C for 30 min. After washing, the cells were resuspended in 250 μl of a solution of azathioprine (The Wellcome Foundation Ltd., London, U.K.) at a concentration of 10 μg/ml; this concentration is able to inhibit the formation of rosettes by T lymphocytes but not by non-T spleen cells[29]. Cell suspensions were then incubated at 37 C for 60 min, after which 250 μl of a sheep red blood cell suspension containing 12.5×10^7/ml were added. After a further 5 min incubation at 37 C, cells were centrifuged in the cold at 100 x g for 5 min, resuspended for 5 min by using a rotating mixer and counted in a hemocytometer chamber. The rosette-forming cells (RFCs) present in 18,000 spleen cells were counted, and values were recorded as RFCs per 1×10^6 cells. The maximal dilution that induced azathioprine sensitivity in 50% of RFCs from thymectomized mice was taken as the thymulin titer. This procedure will be indicated thereafer as "conventional method".

To overcome the possible interference of zinc deficiency, occurring either in vivo[30] or resulting in vitro from dilution of the plasma filtrate by zinc-free medium, thymulin activity was also measured in duplicate using Hank's medium containing 200 nM zinc sulfate. This zinc concentration was chosen on the basis of preliminary experiments performed with graded concentrations ranging from 1 pM to 10 μM. This procedure will be indicated in the following paragraph as the "modified assay".

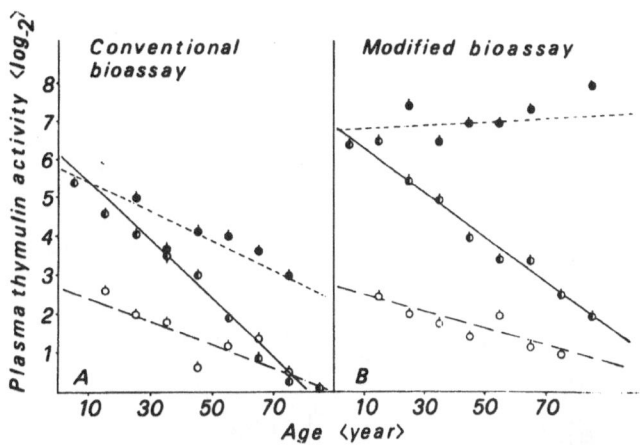

Fig. 1. Plasma thymulin levels measured by the conventional assay (A) and by the modified zinc-supplemented assay (B)in 36 hyperthyroidpatients (●), 28 hypothyroid patients (O) and 88 normal subjects of different ages (◐). Data are reported as means ± SEM of thymulin titers in each age group (from 7, with Publisher's permission).

Circulating thymulin concentrations in hypothyroid and hyperthyroid patients

Fig. 1A shows the change in the circulating thymulin titers as measured with the conventional method in normal subjects and in hypo- or hyperthyroid patients in relation to their age. In normal subjects, thymulin concentrations progressively declined, reaching nearly undetectable levels by the seventh decade of life. A progressive decline was also found in hypo- and hyperthyroid patients, but the former had lower levels of thymulin in all age groups compared to normal controls. The difference was more evident in young than in older subjects. On the other hand, thymulin levels higher than those found in age-matched normal controls were observed in hyperthyroid patients. The difference was much more evident in the older age groups.

The results obtained using the modified assay containing zinc-supplemented medium are shown in Fig. 1B. A progressive decline in thymulin activity was clearly detectable up to the ninth decade. No difference between the results of conventional and modified assays were found in the hypothyroid patients. On the other hand, in hyperthyroid patients, thymulin levels measured by the conventional assay, did not decline with age, and were clearly higher than those of age-mathched normal subjects in all age groups after the first decade.

Correlation between circulating thymulin and thyroid hormones

The correlation between plasma thymulin (as assessed by the modified assay) and serum concentration of T3 and T4 is illustrated in Fig. 2. Significant positive correlations were found (r=0.80 for thymulin vs. T3, p<0.001; r=0.78 for thymulin vs. T4, p<0.001). Similar results were obtained when the thymulin values were assessed by the conventional method (data not shown).

Analysis of the data with respect to the type of hyperthyroidism and hypothyroidism showed no relationship of thymulin activity to thyroid autommune disoders. Similarly, there was no correlation between thymulin activity and titers of anti-thyrogobulin or anti-thyroid microsomal antibodies.

Effect of therapy

The effect of therapy on thymulin levels in hypothyroid and hyperthyroid patients is shown in Fig. 3. Antithyroid drug treatment in hyperthyroid patients was associated with a decrease in thymulin concentrations toward normal values. Administration of L-T4 in doses able to suppress thyrotropin levels in thyroid cancer patients was followed by an increase in thymulin titers to normal or supranormal values.

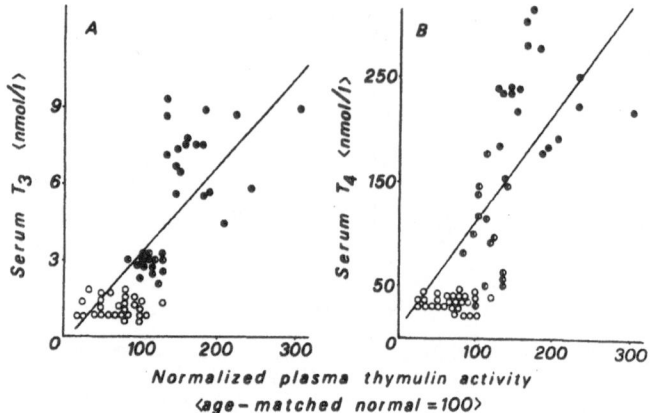

Fig. 2. Correlation between serum T3 (A) or T4 (B) and circulating thymulin by modified bioassay in hypothyroid (O), hyperthyroid (●) and euthyroid (◐) subjects. The age-dependent variations of thymulin activity are normalized for age-matched normal controls (From 7, with Publisher's permission).

PLASMA THYMULIN IN INFANTS WITH LOW-BIRTH-WEIGHT AND LOW T3 SYNDROME

The development and maturation of the immune system is almost complete at birth in humans, and its functions become wholly effective in the early post-natal life[31-34]. Alterations of cell-mediated immunity and other immunological abnormalities have been reported during the first weeks of life in premature and/or low-weight newborns[35,36]. Impaired thymic function might be implicated in this immunodeficiency. In keeping with this concept, low circulating levels of thymulin have been reported in premature and small for gestational age (SGA) infants[36].

As discussed before, thymic endocrine activity appears to be modulated by thyroid function both in experimental animals and in adult humans with hypothyroidism and hyperthyroidism. Several studies have shown that premature or SGA infants have reduced serum thyroid hormone concentrations during the first post natal weeks, when compared to healthy full term newborns[37-42]. To answer the question of whether in premature newborns the impaired thymic activity and thyroid function abnormalities are related, we carried out further studies by performing serial and parallel measurements of thymulin, T3 and T4 during the first weeks of life in full term infants and in preterm newborns with various conditions.

Study groups

Circulating thymulin (measured by the modified bioassay described before) and serum T4 and T3 concentrations were measured in 131 newborns incuding: 26 healthy full term, 23 full term small for gestational age (SGA), 30 preterm appropriate for gestational age (AGA), 22 preterm SGA and 30 with respiratory distress syndrome (RDS) of whom 15 were full term and 15 preterm AGA. Blood samples were obtained 3, 5, 10, 20, and 40 days after delivery.

Plasma thymulin and thyroid hormone concetrations during early post natal life

In healthy full term newborns circulating thymulin concentrations were low during the first days of life and subsequently reached normal values for children aging 1 - 12 months by the tenth day after birth. Persistently low circulating thymulin and T3 were observed in the majority of newborns with pathological conditions, the lowest values being observed in infants with RDS. A high significant positive correlation was present in all groups of newborns between mean circulating thymulin and T3, but not T4. Short-term T3 administration in 6 selected additional preterm AGA newborns caused a significant increase of plasma thymulin levels when compared to 6 untreated controls.

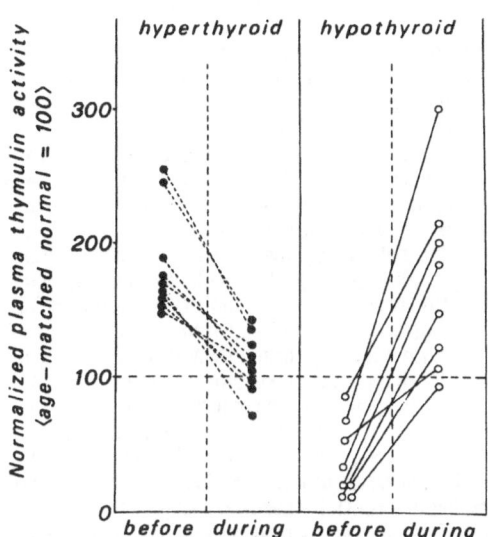

Fig. 3. Normalized plasma thymulin levels as assessed by the modified bioassay after antithyroid drug treatment in 9 hyperthyroid patients and after L-T4 administration in 8 hypothyroid patients. (From 7, with Publisher's permission).

DISCUSSION

The data obtained in hyperthyroid and hypothyroid patients provide, to our knowledge, the first evidence in humans that thymic endocrine function, as assessed by measurement of circulating thymulin activity, is influenced by thyroid status. Using a conventional bioassay, an age-dependent decline of thymulin activity was found both in hypo- and hyperthyroid patients, as previously reported in normal subjects[22,30]. However, comparison with age-matched normal controls revealed that thymulin activity was increased in hyperthyroidism and decreased in hypothyroidism. These changes were reversed by appropriate treatment in both groups of patients.

These results are in agreement with previous observations in mice that circulating thymulin declines after thyroidectomy[4,5] or antithyroid drug treatment and increases after thyroid hormone administration . Further support for an influence of thyroid hormones on thymic endocrine activity derives from the demonstration that exogenous T4 administration to experimental animals resulted in enlargement of both cortical and medullary components of the thymus[43,44], while thyroidectomy was followed by a reduction of the thymic size up to near-complete atrophy[15]. Moreover, the occurrence of an enlarged thymus in human hyperthyroidism has long been recognized[16,45].

The mechanism by which thyroid status affects circulating thymulin is presently unknown. The possibility that it was due to an underlying autoimmune disorder is not supported by the finding that the changes occurring in hypo- and hyperthyroid patients were unrelated to the clinical and humoral evidence of thyroid autoimmunity, while there was a significant correlation with serum thyroid hormone concentrations. We also could rule out the possibility that thyroid hormones *per se* might interfere with the bioassays used to measure thymulin activity, since the *in vitro* addition of either T4 or T3 did not alter the sensitivity of the bioassay[7].

Recent findings have shown that marginal zinc deficiency may account for the reduced circulating thymulin activity occurring in advanced age and in Down's syndrome[30]; in these conditions FTS is still produced, but it does not contain zinc (Zn-FTS, thymulin) and, therefore, remains biologically inactive. The increased thymulin activity found in hyperthyroid by the conventional method was further emphasized by the modified bioassay which employed optimal zinc concentration in the assay mixture. In hypothyroid patients, thymulin activity was decreased in both assays, thus increasing the difference between hypothyroid and age-matched normal subjects. In this respect, hypothyroid patients appeared to differ from patients with Down's syndrome, in whom reduced thymulin activity is partially restored by addition of zinc ions[30]. Since both *in vivo* forms of thymulin (i.e. zinc bound and zinc unbound) should be detected by the modified bioassay, our data indicate that the total concentration of circulating thymulin is increased in hyperthyroidism and decreased in hypothyroidism.

This concept is further supported by the data obtained in premature newborns with the low T3 syndrome. In these conditions plasma thymulin titers remain persistently lower that those of healthy full term infants from birth to 40 days of life. Although the precise mechanism responsible for such phenomenon cannot be definitively established on the basis of our results, this finding is in agreement with the notion that the complex thyroid function abnormalities present in prematurity[37-42] might play an important role in the impairement of thymic endocrine function. In keeping with this notion, when circulating thymulin and T3 concentrations of all groups of newborns were compared, a highly significant positive correlation was found between the two parameters. At variance with T3, plasma thymulin titers were not correlated in newborns with circulating T4. This finding is in keeping with the concept that T3 is the metabolically active hormone[46], but it is apparently in contrast with our data in adults showing a positive correlation between both serum T3 and T4 and plasma thymulin in hypothyroid and hyperthyroid patients. It should be noted, however, that the abnormal thyroid hormone concentrations in hyperthyroid and hypothyroid adults were due to increased or reduced hormonal secretion by the thyroid gland leading to essentially parallel changes of both serum T4 and T3. On the other hand, the main alteration of the thyroid hormone metabolism in sick newborns is reduced peripheral conversion of T4 to T3.

In all the above the conditions studied, changes in circulating thymulin could be due either to altered synthesis and/or release form the thymus or to alterations of its metabolic clearance rate (MCR). The notion that MCRs of many substances are increased in hyperthyroidism and decreased in hypothyroidism lends indirect support to the concept that thyroid hormones affect thymic secretion by increasing either the number[6] or the secretory activity[47] of thymic epithelial cells. In light of this interpretation, the changes in thymulin level in hyperthyroid and hypothyroid patients could reflect an increased or decreased hormonal stimulus on the thymus itself. It is more difficult to explain why hyperthyroidism prevents the age-dependent decline in thymulin concentrations.

The recent demonstration of a feedback mechanism by which the circulating level of thymulin stimulates the rate of thymulin secretion by epithelial cells[48] might, however, explain the findings in hyperthyroid patients. In other words, the excess of thyroid hormones induces, regardless of the age of the patients, increments in thymulin to the maximum compatible with the feedback mechanism.

Regardless of the mechanism involved, our studies provide clear evidence that thyroid status modulates thymic endocrine function, as expressed by thymulin secretion. The question of whether and to what extent such modulation is relevant to the peripheral efficiency of the immune system remains to be elucidated.

AKNOWLEDGEMENTS

This work was partially supported by C.N.R. (Rome, Italy), Target Project "Preventive Medicine and Rehabilitation" Subproject "Mechanisms of aging", Grant n° 86.01899.56.

REFERENCES

1. A. Pinchera, S. Mariotti, L. Chiovato, and C. Marcocci, Influence of thyroid status on thyroid immune surveillance and immunological implications of the low T3 syndrome, in: "The low T3 Syndrome", R.-D. Hesch, ed., Academic Press, London (1981).
2. A. Pinchera, and G.F. Fenzi, Endocrine autoimmune diseases, in: "Endocrinology", L.J. DeGroot, ed., Grune & Stratton, New York (1979).
3. R. Volpé, Autoimmune thyroid disease. A perspective, Mol. Biol. Med. 3:25 (1986).
4. N. Fabris, and E. Mocchegiani, Endocrine control of thymic serum factor production in young-adult and old mice, Cell. Immunol. 91:325 (1985).
5. N. Fabris, E. Mocchegiani, and M. Muzzioli, Thyroid-dependence of age-related decline of FTS production, in: "Immunology and Ageing", N. Fabris, ed., Martinus Nijhoff, The Hague (1982).
6. W. Savino, B. Wolf, S. Aratan-Spire, and M. Dardenne, Fluctuations in the thyroid hormone levels "in vivo" can modulate the secretion of thymulin by the epithelial cells of young mouse thymus, Clin. Exp. Immunol. 55:629 (1984).
7. N. Fabris, E. Mocchegiani, S. Mariotti, F. Pacini, and A. Pinchera, Thyroid function modulates thymic endocrine activity, J. Clin. Endocrinol. Metab. 62:474 (1986).
8. N. Fabris, Influence of thyroid hormones on the immune system, in: "The low T3 Syndrome", R.-D. Hesch, ed., Academic Press, London (1981).
9. D. Keast, and D.Y. Ayre, Antibody regulation in birds by thyroid hormones, Dev. Comp. Immunol. 4:323 (1980).
10. M. Bonnyns, P. Cano, and K. Osterland, Lymphocytes function in the course of Graves' disease, Acta Endocrinol. (Copenh.)(Suppl 204):13 (1976).
11. F. Pacini, H. Nakamura, and L.J. DeGroot, Effect of hypo- and hyperthyroidism on the balance between helper and suppressor T cells in rats. Acta Endocrinol. (Copenh.) 103:528 (1983).
12. V. Sridama, F. Pacini and L.J. DeGroot, Decreased suppressor T lymphocytes in autoimmune thyroid disease detected by monoclonal antibodies, J. Clin. Endocrinol. Metab. 54:316 (1982).
13. N. Aoki, G. Wakisaka, and I. Nagata, Effects of thyroxine on T-cell counts and tumour cell rejection in mice. Acta Endocrinol. (Copenh.) 81:104 (1976).
14. A. Basso, E. Mocchegiani, and N. Fabris, Incresed immunological efficiency in young mice by short-term treatment with L-thyroxine, J. Endocrinol. Invest. 4:431 (1981).
15. N. Fabris, Immunodepression in thyroid-deprived animals, Clin. Exp. Immunol. 15:601 (1983).
16. J.G. Simpson, E.S. Gray, W. Michie, and J.S. Beck, The influence of preoperative drug treatment on the extent of hyperplasia of the thymus in primary thyrotoxicosis, Clin. Exp. Immunol. 22:249 (1975).
17. A.L. Goldstein, T.K.L. Low, M. McAdoo, J. McClure, G.B. Thurman, C.Y. Lay, D. Chang, S.S. Wang, C. Harvey, A.H. Ramel, and J. Meinhofer, Thymosin. I. Isolation and sequence analysis of an immunologically active thymic polypetide. Proc. Natl. Acad. Sci. U.S.A. 74:711 (1977).
18. G. Goldstein, M. Scheid, U. Hammertring, E.A. Bose, D.H. Schlesinger, and H.D. Niall, Isolation of a polypeptide that has lymphocytes-differentiating properties and is probably represented universally in living cells, Proc. Natl. Acad. Sci. U.S.A. 72:11 (1976).
19. J.F. Bach, M. Dardenne, J.M. Pleau, and A.M. Bach, Isolation, biochemical characteristics and biological activity of a circulating thymic hormone in the mouse and in the human. Ann. N.Y. Acad. Sci. 249:186 (1975).
20. M. Dardenne, J.M. Pleau, B. Nabama, P. Lefancier, M. Derrien, J. Choay, and J.F. Bach, Contribution of zinc and other metals to the biological activity of the serum thymic factor. Proc. Natl. Acad. Sci. U.S.A. 79:5370 (1982).
21. W. Savino, and M. Dardenne, Thymic hormone-containing cells. VI. Immunohistologic evidence for the simultaneous presence of thymulin, thymopoietin and thymosin alpha1 in normal and pathological human thymuses. Eur. J. Immunol. 14:987 (1984).
22. J.F. Bach, M. Dardenne, M. Papiernik, A. Barois, P. Levasseur, and H. LeBrigant, Evidence for a serum thymic factor produced by the human thymus, Lancet ii:1056 (1972).
23. V.M. Lewis, J.J. Twomey, P. Bealmear, G. Goldstein, and R.A. Good, Age, thymic involution, and circulating thymic hormone activity, J. Clin. Endocrinol. Metab. 47:145 (1978).

24. J.F. Simpson, E.S. Gray, and J.S. Beck, Age involution in the normal adult thymus. Clin. Exp. Immunol. 19:261 (1975).

25. M.E. Weksler, J.B. Innes, and G. Goldstein, Immunological studies of aging. IV. The contribution of thymic involution to the immune deficiencies of aging mice and reversal with thymopoietin. J. Exp. Med. 148:996 (1978).

26. N. Fabris, M. Muzzioli, and E. Mocchegiani, Recovery of age-dependent immunological deterioration in BALB/c by short-term treatment with L-thyroxine, Mech. Ageing Dev. 18:327 (1982).

27. S. Mariotti, S. Pisani, A. Russova, and A. Pinchera, A new solid-phase immunoradiometric assay for anti-thyroglobulin autoantibody. J. Endocrinol. Invest. 5:227 (1982).

28. S. Mariotti, A. Russova, S. Pisani, and A. Pinchera, A new solid-phase immunoradiometric assay for anti-thyroid microsomal antibody. J. Clin. Endocrinol. Metab. 56:467 (1983).

29. M. Dardenne, and J.F. Bach, The sheep cell rosette assay for the evaluation of thymic hormones, in: "Biological activity of thymic hormones," D. Van Bekkun, ed., Kooyeker, Rotterdam (1975).

30. N. Fabris, E. Mocchegiani, L. Amadio, M. Zannotti, F. Licastro, and C. Franceschi, Thymic hormone deficiency in normal ageing and Down's syndrome: is there a primary failure of the thymus? Lancet i:983 (1984).

31. M.D. Cooper, B-cell differentiation, Birth Defects 19:25 (1983).

32. U. Anderson, A.G. Bird, S. Britton, R. Palacios, Humoral and cellular immunity in humans studied at the cell level from birth to two years of age, Immunol. Rev. 57:5 (1981).

33. A.R. Hayward, Development of lymphocyte responses and interactions in the human fetus and newborn, Immunol. Rev. 57:39 (1981).

34. T. Miyawaki, N. Moriya, T. Nagaoki, N. Tanigichi, Maturation of B-cell differentiation ability and T-cell regulatory function in infancy and childhood. Immunol. Rev. 57:61 (1981).

35. A.C. Fergusson, Prolonged impairement of cellular immunity in children with intrauterine growth retardation. J. Pediatr. 93:52 (1978).

36. R.K. Chandra, Serum thymic hormone activity and cell mediated immunity in healthy neonates, preterm infants, and small-for-gestational age infants. Pediatrics 67:407 (1981).

37. D.A. Fisher, and A.H. Klein, Thyroid development and disorders of thyroid function in the newborn, N. Engl. J. Med. 304:702 (1981).

38. A.H. Klein, T.H. Oddie, M. Parislow, T.P. Faclay Jr., and D.A. Fisher, Developmental changes in pituitary-thyroid function in the human fetus and newborn, Early Hum. Dev. 6:321 (1982).

39. D.A. Fisher, A.H. Klein, and A. Hadeed, Normal and abnormal thyroid function in premature infants: the low T3 syndrome, in: "The low T3 Syndrome", R.-D. Hesch, ed., Academic Press, London (1981).

40. D.A. Fisher, Ontogenesis of hypothalamic-pituitary-thyroid function in the human fetus, in: "Pediatric Thyroidology", F. Delange, D.A. Fisher, and P. Malvaux, eds., Karger, Basel (1985).

41. P. Malvaux, Thyroid function during the neonatal period, infancy and childhood, in: "Pediatric Thyroidology", F. Delange, D.A. Fisher, and P. Malvaux, eds., Karger, Basel (1985).

42. F. Delange, P. Bourdoux, and A.-M. Ermans, Transient disorders of thyroid function and regulation in preterm infants, in: "Pediatric Thyroidology", F. Delange, D.A. Fisher, and P. Malvaux, eds., Karger, Basel (1985).

43. V. Ernstrom, and B. Larsson, Thymic and thoracic duct contribution to blood lymphocytes in normal and in thyroxine treated guinea-pig. Acta Physiol. Scand. 66:189 (1966).

44. W. Michie, J.S. Beck, R.G. Mahafffy, E.F. Honein, and G.B. Fowler, Quantitative radiological and histological studies of the thymus in thyroid disease. Lancet ii:691 (1967).

45. K. Ohga, G.S. Incefy, K.F. Fok, B.W. Erickson and R.A. Good, Radioimmuno-assay for the thymic hormone serum factor (FTS), J. Immunol. Methods 57:171 (1983).

46. P.R. Larsen, J.E. Silva, and M.M. Kaplan, Relationship between circulating and intracellular thyroid hormones: physiological and clinical implications. Endocr. Rev. 2:87 (1981).

47. J.M. Scheiff, A.C. Cordier, and S. Hammount, Epithelial cell proliferation in thymic hyperplasia induced by triiodothyronine, Clin. Exp. Immunol. 27:216 (1977).

48. W. Savino, M. Dardenne, and J.F. Bach, Thymic hormone containing cells. III. Evidence for a feed-back regulation of the secretion of the serum thymic factor (FTS) by thymic epithelial cells. Clin. Exp. Immunol. 52:7 (1983).

THE BB/W RAT, A MODEL FOR "TGI-ASSOCIATED GOITRE"

H.A.M. Voorbij, R.D. van der Gaag, and H.A. Drexhage

Lab. for Clinical Immunology, Dept. of Pathology
Free University Hospital, 1007 MB Amsterdam

ABSTRACT

The presence of circulating thyroid growth stimulating immunoglobulins (TGI) was determined in 12-16 weeks old BB/W rats and in control Wistar rats. Thyroid weights of the BB/W rats were significantly raised in comparison to those of Wistar controls, and on morphology BB/W thyroids showed a strong similarity to human colloid goitre (active high columnar epithelium, branching and budding, absent signs of thyrocyte destruction and organized lymphoid tissue in about 30-40% of animals). Of 5 tested BB/W rats all were positive for TGI when protein-A-sepharose purified serum IgG was used in Feulgen densitometry. Although 50% of BB/W rats had elevated serum TSH levels, it is unlikely that TSH is directly involved in the glandular weight increase since TSH values did not correlate with goitre size. The data show that the BB/W rat may serve as a model for "TGI-associated" nontoxic goitre. This model will have great implications for the study on the pathogenic role of TGI in sporadic and endemic goitre and on studies aiming on receptor purification.

INTRODUCTION

In recent years we have described that some forms of goitres (Drexhage and Van der Gaag, 1986), such as large Graves' goitres, the majority of sporadic nontoxic goitres, and T4-therapy resistant Hashimoto goitres, are associated with the presence in serum of immunoglobulins (Ig's) stimulating the DNA-synthesis of guinea-pig thyroid glands kept in organ culture. Others (Chiovato et al., 1983; Schatz et al, 1983; Valente et al., 1983; McMullan and Smyth, 1984; Rotella et al., 1986) have now confirmed the presence of similar Ig's in the above listed groups of goitrous patients and found circulating Ig's stimulating metabolic processes related to growth, f.i. 3H-thymidine incorporation in isolated thyroid follicles or FRTL5 cells, or G6-PD increase in thyroid explants kept in organ culture. The Ig's thus detected are generally referred to as "thyroid growth stimulating Ig's" (TGI), and it is hypothetically thought that these TGI's might be responsible for the glandular weight increase found in the patients. However, many questions still remain on a) the exact character of TGI; b) the antigen specificity or the receptors to which these Ig's are directed; c) the relationship to Ig's stimulating other metabolic processes in thyroid cells, f.i. the c-AMP pathway; and d) the in vivo relevance to goitre development.

257

Since an experimental animal model for "TGI-associated goitre" would clearly be of advantage to clarify these issues, we have looked for the presence of TGI in the autoimmune-prone Bio Breeding/Worcester (BB/W) rat.

RATIONALE FOR STUDYING TGI IN THE BB/W RAT

The Bio Breeding/Worcester (BB/W) rat is an established model for the study of organ-specific autoimmune disease, and has particularly been useful to investigate a form of insulin dependent diabetes positive for auto-antibodies against the cells of the islets of Langerhans (Seemayer et al., 1982; Martin et al., 1984). Besides this pancreatic lesion a high proportion of BB/W rats develop a form of thyroid autoimmune disease; in 30-40% of animals the thyroid is infiltrated by lymphocytes (Sternthal et al., 1981; Allen et al., 1986) and autoantibodies against the colloid can be demonstrated in 70-80% of animals from the 9th week of age onwards (Like et al., 1982, Voorbij et al., 1986). The presence and titre of these antibodies is, however, not related to the presence of the lymphocytic cell infiltrations (Like et al., 1982, Allen et al., 1986).

The BB/W rat also shows an increase in the thyroid weight (Allen et al., 1986); this thyroid hyperplasia was thought to be a compensatory reaction to the subclinical hypothyroidism caused by the lymphoid cell infiltrations. Puzzling remains, however, in such a concept that only a minority of animals show lymphocytic infiltrations with borderline low serum thyroid hormone levels and raised serum TSH, and this low prevalence of subclinical hypothyroidism can not likely account for the thyroid weight increase found in practically all animals. The goitre development in the BB/W rat is also peculiar in comparison to the lack of glandular weight increase in other established animal models where lymphocytic infiltration of the thyroid occurs and animals are found positive for α-Tg antibodies. The Obese strain chicken for instance shows a progressive destruction and fibrosis of the thyroid gland despite the high levels of serum TSH found in these birds (Wick et al., 1985).

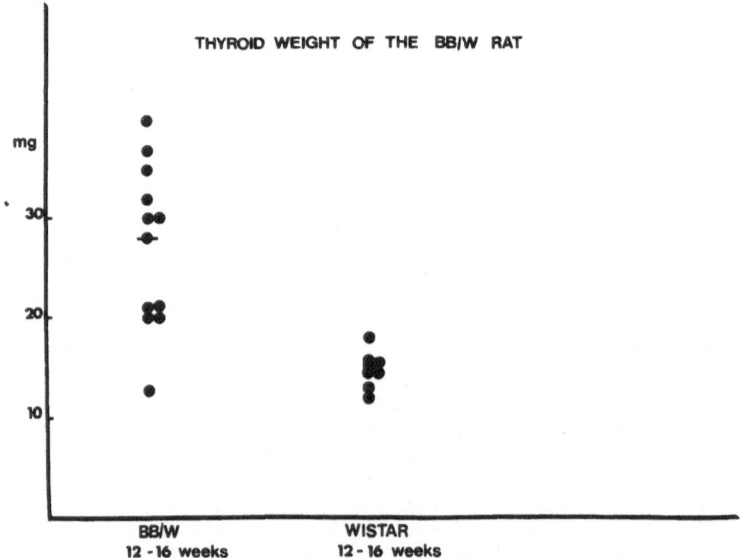

Fig. 1. The thyroid weight of BB/W rats vs. that of Wistar rats of the same age. All but one of 12 BB/W rats show higher glandular weights (p<0.05; Student's t-test)

We have now studied the presence of TGI in the circulation of the BB/W
rat to see whether the occurrence of an immune growth stimulator might
coincide with the glandular enlargement of the animal. BB/W rats (both sexes,
obtained from Organon, Oss, The Netherlands), aged 12-16 weeks, were killed
by asphyxiation. Diabetes in the BB/W rat only develops after the 9th-16th
week of age, whenever rats are diabetic in the breeding colony they are
maintained on daily Protamine-Zinc-Insulin (Organon) injections. Thyroids of
the killed animals were removed and weighed. The weights appeared significantly higher as compared to those of control Wistar rats (R-Amsterdam,
Breeding colony Free University) of the same age and total body weight
(fig. 1): 28.0 mg (mean, s.d. 7.5, n=12) for BB/W rat thyroids vs. 15.6 mg
(mean, s.d. 3.5, n=9) for Wistar controls (p<0.01, Student's t-test). In
three of the animals only a minor infiltration of the thyroid by lymphoid
cells could be observed (histological examination, sublimate-formol fixation,
6μ paraffin sections, haematoxylin-eosin staining). In or near these
lymphocytic infiltrations signs of thyrocyte destruction - macrophage
infiltration, colloidophagy, follicle cell decay - were absent. On the
contrary the follicular epithelium of the BB/W rat was active and high
columnar cells lined the follicles. Occasionally branching and budding of the
epithelial cells was observed. The lymphoid cell accumulations were, in
comparison to destructive inflammatory reactions, actually of a totally
different character. They were highly organized, showing T cell zones with

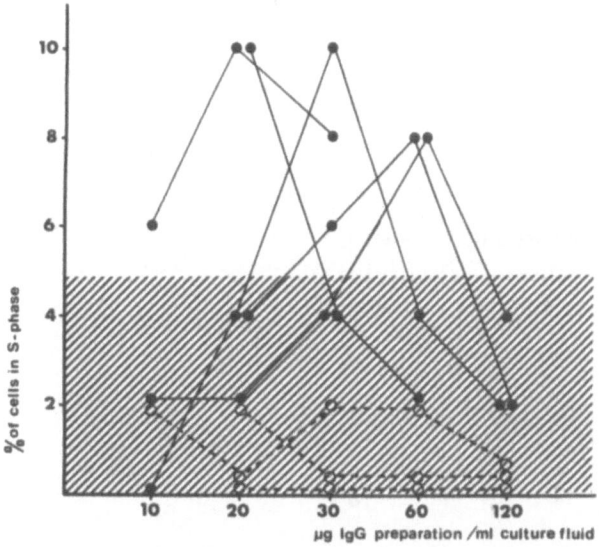

Fig. 2. The results of protein-A-sepharose purified
serum IgG in Feulgen densitometry of BB/W rats (●) and
Wistar controls (o). IgG's were tested for their ability
to induce DNA-synthesis (% of cells in S-phase) in
guinea pig thyroid explants kept in organ culture. The
IgG's of BB/W rats stimulate DNA-synthesis in biphasic
dose-response which pattern is a normal feature of
Feulgen densitometry. Wistar control IgG had no such
effect. The hatched area represents the range of
DNA-synthesis found in non stimulated control guinea pig
thyroid.

interdigitating cells and epitheloid venules, adjacent B cell follicles and cords of plasma cells. This architecture reflects local immune responsiveness and antibody production and is very similar to the architecture seen in mucosa-associated lymphoid tissues (Peyer's patches, bronchus-associated lymphoid tissue).

Five of the twelve BB/W rats were tested for circulating TGI. IgG preparations were prepared by protein-A-sepharose purification from serum, and these were tested in dose-response in the cytochemical bioassay based on Feulgen densitometry (details Drexhage and Van der Gaag, 1986). All five IgG preparations were clearly positive for TGI, and biphasic dose-response curves - a well-known feature of all yet known cytochemical bioassays for polypeptide hormones and their mimicking Ig's - were obtained (fig. 2). Optimal stimulation of DNA-synthesis occurred at concentrations ranging from 10 to 60 µg IgG per ml culture fluid. Two IgG preparations tested as control and prepared from Wistar serum were negative for immune stimulators of DNA-synthesis. With regard to hormonal stimulators of thyroid growth 50 percent of animals showed an elevated level of s-TSH (fig.3, as measured with a RIA, >550 ng/ml; Dr. D. v.d. Heide, Leiden University); as a group the BB/W rats showed borderline-low normal s-T3 and T4 levels compared to the levels found in the Wistar control group (1.95 vs. 3.0 nmol T3/l, and 74.3 nmol vs. 96.1 nmol T4/l respectively). When we tried to correlate the actual weight of the thyroid gland of a given animal with its s-TSH, significant correlations could not be established (fig. 3). This makes it not very likely that TSH plays a significant role in the goitrogenesis of the BB/W rat. Our data on the lack of correlation between thyroid weight and s-TSH are in accordance with earlier reported data on this subject (Allen et al., 1986).

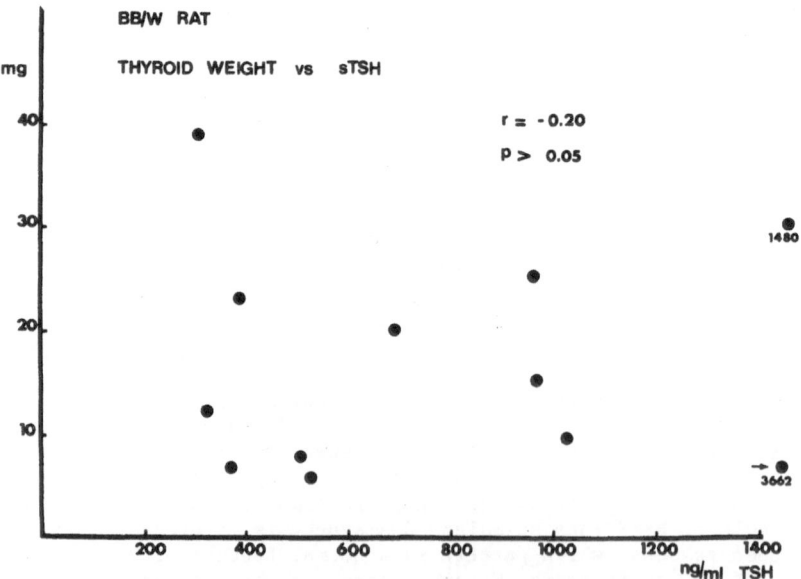

Fig. 3. The lack of correlation between glandular weight increase in the BB/W rat and its serum TSH, as measured by RIA (normal <550 mg/ml).

FURTHER REFLECTIONS

The data listed above imply that the BB/W rat can serve as an animal model for the study of "TGI-associated goitre". Employing cloning and hybridization techniques monoclonal TGI's can now be developed which may elucidate the pathogenic role - if any - of TGI in goitrogenesis, and may serve as tools for the purification and identification of thyrocyte membrane components (receptors) involved in TGI-induced DNA-synthesis.

Two independent groups (Schatz et al., 1983; Medeiros-Neto et al., 1986) have recently reported that also in area's of iodine deficiency goitre development may be associated with the presence of circulating TGI. Moreover - in contrast to the prevailing concept - the Chinamora Research Team (1986) reported that elevated levels of s-TSH do not correlate to goitre size in severe iodine deficiency. Allen et al. (1986) showed that disturbances in iodine intake in the BB/W rat lead to alterations in the frequency of intrathyroidal lymphocytic infiltrations. It might be that the BB/W rat as a model for TGI-associated goitre will also serve to unravel the intriguing relationships between metabolic disturbances due to iodine intake abnormalities, goitrogenesis and thyroid autoimmunity.

Another interesting aspect of the BB/W rat is its marked defect in the T cell system. Most noteworthy young rats show clear T-suppressor cell defects, particularly in total numbers (phenotypically; Woda et al., 1986). Older rats additionally show T-helper/effector defects (Elder et al., 1986). In the human disease entity "TGI-associated sporadic nontoxic goitre" we observed similar generalized T-suppressor cell defects (van der Gaag et al, 1986); it is, however, difficult to visualize how such generalized defects lead to organ-specific autoimmune diseases. The rat model may also prove to be of value to study this problem.

ACKNOWLEDGEMENTS

Our studies were supported by grants of "De Drie Lichten", the Prevention Fund (28-1120) and the Netherlands Organization for the Advancement of Pure Research (ZWO-FUNGO 945-040). We would like to express our sincere thanks to Drs Schot and Schuurman at Organon for their continuing generosity to enable us to study the BB/W rat. Dr. v.d. Heide measured s-TSH; Dr. de Baets performed α-Tg antibody estimations. Mrs. C. van Rijn typed the manuscript.

REFERENCES

Allen, E.M., Appel, M.C., Braverman, L.E., 1986. The effect of iodide ingestion on the development of spontaneous lymphocytic thyroiditis in the diabetes-prone BB/W rat. Endocrinology, 118: 1977-1981.

The Chinamora Research Team, 1986. Endemic goitre in Chinamora, Zimbabwe. Lancet, i: 1198-1200.

Chiovato, L., Hammond L.J., Hanafusa, T., Pujol-Borell, B., Doniach, D., and Bottazzo, G.F., 1983. Detection of thyroid growth immunoglobulins (TGI) by 3H-thymidine incorporation in cultured rat thyroid follicles. Clin. Endocrinol. (Oxf.), 19, 581-590.

Drexhage, H.A., Gaag, R.D. van der, 1986. Immunoglobulins affecting thyroid growth. In: Immunology of Endocrine Diseases (ed. A.M. McGregor), MTP Press Ltd, Lancaster, pp. 51-71.

Drexhage, H.A., Gaag, R.D. van der, 1986. Thyroid growth stimulating immunoglobulins (TGI) and goitre. In: The thyroid and autoimmunity (eds. H.A. Drexhage, W.M. Wiersinga), Elsevier Science Publishers, Amsterdam, pp. 173-186.

Elder, M.E., MacLaren, N.K., 1983. Identification of profound peripheral T-lymphocyte immunodeficiencies in the spontaneously diabetic BB rat. J. Immunol. 130: 1723.

Gaag, R.D. van der, Blomberg-van der Flier, B.M.E., Plassche-Boers, E. van de, Kokjé-Kleingeld, M., Drexhage, H.A., 1986. T-suppressor cell defects in euthyroid nonendemic goitre. Acta Endocrinologica 112: 83-88

Kabel, P.J., Voorbij, H.A.M., Gaag, R.D. van der, Wiersinga, W.M., Haan, M. de, Drexhage, H.A. Dendritic cells in autoimmune thyroid disease. Acta Endocrinologica (in press).

Like, A.A., Appel, M.C., Rossini A.A., 1982. Autoantibodies in the BB/W rat. Diabetes 31: 816-820.

Martin, D., Logothatopoulos, J., 1984. Complement fixing islet cell antibodies in the spontaneously diabetic BB rat. Diabetes 33: 93-96.

McMullan, N.M., Smyth, P.P.A., 1984. In vitro generation of NADPH as an index of thyroid stimulating immunoglobulins (TGI) in goitrous disease. Clin. Endocrinol. (Oxf.) 20: 269-280.

Medeiros-Neto, G.A., Halpern, A., Cozzi, Z.S., Lima, N., Kohn, L.D., 1986. Thyroid growth immunoglobulins in large multinodular endemic goiters: effect of iodized oil. J. Clin. Endocrinol. Metab. 63: 644-650.

Rotella, C.M., Mavilia, C., Kohn, L.D., Toccafondi, R., 1986. Thyroid growth promoting antibody in patients with nontoxic goitre. In: The thyroid and autoimmunity (eds. H.A. Drexhage, W.M. Wiersinga), Elsevier Science Publishers, Amsterdam, pp. 198-201.

Schatz, H., Beckman, F.H., Floren, M., 1983. Radioassay for thyroid growth stimulating immunoglobulins (TGI) with cultivated porcine thyroid follicles. Horm. Metab. Res. 15: 626-627.

Seemayer, T.A., Tannenbaum, G.S., Goldman, H., Colle, E., 1982. Dynamic time course studies of the spontaneously diabetic BB Wistar rat . III. Light microscopy and ultrastructural observations of pancreatic islets of Langerhans. Am. J. Pathol. 106: 237.

Sternthal, E., Like, A.A., Sarantis, K., Braierman, L.E., 1981. Lymphocytic thyroiditis and diabetes in the BB/W rat. Diabetes 30: 1058-1061.

Valente, W.A., Vitti, P., Yavin, E., Rotella, C.M., Grollman, E.F., Toccafondi, R.S., Kohn, L.D., 1982. Monoclonal antibodies to the thyrotropin receptor; stimulating and blocking antibodies derived from the lymphocytes of patients with Graves' disease. Proc. Natl. Acad. Sci. USA, 79, 6680-6684.

Voorbij, H.A.M., Kabel, P.J., Drexhage, H.A., 1986. Antigen-presenting cells and the thyroid autoimmune response in the BB/W rat. In: The Thyroid and Autoimmunity (eds. H.A. Drexhage, W.M. Wiersinga), Elsevier Science Publishers, Amsterdam, pp. 166-169.

Wick, G., Möst, J., Schauenstein, K., Krömer, G., Dietrich, H., Ziemiecki, A., Fässler, R., Schwartz, S., Neu, N., Hala, K., 1985. Spontaneous autoimmune thyroiditis, a bird's eye view. Immunology Today, 6: 359-364.

Woda, B.A., Like, A.A., Padden, C., McFadden, M.L., 1986. Deficiency of phenotypic cytotoxic-suppressor T-lymphocytes in the BB/W rat. J. Immunol., 3: 856-859.

NON-THYROIDAL COMPLICATIONS OF GRAVES' DISEASE:

PERSPECTIVE ON PATHOGENESIS AND TREATMENT

Joseph P. Kriss[*], I. Ross McDougall[*], Sarah S.
Donaldson[+], and Helena C. Kraemer[o]

Departments of Diagnostic Radiology and Nuclear Medicine[*],
Therapeutic Radiology[+] and Psychiatry[o], Stanford University
School of Medicine, Stanford, CA 94305 USA

A substantial number of patients with Graves' disease have significant and sometimes disabling abnormalities in sites anatomically remote from the thyroid, such as in orbital tissues (ophthalmopathy), pretibial skin (dermopathy), and bones of the extremities (acropachy).

The major disorder in Graves' disease is hyperthyroidism. It is now generally accepted that hyperthyroidism results from an interaction of autoantibodies to the TSH-receptor (TSH-R) on thyroid cells, generating events that mimic TSH in stimulating the cells to synthesize and release thyroid hormone[1-5]. Different species of anti-TSH-R have been described, varying in determinant specificity, ability to block TSH-binding, stimulate thyroid hormone synthesis, or increase growth of thyroid cells[4-8]. On the other hand, the pathogenesis of the disorders affecting non-thyroidal tissues is poorly understood. The primary pathological events are unclear, the specific cellular targets have yet to be identified, and the effectors which trigger the cascade of abnormal cellular responses are unknown.

Ophthalmopathy (O) has been the most widely studied of the non-thyroidal disorders mentioned above; two main theories of pathogenesis for Graves' ophthalmopathy have been proposed:

Theory 1. Ophthalmopathy is an autoimmune disorder which bears no relationship to Graves' disease and is causally related to antibodies interacting with unique orbital antigens.

Evidence for
· Sera of O patients contain antibodies to a soluble human eye muscle (EM) antigen[9], to human EM membranes[10], or to "retro-orbital antigens" of guinea pig Harderian gland and porcine EM[11,12].
· Sera of O patients inhibit competitively the binding of affinity-purified, non-protein antigens obtained from solubilized human EM and orbital tissue membranes[13].
· Immunoglobulins which bind to a 100,000x g pellet of porcine EM protein are found more often in sera of O patients than of patients with other thyroid disease or normals[14].
· Antibody dependent cell-mediated cytotoxicity with monoclonal antibodies to EM antigens has been reported[15].

Arguments against:
· Binding of antibodies to orbital cell antigens does not explain the development of the disease; it could reflect the result of prior muscle damage rather than its cause.
· Reference 10 lacks non-eye muscle controls; data not confirmed[16].
· Small difference between O patients and control[13].
· Relevance of non-human test systems can be questioned.
· The observations fail to account for the strong association between ophthalmopathy and autoimmune thyroid disease.

Theory 2. Ophthalmopathy is an autoimmune complication of Graves' disease. The thyroid gland and some orbital tissues share common antigenic determinants. Antibodies formed against the determinant of one site cross-react with that of the other site, and initiate different cellular events at these sites.

Evidence for
· An ipsilateral lymphatic thyroidal-orbital connection via the anterior deep cervical system in thyrotoxic subjects has been demonstrated; cephalad flow of lymph from the thyroid occurs commonly[17].
· Human Tg and Tg-anti-Tg complex bind more to human and bovine EM membranes than to other membranes[18,19], and also to lipid vesicles containing human EM protein[20].
· Tg-anti-Tg complex may be detected in sera of patients with autoimmune thyroid disease, including those with O[21,22].
· Serum Tg is high in Graves' hyperthyroidism[23] and rises further after ^{131}I therapy or thyroidectomy[23,24]; these therapies are sometimes followed by onset or worsening of O[24-26].
· There are Tg-like determinants in normal human EM[27,28].
· After removal of half of an enlarged thyroid, protrusion, which previously was bilateral, disappeared on the operated side, but persisted on the other[29].
· Monoclonal anti-Tg, and anti-Tg in patient sera react with a Tg determinant in human orbital connective tissue membranes[30]
· Retro-orbital tissues contain TSH-receptors (TSH-R)[31,32] Binding of TSH is augmented by serum/Ig from O patients[33,34].
· Monoclonal antibodies to bovine and human TSH-R, and IgG from O patients stimulate collagen synthesis in human forearm fibroblasts; response correlates with disease severity[35].
· Ig of Graves' patients binds to a 23 KD protein, which is found in normal thyroid tissue and in "retro-ocular connective tissue" obtained from an O patient[36].

Arguments against:
· No direct evidence that thyroidal antigens or humoral or cellular effectors reach the orbit via cervical lymphatics.
· Monoclonal anti-Tgs do not bind to EM[28,37]. Tg cannot be demonstrated immunohistochemically in human EM[28].
· Presence and level of anti-Tg and Tg-anti-Tg complex in serum are not correlated with O[22]. Incidence of O is low in Hashimoto's patients, whose sera often contain these substances.
· Stimulation of collagen synthesis is observed with forearm skin fibroblasts[35]; relevance of the observation can be questioned.
· No agreement on the autoantibodies and antigens involved.

Analysis of these published studies reveals collectively (a) a multiplicity of postulated mechanisms, (b) lack of agreement or information on the cellular targets, (c) conflicting or nonreproducible results, (d) lack of distinction between cause and effect, or (e) lack of apparent relevance of an observation to the disease state in man.

Table 1. Demographic Data on Treated Patients

Total Patients   156 (M 53; F 103) lost 8
  Median Age   52 yr
  Age <40 yr   18 (12%)
  Median duration eye signs pre-treatment   11 mo
  Median duration follow-up   34 mo

Description	No. Pts.	%
Previous thyroid disease	152	97
Hyperthyroidism	119	76
Hypothyroidism	16	10
Hashimoto's thyroiditis	14	9
X-ray therapy to the neck	3	2
Active hyperthyroidism, concomitant Rx	14	9
Dermopathy	23	15
Previous orbital decompression	8	5
Eye signs started or worsened after ^{131}I Rx	52	33
after thyroidectomy	6	4
On oral prednisone	46	29
prednisone stopped post-treatment	37	80
Eye surgery post-treatment	48	31

On the premise that ophthalmopathy is an autoimmune disorder, and that lymphocytes infiltrating the eye muscles may be effectors, in 1968 we began treating patients with progressive ophthalmopathy with supervoltage orbital radiotherapy using a 6-mev linear accelerator, delivering a well-collimated, high energy x-ray beam to the extraocular muscles[38]. To date we have treated 270 patients. Eye muscle or eyelid surgery has been done after the radiotherapy in about a third of the patients. Since, in some of these, most of the improvement may be attributed to the surgery, it is important to know what may be achieved by supervoltage radiation alone. Thus, in this analysis of our results, we have excluded all observations made after surgical intervention.

We assessed severity of disease by numerically rating each of 5 signs: soft tissue, proptosis, eye muscle, cornea, and sight loss, and then summing the scores to derive an ophthalmic index[38]. We present here the results on the first 156 patients, for whom the follow-up is the longest and most complete; demographic data are shown in Table 1.

Each of our patients had progressively worsening signs over a period of weeks or months before receiving radiotherapy. The over-all results of treatment are shown in Figure 1 which compares the pre-treatment index with that after treatment. Note (a) the marked shift toward lower index scores including a substantial number at 0 and 1, but (b) evidence of some residual abnormality in the majority.

Analysis according to disease manifestation revealed significant differences in response (Fig. 2). For example, before treatment 91% of all patients had soft tissue signs; in 68% of these, these signs resolved completely, 18% improved, 13% showed no response, and 1% worsened. The results for eye muscle signs were not as good: 1/3 resolved completely, but >1/3 showed no response.

In Figure 3 the responses by sign are examined according to the initial severity of each sign. For example, the severer grades of soft tissue resolved completely in 2/3 of the cases; very few had no response. Grade 1 proptosis resolved completely in half the patients; however, higher grades resolved infrequently, although many improved to

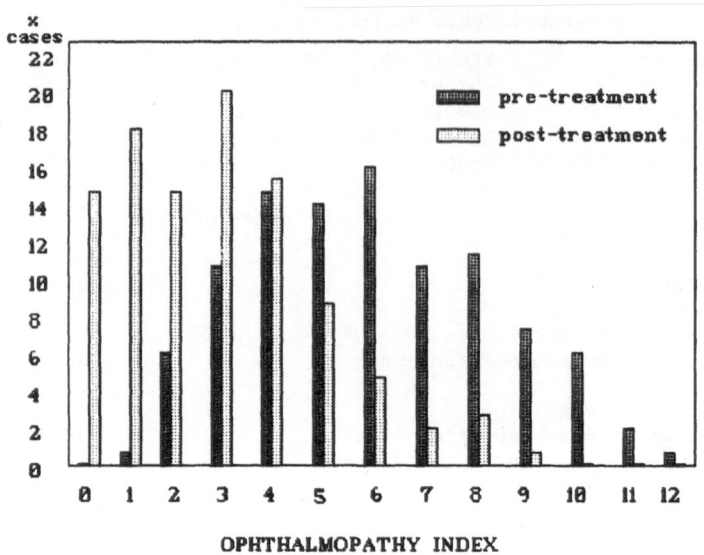

OPHTHALMOPATHY INDEX

Figure 1. Pre- and Post-Treatment Ophthalmopathy Indices

sign	PRE-TREATMENT		POST-TREATMENT [*]				
	no. cases	% of total	no. follow	worse	no response	improved	complete resolution
soft tissue	142	91	135	1	13	18	68
proptosis	118	76	111	6	47	16	31
eye muscle	147	94	139	1	37	28	33
cornea	38	19	27	4	22		74
sight loss	85	54	81	2	27	15	56

[*] results given as % of those involved and followed

Figure 2. Response to Treatment According to Manifestation

a lower grade. About 1/3 of those with eye muscle involvement did not
improve, regardless of initial grade; here the frequency of complete
resolution varied inversely with the severity of involvement. Severer
grades of sight loss responded favorably. The higher failure rate in
those with mild visual acuity loss probably reflects the frequency of
pre-existing cataract and/or retinal disease.

Sign	PRE-THERAPY Grade	POST-THERAPY [*] No.	Worse	No response	Improved	Complete resolut'n
Soft tissue	3	18		6	38	65
	2	63		2	32	67
	1	61	2	28		71
Proptosis	3	15		33	58	8
	2	44	5	59	25	11
	1	59	9	48		51
Eye muscle	3	57		39	41	19
	2	58	2	37	31	29
	1	32		37		63
Cornea	1.2	30	4	22		74
Sight loss	3	7			58	58
	2	25	4	16	36	44
	1	53	2	36		62

[*] results given as × of those involved and followed

Figure 3. Response to Treatment According to Sign and Grade

From a step-wise linear regression analysis of our data we derived formulae for predicting the final post-treatment scores for any affected individual:

r

$$\hat{S}_{final} = 0.088 + 0.124 S_{initial} + 0.495 \text{ Hashimoto} \qquad 0.33$$

$$\hat{P}_{final} = -0.051 + 0.711 P_{initial} + 0.572 \text{ concomitant Rx} \qquad 0.74$$

$$\hat{E}_{final} = -0.086 + 0.652 E_{initial} - 0.370 \text{ female} + 0.884 \text{ Hash.} \qquad 0.62$$

$$\hat{C}_{final} = 0.022 + 0.252 C_{initial} \qquad 0.40$$

$$\hat{Si}_{final} = -0.409 + 0.310 Si_{initial} + 0.009 \text{ age in years} \qquad 0.50$$

The predicted final score is related directly to the initial score, but there are several other significant correlations. The presence of Hashimoto's thyroiditis adversely affects the final score for soft tissue or eye muscle involvement. Proptosis response is less for patients receiving treatment for hyperthyroidism at the time of radiotherapy. Eye muscle response is better for females than for males. Sight loss is related to age.

Most of the non-responses associated with decreased visual function were due to persistence of eye muscle signs. Most of these subsequently were operated on, with 96% of those patients getting a good result. We conclude that sequential treatment by orbital radiotherapy followed by eye muscle or eyelid surgery, if necessary, is a reasonable treatment strategy for progressive ophthalmopathy, considering our current lack of information concerning its pathogenesis.

REFERENCES

1. Adams DD, Purves HD, Abnormal responses in the assay of thyrotropin, Proc Univ Otago Med School 34:11-12, 1956.
2. McKenzie JM, Delayed response to serum from thyrotoxic patients, Endocrinology 62:865-868, 1958.
3. Kriss JP, Pleshakov V, Chien JR, Isolation and identification of the long-acting thyroid stimulator and its relation to hyperthyroidism and circumscribed pretibial myxedema, J Clin Endocrinol Metab 24:1005-1028, 1964.
4. McKenzie JM, Zakarija M, LATS in Graves' disease, Recent Prog Horm Res 33:29-53, 1977.
5. Yavin E, Yavin Z, Schneider MD, Kohn LD, Monoclonal antibodies to the thyrotropin receptor: implications for receptor structure and the action of autoantibodies in Graves' disease, Proc Natl Acad Sci USA 78:3180-2184, 1980.
6. Matsukura N, Yamada Y, Nohara Y, Konishi J, Kasagi K, Kojima H, Wataya K, Familial neonatal transient hypothyroidism due to maternal TSH-binding inhibitor immunoglobulins, New Engl J Med 303:738-741, 1980.
7. Valente WA, Vitti P, Yavin Z, Yavin E, Rotella CM, Grollman EF, Toccafondi RS, Kohn LD, Monoclonal antibodies to the thyrotropin receptor: Stimulating and blocking antibodies derived from the lymphocytes of patients with Graves' disease, Proc Natl Acad Sci USA 79:6680-6684, 1982.
8. Atkinson S, Kendall-Taylor P, The stimulation of thyroid hormone secretion in vitro by thyroid-stimulating antibodies, J Clin Endocrinol Metab 53:1263-1266, 1981.
9. Kodama K, Sikorska P, Bandy-Dafoe K, Wall JR, Demonstration of a circulating autoantibody against soluble eye-muscle antigen in Graves' ophthalmopathy, Lancet ii:1353-1356, 1982.
10. Faryna M, Nauman J, Gardos A, Measurement of autoantibodies against human eye muscle membranes in Graves' ophthalmopathy, Brit Med J 290:191-192, 1985.
11. Atkinson S, Holcombe M, Kendall-Taylor P, Ophthalmopathic immunoglobulin in patients with Graves' ophthalmopathy, Lancet 11:374-376, 1984.
12. Kendall-Taylor P, Atkinson S, Holcombe M, A specific IgG in Graves' ophthalmopathy and its relation to retro-orbital and thyroid autoimmunity, Brit Med J 288:1183-1186, 1984.
13. Salvi M, How JS, Wall JR, Detection of autoantibodies against affinity purified orbital membrane antigens in Graves' ophthalmopathy using a competitive binding ELISA, 61st Meeting, Am Thy Assoc, Abst T-8, 1986.
14. Baker JR, Weetman AP, Wartofsky L, Nutman T, Burman KD, Serum immunoglobulins in patients with Graves' ophthalmopathy directed against unique determinants of porcine eye muscle, Clin Res 34:420A, 1986.
15. Wang, PW, Hiromatsu Y, Laryea E, Sosu L, How J, Wall JR, Immunologically mediated cytotoxicity against human eye muscle cells in Graves' ophthalmopathy, J Clin Endocrinol Metab 63:316-322, 1986.
16. Sikorska H, Wall JR, Failure to detect eye muscle membrane specific antibodies in Graves' ophthalmopathy, Brit Med J 291:604, 1985.
17. Kriss JP, Radioisotopic thyroidolymphography in patients with Graves' disease, J Clin Endocrinol Metab 31:315-324, 1970.
18. Konishi J, Herman MM, Kriss JP, Binding of thyroglobulin and thyroglobulin-antithyroglobulin immune complex to extraocular muscle membrane, Endocrinology 96:434-446, 1974.
19. Kriss JP, Konishi J, Herman MM, Studies on the pathogenesis of Graves' ophthalmopathy (with some related observations regarding therapy), Recent Prog Hormone Res 31:533-566, 1975.

20. Kriss JP, Mehdi SQ, Cell mediated lysis of lipid vesicles containing eye muscle proteins: implications regarding pathogenesis of Graves' ophthalmopathy, Proc Natl Acad Sci USA 76:2003-2007, 1979.
21. Takeda Y, Kriss JP, Radiometric measurement of thyroglobulin-antithyroglobulin immune complex in human serum, J Clin Endocrinol Metab 44:46-55, 1977.
22. Ohtaki S, Endo Y, Horinouchi K, Yoshitake S, Ishikawa E, Circulating thyroglobulin-antithyroglobulin immune complex in thyroid diseases using enzyme-linked immunoassays, J Clin Endocrinol Metab 52:239-246, 1981.
23. Izumi M, Larsen PR, Correlation of sequential changes in serum, thyroglobulin, triiodothyronine, and l-thyroxine in patients with Graves' disease and subacute thyroiditis, Metabolism 27:582-593, 1967.
24. Kriss JP, Pleshakov V, Rosenblum AL, Holderness M, Sharp G, Utiger R, J Clin Endocrinol Metab 27:582-593, 1967.
25. Naffziger HC, Jones OW Jr, Surgical treatment of progressive exophthalmos following thyroidectomy, J Am Med Assoc 99:638-642, 1932.
26. Kriss JP, Pathogenesis and treatment of Graves' ophthalmopathy, Thyroid Today 7, 1984.
27. Mullin BR, Levinson RE, Friedman A, Henson DE, Winand RJ, Kohn LD, Delayed hypersensitivity in Graves' disease and exophthalmos: identification of thyroglobulin in normal human orbital muscle, Endocrinology 100:351-366, 1979.
28. Tao TW, Cheng P, Pham H, Leu SL, Kriss JP, Monoclonal antithyroglobulin antibodies derived from immunization of mice with human eye muscle and thyroid membranes, J Clin Endocrinol Metab 63:577-582, 1986.
29. Sattler H, Basedow's Disease (translated by Marchand GW, Marchand JF), Grune and Stratton NY, pp 27-41, 1952.
30. Kuroki T, Ruf J, Whelan L, Miller A, Wall JR, Antithyroglobulin monoclonal and autoantibodies cross-react with an orbital connective tissue membrane antigen: a possible mechanism for the association of ophthalmopathy with autoimmune thyroid disorders, Clin Exp Immunol 62:361-370, 1985.
31. Winand RJ, Kohn LD, The binding of ^{3}H-labeled exophthalmogenic factor by plasma membranes of retro-orbital tissue, Proc Natl Acad Sci 69:1711-1715, 1972.
32. Winand RJ, Kohn LD, Stimulation of adenylate cyclase activity in retro-orbital tissue membranes by thyroglobulin and exophthalmogenic factor derived from thyrotropin, J Biol Chem 250:6522-6526, 1975.
33. Bolonkin D, Tate RL, Luber JH, Kohn LD, Experimental exophthalmos binding of thyrotropin and an exophthalmogenic factor derived from thyrotropin to retro-orbital tissue plasma membranes, J Biol Chem 250:6516-6521, 1975.
34. Kohn LD, Winand RJ, Pathogenesis of human and experimental exophthalmos, In Proceedings of the Fourth International Congress of Endocrinology (ed. Scow RO), Excerpta Medica, Amsterdam, p 1150, 1982.
35. Rotella C, Zonefrati R, Toccafondi R, Valente WA, Kohn LD, Ability of monoclonal antibodies to the thyrotropin receptor to increase collagen synthesis in human fibroblasts: an assay which appears to measure exophthalmogenic immunoglobulins in Graves' sera, J Clin Endocrinol Metab 62:357-367, 1986.
36. Bahn RS, Gorman CA, Woloschak GE, Johnson CM, Serum IgG from patients with Graves' disease binds to a 23 KD protein from human retro-ocular connective tissue, 61st Meeting, Am Thy Assoc, Abst T9, 1986.
37. Kodama K, Sikorska H, Bayly R, Bandy-Dafoe P, Wall JR, Use of monoclonal antibodies to investigate a possible role of thyroglobulin in the pathogenesis of Graves' ophthalmopathy, J Clin Endocrinol Metab 59:67-73, 1984.
38. Donaldson SS, Bagshaw MA, Kriss JP, Supervoltage orbital radiotherapy for Graves' ophthalmopathy, J Clin Endocrinol Metab 37:276, 1973.

CROSS-REACTIVITY BETWEEN ANTIBODIES TO HUMAN THYROGLOBULIN AND TORPEDO
ACETYLCHOLINESTERASE IN PATIENTS WITH GRAVES' OPHTHALMOPATHY

M. Ludgate[1], C. Owada[2], R. Pope[3], P. Taylor[2], and G. Vassart[1]

IRIBHN, ULB, Brussels[1]; Dept. Pharmacology, University
of San Diego, California[2]; Dept. Medicine, UWCM, Cardiff[3]

INTRODUCTION

     The pathogenesis of Grave's ophthalmopathy (GO) remains an enigma
although there is some evidence for autoimmune mechanisms and also for
antigens shared by the thyroid and eye orbit (1,2). The extra-ocular
muscles seem to be the primary target for the disease process, being
heavily infiltrated by lymphocytes. To date a plausible explanation for
this has been wanting but thyroglobulin (Tg) has been proposed as the
"common link" (3). The recent demonstration of a significant homology
between bovine Tg and torpedo acetylcholinesterase (TAche) (4) and subsequently the comparison of their hydropathy profiles and conservation of
cysteine residues involved in disulphide bonds implies that the two proteins may share common epitopes (5). This led us to propose that some
antibodies or T lymphocytes sensitized to human Tg might recognize and
cross-react with human Ache and the extra-ocular muscles with their
abundant nerve supply would be more affected than skeletal muscle (6).

     To test this hypothesis we have performed enzyme linked immunosor-
bent assays (ELISA) to investigate the binding of GO patients sera to
human Tg and torpedo Ache.

METHODS

     Subjects : - Eight patients with severe GO (at least stage 4 by the
American Thyroid Association Classification) were studied at a time when
they were euthyroid following various treatment regimens and also five
patients with Hashimoto's thyroiditis (HT) receiving thyroxine and seven
normal controls.

     Antigens : - Human thyroglobulin was prepared from thyroids of
patients with Graves' disease. Affinity purified acetylcholinesterase was
prepared from the electric organ of Torpedo Californica.

<u>ELISA :</u>   96 well plates coated in carbonate/bicarbonate buffer
pH 9.6 at 4°C overnight with 10 µg/ml antigen

$\downarrow$

At each stage   Serum samples diluted 1:100 in PBSN-1 % BSA, applied for
plates were   2 hours at room temperature
washed x 3 in
phosphate $\downarrow$
buffered saline   Anti-human IgG conjugated with alkaline phosphatase
.05 % nonidet   1:7500 dilution (Promega) for 2 hours at room
(PBSN).   temperature

$\downarrow$

pNPP substrate (Sigma) in diethanolamine buffer pH 9.8
colour developed and absorbance read at 405 nm.

RESULTS

	HTg	TAche
Normals (n=7)	$\bar{x}$ = .303 SD = .052	$\bar{x}$ = .320 SD = .062
GO patients (n=9)	$\bar{x}$ = .704 SD = .234**	$\bar{x}$ = .626 SD = .210*
Haschimoto's thyroiditis (n=5)	$\bar{x}$ = 1.033 SD = .481	$\bar{x}$ = .690 SD = .111

*The difference between the response of GO patients and that of normals is
significant (p < .005) as assessed by Students "t" test **(p < .001)

Based on the mean + 2SD of the control group 6/9 and 8/9 GO patients gave
positive responses to TAche and HTg respectively. Preincubation of sera
with TAche before performing the ELISA significantly reduced the level of
binding to both antigens, HTg also reduced the level of binding but was
not significant for TAche.

CONCLUSIONS

The experiments, although preliminary, indicate that there is
significant binding of GO patients sera to TAche and that this correlates
strongly with binding to human Tg.

However, there are many points which remain to be explained :
(i) why do Hashimoto's thyroiditis patients whose sera bind to TAche in an
ELISA not have eye disease ? We suggest that this may be a quantitative
effect since serum cholinesterase levels have been shown to be increase
during thyrotoxicosis thus it seems plausible that acetylcholinesterase at
nerve/muscle interfaces would also be elevated and most patients with GO
have had an episode of hyperthyroidism before the onset of eye signs.
(ii) not all patients with GO have detectable levels of antibody to
thyroglobulin. It is conceivable that thyroid infiltrating lymphocytes
include T cells sensitized to Tg even in the absence of circulating
antibody.

We do not propose that antibodies which recognise acetylcholinesterase are pathogenic "per se" but the demonstrated cross-reactivity
between them and Tg supports the hypothesis that the "antigenic
similarity" between Tg and Ache may play a role in the aetiology of GO.
Further experiments are required to investigate the contributions made by
humoral and/or cell mediated immune mechanisms in the disease process.

REFERENCES

1. P. Kendall-Taylor, <u>Clinics in Endocrinology and Metabolism</u>, 14:331 (1985).
2. T.W. Tao, P.J. Cheng, H. Pham, S.L. Len and J.P. Kriss, <u>J. Clin. Endocrinol. Metab</u>., 63:577 (1986).
3. B.R. Mullin, R.E. Levinson, A. Friedman, D.E. Henson, R.J. Winand and L.D. Kohn, <u>Endocrinology</u>, 100:351 (1976).
4. M. Schumacher, S. Camp et al., <u>Nature</u>, 319:407 (1986).
5. S. Swillens, M. Ludgate, L. Mercken, J.E. Dumont and G. Vassart, <u>Biochem. Biophys. Res. Comm</u>., 137:142 (1986).
6. M. Ludgate, S. Swillens, L. Mercken and G. Vassart, <u>Lancet</u>, II:219 (1986).

MULTIPLE AUTOANTIGENIC DETERMINANTS IN

THYROID AUTOIMMUNITY

A.P. Weetman, R. Smallridge, C. Hayslip, and K.D. Burman

Dept of Medicine, Royal Postgraduate Medical School
London W12 OHS, UK. and
Walter Reed Army Medical Center
Washington DC 20307, USA

INTRODUCTION

Autoantibodies directed against thyroglobulin (Tg), microsomes
(Mic) and the TSH receptor (TSH-R) are well recognised in thyroid
autoimmunity. Both Tg and Mic antibodies are found in Hashimoto's
thyroiditis (HT) and Graves' disease (GD) while Mic antibodies are
strongly associated with post-partum thyroiditis (PPT). However in
subacute granulomatous thyroiditis (SAT) and subacute lymphocytic or
"silent" thyroiditis (ST), these antibodies are infrequent, transient
and of low titre (Hay, 1985).

The lack of correlation between thyroid membrane (TMEM) binding
antibodies and those detected by assays for Tg, Mic and TSH-R antibodies
in Graves' disease (Gardas et al 1984) suggests the presence of
additional autoantibodies in thyroiditis. We have assessed this
possibility by qualitative immunoblotting.

METHODS

Materials

TMEM consisted of the 2000g supernatant of an homogenate of three
pooled Graves' thyroids. Tg and Mic were prepared as detailed elsewhere
(Weetman et al 1984).

Sera. Samples were obtained from 20 patients with GD, 17 with PPT, 15
with HT, 9 with SAT and 6 with ST. These were compared with sera from
11 healthy laboratory staff. Serum samples from SAT and ST patients
were obtained within a month of disease onset; those from patients with
PPT were taken between one and two months after delivery.

Immunoblotting

TMEM were run on SDS-PAGE (sodium dodecyl sulphate-polyacrylamide
gel electrophoresis) under reducing conditions on a 5 - 15% gradient gel
and the fractionated antigen transferred electrophoretically to
nitrocellulose paper (Towbin et al 1979). Strips were then incubated
with sera, 1:50 dilution, and bound antibody visualised by incubation
with ^{125}I-protein A and autoradiography.

RESULTS

Over 50 protein bands were found on Coomassie blue staining of
TMEM after SDS-PAGE. From experiments with purified antigens, these
included bands at 200 – 300 kd (Tg) and 100 – 105 kd (Mic). However,
immunoblotting of all five groups of thyroiditis sera onto TMEM revealed
antibody binding to determinants at other molecular weights (Fig 1).

The control sera bound to two bands at 30 kd and 50 kd, which may
be regarded therefore as non-specific in considering the disease groups.
In the GD and HT groups, over half the sera reacted with determinants at
200 – 300 kd (Tg) and 105 kd (Mic) but in addition 18 GD and 13 HT sera
also identified at least one other determinant in the range 15 – 160 kd.
The binding of the GD sera was not blocked by TSH (1u/ml) and the
patterns did not correlate with the level of Mic or Tg antibodies.

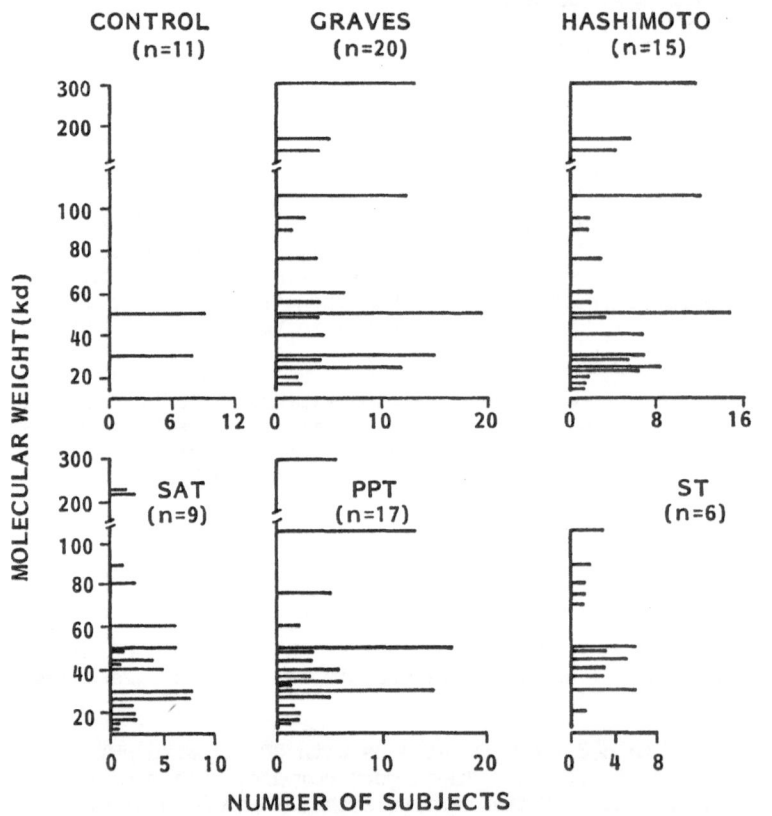

Fig. 1. Frequency distribution of serum reactivity with TMEM
         determinants in normals and patients with thyroid
         auto-immunity. The number of subjects in each group is
         given in parentheses. The length of each line for a
         given molecular weight shows the number of reactive sera
         in each group.

The other patient groups, SAT, ST and PPT, also reacted with determinants at 15 - 120 kd (Fig 1). It was striking that all eight of the SAT patients and three of the six ST patients, whose sera reacted with one or more of these determinants, did not have Tg or Mic antibodies detectable by haemagglutination or ELISA. Several determinants were recognised by sera in all five disease groups, particularly those at 60, 40 and 25 kd.

DISCUSSION

A number of new thyroid autoantigenic determinants in TMEM have been identified by immunoblotting which do not appear to be related to Tg, Mic or TSH-R. Our data explain the lack of correlation between the results of tests for autoantibodies against these established antigens and those obtained with a radioimmunoassay employing TMEM (Gardas et al 1984). Such a complex antigen preparation would also seem likely to engender a heterogenous response when used to stimulate lymphocytes in vitro (Okita et al 1981).

The localisation of these antigens remains to be established. However a recent report has confirmed the present findings in GD using TMEM from FRTL$_5$ cells, so that at least some of the determinants are not species specific (Cohen and Ladenson 1985). Finally it is of interest that patients with ST, PPT and SAT, as well as GD and HT, had antibodies against these novel determinants, suggesting shared immunopathogenic mechanisms in all five types of thyroiditis.

REFERENCES

Cohen J.L., Ladenson P.W., 1985, Identification of thyroid antigens recognised by Graves' autoantibodies. Clin.Res. 33: 303A.
Gardas, A., Czarnocka, B., Faryna, M. et al., 1984, Simple and sensitive method for estimation of antithyroid plasma membrane antibodies in the serum of patients with autoimmune thyroid diseases; comparison with other assays. Acta Endocrinol.,105:492.
Hay, I.D., 1985, Thyroiditis: a clinical update. Mayo Clin.Proc. 60: 836.
Okita, N., Row V.V., Volpé R., 1981, Suppressor T lymphocyte deficiency' in Graves' disease and Hashimoto's thyroiditis. J. Clin. Endocrinol.metab. 52:528.
Towbin, H., Staehelin, T. and Gordon, J., 1979, Electrophoretic transfer of proteins from polyacrylamide gels to nitrocellulose sheets: procedures and some applications. Proc. Natl. Acad. Sci. U.S.A., 76:4350.
Weetman, A.P., McGregor, A.M., Wheeler, M.H. and Hall, R., 1984, Extrathyroidal sites of autoantibody synthesis in Graves' disease. Clin. Exp. Immunol. 56:330.

FURTHER CHARACTERIZATION OF THE THYROID MICROSOMAL ANTIGEN

BY MONOCLONAL ANTIBODIES

Luc Portmann, Noboru Hamada,
Wilfred A. Franklin*, and Leslie J. DeGroot

Thyroid Study Unit, Department of Medicine and *Pathology
The University of Chicago
Chicago, IL 60637, USA

INTRODUCTION

The thyroid microsomal antigen has been recently identified as a 107 kD protein (1) by Western blot and immunoprecipitation using sera of patients with thyroid autoimmune disease. In addition other studies have reported the presence of antibodies in those sera against human thyroid peroxidase (2), and a coelution during gel filtration of peroxidase enzymatic activity and microsomal antigenicity (3) suggesting an identity between microsomal antigen and thyroid peroxidase. We developed monoclonal antibodies against this 107 kD antigen to better characterize its nature and relationship to thyroid peroxidase.

MATERIALS AND METHODS

Immunization protocol: The 107 kD gel-purified antigen was injected to Balb/c female mice intraperitoneally every four weeks until the sera were positive for the presence of binding by Western blot to the 107 kD band. Fusion was done as previously described (4) and after appropriate screening, hybridomas were subcloned and expanded.

Immunoprecipitation study and Western blot: Thyroid microsomes were immunoprecipitated using a human sera with a high MCHA titer but TGHA(-) and TRAb(-), and addition of Pansorbin (Calbiochem, La Jolla, CA). After appropriate washing, proteins were eluted and submitted to Sodium Dodecyl Sulfate-Polyacrylamide Gel Electrophoresis (SDS-PAGE) (1). After blotting, nitrocellulose sheets were incubated with monoclonal antibodies and binding was visualized using peroxidase conjugated antibody.

Proteolysis of microsomal antigen: Microsomal antigen was incubated with either trypsin, type III-S, from bovine pancreas (Sigma, St.Louis, Mo) or V8-protease, Staphylococcus aureus (Miles Scientific, Elkhart, IN) in a shaking waterbath at 37 C. Reaction was stopped by addition of chromatographically purified soybean trypsin inhibitor (Sigma) or/and boiling the samples. After electrophoresis, the proteins were blotted into nitrocellulose sheets and incubated with human sera and monoclonal antibodies.

Enzyme-Linked Immunoabsorbent Assay (ELISA). Thyroid microsomal fraction was coated onto ELISA-plates, and binding of antibodies (monoclonal anti-

antibodies & human sera) was measured using peroxidase-linked second antibody as previously described (2).

Binding to Thyroid Peroxidase: Binding of monoclonal antibodies and human sera to hog highly purified thyroid peroxidase (5) as well to human immunopurified thyroid peroxidase (6) was determined after Western blot. In addition immunoprecipitation of thyroid peroxidase enzymatic activity by human sera and monoclonal antibodies was determined, after incubation of solubilized thyroid peroxidase with antibodies and Protein A-Sepharose 4B (2).

Immunohistochemical Studies: Binding of monoclonal antibodies to various thyroid tissues (nodules, carcinomas) was studied using an alkaline phosphatase anti-alkaline phosphatase method (7).

RESULTS

Microsomal Antigen: Six monoclonal antibodies were obtained after four fusions. They all bound to 101 and 107 kD proteins, when either total microsomal proteins or immunopurified microsomal antigen were applied to SDS-PAGE and blotted. In the absence of reducing agent these antibodies were found to bind to higher molecular weight bands, but less strongly. Trypsinization of the microsomal antigen produced a doublet of new polypeptides of 84 and 88 kD, which were antigenic for all monoclonal antibodies, but only a few of the human polyclonal antibodies tested, previously shown to bind to 101 and 107 kD proteins.

TABLE 1. Binding of antibodies to microsomal antigen/thyroid peroxidase

	Three different human antibodies MCHA(+), TGHA(-)			Monoclonal antibodies (anti-107 kD)
	a	b	c	
Microsomal antigen				
1) antigen coated on ELISA-plates	+	+	+	+
2) antigen after Western blot	-	+	+ (101-107 kD)	+
3) + trypsin	-	-	+ (84-88 kD)	+
4) + V8-protease	-	+	+ (101 kD)	+
Thyroid peroxidase				
1) human immunopurified	+	+	+	+
2) hog highly purified	-	-	ND	+
3) immunoprecipitation of peroxidase enzymatic activity	+	+	ND	-

presence of binding of antibodies: +   absence of binding: -
ND : not determined

Addition of V8-protease led to a disappearance of the 107 kD band by protein staining of the gel as well as by immunoreactivity after blotting using either monoclonal or human polyclonal antibodies; the pattern of the 101 kD band remained unchanged. All antibodies had a strong binding to microsomal antigen coated on ELISA plates, no difference was observed between monoclonal and patients with MCHA (+) sera. This suggests that the thyroid microsomal fraction contains native as well as denatured thyroid peroxidase.

Thyroid Peroxidase: No immunoprecipitation of thyroid peroxidase activity was observed when using monoclonal antibodies. This may be because we used a fully denatured and reduced antigen in the immunization protocol or because binding of one monoclonal antibody may be insufficient to cause immunoprecipitation. However the monoclonal antibodies bound well to purified human (6/6 mAb) and to hog thyroid peroxidase (5/6). The antigenic regions recognized by monoclonal antibodies are probably present only in a denatured thyroid peroxidase.

Immunohistochemical Studies: All monoclonal antibodies demonstrated strong and similar binding to colloid nodule or hyperplastic thyroid tissue. Binding was seen only to thyroid acinar cells, not to colloid or interstitium in opposition to monoclonal antibodies against thyroglobulin. Binding was almost as strong to follicular and Huerthle cell carcinomas but was weak or absent to papillary carcinomas.

CONCLUSIONS

Monoclonal antibodies were developed against a well defined microsomal antigen, and demonstrate that the microsomal antigen and the thyroid peroxidase are identical. This antigenic molecule is constituted by two related but different polypeptides, having trypsin-sensitive immunoreactive domains. The variability of binding of patients' antibodies to trypsinized microsomal antigen (thyroid peroxidase) may be useful for correlating epitopes recognized by various autoantibodies with the natural course of autoimmune thyroid disease. The expression of microsomal antigenicity or thyroid peroxidase is not homogeneous in thyroid carcinomas which may reflect a difference of carcinogenetic factors involved.

REFERENCES

1. N. Hamada, C. Grimm, H. Mori, and L.J. DeGroot, Identification of a thyroid microsomal antigen by Western blot and immunoprecipitation, J Clin Endocrinol Metab 61:120 (1985).
2. L. Portmann, N. Hamada, G. Heinrich, and L.J. DeGroot, Anti-thyroid peroxidase antibody in patients with autoimmune thyroid disease: possible identity with anti-microsomal antibody, J Clin Endocrinol Metab 61:1001 (1985).
3. B. Czarnocka, J. Ruf, M. Ferrand, and P. Carayon, Parenté antigénique entre la peroxydase thyroïdienne et l'antigène microsomal impliqué dans les affections autoimmunes de la thyroïde, CR Acad Sc Paris 300, III, 15:577 (1985).
4. T. J. McKearn, F.W. Fitch, and D.E. Smilek, Properties of rat anti-MCH antibodies produced by cloned rat-mouse hybridomas, Immunol Rev 47:91 (1979).
5. A. B. Rawith, A. Taurog, S.B. Chernoff, and M.L. Dorris, Hog thyroid peroxidase: physical, chemical, and catalytic properties of the highly enzyme, Arch Biochem Biophys 194:244 (1979).
6. B. Czarnocka, J. Ruf, M. Ferrand, P. Carayon, and S. Lissitzky, Purification of the human thyroid peroxidase and its identification as the microsomal antigen involved in autoimmune thyroid disease, FEBS letters 190:147 (1985).
7. J. L. Cordell, B. Falini, W.N. Erber et al, Immunoenzymatic labeling of monoclonal antibodies using immune complexes of alkaline phosphatase and monoclonal anti-alkaline phosphatase (APAAP complexes), J Histochem and Cytochem 32:219 (1984).

MOLECULAR CLONING OF A THYROID PEROXIDASE cDNA FRAGMENT ENCODING
EPITOPES INVOLVED IN HASHIMOTO'S THYROIDITIS [HT].

C. Dinsart, F. Libert, J. Ruel*, M. Ludgate, J.
Pommier**, J. Dussault*, and G. Vassart

IRIBHN, U.L.B. Bruxelles and *INSERM, Bicêtre
France and **Université Laval, Québec

INTRODUCTION

     Measurement of "anti microsome" antibodies in patients with thyroid
diseases is part of the routine diagnostic procedures involved in the
evaluation of their status. These auto-antibodies may reach extremely
high titers and are responsible for the tissue destruction observed in
Hashimoto thyroiditis. Until very recently the "microsomal antigen" was
defined solely as an unidentified component of thyroid microsomes,
different from thyroglobulin. During the last year, strong indications
have been obtained in favor of the identity between the microsomal
antigen and thyroid peroxydase (TPO)(1-2). However, standard antimicrosome
antibody assays still use a rather crude thyroid microsome preparation
as their antigen. While it would certainly be preferable to use
purified TPO in such assays, the continuous preparation of purified
enzyme is time consuming and expensive. Use of the recombinant DNA
methodology would obviate this difficulty and provide us with unlimited
amounts of clonally pure TPO antigens involved in the auto-immune
process.

Molecular cloning of antigens involved in thyroid autoimmunity.

     With the aim of identifying and cloning antigens involved in
thyroid autoimmunity, we have exploited the power of the λgtll cloning
system to isolate and identify antigens involved in Hashimoto's
thyroiditis (3).

     A cDNA library has been prepared from a normal human thyroid in
this vector. Individual phages harbor and express as a fused protein
segments of the whole coding information expressed in thyroid tissue.
Recombinant phages encoding epitopes involved in autoimmune phenomena
were identified by screening the library with serum from patients with
Hashimoto thyroiditis. A variety of clones were identified in this
manner. A fraction of them was found to react with antibodies directed
against purified TPO and a subfraction of these were recognized by sera
from 19 out of 19 patients with Hashimoto thyroiditis. This subset of
clones thus express TPO epitope(s) commonly involved in the disease.
Some of the clones have also been screened using two murine monoclonal
antibodies to the human thyroid microsome [MAHM].

Isolation of human thyroid mRNA

Synthesis of ds cDNA

Insertion in lambda gt11 vector

Thyroid cDNA expression library (2.10^7 clones)

Screening with autoantibodies and with TPO antibodies

Identification of TPO clones bearing auto-antigens

Preparation of the recombinant antigen

Development of a recombinant TPO antibody assay

Development of a recombinant TPA autoantibody assay

The recombinant phages described hereabove and harboring DNA segments which code for TPO epitopes involved in autoimmunity allow preparation in E.coli of large amounts of antigens uncontaminated with any other thyroid protein. They have been used to develop a model assay where the recombinant antigen is fixed onto nitrocellulose paper and incubated with the sera to be tested. Reactive autoantibodies are detected by a colorimetric reaction involving anti human IgG coupled to alkaline phosphatase.

It is expected that other auto-antigens will be cloned in this manner and lead to the development of a new generation of assays involved in the evaluation of autoimmunity.

REFERENCES

1) Czarnocka B., Ruf J., Ferrand M., Carayon P., Lissitzky S. (1985), FEBS Lett 190: 147.
2) Portmann L., Hamada N., Heinrich G., DeGroot L.J. (1985) J. Clin. Endocrinol. Metab. 61: 1001.
3) Young R. and Davis R.W. (1983) Proc. Natl. Acad. Sci. USA 80: 1194.

FURTHER EVIDENCE THAT THYROID PEROXIDASE AND THE "MICROSOMAL ANTIGEN" ARE THE SAME ENTITY

B. Czarnocka, J. Ruf, C. Alquier*, M.E. Toubert, C. Dutoit, M. Ferrand and P. Carayon

U 38 INSERM - UA 178 CNRS and (*) U 172 INSERM - UA 1179 CNRS
University of Aix-Marseille Medical School, Marseille, France

INTRODUCTION

The first hint to the nature of the thyroid microsomal antigen was provided by the observation that TPO was antigenically related to the microsomal antigen [1]. Then TPO was purified by monoclonal antibody (mAb) assisted affinity chromatography and shown to react with autoimmune antibodies (aAb) in serum of patients with autoimmune thyroid diseases [2]. Titers of anti-TPO and anti-microsomal aAb in serum were found significantly correlated [3] which suggested that TPO effectively was the microsomal antigen. Other groups of investigators confirmed that anti-thyroid aAb reacted with TPO, but proposed that TPO was only a part of a putative microsomal antigen complex [5-8]. To answer the question whether TPO effectively was the microsomal antigen or only a part of it we undertook different experiments based on the use of highly purified human TPO and mAb to it [9-11]

1 - COLOCALIZATION OF THE MICROSOMAL ANTIGEN AND TPO

The localisation on ultrathin tissue sections and isolated follicles of the binding sites of 5 anti-TPO mAb correlated well with the distribution of endogeneous peroxidase i.e. apical cell surface labelling and intracellular localization in perinuclear cisternae, rough endoplasmic reticulum and vesicles. Furthermore the anti-microsomal aAb labelled the same regions of the cell surface and the same intracellular organelles. Control with preparations of anti-microsomal aAb depleted in anti-TPO were negative.

2 - COPURIFICATION OF ANTI-TPO AND ANTI-MICROSOMAL aAb

IgG from patients with AITD were put onto a Tg-Sepharose column. Anti-TPO and anti-microsomal activity were present in the filtrate and the washing fraction but not in the eluate. An aliquot of IgG depleted in anti-Tg aAb was put onto a TPO-Sepharose column. The filtrate and the washing fraction did not contain anti-microsomal and anti-TPO activities which were recovered after

Address correspondence to Dr Pierre Carayon U 38 INSERM, Faculté de Médecine, F-13385 Marseille Cedex 5, France.

elution with glycine-HCl buffer. The different affinity
chromatography fractions were analyzed by Western blot. Typical
scannergrams are presented Fig.1.

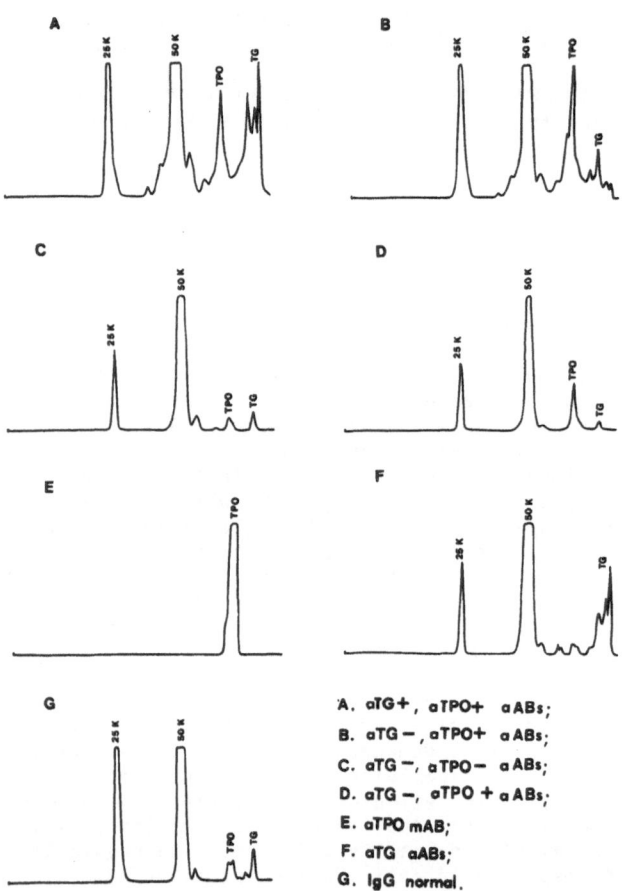

A. aTG+, aTPO+ aABs;

B. aTG −, aTPO+ aABs;

C. aTG −, aTPO− aABs;

D. aTG −, aTPO + aABs;

E. aTPO mAB;

F. aTG aABs;

G. IgG normal.

Fig. 1. Scannergrams of anti-thyroid antibodies IgG from a pool of
sera from patients with autoimmune thyroid diseases (A) were
depleted in anti-Tg aAb (B) and, next, in anti-TPO aAb (C).
Affinity-purified anti-TPO aAb (D) were recovered. The different
preparations were incubated with microsomes transfered to
nitrocellulose and the bound IgG were visualized by anti-human IgG
labelled with horse radish peroxidase. Anti-TPO mAb (E), anti-Tg aAb
(F) and normal IgG (G) were used as a control.

3 - HETEROGENEITY OF ANTI-TPO aAb

Preliminary mapping of the antigenic surface of TPO with mAb distinguished five different antigenic regions. Experiments with pooled or individual sera from patients with AITD showed that anti-TPO aAb reacted strongly with two antigenic regions. This suggested that the heterogeneity of anti-TPO aAb was restricted. However, anti-TPO aAb at high concentration inhibited the binding to TPO of the whole set of 66 mAb. Furthermore, anti-TPO aAb at high concentration inhibited the binding of anti-TPO pAb. These results indicated that aAb recognized many antigenic sites on TPO.

CONCLUSION

Copurification of anti-TPO and anti-microsomal aAb and colocalization of TPO and the microsomal antigen provide further evidence that TPO effectively is the microsomal antigen. Furthermore, the heterogeneity of anti-TPO aAb, taken together with the sensitivity of TPO to denaturation, may explain that the TPO activity and the microsomal antigen immunoactivity could appear dissociated.

REFERENCES

1. B. Czarnocka, J. Ruf, M. Ferrand and P. Carayon, Antigenic relationship between thyroid peroxidase and the microsomal antigen involved in thyroid auto-immune diseases, C.R. Acad. Sci. (Paris) 300 : 577 (1985)
2. B. Czarnocka, J. Ruf, M. Ferrand, P. Carayon and S. Lissitzky, Purification of the human thyroid peroxidase and its identification as the microsomal antigen involved in autoimmune thyroid diseases, FEBS Lett. 190 : 147 (1985)
3. B. Czarnocka, J. Ruf, M. Ferrand, S. Lissitzky and P. Carayon, Interaction of highly purified thyroid peroxidase with anti-microsomal antibodies in autoimmune thyroid diseases. J. Endocrinol. Invest. 9 : 135 (1986)
4. S. Mariotti, R. Bechi, S. Anelli, J. Ruf, A. Lombardi, L. Chiovato, B. Czarnocka, P. Carayon and A. Pinchera, Evidence for identity of serum thyroid microsomal and anti-human thyroid peroxidase autoantibodies, in :"The Thyroid and Autoimmunity", H.A. Drexhage and W.M. Wiersinger eds., Elsevier Science, Amsterdam pp 86 (1986)
5. L. Portmann, N. Hamada, G. Heinrich and L.J. DeGroot, Anti-thyroid peroxidase in patients with autoimmune thyroid disease : possible identity with anti-microsomal antigen, J. Clin. Endocrinol. Metab. 61 : 1001 (1985)
6. L. Portmann, N. Hamada and F. Fitch, Characterization of monoclonal antibody to a thyroid microsomal antigen, Proceedings of 68th Annual Meeting of the American Endocrine Society, Anaheim, Abstract 831 (1986)
7. T. Kotani, K. Umaki, S. Matsunaga, E. Kato and S. Ohtaki, Detection of autoantibodies to thyroid peroxidase in autoimmune thyroid diseases by micro-ELISA and immuno-blotting , J. Clin. Endocrinol. Metab. 62 : 928 (1986)
8. S. Ohtaki, T. Kotani and Y. Nakamum, Characterization of human thyroid peroxidase purified by monoclonal antibody-assisted chromatography, J. Clin. Endocrinol. Metab. 63 : 570 (1986)

9. J. Ruf, B. Czarnocka, M.E. Toubert, M. Ferrand and
    P. Carayon, Characterization of monoclonal, polyclonal
    and autoimmune antibodies to thyroid peroxidase,
    Submitted for publication
10. B. Czarnocka, J. Ruf, C. Alquier, C. Dutoit, M. Ferrand
    and P. Carayon, Co-purification of anti-thyroid
    peroxidase and microsomal autoantibodies by thyroid
    peroxidase-affinity chromatography, submitted for publication
11. C. Alquier, J. Ruf and P. Carayon, Co-localization of
    thyroid peroxidase and the binding sites for anti-
    microsomal and anti-peroxidase antibodies, submitted for
    publication

COMPETITIVE AND IMMUNOMETRIC RADIOASSAYS FOR THE MEASUREMENT OF ANTI-THYROID

PEROXIDASE AUTOANTIBODIES IN HUMAN SERA

Stefano Mariotti, Stefano Anelli, Jean Ruf*, Riccardo Bechi, Antonio Lombardi, Pierre Carayon*

Cattedra di Endocrinologia, Università di Pisa and (*) Biochimie Médicale Université Aix-Marseille II
Pisa, Italy and Marseille, France

INTRODUCTION

Thyroid autoimmune disorders are associated with the presence of circulating autoantibodies reacting with the thyroid microsomal antigen (M-Ag), a membrane protein mainly localized in the apical cytoplasm and in the microvillar plasma membrane of thyroid follicular cells (1-4). Most recently, evidence has been obtained that M-Ag is actually represented by human thyroid peroxidase (TPO) (5,6). Accordingly, autoantibodies reacting with highly purified TPO (anti-TPO Ab) were detected in selected sera from patients with autoimmune thyroid diseases containing anti-M-Ag autoantibodies (anti-M Ab), and a significant correlation between the two antibodies was generally observed (5-8). However, the precise prevalence of anti-TPO Ab in thyroid diseases is still poorly known.

Taking advantage of the availability of highly purified TPO and of a monoclonal anti-TPO antibody, in the present study we developed two radioimmmunological methods for anti-TPO determinations which appear particularly suitable for clinical applications.

MATERIALS AND METHODS

Antigenic preparations

Human thyroid microsomes were prapared by differential centrifugation from surgical specimens of toxic diffuse goiter, as detailed elsewhere (9). TPO was immunopurified on anti-TPO monoclonal antibody affinity column, as previously described (6).

Serum samples

Sera were obtained form 34 patients with Hashimoto's thyroiditis, 13 with idiopathic myxedema, 45 with Graves' disease, 10 with miscellaneous nonautoimmune thyroid disorders and from 29 normal control subjects. In all samples anti-M Ab were assayed by passive hemagglutination (PH).

Preparation and radioiodination of antibodies

Human immunoglobulins G (IgG) preparations and affinity chromatography purified anti-IgG antibody were prepared and radioiodinated as previously described (9,10). Anti-TPO monoclonal antibody was obtained by fusing spleens of mice immunized with human thyroid membrane preparations as detailed elsewhere (5,6). Anti-TPO monoclonal antibody was labeled with 125-I using the chloramine T method.

Radioassays of anti-M Ab

In some experiment anti-M Ab were also measured by competitive binding radioassay (CR)(10) and by immunoradiometric assay (IRMA) (9), as previously described.

To this purpose, we developed two radioassays with similar design to those used for anti-MAb.

In the CR, anti-TPO Ab was detected by its ability to inhibit 125-I-anti-TPO monoclonal antibody binding to wells coated with thyroid microsomes. Briefly, 0.5 µl of the test sera were incubated within the coated wells overnight at room temperature with 125-I-anti-TPO monoclonal antibody. After removal of the unbound material by washing, the radioactivity fixed to the wells was counted. Results were expressed as percent inhibition of the maximal specific radioantibody binding. Values exceeding 11.6% (i.e. mean + 2 SD of the results obtained in the normal controls) were considered as indicative of positive anti-TPO by CR.

IRMA was carried out by incubating for 2 h at 45°C 1.0 µl of the test sera within microtiter plates coated with purified TPO. After removal of unbound material by washing, anti-TPO Ab were detected by adding overnight at room temperature 125-I-anti-IgG antibody. Results were expressed as percent of the specific radioantibody binding obtained in each assay with a standard reference serum containing a large excess of anti-TPO Ab ("normalized 125-I-anti-IgG binding"). Values >11.7% (i.e. exceeding 2 SD the mean of controls) were considered as positive anti-TPO Ab by IRMA.

RESULTS

The results obtained by CR are summarized in Fig. 1. Anti-TPO Ab were detected by both radioassays in most patients with Hashimoto's thyroiditis, idiopathic myxedema and Graves' disease. Anti-TPO Ab were in general undetectable in normal subjects and in patients with miscellaneous non-autoimmune thyroid diseases, with the exception of some cases showing positive anti-M Ab by PH. Similar results were observed by IRMA. When the results obtained in all the above determinations were grouped together, a highly significant correlation between anti-TPO Ab as assessed by CR (r=0.920, p<0.00001) or IRMA (r=0.915, p<0.00001) was found with the anti-M Ab titers by PH.

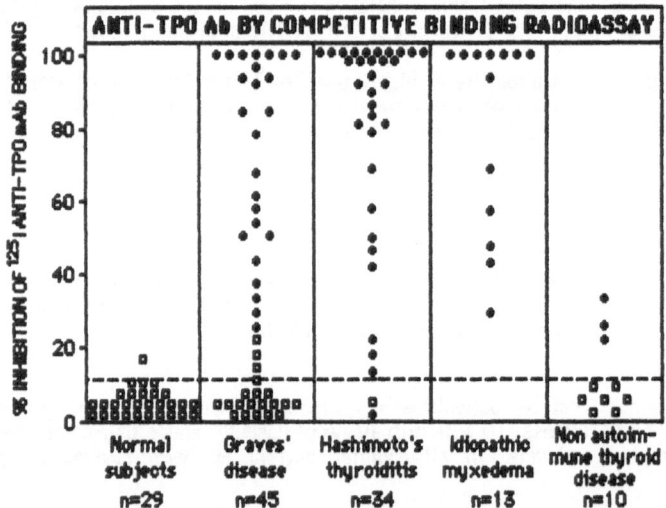

Fig. 1. Anti-TPO Ab by CR in 131 subjects with or without thyroid disease. Results are expressed as percent inhibition of 125-I-anti-TPO monoclonal antibody (mAb) binding to thyroid microsomes coated on microtiter wells. (●) Positive and (□) negative anti-M Ab by PH

To assess the specificity of the radioassays, anti-TPO Ab were assayed in several sera containing different organ specific and nonorgan-specific autoantibodies. Negative results were consistently obtained with each serum, with the exception of the samples that also contained anti-M Ab detected by PH or radioassays.

The procedure previously illustrated for anti-TPO Ab allows only semi-quantitative estimation of the antibody levels. Preliminary experiments showed that a standard calibration curve could be obtained in both radioassays by adding progressive amounts of a human IgG preparation containing high titres of anti-TPO Ab. Dilution curves of anti-TPO Ab positive sera were found to be parallel to the standard curve, indicating the possibility to express the levels of anti-TPO Ab in quantitative units.

CONCLUSIVE REMARKS

In the present investigation we developed two radioassays for detection of anti-TPO Ab in human sera. Both methods appeared to be simple, sensitive and potentially able to provide quantitative data. The specificity of the assays was proved by the negative results obtained with sera containing several unrelated autoantibodies.

Using these techniques we confirmed and extended previous limited observations indicating the presence of circulating anti-TPO Ab in autoimmune thyroid diseases (5-8). Anti-TPO Ab were strictly correlated to anti-M Ab, irrespective of the nature of primary thyroid disease. This finding provides further support to the concept of the identity of M-Ag and TPO.

The availability of simple assays for anti-TPO Ab determination will allow extensive clinical investigations to clarify the role of these antibodies in thyroid autoimmunity.

AKNOWLEDGEMENTS

This work was partially supported by C.N.R. (Rome, Italy), Target Project "Preventive Medicine and Rehabilitation" Subproject "Mechanisms of aging", Grant n° 86.01899.56.

REFERENCES

1. I. M. Roitt, N. R. Ling, D. Doniach, and K. G. Couchman, The cytoplasmic auto-antigen of the human thyroid. I. Immunological and biochemical considerations. Immunology 7:375 (1964).
2. E. L. Khoury, L. Hammond, G. F. Bottazzo, and D. Doniach, Presence of the organ-specific "microsomal" autoantigen on the surface of human thyroid cells in culture: its involvement in complement-mediated cytotoxicity. Clin. Exp. Immunol. 45:316 (1981).
3. G. F. Fenzi, L. Bartalena, L. Chiovato, C. Marcocci, C. M. Rotella, R. Zonefrati, R. Toccafondi, and A. Pinchera, Studies on thyroid cell surface antigens using cultured human thyroid cells. Clin. Exp. Immunol. 47:336 (1982).
4. E. L. Khoury, G. F. Bottazzo, and I. M. Roitt, The thyroid "microsomal" antibody revisited. Its paradoxical binding in vivo to the apical surface of follicular epithelium. J. Exp. Med. 159:577 (1984).
5. B. Czarnocka, J. Ruf, M. Ferrand, and P. Carayon, Antigenic ralationship between thyroid peroxidase and the microsomal antigen involved in thyroid auto-immune diseases. C. R. Acad. Sc. Paris 300:577 (1985).
6. B. Czarnocka, J. Ruf, M. Ferrand, P. Carayon, and S. Lissitzky, Purification of the human thyroid peroxidase and its identification as the microsomal antigen involved in autoimmune thyroid disease F F B S left 190·147 (1985)

THYROID PEROXIDASE AND THE "MICROSOMAL ANTIGEN" CANNOT BE DISTINGUISHED BY IMMUNOFLUORESCENCE ON CULTURED THYROID CELLS

L.Chiovato, P.Vitti, C.Mammoli, G.Lopez, P.Cucchi, S.Battiato, P. Carayon*, G.F.Fenzi, and A.Pinchera

Cattedra di Endocrinologia, University of Pisa, Pisa Italy, and* Biochimie Mèdicale, University of Aix-Marseille II, France

INTRODUCTION

Recent evidence indicates that human thyroid peroxidase (TPO) shares most of the characteristics of the thyroid microsomal autoantigen (MAg)(1, 2). The question of whether TPO accounts for a part or all the antigenic activity recognized by circulating anti-MAg autoantibody (anti-MAb) is still unsolved. Using an indirect immunofluorescence technique MAg can be identified in the cytoplasm and on the surface of human thyroid cells (3). More recently we have shown that in the differentiated rat thyroid cell strain FRTL-5 the expression of MAg is modulated by TSH added in the culture medium (4). In this study a four-layer IFL technique was applied to human thyroid cells in primary culture in order to obtain a simultaneous staining of the antigen(s) recognized by autoimmune sera containing anti-MAb and by a monoclonal anti-TPO antibody (1). Experiments were performed with cells cultured in the presence or in the absence of TSH.

MATERIALS AND METHODS

Human thyroid cells were obtained by collagenase digestion from surgical specimens of nontoxic goiters and cultured on glass coverslips in Coon's medium supplemented with 5% calf serum and a 6-hormone mixture (insulin, 10 µg/ml; hydrocortisone, 10 pM; transferrin, 5 µg/ml; 1-glycyl-histidyl-lysine, 10 ng/ml; somatostatin, 10 ng/ml and TSH 300 µU/ml).In some experiments cells were deprived of TSH for 7-8 days.

Sera containing anti-MAb, but negative for anti-thyroglobulin antibodies as assessed by passive hemagglutination were obtained from Hashimoto's patients.

In the four-layer IFL procedure, human thyroid cells were incubated in the sequence with: 1) an anti-TPO monoclonal Ab (100 ng/ml); 2) a rhodaminated goat anti-mouse Ig conjugate (Kappel, 1/30); 3) an anti-MAb positive serum (1/16); 4) a fluoresceinated sheep anti-human Ig conjugate (Wellcome, 1/30). Viable cells were used for surface staining, while acetone fixed cells were employed to expose cytoplasmic antigens. After extensive washing coverslips were mounted in glycerol and examined by UV microscope.

Single exposure and double exposure color microphotographs were obtained.

RESULTS

Both human anti-MAb and the anti-TPO monoclonal antibody produced a typical dotted surface staining when applied on viable cells cultured in medium containing TSH. The same cells were stained by the two antibodies and in no case a dissociation of the green and the red layer was observed. When thyroid cells were fixed before the IFL procedure, human anti-MAb sera and the monoclonal anti-TPO antibody gave a positive fluorescence of the cytoplasm. As in the case of the surface fluorescence both antibodies stained the same type of cell. Double exposure microphotographs revealed a complete overlap of the green and the red fluorescence, resulting in a yellow staining of the surface and of the cytoplasm of human thyroid cells (Fig.1). Cross reactivity between the four layers was excluded by appropriate control experiments.

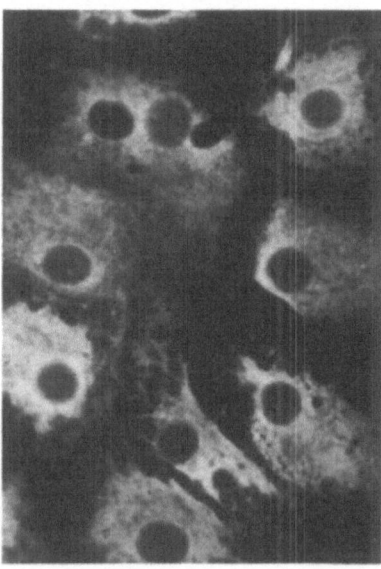 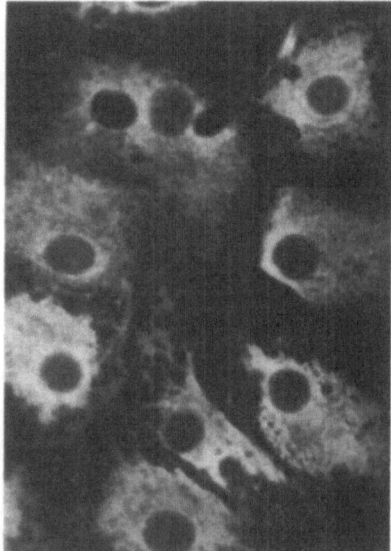

Fig.1

Double indirect IFL staining of human thyroid cells cultured in the presence of TSH. Cells were fixed with acetone before the IFL procedure performed as detailed under Materials and Methods. Left:
cytoplasmic staining produced by the anti-TPO monoclonal antibody; right:cytoplasmic fluorescence produced by a human anti-MAb serum. The same cells are stained with an identical pattern by both antibodies.(original magnification x 100).

TSH withdrawal from the culture medium was followed by a progressive disappearance of the antigen recognized on the cell surface and in the cytoplasm by human anti-MAb and by the monoclonal anti-TPO antibody. Even in these experiments it was impossible to separate the green and the red fluorescence.

DISCUSSION

Using an indirect IFL procedure thyroid peroxidase could be identified in the cytoplasm and on the surface of human thyroid cells cultured in the presence of TSH. The distribution and the pattern of fluorescence obtained with the monoclonal anti-TPO antibody was undistinguishable from that found with human sera containing anti-MAb. The same cells were stained by the two antibodies and the red and green fluorescence obtained in the four-layer IFL technique were completely overlapped. TSH withdrawal from the culture medium was followed after 7-8 days by a complete disappearance of the antigen recognized in the cytoplasm and on the surface of human thyroid cells by human anti-MAb and by the monoclonal anti-TPO antibody. Therefore, our results provide further evidence for the identity of the so called microsomal antigen and thyroid peroxidase.

REFERENCES

1. B.Czarnocka, M. Ferrand, P. Carayon, and S. Lissitzky, Purification of the human thyroid peroxidase and its identification as the microsomal antigen involved in autoimmune thyroid diseases.FEBS Lett. 190:147 (1985).
2. S.Mariotti, R. Bechi, S. Anelli, J. Ruf, A. Lombardi, L. Chiovato, B. Czarnocka, P. Carayon, and A. Pinchera, Evidence for identity of serum thyroid microsomal and anti-human thyroid peroxidase autoantibodies, in: "The Thyroid and Autoimmunity", H.A. Drexhage, W.M. Wiersinga, eds., Elsevier Science Publisher, Amsterdam (1986).
3. E.L. Khoury, L. Hammond, G. F. Bottazzo, and D. Doniach, Presence of organ-specific microsomal autoantigen on the surface of human thyroid cells in culture: its involvement in complement-mediated cytotoxicity, Clin. Exp. Immunol. 43:316 (1981).
4. L.Chiovato, P. Vitti, A. Lombardi, L. D. Kohn, and A. Pinchera, Expression of the microsomal antigen on the surface of continuously cultured rat thyroid cells is modulated by thyrotropin, J. Clin. Endocrinol. Metab. 61:12 (1985).

MEASUREMENT OF ANTI-α-GALACTOSYL ANTIBODIES IN THE COURSE OF VARIOUS THYROID DISORDERS AND ISOLATION OF AN ANTIGENIC GLYCOPEPTIDE FRACTION

J. Etienne-Decerf, P. Mahieu, M. Malaise and R. Winand

Université de Liège, Institut de Pathologie, C.H.U., B. 23

4000 Sart-Tilman par Liège 1, Belgium

INTRODUCTION

Galili et al.[1] recently described the presence of a natural anti-α-galactosyl IgG antibody (a-Gal-Ab) in the serum of all normal subjects. This antibody specifically recognizes terminal Gal α(1⟶3) structures[2]. In auto-immune thyroid disorders, an overall B cell activation occurs, as reflected by the appearance of various IgG autoantibodies. We have therefore tested the possibility that a-Gal-Ab titers could be enhanced in those diseases. Using an indirect immunofluorescence technique, we previously showed the binding of purified a-Gal-Ab to the surface of trypsinized thyroid cells[3]. In the present work, we purify a thyroid glycopeptidic fraction which recognizes the a-Gal-Ab.

MATERIAL AND METHODS

The titers of a-Gal-Ab were measured by passive hemagglutination of rabbit red blood cells (RBC) according to a technique previously described[4]. Thyroid glycopeptides were prepared from a Graves'disease thyroid gland after disruption of the tissue in 0.25 M sucrose, 20 mM Tris acetate pH 7.4. Glycopeptide fractions were obtained by digestion of the homogenate with pronase at 37°C during 72 h in 0.15 M Tris acetate pH 7.8, 0.1 % sodium azide[5]. Glycopeptides were isolated by gel filtration on Sephadex G 200. The excluded material was divided in 2 fractions : the first (I) was stored at -70°C whereas the second one (II) was submitted to affinity chromatography on a column of a-Gal-Ab linked by a CNBr bridge to Sephadex G 200. Anti-Gal-Ab were purified by affinity chromatography on milibiose-agarose column[4]. The presence of Gal α(1⟶3) structures in the fractions was tested by the inhibition of hemagglutination.

RESULTS AND DISCUSSION

The titers of a-Gal-Ab in 50 control sera ranged from 1/10 to 1/80. Elevated titers are observed in 6/6 patients with progressive exophthalmos, in 5/5 patients with untreated Graves'disease, in 11/12 patients with progressive non toxic goitre and in 3/7 patients with autoimmune thyroiditis (Fig. 1).

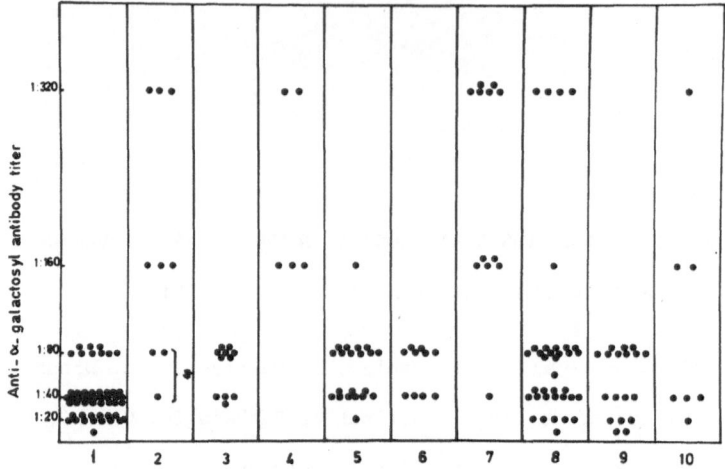

Fig. 1. Titers of anti-α-galactosyl antibody in control subjects and in different thyroid disorders. Elevated titers are 1:80. 1. Control subjects; 2. Progressive exophthalmos (*Prednisolone 30 mg/day); 3. Residual exophthalmos; 4. Untreated Graves'disease; 5. Treated Graves'disease; 6. Cured Graves'disease; 7. Progressive non toxic goitre; 8. Non progressive non toxic goitre; 9. Primary myxoedema; 10. Autoimmune thyroiditis.

Table 1. Inhibition of anti-galactosyl[a]-mediated rabbit RBC agglutination by glycopeptides[b] isolated from human thyroid gland.

Glycopeptides	Concentration (µg/ml)	Anti-gal dilution			
		1:20	1:40	1:80	1:160
I	20	+	+	+	–
IIa	20	+	–	–	–
IIb	20	+	+	+	–
	40	+	+	+/–	–
No	–	+	+	+	–

[a]25 µg of anti-α-galactosyl antibody.
[b]Glycopeptides are obtained by pronase digestion of human thyroid tissue.

By contrast, the titers are within the normal range in primary myxoedema (17 cases) and in residual exophthalmos (11 cases) whereas they are only increased in 1/31 patients with treated or cured Graves'disease and in 5/36 patients with non progressive non toxic goitre. The a-Gal-Ab mainly belong to the IgG class. The hemagglutination of rabbit RBC was decreased by D-galactose (100 mM) and completely inhibited by 2 µg of pentahexosyl ceramide with terminal Gal $\alpha(1 \longrightarrow 3)$ structures. On the contrary, 20 µg of trihexosyl ceramide with terminal Gal $\alpha(1 \longrightarrow 4)$ residues had no effect on the hemagglutinating titers. These data confirm the results of Galili et al.[2]. Since thyroid tissue does not possess pentahexosyl ceramide, we have tested the possibility that Gal $\alpha(1 \longrightarrow 3)$ stuctures are present in glyco-

peptides purified from a thyroid gland obtained after surgery in a Graves'
disease patient. The crude glycopeptide preparation (I) did not inhibit
the hemagglutination of rabbit RBC (Table 1). After affinity chromatography
on a-Gal-Ab column, unadsorbed glycopeptidic fraction (IIb) (70 % of starting material) did not decrease the hemagglutinating titers (Table 1).
On the contrary, the adsorbed fraction (IIa), eluted in acidic buffer and
immediately neutralized with Tris-base, strongly inhibited the hemagglutination at a concentration of 20 µg/ml (Table 1).

It is therefore likely that this fraction contains (a) glycopeptide(s) with
terminal Gal $\alpha(1\longrightarrow 3)$ residues. Kress et al.[5] did not observe glycopeptides
with such terminal structures in normal human thyroid tissue. Since our
starting material is a thyroid from Graves'disease, an attractive hypothesis
should be that normally hidden Gal $\alpha(1\longrightarrow 3)$ structures are "unmasked" in
pathological conditions at the surface of thyroid cells, as has been already
shown after a prior, very mild trypsin treatment of normal human thyroid
cells[3]. It is also tempting to speculate that such exposure might be responsible, at least in part, for the increase in a-Gal-Ab titers observed
in patients with various autoimmune thyroid disorders.

REFERENCES

1. U. Galili, E.A. Rachmilewitz, A. Peleg, I. Flechner, A unique natural
    human IgG antibody with anti-α-galactosyl specificity, J. Exp. Med.
    160:1519 (1984).
2. U. Galili, B.A. Macher, S.B. Shohet, Human natural anti-α-galactosyl
    IgG. The specific recognition of $\alpha(1\longrightarrow 3)$-linked galactose resi-
    dues, J. Exp. Med. 162:573 (1985).
3. J. Etienne-Decerf, M. Malaise, P. Mahieu, R. Winand, Elevated anti-α-
    galactosyl antibody titers : a marker of progression in autoimmune
    thyroid disorders and in endocrine ophthalmopathy ? Acta Endocr.
    In Press.
4. M.G. Malaise, J.C. Davin, P. Mahieu, P. Franchimont, Elevated anti-
    galactosyl antibody titers reflect a renal injury after gold or
    D. Penicillamine in rhumatoid arthritis. Clin. Immunol. Immunopathol.
    40:356 (1986).
5. B.C. Kress, R.G. Spiro, Studies on the glycoprotein nature of the thy-
    rotropin receptor : interaction with lectins and purification of
    the bovine protein with the use of Bandeiraea (Griffonia) Simplici-
    folia I affinity chromatography, Endocrinology 118:974 (1986).

THE IgG SUBCLASS DISTRIBUTION OF THYROID AUTOANTIBODIES IN GRAVES' DISEASE

Anthony P. Weetman and Shara Cohen

Department of Medicine
Royal Postgraduate Medical School
London W12 OHS, UK

INTRODUCTION

There have been conflicting reports on the IgG subclass distribution of thyroglobulin (Tg) and microsomal (Mic) autoantibodies in Hashimoto's thyroiditis. Early studies showing no restriction of subclass used polyclonal anti-subclass antibodies (1,2). Recently assays with monoclonal reagents have shown relative (3) or complete (4) subclass restriction of the response to IgG_1 and IgG_4. The position for Graves' disease is not clear. We have therefore examined the IgG subclass distribution of Tg and Mic antibodies using monoclonal reagents evaluated for their binding to immobilised IgG.

PATIENTS AND METHODS

Thirty one Graves' patients were studied before and after 6 months treatment with carbimazole 40mg daily, supplemented with T3 20ug qds. Fifteen patients were in remission one year after stopping treatment.

Monoclonal antibodies against IgG subclasses detailed elsewhere (5) and obtained from Unipath or Dr. C.B. Reimer, were evaluated in an ELISA for binding to WHO 67/97, a serum of known subclass composition (Fig. 1). These results, clearly show that, of the monoclonals used in other studies (3,4), HP 6009 and HP 6010 are likely to under-represent, and HP 6011 over-represent, the amount of IgG_2-IgG_4 subclasses when directly compared with HP 6012 (against IgG_1) in an ELISA.

To assess IgG_1-IgG_4 subclasses in Tg and Mic antibodies for the present study, we used HP 6069, HP 6002, HP 6047 and HP 6025 as second antibodies in an ELISA similar to that used previously (3,4). Results were expressed as a percentage absorbance for each subclass of the sum of absorbances for IgG_1-IgG_4.

RESULTS

There was a relative preponderance of the IgG_4 subclass in both antibodies (Table 1); however seven patients had no IgG_4 Tg antibody and nine had no IgG_4 Mic antibody. There were significant differences between Tg and Mic antibodies in distribution of the other subclasses, shown in Table 1.

Table 1. Percentage Distribution of IgG Subclasses in Tg and Mic antibodies before treatment.

	IgG_1	IgG_2	IgG_3	IgG_4
Tg Ab	35	30	17	15
Mic Ab	26*	57**	2**	16

* P< 0.05, ** P < 0.001 compared to Tg Ab.

Sixteen patients (52%) were HLA–DR3 positive, seven of whom relapsed. For Mic antibodies, the amount of IgG_4 subclass was significantly greater in the DR3–negative than the DR3–positive group (20 vs 11%, P < 0.01).

Furthermore there were significant changes after treatment in the subclass distribution. The most striking of these (Table 2) was a rise in IgG_2 and fall in IgG_4 percentage of Mic antibodies as patients entered remission: this was not seen in the relapse group.

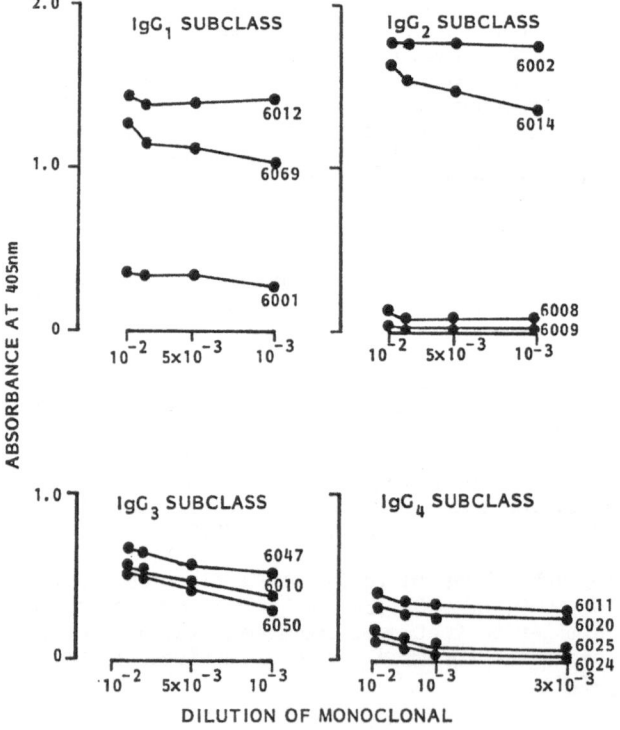

Fig. 1. Dilution curves of monoclonal antibody binding to WHO67/97 coated at 10^{-4} dilution onto an ELISA plate. WHO67/97 contains 5 g/l IgG_1, 2.6g/l IgG_2, 0.4g/l IgG_3 and 0.5 g/l IgG_4. The numbers given to each monoclonal refer to the code agreed by the WHO/IUIS joint committee(5).

Table 2. Percentage Distribution of Subclasses in Mic
Antibodies with Remission (n = 15)

	IgG_1	IgG_2	IgG_3	IgG_4
Untreated	22	59	2	17
6 mo. on CBZ	16	66*	4	16
12 mo. off CBZ	18	71**	2	9**

*P <0.05, ** P<0.01 compared to untreated values.
CBZ = carbimazole

DISCUSSION

These results show an excess of IgG_4 in Tg and Mic antibodies in
Graves' disease. Unlike studies on Hashimoto's thyroiditis (3,4) we
found considerable activity in the IgG_2 and IgG_3, as well as IgG_1,
subclasses. This is due to the selection of monoclonals which bind more
strongly to IgG_2 and IgG_3 in the present study (Fig 1). We would stress
that the percentage values given in this and previous studies (3,4)
cannot be taken as exactly reflecting true serum concentration, in view
of the differences between monoclonals in avidity. The reasons for
these disturbances in subclass distribution are currently unknown
although IgG_4 subclass antibodies are associated with a chronic immune
response. Antithyroid drug therapy produced an alteration in the
subclass distribution of the thyroid autoantibodies, compatible with the
known immunological effects of this treatment, but there was no shift in
the proportion of the non-complement fixing IgG_4 subclass making up Mic
antibodies. However, IgG_2 only fixes complement weakly and fails to
bind to monocyte Fc receptors so that the changes seen in the Mic IgG_2
subclass may have some immunological consequences.

REFERENCES

1.   E. A. Lichter Thyroglobulin antibody activity in the γ- globulins
     γ- A, γ-B and γ-C of human serum. Proc. Soc. Exp. Biol. Med.
     116:553 (1964).
2.   F. C. Hay and G. Torrigiani, The distribution of
     anti-thyroglobulin antibodies in the immunoglobulin G subclasses.
     Clin. Exp. Immunol. 16:517 (1974).
3.   A. B. Parkes, S. M. McLachlan, P. Bird and B. Rees Smith, The
     distribution of microsomal and thyroglobulin antibody activity
     among the IgG subclasses. Clin. Exp. Immunol. 57:239 (1984).
4.   T. F. Davies, C. M. Weber, P. Wallack and M. Platzer, Restricted
     heterogeneity and T cell dependence of human thyroid autoantibody
     immunoglobulin G subclasses. J. Clin. Endocrinol. Metab. 60:945
     (1986).
5.   R. Jefferis, C. B. Reimer, F. Skvaril et al., Evaluation of
     monoclonal antibodies having specificity for human IgG subclasses:
     results of an IUIS/WHO collaborative study. Immunol. Letters
     10:223 (1985).

THYROID HORMONE BINDING AUTOANTIBODIES (THBA) IN HUMANS AND
ANIMALS

Salvatore Benvenga* and Jacob Robbins

Clinical Endocrinology Branch, NIADDK

National Institutes of Health, Bethesda, Md 20892

INTRODUCTION

This paper refers to the 197 cases of THBA reported up to
now in the North American, European and Japanese literature, and
to the relevant data on THBA in animals.

CHARACTERISTICS OF THBA IN HUMANS

Prevalence

THBA are absent in newborns. In the general adult population
THBA are found in fewer than one per thousand persons, whereas in
thyroid diseases the prevalence averages 14 %. THBA are most frequently detected in patients with autoimmune thyroid diseases, in
females (71/93) and are frequently associated with significant
titers of thyroglobulin antibodies (Tg-Ab) (78/117).

Specificity

THBA may be directed against: 1. T3; 2. T4; 3. T3+T4; 4. T4+
rT3; 5. T3+T4+rT3 -the former being the most commonly reported.

Class, subclass, typing and binding constants

THBA are immunoglobulins of the IgG class, though there are
cases in which IgG were accompanied by IgM (n=2), IgA (n=1) or IgM +
IgA (n=1). There is a unique instance of THBA of the IgE class.
IgG subclasses were studied in 3 cases, with these results: G1=3/3,
G2=1/3, G3=3/3, G4=0/3. Light chain specificity is known for 9 cases:
λ =4, k=2, λ + k=3. As to the binding constants, Ka ranges 1.8 x
10^8 M^{-1} to 8.7 x 10^{10} M^{-1}(Ab to T4) and 1.7 x 10^8 M^{-1} to 8.4 x 10^{10}
M^{-1}(Ab to T3), and the respective Bmax from 0.12 to 140·µg T4/dl
and from 0.007 to 13 µg T3/dl.

---

* Permanent address: Istituto Pluridisciplinare di Clinica e Terapia
  Medica, University of Messina, School of Medicine, Policlinico
  Universitario, 98100 Messina, Italy.

Interference in the RIAs for thyroid hormones (TH)

Given that: 1. nonspecific methods to separate bound from free radioactivity do not distinguish the endogenous (human) from the exogenous (animal) TH-Ab; 2. specific methods, instead, produce precipitation of the radioactivity bound to the exogenous TH-Ab; 3. in the solid phase RIA, radioactivity is sequestred by the endogenous Ab coated covalently to the tube wall, the plasma level of TH is underestimated in case #1, and overestimated in cases #2 and #3. Whichever the method used, no interference occurs if TH is/are measured in the ethanol extract of the serum. Valid methods to measure free TH are those in which the free TH are physically separated from the serum proteins before the assay procedure. It is obvious that the extent of interference in any method depends on the intrinsic features of THBA (concentration, Ka, Bmax).
THBA having not very high binding potential for T4 do not affect the immunoradiometric assay for thyroxine-binding globulin (TBG) Preliminary data by Benvenga & Trimarchi (unpublished) indicate that THBA provoke underestimation of serum Tg, when assessed with an immunoradiometric assay, and that THBA exist which are capable of binding Tg but are unable to agglutinate tanned red cells coated with human Tg.

Detection of THBA

Methods include electrophoresis, gel-filtration, affinity chromatography, immunoprecipitation (RIA)

Effects on thyroid status and treatment

Unless a concomitant disease implying thyroid failure is operating, thyroid may respond to the neutralization of the circulating TH by THBA through the temporary TSH-stimulated secretion of TH. THBA *per se* do not call for any particular therapy.No explanation has been offered for the difference between THBA, which tend to persist during and after therapies for the associated thyroid diseases, and the other Ab (TGHA, MCHA, TSI) which, instead, decrease in response to the therapy.

THBA IN ANIMALS

Spontaneously occurring THBA have been demonstrated in the obese strain (OS) and the Cornell strain (CS) of the White Leghorn chickens, and recently in dogs Other subprimates such as guinea pigs, rabbits, mice and rats, and primates such as baboons and monkeys have been used experimentally to raise THBA. Taken together, data in animals indicate that is Tg the antigen that stimulates the immune system to produce THBA. Tg needs to be associated with Freund's adjuvant to exert this stimulus; the requirement in humans in not known THBA in animals are transient.

PATHOGENESIS [MECHANISM(S) OF THBA SYNTHESIS]

Several findings point to the thyroid as the source of the antigen responsible for the production of THBA :
1. THBA occur more frequently in subjects with (autoimmune) thyroid diseases than in subjects with nonthyroid diseases or healthy ;
2. in certain animals (OS and CS, *vide supra)* THBA are associated with an underlying autoimmune thyroiditis; 3. THBA tend to decrease after subtotal thyroidectomy; 4. THBA have been reported in persons and dogs previously treated with desiccated thyroid , indicating that partially absorbed thyroid fragments may be immunogenic.

Other data suggest that the responsible antigen should be Tg:
1. Tg can serve as an iso- or hetero-antigen for eliciting THBA in various animals, and injected in Freund's adjuvant is the most potent antigen; 2. Tg naturally contains TH and it is the most important iodinated (macro)molecule of the thyroid; 3. iodinated Tg is not present in the blood stream, and thus it may be a foreign substance for the immune competent cells; 4. THBA are associated frequently with TGHA, and in primates as well as in subprimates titers of TGHA usually correlate with levels of THBA; 5. THBA cross-react with Tg and actually THBA may be Tg-Ab capable of binding TH. Other theories about the pathogenesis of THBA have been put forward: (i) the physiological TH binding proteins may serve as immunogens; (ii) a non-immune interaction of TH with circulating immunoglobulins could result in the synthesis of other IgG that bind TH; (iii) THBA may represent an inherited disorder or a benign gammopathy. A disorder of the immune system do not seem to be a pre-requisite for the production of THBA, since: 1. only 3 cases of THBA have been detected in patients with such disturbances. Moreover, the frequence of THBA in a series of patients with various diseases of the lymphoretycular system was 0/32 ; 2. THBA have been found in entirely normal individuals; 3. THBA remained persistently undetectable during the 3 year follow-up of a patient with diffuse lymphocytic lymphoma (in remission) and subsequent development of Hashimoto's thyroiditis .
In conclusion, THBA represent an additional carrier for TH in plasma. In all probability, THBA are Tg-Ab directed against regions of the Tg molecule containing thyroxyl residues. At least 2 such residues are sufficiently exposed to interact with THBA and sufficiently apart to allow the binding of 2 IgG molecules simultaneously.

REFERENCES

Benvenga, S., 1983 , Quantitative and qualitative genetically determined variations in thyroid hormone transport, Min. Endocrinol., 8: 117.

Benvenga, S., Trimarchi, F., Barbera, C., Costante, G., Morabito, S., Barberio, C., and Consolo, F., 1984, Circulating immunoglobulin E (IgE) antibodies to L-thyroxine in a euthyroid patient with multinodular goiter and allergic rhinitis, J. Endocrinol. Invest., 7: 47 .

Benvenga, S., Sobbrio, G., Vermiglio, F., Costante, G., Trimarchi, F., 1985, T4 antibodies and thyroxine-binding globulin (TBG) immunoradiometric assay, in: "Auto-immunity and the thyroid," Walfish, P.G., Wall, J.R., and Volpe, R., eds., Academic Press, Orlando.

Benvenga, S., Barresi, G., Mazzeo, R.S., Turiano, S., Micali, B., Arrigo, F., and Trimarchi, F., 1983, Tiroidite di Hashimoto manifestatasi clinicamente dopo stabile remissione di linfoma linfocitico diffuso, Min. Endocrinol., 8:45 .

Trimarchi, F., Benvenga, S., Costante, G., Barbera, C., Melluso, R., Marcocci, C., Chiovato, L., De Luca, F., and Consolo, F.,1983, Identification and characterization of circulating thyroid hormone autoantibodies in thyroid diseases, in autoimmune nonthyroid illnesses and in lymphoretycular system disorders, J. Endocrinol. Invest., 6: 203.

Byfield, P.G.H., Clinghan, D., and Himsworth R.L., 1984,Exposure of thyroxine residues in human thyroglobulin. Two binding sites, Biochem. J.,219: 405.

HIGH FREQUENCY OF INTERFERON-γ PRODUCING T CELLS IN THYROID INFILTRATES OF PATIENTS WITH HASHIMOTO'S THYROIDITIS

A. Tiri, G.F. Del Prete, S. Mariotti, A. Pinchera,
S. Romagnani and M. Ricci

Allergology Clinical Immunology, University of Florence
and ( ) Endocrinology, University of Pisa
Policlinico Careggi, 50134 Florence, Italy

In the last few years, some phenotypic and functional aspects of thyroid infiltrating T lymphocytes in Hashimoto's thyroiditis (HT) have been defined[1-5]. Most thyroid T cells have the CD8+ cytotoxic/suppressor phenotype and a proportion of them express receptors for IL-2, suggesting their in vivo activation[4]. In addition, most of T-cell clones established from HT infiltrates appeared to be progenies of CD8+ T cells with natural killer (NK) activity. Here we report an analysis at clonal level of T lymphocytes infiltrating HT glands in which their ability to produce interleukin-2 (IL-2) and interferon-gamma (IFN-γ) was evaluated.

Patients. Thyroid specimens and peripheral blood (PB) were obtained from four women with HT (mean age 43, range 32–48) who had subtotal thyroidectomy because of obstructive symptoms. Two patients with HT were euthyroid and two slightly hypothyroid at the time of surgery. Four healthy women and two subjects who underwent splenectomy after trauma also provided cells for clonal analysis.

T cell cloning system. Thyroid, PB or spleen cell suspensions were seeded in limiting number (0.3 cells/well) in round-bottomed microwells containing 10^5 irradiated spleen feeder cells and 1% phytohemagglutinin (PHA), as detailed elsewhere[2]. After 48 hr and then weekly, microcultures were supplemented with 10^5 irradiated feeder cells in 0.1 ml recombinant IL-2 (rIL-2, Biogen, Geneva) until a suitable number of cells for phenotypic and functional studies was available.

Assay for natural killer (NK) activity. T blasts from each clone were washed, resuspended, counted and tested against the human K562 cell line (E/T ratio 4:1)[2,4]. ^{51}Cr release exceeding the mean spontaneous release by more than 5 SD was considered positive for NK activity.

Induction of IFN-γ and IL-2 production by T-cell clones. To evaluate the ability of single T-cell clones to produce IFN-γ and/or IL-2, T blasts were washed 4 times, counted and resuspended at 10^5/0.2 ml medium containing 1% PHA. Cultures were incubated for 40 h at 37 C and supernatants (SN) removed and tested for IFN-γ or IL-2 content.

Quantitation of IFN-γ . For the quantitative measurement of IFN-γ in culture SN, the IMRX Interferon-gamma RIA (Centocor Inc., Malvern, PA) was used. Culture SN showing IFN-γ levels 5 SD over those of control SN derived from irradiated feeder cells alone were regarded as positive.

Measurement of IL-2. To evaluate the ability of T-cell clones to produce IL-2, 0.2 ml SN were added at different concentrations to 4×10^3 mouse CTLL cells. SN able to induce ^{3}H-TdR uptake in CTLL cells 3 SD over that of control SN derived from irradiated feeder cells alone were considered as positive. An estimate of IL-2 produced by single T-cell clones was performed with known concentrations of rIL-2.

Results

A total number of 623 clones was examined for their ability to produce IFN-γ and IL-2 following PHA stimulation. The clonal analysis included 69 CD4[+] and 104 CD8[+] clones from thyroid infiltrates, 170 CD4[+] and 61 CD8[+] clones from patient PB, 108 CD4[+] and 40 CD8[+] clones from normal PB and 53 CD4[+] and 18 CD8[+] clones from normal spleen. As shown in Table 1, the proportion of IFN-producing (IFN-P) clones derived from HT infiltrates was significantly higher ($p < 0.0005$) than that of IFN-P clones established from normal spleen or PB of both patients and controls. In contrast, no significant difference was found in the proportion of IFN-P clones between patient and normal PB. Both CD4[+] and CD8[+] thyroid-derived IFN-P clones usually released higher amounts of IFN-γ than did control clones with the same phenotype. In contrast, among clones established from the PB of HT patients only CD4[+], but not CD8[+], clones showed a mean IFN-γ production significantly greater ($p < 0.002$) than that of control clones. It is of note that, in the absence of previous activation with PHA, none of the clones tested showed detectable secretion of IFN-γ. We then asked whether modulation of the CD3 complex could actually trigger thyroid-derived clones to an IFN-γ production as high as that obtained with PHA. As shown in Table 2,

Table 1. PHA-induced production of IFN-γ and IL-2 by T cell clones from thyroid infiltrates and PB from patients with HT

Source of T cells	Phenotype	IFN-γ production		IL-2 production	
		%	U/ml	%	U/ml
HT Infiltrate	CD4	88	125 + 18	64	2.4 + 0.4
	CD8	84	117 + 15	53	2.1 + 0.5
HT PB	CD4	61	78 + 6	64	3.2 + 0.3
	CD8	67	50 + 4	59	2.7 + 0.4
Normal Lymphoid tissue	CD4	60	45 + 4	53	2.3 + 0.3
	CD8	50	34 + 4	56	2.6 + 0.5
Normal PB	CD4	53	35 + 2	68	2.7 + 0.5
	CD8	65	33 + 2	52	2.2 + 0.4

Table 2. IFN-γ production by T cell clones following activation with PHA
or anti-CD3 (OKT3) monoclonal antibody

Clone (phenotype)	IFN-γ production (U/ml)		
	Medium	PHA	OKT3
HTIn 2.2 (CD8)	< 10	224	79
HTIn 2.14 (CD8)	< 10	126	64
HTIn 2.31 (CD4)	< 10	150	93
HTPB 2.17 (CD4)	< 10	356	84
HTPB 2.3 (CD4)	< 10	96	54
HTPB 2.28 (CD8)	< 10	< 10	< 10
NCPB 4.29 (CD4)	< 10	46	28
NCPB 4.11 (CD4)	< 10	26	19
NCPB 4.7 (CD4)	< 10	< 10	< 10

IFN-γ production by 9 representative clones obtained from HT thyroid
infiltrate (HTIn) and PB (HTPB) or from normal PB (NCPB).

maximum IFN-γ production was observed when clones were stimulated with
PHA, but OKT3 MoAb, at doses optimal for for clonal proliferation, was
also effective in triggering thyroid-derived clones to high IFN-γ
secretion. All clones were also assayed for their ability to produce
IL-2 following PHA stimulation. As shown in Table 1, there was no
significant difference between infiltrates or PB of HT patients and
normal spleen or PB.

In previous studies we showed that a considerable proportion of
clones derived from HT thyroid T lymphocytes were the progeny of
activated CD8 cytolytic T cells with NK activity[2,4]. Thus, the
possible relationship between high IFN-γ production and NK activity of
T-cell clones from HT patients was investigated. Among clones
established from thyroid infiltrates, the proportion of IFN-P clones
showing NK activity (NK+) was much higher (> 70%) than that found in
clones from normal spleens (29%) or PB (36%) (p < 0.0005).
The percentage of IFN-P NK clones established from patient PB was also
significantly increased, even though to a lower extent (52 % - p < 0.02).
However, unlike thyroid-derived IFN-P NK clones, the majority of which
(82/117) were CD8+, most patient PB-derived NK+ clones showing IFN-γ
production (42/76) were CD4+. Almost all NK+ thyroid-derived clones
(117/131) could be triggered to high IFN-γ secretion (Table 3). Among
clones derived from patient PB, the majority of those with NK activity
(76/107) were IFN-P and their mean IFN-γ production was significantly
higher (p <0.0005) than that of NK⁻ clones from either patient or normal
PB. In contrast, only a few clones from normal PB or spleen showed the
capacity to produce high levels of IFN-γ, irrespective of their
potential to kill NK-sensitive targets, and there was no difference in
the mean IFN-γ production between control NK+ or NK⁻ clones.

Abnormal IFN-γ secretion by thyroid infiltrating T cells might play
a role in the expression and/or maintenance of HT. IFN-γ production

Table 3. Association between NK activity and high production of IFN-γ
in T cell clones from HT thyroid infiltrates and PB.

Source of T cells	IFN-γ production (U/ml)			
	CD4$^+$NK$^+$	CD4$^+$NK$^-$	CD8$^+$NK$^+$	CD8$^+$NK$^-$
HT Infiltrate	173 ± 29	60 ± 10	125 ± 16	41 ± 9
HT PB	104 ± 11	47 ± 4	59 ± 14	24 ± 2
Normal Lymphoid tissue	58 ± 18	44 ± 4	34 ± 4	31 ± 7
Normal PB	34 ± 4	36 ± 2	34 ± 3	30 ± 3

(For underlined values p < 0.0005)

during T cell responses has been considered necessary for the maturation of antigen-specific T cells and concomitant with the generation of cytotoxic T lymphocytes[6-8]. Since IFN-γ is a promoter of NK function[9], the increased NK activity shown by clones derived from HT infiltrates could be due to their concomitant ability to secrete high concentrations of IFN-γ. In addition, since IFN-γ may exert a B cell growth factor activity and act synergistically with IL-2 and other helper factors in B-cell differentiation[10-12], the presence of activated B lymphocytes that easily differentiate into spontaneously autoantibody-producing cells[13] might be related to the high intrathyroidal potential of IFN-γ secretion. Whether IFN-γ production in thyroid infiltrates is related to MHC class II antigen expression on thyrocytes[5,14,15] which activate high IFN-P autoreactive T cells, or it is an inherent feature of a proportion of T cells from subjects undergoing autoimmunity remains to be established.

References

1. M.C. Bene et al., - Clin exp Immunol 52:311 (1983).
2. G.F. Del Prete et al., - J Clin Endocrinol Metab 62:52 (1986).
3. M. Bagnasco et al., - Int Archs Allergy appl Immunol (in press).
4. G.F. Del Prete et al., - Clin exp Immunol 64:140 (1986).
5. Y. Iwatani et al., - J Clin Endocrinol Metab 63:695 (1986).
6. W.L. Farrar et al., - J Immunol 126:1120 (1981).
7. J.Y. Djeu et al., - J Exp Med 156:1222 (1982).
8. J.R. Klein and M.J. Bevan - J Immunol 130:1780 (1983);
9. G. Trinchieri and B. Perussia - Immunol Today 6:131 (1985).
10. S. Romagnani et al., - J Immunol 136:3513 (1986).
11. H.J. Leibson et al., - Nature 309:799 (1984).
12. M. Brunswick and P. Lake - J Exp Med 161:953 (1985).
13. S.M. McLachlan et al., - Clin exp Immunol 52:45 (1983).
14. G.F. Bottazzo et al., - Lancet 2:1115 (1983).
15. T.F. Davies - J Clin Endocrinol Metab 61:418 (1985).

LYMPHOKINE PRODUCTION AND FUNCTIONAL ACTIVITIES OF T CELL CLONES

FROM THYROID GLAND OF HASHIMOTO'S THYROIDITIS

M. Bagnasco, S. Ferrini, D. Venuti, I. Prigione, G. Giordano,
and G.W. Canonica

I.S.T.-Endocrinologia & Semeiotica Medica III (I.S.M.I.)Genoa University
V.le Benedetto XV n.6 - 16132 Genoa Italy

Many investigationshave been directed to elucidate the possible patogene-
thical role of T cells in autoimmune thyroid   diseases, namely Hashimoto's thyroiditis (HT) and Graves' diseases (GD). Phenotypic and functional analysis of T cells at the clonal level, using high-efficiency cloning
techniques (1), proved to be the most reliable method for characterizing
T cell functional repertoire at the level of the target organ. We thus
employed such a technique to study T cells derived from thyroid infiltrates (and for comparizon, peripheral blood) of patients with HT or GD. The
results obtained demonstrated major differences between the two disease,
as far as both lymphokine (namely, γ-interferon γIFN) production and
cytolytic capabilities are concerned.

Materials and Methods: T cells were isolated from both thyroid tissue and
peripheral blood of two patients with HT and two patients with GD, as
previously described. (2). The cells thus obtained were cloned, according to the method of Moretta et al. (1). The theoretical cell concentra
tion plated ranged from two to 0,5/microwell. Control wells with feeder
cells alone were also set up. The clonal efficiences were calculated from
limiting dilution analysis (3). The proliferating microcultures containing 1 or less cells/well (operationally regarded as clones) were expanded for phenotypic and functional analysis. Lymphokine production was
evaluated on 24 h supernatants after 1% PHA stimulation: IL-2 was assayed
using the IL-2 dependent CTLL line, γIFN by immunoradiometric assay (Centocor Medical System Italy). Cytolytic activites were evaluated by ^{51}Cr
release assay against P815 cell line in the presence of PHA (lectin-depen
dent cytotoxicity, which allows to evaluate cytolytic T cells of any specificity) and against the NK sensitive K562 line. T3, T4, T8 surface antigen expression was evaluated by indirect immunofluorescence using appropriate monoclonal antibodies.

Results and discussion: T cell clones were raised from thyroid infiltrating and peripheral blood T cells of HT and GD patients. The clonal efficiences ranged from 39 to 100% (peripheral blood) and from 24 to 40%
(infiltrates). The results of phenotypic and functional analysis of the

clones are shown in the table. In both HT patients, a significant increase of T cell clones with cytolytic (LDCC) capability was observed in Ti-derived vs. PB-derived microcultures: in addition a significant increase of Ti-derived clones with NK-like activity was observed in 1 HT patient. Note that, in addition to cytoytic clones expressing the thypical T3$^+$ T4$^-$ T8$^+$ phenotype, a remarkable proportion (6/11 in patient HT 1) of T3$^+$ T4$^+$ T8$^-$ cytolytic clones were observed. By contrast the proportion of cytolytic clones was minimal in thyroid infiltrates of GD significantly lower than in peripheral blood: this finding strongly suggests major differences between HT and GD, as far as the functional repertoire of thyroid infiltrating T cells is concerned. Moreover, differences have been observed in lymphokine production: first of all, the frequency of γIFN producer clones seems to be greater in HT TI with respect to PB, but similar in TI and PB of GD. Further, in HT, a relevant proportion (the large majority in pt. HT 2) of cytolytic T cell clones are also able to produce IL-2 (and γ-IFN), i.e. they may exert both inducer and effector functions: this fenomenon is not apparent in GD: further more, in the latter disease a proportion of TI derived T3$^+$ T4$^+$ T8$^-$ non cytolytic clones are also inable to produce IL-2 or γ-IFN under mitogenic stimulation.

Taken together, all this data strongly support our previous hypothesis based on other experimental evidences concerning major differences in the pathogenetical role of T cells between GD and HT (5). In fact, in HT infiltrates a great number of T cells are able to display cytolytic activity and also to release IL-2 and γ-IFN (known to be an adequate stimulus for MHC class II antigen expression by thyroid epithelial cells) (4): thus, a major role of these cells in both producing thyroid damage and perpetuating the autoimmune process is likely. In GD this is not the case, in that only few T cells with the cytolytic programm are detectable in the thyroid the other being IL-2 producer or having no known lymphokine production. (possible production of B cell growth factor(s) different from IL-2 or γIFN?).

Table I   AUTOIMMUNE THYROID DISEASE

Thyroid T cell clones

	Hashimoto's T.	Graves' D.
T4$^+$	10%	84%
T8$^+$	80%	16%
LDCC	89%	16%
NK	53%	10%
IL-2 prod.	95%	35%
γ-IFN prod.	63%	53%

References

1) Moretta, A. et al. J. Exp. Med., 1983, 157, 743.
2) Bagnasco et al., Int. Arch. Allergy Appl. Immunol. 1986 in press
3) Taswell C., J. Immunol. 1981, 126, 1614.
4) Todd I. et al. clin. Exp. Immunol. 1985, 61, 265
5) Canonica G.W. et al., Clin. Immunol. Immunopathol., 1985, 36, 40.

CIRCULATORY THYROGLOBULIN THRESHOLD IN SUPPRESSOR ACTIVATION

Yi-chi M. Kong, Mark Lewis, Alvaro A. Giraldo* and
Brian E. Fuller

Department of Immunology and Microbiology, Wayne State Univ.
Sch. of Med. and *Div. of Immunopathol., St. John Hosp.
Detroit, Mich. U.S.A.

INTRODUCTION

Murine experimental autoimmune thyroiditis (EAT) has served as a
model for Hashimoto's thyroiditis, and mouse thyroglobulin (MTg) as a
model for self antigen of the thyroid in genetically susceptible
(MHC-associated) individuals[1]. EAT is induced readily when autoreactive
inducer/helper T cells (T_I) are stimulated by MTg given repeatedly[2] or
with an adjuvant, such as lipopolysaccharide (LPS)[3]. However, the pre-
injection of 100-200 µg MTg or thyroid-regulating hormones (TSH or TRH)
activates suppressor mechanisms which interfere with EAT induction[4].
Both regimens elevate the levels of circulating MTg for a short interval.

We hypothesize that circulatory Tg plays an important role in maintaining self tolerance in susceptible individuals by preserving the dominance of suppressor T cell (T_S) over T_I, which otherwise would (could)
respond to the constant stimuli of fluctuating autoantigen concentrations
plus various environmental activators[5]. Moreover, this tolerance can be
strengthened by a modest increase in circulating MTg level for a critical
interval to withstand strong challenge in the form of MTg + potent adjuvant.

We have tested this hypothesis by monitoring the concentration of
MTg and duration of its increase in the blood after raising its level
with exogenous MTg in tolerogenic doses, or with endogenous MTg released
by TSH stimulation[5,6]. The results show that increases above normal
limits and for at least 2-3 days are critical in activating mechanisms
suppressive to EAT induction. Additional data are presented briefly
here.

MATERIALS AND METHODS

Animals. Female CBA/J ($H-2^k$) mice, age 6-10 weeks, were used.

Thyroglobulin. MTg was purified by column chromatography on
Sephadex G-200 and injected i.v.[7] For use in tolerance enhancement, it
was ultracentrifuged to remove aggregates immediately before injection[5].
Ovalbumin (OVA), 100 µg i.p., served as control immunogen.

Adjuvant. LPS prepared from Salmonella enteritidis was injected i.v.
for challenge in combination with MTg, and LPS prepared from Escherichia

coli for modification of MTg clearance rate.

Thyrotropin. Bovine TSH (Sigma Chemicals) was given by mini-osmotic pumps (Alza Corp.) in the peritoneal cavity at a dose of 0.25 IU/day for $3\frac{1}{2}$ or 7 days.

MTg and thyroxine assays. A sandwich ELISA, using two monoclonal antibodies to MTg, one labeled with alkaline phosphatase, was performed in microtiter plates (sensitivity about 25 ng/ml)[5]. T4 was measured by RIA with a single antibody, charcoal separation technique[8].

Assays for EAT. Autoantibody titers were measured by hemagglutination with human group O erythrocytes coupled to MTg or OVA with chromic chloride[7]. Mice were killed 28 days after initial challenge. Serial thyroid sections were examined, lesions graded on a scale of 0 to 4 and compared by nonparametric statistics.

RESULTS AND CONCLUSIONS

We have injected graded doses (20-100 µg) of exogenous MTg 7 days apart (day -10, -3) and then challenged the animals on day 0 with MTg + LPS. Doses that strengthen self tolerance, $\not> 50$ µg, sustained circulatory MTg levels above normal limits for >35 h[5]. To determine if LPS, an agent also known to interfere with clearance by the mononuclear phagocytic system, could alter the MTg levels and resistance to EAT, we injected 20 µg MTg 24 h after 20 µg LPS. Clearance of circulating MTg was extended from a $t\frac{1}{2}$ of 3 h to 5 h. Table 1 shows that both anti-MTg titers and severity of thyroiditis were significantly reduced. Thus, delayed clearance of MTg enabled a subtolerogenic dose to activate suppressor cells[4], which may partly explain the suppression by LPS on antibody response to a foreign antigen when given a day before antigen, as noted by others[9]. In contrast, antibody titers to OVA, given only at challenge, were comparable in all groups.

Table 1. LPS Given 24 Hours before MTg Enhances Tolerogenicity

Treatment[a]		IgG Antibodies to MTg[b]		Thyroid Pathology[b]	
LPS	MTg				
d -11, -4	d -10, -3	Pos./Total	Log$_2$ titer $\pm$ SE	Pos./Total	Index $\pm$ SE
+	−	6/6	12.5 $\pm$ 0.4	6/6	0.9 $\pm$ 0.06
−	−	5/5	15.4 $\pm$ 0.7	5/5	1.0 $\pm$ 0.0
+	+	6/6	6.5 $\pm$ 0.6	4/6	0.5 $\pm$ 0.2[c]
−	+	5/5	10.8 $\pm$ 2.0	5/5	1.4 $\pm$ 0.3

[a]All animals were challenged with MTg, OVA and LPS d 0, 7 (see methods).
[b]Data from d 28 after challenge; anti-OVA titers averaged 10-12 in all groups.
[c]Significantly different from untreated (p = 0.041) and MTg-pretreated p = 0.015) groups.

Another regimen to raise circulating MTg level is by TSH stimulation. TSH was infused via osmotic pump for 7 days. MTg concentrations increased for 2-3 days and resistance to EAT induction was significantly enhanced[5]. The presence of TSH pump after $3\frac{1}{2}$ days in the peritoneal cavity was sufficient to increase the MTg concentration, which peaked in 3 days; LPS given before the rise increased the MTg level even higher without altering the overall kinetics. The results after challenge are presented in Table 2. Both anti-MTg titers and thyroid damage were reduced, but anti-OVA titers were not affected.

Table 2. Resistance to EAT Induction Enhanced by TSH Infusion and LPS Treatment

Treatment[a] d -10	IgG Antibodies to MTg[b]		Thyroid Pathology[b]	
	Positive/Total	Log$_2$ titer ± SE	Positive/Total	Index ± SE
Sham	14/14	15.0 ± 0.9	14/14	1.5 ± 0.1
TSH pump LPS + 6 h	12/12	10.4 ± 0.8	10/12	0.8 ± 0.1[c]

[a]All animals were challenged with MTg, OVA and LPS d 0, 7 (see methods).
[b]Data from d 28 after challenge; anti-OVA titers averaged 11-12 in both groups.
[c]Significance, $p < 0.001$.

The involvement of T_S has been shown after introducing tolerogenic doses of exogenous MTg[4], but their role following TSH stimulation is unknown. Nevertheless, both schemes show a correlation between strengthened self tolerance and enhanced MTg level and duration. This raises an interesting role for circulating Tg in normal regulation.

This work was supported by grants from the National Institutes of Health AM 30975 and AM 31827.

REFERENCES

1. Y.M. Kong, The mouse model of autoimmune thyroid disease, in: "Immunology of Endocrine Diseases". A.M. McGregor, ed., MTP Press Ltd., Lancaster (1986).
2. M. ElRehewy, Y.M. Kong, A.A. Giraldo, and N.R. Rose, Syngeneic thyroglobulin is immunogenic in good responder mice, Eur. J. Immunol. 11:146 (1981).
3. P.S. Esquivel, N.R. Rose, and Y.M. Kong, Induction of autoimmunity in good and poor responder mice with thyroglobulin and lipopoly-saccharide, J. Exp. Med. 145:1250 (1977).
4. Y.M. Kong, I. Okayasu, A.A. Giraldo, K.W. Beisel, R.S. Sundick, N.R. Rose, C.S. David, F. Audibert, and L. Chedid, Tolerance to thyroglobulin by activating suppressor mechanisms. Ann. N.Y. Acad. Sci. 392:191 (1982).
5. M. Lewis, A.A. Giraldo, and Y.M. Kong, Resistance to experimental autoimmune thyroiditis induced by physiologic manipulation of thyroglobulin level, Submitted (1986).
6. M. Lewis, A.A. Giraldo, and Y.M. Kong, The crucial role of circulatory thyroglobulin in activation of suppressor mechanisms, Immunobiol. 167:44 (1984).
7. Y.M. Kong, C.S. David, A.A. Giraldo, M. ElRehewy, and N.R. Rose, Regulation of autoimmune response to mouse thyroglobulin: Influence of H-2D-end genes, J. Immunol. 123:15 (1979).
8. M. Lewis, J.R. Bourke, P. Conn, and D.C. Evered, in: "Thyroid Research VIII", J. R. Stockigt and S. Nagataki, eds., Aust. Acad. Sci., Canberra (1980).
9. G.P. Haas, A.G. Johnson, and A. Nowotny, Suppression of the immune response in C3H/HeJ mice by protein-free lipopolysaccharides, J. Exp. Med. 148:1081 (1978).

THYROGLOBULIN AUTOANTIBODY IgG SUBCLASSES; REGULATION BY T CELLS

Nita Forouhi, Sandra M. McLachlan, Shirley L. Middleton,
Marian Atherton, Peter H. Baylis, Fred Clark and Bernard
Rees Smith

Departments of Pathology and Medicine, University of
Newcastle upon Tyne and Endocrine Immunology Unit
Department of Medicine, University of Wales College of
Medicine, Cardiff, U.K.

Microsomal and thyroglobulin (Tg) antibodies in patients with autoimmune thyroid disease are usually restricted to subclasses IgG1 and/or
IgG4 (1,2) and this distribution is likely to reflect the capacity of
these antibodies to induce thyroid damage (3). Using an in vitro system
we have investigated the role of T cells in determining the IgG subclass
distribution of Tg antibodies synthesised by peripheral blood lymphocytes
from 7 Hashimoto patients with high circulating titres of Tg antibodies
(>1:10,000 by haemagglutination tests). The IgG subclass distribution of
Tg antibodies present in serum and synthesised in culture was analysed by
an ELISA technique (1,4) using murine monoclonal antibodies to human IgG
subclasses 1 to 4.

In the presence of the T cell dependent activator Pokeweed mitogen,
unfractionated blood lymphocytes synthesised Tg antibodies which were 87%
IgG1 in 1 patient, 57 ± 4% IgG1 and 39 ± 4% IgG4 in 5 patients (mean ± SEM)
and 90% IgG4 in 1 patient; these in vitro subclass patterns were comparable
with the subclass distribution obtained for serum Tg antibody in each
individual as we observed previously (4). B cells, isolated by removal of
T lymphocytes rosetting with neuraminidase treated sheep erythrocytes (5),
lacked the ability to secrete Tg antibodies of subclass IgG1 and/or IgG4.
However, as illustrated for patient MF (Fig 1), the response could be
restored to the original levels and proportions of IgG1 and/or IgG4 Tg
antibody by the addition of T cells. Synthesis of Tg antibody of both
subclasses was affected by the length of time for which unfractionated
lymphocytes or B and T cell fractions were cultured, higher amounts of Tg
antibody of subclasses IgG1 and particularly IgG4 being secreted after 14
days compared with 7 days. Further removal of suppressor T cells by pretreatment of the T cell fraction with Mitomycin C, MMC (6) had little effect
on the proportions of IgG1 and IgG4 Tg antibody although the total amounts
of Tg antibody of both subclasses were sometimes increased (Fig.1).

The ability of the B cell fraction (cultured with Pokeweed mitogen)
to synthesise Tg antibody was independent of the donor of the T cells.
For example, B cells from a patient with 85% IgG4 antibody in serum
secreted antibody of this subclass when cultured with autologous T cells
or with T cells from a patient whose serum Tg antibodies were 93% IgG1.

319

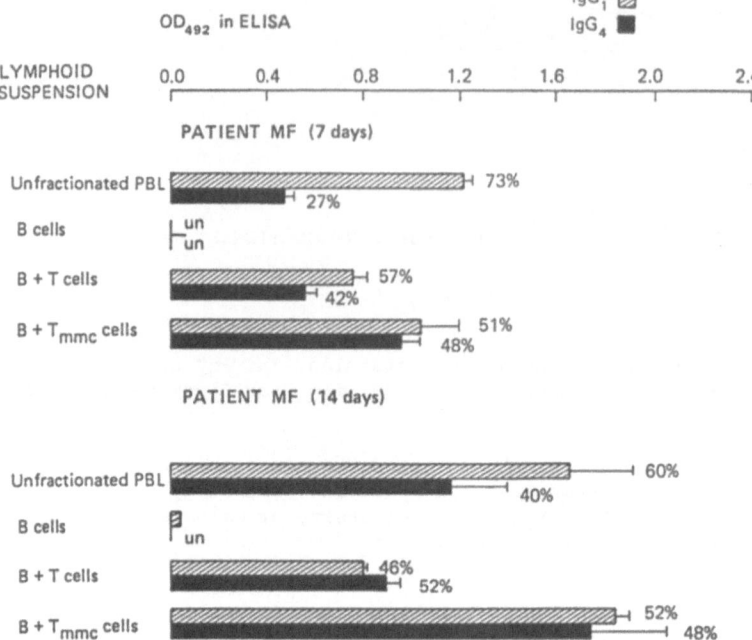

Fig. 1. Synthesis of Tg antibody of subclasses IgG1 and IgG4 by lymphocytes from patient MF cultured with Pokeweed mitogen for 7 or 14 days. Results are given as the Optical Density at 492 nm (OD_{492}) in the ELISA and as the % contribution made to total Tg antibody by subclasses IgG1 and IgG4. The contributions made to Tg antibody by IgG2 and IgG3 were negligible.

Conversely, Tg antibodies from another patient were over 80% IgG1 whether the B cells were incubated with her own T cells or with T cells from a normal donor without detectable serum autoantibodies.

These studies indicate that the IgG subclass distribution of Tg antibodies (and probably other thyroid antibodies as well) is determined at the level of the B cells. However, T cells are required to elicit the synthesis of Tg antibody by B cells and they also regulate the overall autoantibody level, at least in vitro, and it seems likely that this will also be the case in vivo.

ACKNOWLEDGEMENTS

These studies were supported by the Medical Research Council and the Newcastle Health Authority, U.K.

REFERENCES

1. A.B. Parkes, S.M. McLachlan, P. Bird and B. Rees Smith, The distribution of microsomal and thyroglobulin antibody activity among the IgG subclasses, Clin Exp Immunol 57: 239 (1984).
2. T.F. Davies, S.M. Weber, P. Wallack and M. Platzer, Restricted heterogeneity and T cell dependence of human thyroid autoantibody immunoglobulin G subclasses, J Clin Endocrinol Metab 62: 945 (1986).

3. R. Jansson, P.M. Thompson, F. Clark and S.M. McLachlan, Association between thyroid microsomal antibodies of subclass IgG-1 and hypothyroidism in autoimmune postpartum thyroiditis, Clin Exp Immunol 63: 80 (1986).
4. P.M. Thompson, S.M. McLachlan, A. Parkes, F. Clark, D. Howe and B. Rees Smith, The IgG subclass distribution of thyroglobulin antibody synthesized in culture, Scand J Immunol 18: 123 (1983).
5. M.E. Weiner, C. Bianco and V. Nussenzweig, Enhanced binding of neuraminidase-treated sheep erythrocytes to human T lymphocytes, Blood 42: 93 (1973).
6. F.P. Siegal and M. Siegal, Enhancement by irradiated T cells of human plasma cell production:dissection of helper and suppressor functions in vitro, J Immunol 118:642 (1977).

CELLULAR IMMUNITY AND SPECIFIC DEFECTS OF T-CELL SUPPRESSION IN PATIENTS WITH AUTOIMMUNE THYROID DISORDERS

S. Vento, C.J. O'Brien, T. Cundy[+], C. McSorley, E. Macchia*, and A.L.W.F. Eddleston

The Liver Unit and [+]Department of Medicine
King's College School of Medicine & Dentistry
London; *Cattedra di Endrocrinologia, University
of Pisa, Pisa

INTRODUCTION

Graves' disease, Hashimoto's thyroiditis and idiopathic myxoedema are autoimmune thyroid diseases characterised by the production of autoantibodies against the microsomal/ microvillar antigen, thyroglobulin and/or the TSH receptor. Sensitisation of T lymphocytes to antigens contained within crude thyroid homogenates has also been demonstrated and cellular immunity has been proposed as an additional mechanism in the pathogenesis of these disorders,[1] but the determinants to which this response is directed have not been identified.

Recently, it has been shown that a functional TSH receptor is contained in fat cell membrane preparations.[2]

We have used an indirect T lymphocyte migration inhibitory factor (T-LIF) assay in agarose microdroplets, developed in our laboratories,[3] and assessed both T cell sensitisation and specific suppressor T (Ts) lymphocyte activity to thyroid antigens in patients with autoimmune thyroid diseases employing human thyroid plasma membranes and guinea pig fat cell membranes as antigenic preparations (prepared according to Fenzi et al.[4] and Endo et al.,[2] respectively).

PATIENTS

30 patients were studied: 14 had Graves' disease (GD) (1 untreated and hyperthryoid, 8 euthyroid on treatment with carbimazole or propylthiouracil, 5 euthyroid off-treatment), 10 had Hashimoto's thyroiditis (HT) (2 untreated and hypothyroid, 6 euthyroid on treatment with thyroxine, 2 euthyroid and untreated) and 6 had idiopathic, agoitrous, autoantibody-associated myxoedema (Myx) (all euthyroid on treatment with thyroxine).

METHODS

The indirect T-LIF assay employed has been described in detail previously.[3,5] To assess antigen-specific Ts cell function, a small number (ratio 1:9) of T cells to be studied for suppressor activity was added to sensitised T cells; the mixture was then incubated with antigen and the supernatants tested for T-LIF activity.

RESULTS

25/27 patients with autoimmune thyroid disease tested had peripheral blood T lymphocytes sensitised to thyroid plasma membranes, the two exceptions being the only two patients studied while being pregnant. In contrast, only patients with Graves' disease had T cells sensitised to fat cell membranes; T-LIF release from T cells of these patients was no longer detectable after preincubation of fat cell membranes with partially purified TSH (Thytropar, Armour) at concentrations ranging from 0.5 to 5 mU/µg membranes, while it persisted after preincubation of thyroid plasma membranes with TSH.

T-LIF release from T cells of patients with GD in response to fat cell membranes was no longer detectable after addition of T cells from normal subjects or patients with either HT or Myx. T-LIF release in response to thyroid membranes was not detectable in co-cultures (ratio 9:1) of T lymphocytes from patients with GD and either normals or patients with Myx, from patients with HT and normals, and from patients with Myx and either normals or patients with GD. In contrast, it persisted in co-cultures of T lymphocytes from patients with GD and HT or from patients with HT and Myx.

DISCUSSION

The results of this study, showing that peripheral blood T lymphocytes from patients with different autoimmune thyroid diseases are sensitised to thyroid plasma membranes, whereas only T cells from patients with Graves' disease show, in addition, sensitisation to fat cell membranes, favour the hypothesis that the TSH receptor is a target of cellular immune reactions in subjects with Graves' disease. This is further supported by the results of the experiments in which preincubation of fat cell membranes with low concentrations of TSH prevented T-LIF release by T cells from these patients, probably interfering with antigenic recognition.

The results of the T lymphocyte co-culture experiments support the hypothesis that circulating Ts lymphocytes capable of recognising thyroid autoantigens are present in normal subjects and defective in patients with autoimmune thyroid diseases.[6] In addition, they suggest that a defect in Ts cells specific for the TSH receptor is restricted to patients with Graves' disease and may determine the persistence of sensitised T lymphocytes specific for the same antigen.

Finally, the results of the T cell mixture experiments in the presence of thyroid plasma membranes suggest that at least two additional thyroid antigens evoke cell-mediated immune responses in autoimmune thyroid diseases, one being recognised by T cells from patients with HT and GD, the other by T lymphocytes from patients with HT and Myx. Further studies using highly purified thyrocyte antigens and cloned T lymphocyte populations from both peripheral blood and thyroid glands of patients with autoimmune thyroid diseases are needed before definitive conclusions can be drawn.

REFERENCES

1. R. Volpè, Autoimmunity in the endocrine system, Monogr. Endocrinol. 20: 19 (1981)
2. K. Endo, S.M. Amir and S.H. Ingbar, Development and evaluation of a method for the partial purification of immunoglobulins specific for Graves' disease, J. Clin. Endocrinol. Metab. 52: 1113 (1981)
3. S. Vento, J.E. Hegarty, G.F. Bottazzo et al, Antigen-specific suppressor cell function in autoimmune chronic active hepatitis, Lancet 1: 1200 (1984)
4. G.F. Fenzi, E. Macchia, L. Bartalena et al, Radioreceptor assay of TSH: its use to detect thyroid-stimulating immunoglobulins, J. Endocrinol. Invest. 1: 17 (1978)
5. S. Vento, C.J. O'Brien, B.M. McFarlane et al, T-lymphocyte sensitisation to hepatocyte antigens in autoimmune chronic active hepatitis and primary biliary cirrhosis: evidence for different underlying mechanisms and different antigenic determinants as targets, Gastroenterology 91: 810 (1986)
6. N. Okita, V.V. Row and R. Volpè, Suppressor T-lymphocyte deficiency in Graves' disease and Hashimoto's thyroiditis, J. Clin. Endocrinol. Metab. 52: 528 (1981)

THE INFLUENCE OF INTERLEUKIN-1 ON THE FUNCTION OF HUMAN THYROID CELLS

Å. Krogh Rasmussen, U. Feldt-Rasmussen, K. Bech, S. Poulsen, and K. Bendtzen

Med. depart. E, Frederiksberg Hospital & Lab. of Med. Immunol. State University Hospital, Copenhagen, Denmark

Interleukin 1 (IL-1) is a T- and B-lymphocyte activating cytokine released primarily by antigen-presenting macrophages (1,2). We have recently found that IL-1 elicited functional impairment of human thyroid cells in monolayers. The aim of the present study was to further elucidate the influence of recombinant IL-1β (rIL-1β) on the secretion of thyroglobulin (Tg) and cAMP from cultured human thyroid cells.

MATERIAL AND METHODS

Fresh normal human thyroid tissue was obtained from thyroid surgery and prepared as reported by Reader et al. (3) with minor modifications. The cells were cultured in Nunclon multidish plates with a suspension of 2×10^5 cells per 1 ml in each well and formed monolayers within 3-4 days. Thyroid monolayers were cultured with or without TSH (100 mU/ml) or insulin (10 µg/ml). The cells were incubated with human rIL-1β (pI7 form) - kindly provided by dr. Ch. A. Dinarello (Boston), and the activity of IL-1 was estimated by a mouse thymocyte costimulatory assay (4). After 2 and 4 days Tg in the cell-free supernatants was measured by a double-antibody radioimmunoassay (5), cyclic AMP (cAMP) was measured by a competitive protein binding assay (6) and the DNA-content of the cells by the diphenylamine method (7).

RESULTS

Addition of TSH and/or insulin to primary thyroid cell cultures potentiated the response of both Tg and cAMP. Typical examples of Tg- and cAMP-values with or without 4 days stimulation of TSH in a primary culture are demonstrated in table 1.

Both primary and secondary thyroid cells secreted increased cAMP into the medium after TSH-stimulation, whereas only primary cultures had preserved the ability to increase Tg-secretion essentially during TSH-stimulation (table 2). Specially the cAMP-secretion was stimulated by TSH. In both primary and secondary cultures rIL-1β in concentrations between 0.01 and 100.0 U/ml inhibited dose-dependently the insulin- and TSH-stimulated Tg-secretion (up to 75%) after 4 days incubation, whereas a concentration of rIL-1β of 0.001 stimulated Tg production (fig. 1). This pattern was found both with and without addition of TSH. The insulin- and TSH-stimulated cAMP-secretion

TABLE 1

INFLUENCE OF TSH AND INSULIN OF SECRETION OF cAMP AND Tg FROM CULTURED HUMAN THYROID CELLS

| | cAMP (pmol/µgDNA) | | Tg (ng/µg DNA) $ | |
	+ Ins	− Ins	+ Ins	− Ins
+ TSH	13.6	15.4	267	170
− TSH	2.8	0	222	103

$ cAMP was investigated after 2 days and Tg after 4 days TSH stimulation.

was similarly dose-dependently inhibited at equal concentrations of rIL-1β. The influence of rIL-1 on Tg and cAMP secretion was most pronounced in secondary cultures.

CONCLUSIONS

Addition of insulin was not necessary for a significant response to TSH stimulation of either primary or secondary cultures, but potentiated the responses. Thyroid cell functions were stimulated by rIL-1 β at very low concentrations. These effects were shown in both primary and secondary cultures and were independent of presence of TSH or insulin.

Il-1 production is usually considered a result of an immune reaction, where the presence of an antigen initiates a series of cellular and humoral interactions leading to activation of specifically reactive T-lymphocytes by the antigen-presenting cell, usually a macrophage. This T-cell activation is dependent upon the production by the macrophage of IL-1. As a result, the T-cells elaborate macrophage-activating factors, whereafter the monocytes increase the secretion of IL-1 (1). This study has shown that IL-1 in pharmacological levels has an inhibitory effect on cultured human thyroid cells, while in physiological levels, it stimulated the cell function. Thus, IL-1 might have an influence on the thyroid gland in vivo and play a role for the development of autoimmune thyroid diseases.

TABLE 2

THE PERCENTAGE INCREASE OF Tg AND cAMP AFTER 4 DAYS TSH-STIMULATION IN INSULIN DEPLETED CELLS

	Tg Median (ranges)	cAMP Median (ranges)
Primary cultures:	39% (15–89) (n=5)	61% (47–100) (n=5)
Secondary cultures:	7% (0–22) (n=7)	94% (91–99) (n=7)

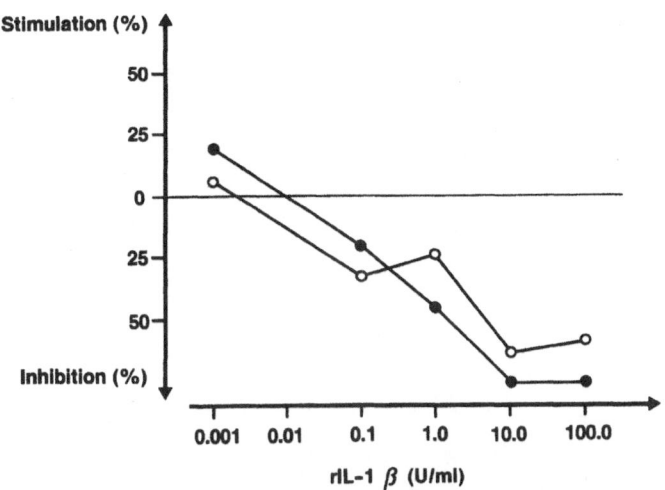

Figure 1. The relative changes of TSH-stimulated Tg and cAMP secretion after incubation with rIL-1β in a secondary culture (a typical example). The closed circles indicate the Tg secre--tion in the medium after 4 days incubation, and the open circles indicate the cAMP secretion in the medium after 2 days incubation.

REFERENCES

1. K. Bendtzen, Biological properties of interleukins, Allergy 38:219 (1983).
2. C. A. Dinarello, Interleukin-1 and the pathogenesis of the acute-phase response, N. Engl. J. Med. 311:1413 (1984).
3. S. C. J. Reader, B. Davison, J. G. Ratchcliffe, W. R. Robertson, Measurement of low concentrations of bovine thyrotrophin by iodide uptake and organification in porcine thyrocytes, J. Endocr. 106:13 (1985).
4. I. Geri, R. K. Gershon, B. H. Waksmann, Potentiation of the T-lymphocyte response to mitogens, J. Exp. Med. 136:128 (1972).
5. U. Feldt-Rasmussen, I. Holten, H. Sand Hansen, Influence of thyroid substitution therapy and thyroid autoantibodies on the value of serum thyroglobulin in recurring thyroid cancer, Cancer 51:2240 (1983)
6. K. Bech, S. N. Madsen, Thyroid adenylate cyclase stimulating immunoglobulins in thyroid diseases, Clin. Endocrinol. (Oxf.) 11:47.
7. K. Burton, A study of the conditions and mechanism of the diphenylamine reaction for the colorimetric estimation of deoxyribonucleic acid, Biochem. Journ. 62:315 (1956).

IMMUNOHISTOCHEMICAL CHARACTERISATION OF LYMPHOCYTES

IN EXPERIMENTAL AUTOIMMUNE THYROIDITIS

A.P. Weetman and S.B. Cohen

Dept. of Medicine
Royal Postgraduate Medical School
London W12 0HS, UK

INTRODUCTION

EAT in the rat is under genetic control, and the Buffalo (Buf) rat appears to be an unusually high responder strain. Spontaneous disease has been reported and appears to represent the action of environmental factors on the genetic background of this strain. This would account for the low incidence in young rats with a maximal prevalence of 48% in ex-breeder females (Silverman and Rose, 1971). However a variety of treatments are known to increase the incidence of EAT, including trypan blue (TB), 3-methylcholanthrene (3-MC), neonatal thymectomy (Tx) and immunisation with thyroglobulin (Tg) in a variety of adjuvants (Glover et al 1968, Reuber 1970, Silverman and Rose 1974, 1975).
We have compared these four models of EAT and sought to identify which most resembles Hashimoto's thyroiditis, with particular reference to the thyroid mononuclear cell infiltrate.

METHODS

Induction of EAT
Neonatal Tx was performed within 24 hr of birth on six animals. At six weeks old, nine animals received 750ug TB sc weekly x 5, nine were given 4mg 3-MC sc weekly x 5 and a further nine were given 1mg rat Tg emulsified in complete Freund's adjuvant (CFA) im/sc twice, a week apart. The animals were all female and were compared with a control untreated group of six animals. All assessments were made at 12 weeks of age.

Measurements

Tg antibodies were measured by ELISA as described elsewhere (Rennie et al, 1983). T4 and TSH levels were measured by radioimmunoassay, for TSH using the kit and protocol of Dr. A.F. Parlow (NIAMDD, NIH, USA). FACS analysis of peripheral blood lymphocytes was performed using the Ox8 (suppressor/cytotoxic T cells) and W3/25 (helper T cells and some macrophages) from Sera-Lab. Additional monoclonal reagents used for immunoperoxidase staining of thyroid frozen sections were Ox6 (anti-Ia, I-A equivalent), Ox17 (anti-Ia, I-E equivalent), Ox12

(kappa chain on B cells), Ox18 (anti-class I), Ox19 (pan T) and an
in-house monoclonal anti-rat Tg.   Severity of thyroiditis and staining
by immunoperoxidase were graded blind.

RESULTS

All Tx, CFA/Tg and TB, but no 3-MC or control rats had Tg
antibodies.   Antibody levels were significantly different in the three
groups; Tx > CFA/Tg (P < 0.001), CFA/Tg > TB (P< 0.01).   TSH levels are
shown in Fig. 1; they were only increased in the Tx group (P< 0.05).
However, free T4 levels were normal (mean $\pm$ SD Tx 62 $\pm$ 14 nmol/l,
controls 63 $\pm$ 19 nmol/l).   Circulating T cell subsets were not different
from controls in the Tx, TB and CFA/Tg groups, the mean ratio of Ox 8:
W3/25 being 1.3 - 1.8.   However in the 3-MC group there were less Ox 8
cells (P< 0.05 compared to controls) with an Ox8: W3/25 ratio of 0.9 .

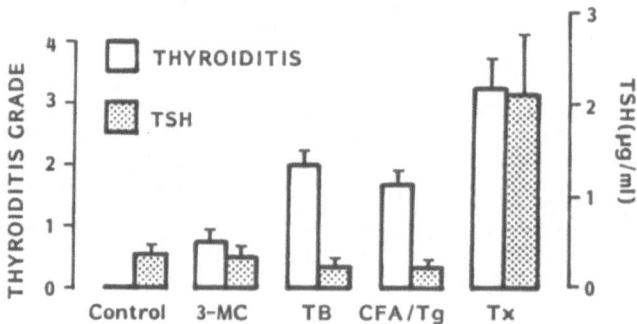

Fig. 1.   Thyroiditis severity (graded 0 - 4) and TSH levels in
           controls and animals with EAT.   The mean $\pm$ SEM is shown
           for each group. The upper limit of normal for TSH is
           1ug/ml.

Thyroiditis was found in all groups except controls (Fig. 1) and
severity was ordered Tx > TB or CFA/Tg (P < 0.01) > TB (P< 0.01). The
immunohistochemical features are shown in Table 1.   A few dendritic
cells (Ox6, Ox17-positive) were found in control thyroids as expected,
but were increased in the CFA/Tg and 3-MC groups.   In the TB group, the
majority of Ox6, Ox17-positive cells were W3/25-positive, Ox19-negative,
i.e. macrophages.   In all three groups T and B cells were infrequent.
However in the Tx group, there was extensive infiltration with Ox12, Ox8
and W3/25 cells.   In four Tx animals there was occasional Ox6 and Ox17
expression by thyroid follicular cells.   Staining with anti-Tg was seen
in the interstitium as well as the remaining follicles in these animals.

Table 1.   Extent of thyroid mononuclear cell infiltration in EAT

	Ox6/Ox17	Ox8	W3/25	Ox12
Control	+	O	O	O
3-MC	++	+	$\pm$	$\pm$
TB	++	++(Ox19⁻)	$\pm$	$\pm$
CFA/Tg	++	+	+	$\pm$
Tx	+++	+++	+++	++

$\pm$ = present in some animals + = mild infiltration
++ = moderate infiltration   +++ = severe infiltration.

DISCUSSION

These results show that EAT in the Buf is heterogenous,
particularly in respect of the thyroid lymphocytic infiltrate. The most
severe thyroiditis was found in Tx animals, which nonetheless showed no
sign of T cell subset alteration in the peripheral blood. This model
closely resembled Hashimoto's thyroiditis; TSH was increased (albeit
with normal T4 levels), the lymphocytic infiltrate resembled the human
disease and some thyroid follicular cells were Ia-positive (Aichinger et
al 1985). This latter feature was also characteristic of spontaneous
thyroiditis in the OS chicken (Wick et al 1984) but was not found in
other forms of Buf EAT. Further understanding of the role of thyroid
cell Ia expression in the development of autoimmunity should come from
study of Tx induced EAT, although the presence of thyroiditis in two Tx
animals without detectable follicular cell Ia expression suggests that
this role may not be crucial to disease initiation.

REFERENCES

Aichinger, G., Fill, H. and Wick, G., 1985, In situ immune complexes,
    lymphocyte subpopulations, and HLA-DR positive epithelial cells in
    Hashimoto's thyroiditis. Lab. Invest., 52:132.
Glover, E.L., Reuber, M.D. and Grollman, S., 1968, Influence of age
    and sex on thyroiditis in rats injected subcutaneously with
    3-methylcholanthrene. Path. Microbiol., 32:314.
Rennie, D.P., McGregor, A.M., Keast, D., Weetman, A.P. and Foord, S.M.,
    Dieguez, C., Williams, E.D. and Hall, R., 1983, The influence of
    methimazole on thyroglobulin-induced autoimmune thyroiditis in the
    rat. Endocrinol., 112:326.
Reuber, M.D., 1970, Influence of age and sex on chronic thyroiditis in
    rats given subcutaneous injections of trypan blue. Toxicol. Appl.
    Pharm., 17:60.
Silverman, D.A. and Rose, N.R., 1971, Autoimmunity in methylcholanthrene
    -induced and spontaneous thyroiditis in Buffalo strain rats. Proc.
    Soc. Exp. Biol. Med., 138:579.
Silverman, D.A. and Rose, N.R., 1974, Neonatal thymectomy increases the
    incidence of spontaneous and methylcholanthrene enhanced
    thyroiditis in rats. Science, 184:162.
Silverman, D.A. and Rose, N.R., 1975, Spontaneous and
    methylcholanthrene-induced thyroiditis in Buf rats. I. The
    incidence and severity of the disease, and genetics of
    susceptibility. J. Immunol., 114:148.

Wick, G., Hala, K., Wolf, H., Boyd, R.L. and Schauenstein, K. 1984,
Distribution and functional analysis of B-L/Ia-positive cells in
the chicken: expression of B-L/Ia antigens on thyroid epithelial
cells in spontaneous autoimmune thyroiditis. Mol. Immunol.,
21:1259

λ LIGHT CHAIN RESTRICTION IN THE DIFFUSE THYROID LYMPHOID INFILTRATE IN UNTREATED GRAVES' DISEASE

Claire A. Smith, Bharat Jasani, and E. Dillwyn Williams

Department of Pathology
University of Wales College of Medicine
Heath Park
Cardiff
Wales, U.K.

INTRODUCTION

It has recently been shown that the pathogenically important TSH receptor antibodies found in Graves' disease are mainly synthesised by lymphocytes closely associated with thyroid follicles.[1] It has also been shown that these antibodies are almost exclusively restricted to the λ light chain type.[2] In this study we have used an immunoperoxidase technique to analyse, in situ, the distribution of the light chain isotypes of plasma cells found within Graves' disease thyroids.

MATERIALS AND METHODS

Patients

Specimens from 7 patients with no pre-operative antithyroid treatment were obtained from archive material (1910-1914) and compared with tissue from 14 patients treated with carbimazole. All tissue used was formalin fixed and paraffin embedded. Sections from one randomly selected block from each patient were analysed.

Antibodies

The antibodies used in this study were a series of monospecific polyclonal antibodies directed against the different light and heavy chain isotypes (BDS Biological Ltd.). Anti-λ, K were used at 1:1000, anti-γ at 1:2000 and anti-α, μ at 1:3200.

Staining Procedure

Sections were cut and endogenous peroxidase blocked by incubation with methanol/H_2O_2. These were trypsinised and subjected to a previously described immunoperoxidase staining procedure.[3]

Counting Procedure

As in previous studies[4,5] the plasma cell population was divided into

3 categories; diffusely scattered (DS), loosely aggregated (LA) and germinal centre associated (G.C.). The D.S. cells were counted in a minimum of 20 non-overlapping high power fields distributed over the entire section and the mean number of cells/field calculated. For the loose aggregates and the germinal centre plasma cell counts the total number of positive cells present were counted and expressed as means for each category.

RESULTS

The immunoperoxidase procedure was validated for specificity and accuracy by comparing the sum of the δ, μ, α counts with that of the λ, K counts. These showed a concordance rate of 98.2%. Table 1 shows the percentage of λ light chain expression (mean $\pm$ S.E.) for each category of cells. The diffusely scattered cells in the untreated glands showed a significant increase in the proportion of cells expressing λ light chain when compared to the L.A. or G.C. cells, or when compared to an equal division of cells ($p<0.005$) or the expected (40%) ratio in simple inflammatory infiltrates ($p<0.001$). There was no significant difference between any of the 3 cell categories in the carbimazole treated thyroids.

COMMENT

These results show that in Graves' disease the diffusely scattered plasma cells are the only group of intrathyroid plasma cells showing a λ chain predominance. The extent of this predominance is significantly different from both random and expected distribution of light chain subclasses of plasma cells. Carbimazole treatment reduces the numbers of λ cells to a greater extent than it reduces the numbers of K cells. It has been shown by others that the cells that produce TSH receptor antibodies are almost exclusively of λ light chain isotype,[2] and that they are synthesised by cells associated with thyroid follicles.[1] We therefore suggest that the diffusely scattered plasma cells are of much more importance in the pathogenesis of Graves' disease than the more obvious germinal centres and lymphoid aggregates, and that carbimazole has a selective effect on the group of plasma cells that includes the TSH antibody producing cells. This study also demonstrates the importance of not regarding the lymphoid infiltrate in Graves' disease as composed of a homogenous population of cells.

Table 1. Mean percentage of λ positive plasma cells in various categories of cell infiltrates

Patient Group	Category of Cell Infiltrate		
	DS	LA	GC
Untreated	63.5 $\pm$ 2.9	50.8 $\pm$ 8.0	45.7 $\pm$ 1.0
Carbimazole treated	54.2 $\pm$ 5.5	39.8 $\pm$ 13.7	48.9 $\pm$ 14.6

REFERENCES

1. S. M. McLauchlan, C.A.S. Pegg, M. C. Atherton, S. L. Middleton, F. Clark and B. Rees Smith, TSH receptor antibody synthesis by thyroid lymphocytes, Clin. Endocrinol. 24:223 (1986).
2. J. Knight, P. Laine, A. Knight, D. Adams and N. Ling, Thyroid stimulating autoantibodies usually contain only λ -light chains: evidence for the "forbidden clone" theory, J. Clin. Endocrinol. Metab. 62:342 (1986).
3. B. Jasani, R. E. Edwards, N. D. Thomas and A. R. Gibbs, The use of vimentin antibodies in the diagnosis of malignant mesothelioma, Virchows Arch. (Pathol. Anat.) 406:441 (1985).
4. C. Smith and B. Jasani, Immunohistochemical definition of lymphocyte subpopulations in autoimmune thyroiditis, J. Path. 143:297A (1984).
5. B. Jasani, C. Smith and E. D. Williams, A high predominance of OKT8[+] and activated leu 3a[+] cells in the scattered lymphocyte population of the Graves disease thyroid, J. Endocrinol. 104 (Supplement), 96:160A (1985).

NATURAL KILLER CELL ACTIVITY IN HASHIMOTO, GRAVES' DISEASE AND EUTHYROID EXOPHTHALMOS

Bente K. Pedersen, Ulla Feldt-Rasmussen, Hans Perrild, Jens Mølholm Hansen, and Tom Christensen

Laboratory of Medical Immunology TTA, Rigshospitalet University Hospital, Department of Medicine E,Frederiksberg Hospital, Department of Medicine F, Herlev County Hospital Department of Ophthalmology, Gentofte County Hospital Copenhagen, Denmark

INTRODUCTION

Natural killer (NK) cells are functionally identified by their ability to lyse a variety of target cells; morphologically they are identified as large granular lymphocytes (LGL). NK cells are augmented by interferon (IF), interleukin 2 (Il-2) and inhibited by various agents including certain prostaglandins (PG), e.g. PGE1, PGE2, PGA1 and PGA2. NK cells are thought to play an important role in immune surveillance against cancer and certain infections. Evidence for a role of NK cells in autoimmune disorders is forthcoming. Significantly reduced NK cell activity has been described in patients with systemic lupus erythematosus, Sjögren's syndrome and multiple sclerosis. In the present study we have characterized the quality and quantity of NK cells in patients with Hashimoto, Graves' disease and euthyroid exophthalmos.

PATIENTS AND METHODS

A total of 43 patients with various thyroid diseases and 22 controls were studied. Patients characteristics are given in Table 1. The diagnosis of Hashimoto's thyroiditis was based on presence of a characteristic goitre, positive antithyroglobulin and/or antimicrosomal antibodies and evidence of thyroid failure with low thyroid hormones and high TSH. All patients - except 3 studied at diagnosis - were euthyroid on L-thyroxine. The patients with Graves' disease all had diffuse uptake on ^{99m}Tc-scintigraphy and both clinical and biochemical evidence of hyperthyroidism. Eight of the patients were studied at the time of diagnosis while still untreated. The remaining 8 were studied after 12 months in average (range: 4-36) of treatment with antithyroid drugs (thiamazole 5 to 10 mg daily). The patients with non-toxic goitre were all euthyroid with a diffuse or multinodular scintigram, and all were untreated. The patients with euthyroid Graves' exophthalmos all had unilateral exophthalmos and evidence of eyemuscle enlargement on a CT-scan of the orbit. The duration of disease was more than 7 years except for one studied 6 months after diagnosis. NK cell activity of mononuclear cells was measured against K 562 targer cells in a 4 h ^{51}Cr release assay,

Table 1. Characteristics of patients with thyroid disease. Median and range are given.

Patients group	n	o/o	Age (years)	Free T4 Index (units)	Free T3 Index (units)	TSH mU/l
Hashimoto's thyroiditis	11	10/1	60 (26-90)	5.9 (1.4-14.7)	84 (60-141)	3.7 (<3 - >80)
Graves' disease (untreated)	8	7/1	61 (20-79)	25.1 (7.4-31.0)	780 (98-934)	<3 (<3 - <3)
Graves' disease (during treatment)	8	6/2	63 (27-70)	7.0 (5.1-8.8)	124 (70-219)	<3 (<3 - 7.5)
Non-toxic goitre	9	9/0	53 (35-78)	7.3 (5.5-10.1)	105 (73-140)	<3 (<3 - 5.0)
Euthyroid exophthalmos	7	5/2	59 (35-78)	9.4 (6.2-11.9)	176 (72-193)	3.0 (<3 - 3.9)

Table 2. NK cell activity of patients with thyroid diseases and controls.

	NK	NK+Il-2	NK+IF	NK+indo	%LGL
Controls	34.7 (11.9-61.1)	41.2 (16.2-65.5)	56.5 (28.9-67.9)	37.5 (15.8-65.0)	4.3 (1.5-8.5)
Hashimoto's disease	25.1 (14.7-44.7)	34.1 (11.6-49.7)	49.7 (20.2-59.6)	32.4 (9.9-50.4)	3.0 (1.5-10.5)
Graves' disease (untreated)	34.4 (5.7-51.4)	50.0 (10.8-62.9)	58.6 (27.3-65.7)	37.5 (15.8-65.0)	4.1 (2.3-8.7)
Graves' disease (treated)	21.8 (12.4-32.4)	27.9 (19.2-44.5)	47.0 (31.3-60.7)	28.0 (17.9-42.1)	3.8 (2.1-10.1)
Non-toxic goitre	37.1 (23.9-60.6)	45.3 (37.0-69.2)	57.9 (47.8-68.7)	42.6 (30.8-64.5)	3.9 (2.0-8.6)
Euthyroid exophthalmos	11.7 (1.0-23.9)	20.6 (0-43.4)	35.3 (3.3-53.7)	15.3 (0-36.8)	3.5 (2.5-5)

E/T ratio=80/1. In vitro incubation of NK cells with -IF, Il-2 and indomethacin (indo) 1 ug/ml was performed. LGLs were identified and enumerated in cytocentrifuge preparations stained with May-Grünwald; all methods have previously been described in detail (2).

RESULTS

The NK cell activity in the different groups of patients with thyroid diseases was compared with the NK cell activity in normal healthy controls. Only patients with euthyroid exophthalmos had significantly suppressed NK cell activity. IF, Il-2 as well as indo significantly enhanced NK cell activity in all groups tested, but neither of these agents fully restored the suppressed NK cell of patients with euthyroid exophthalmos. The quantity of NK cells, estimated as %LGLs. did not differ significantly from that of controls.

DISCUSSION

There are several, but conflicting, studies on NK cell activity in autoimmune thyroiditis (reviewed by Burman and Baker) (3). Both reduced, elevated and normal NK cell activity has been demonstrated in patients with Hashimoto and Graves' disease, but in euthyroid patients or patients in remission NK cell activity seems to be normal. In our study the NK cell activity of patients with Hashimoto or Graves' disease was lower than that of normal healthy controls or atoxic struma, but these differences were not statistically significant. Otherwise the NK cell activity of 7 patients with euthyroid exophthalmos was severely suppressed. The finding that the NK cell activity of patients with euthyroid exophthalmos could not be fully restored by addition of IF, Il-2 or indomethacin indicates that the NK cell activity was not suppressed because of low production of IF or Il-2 or high PG production. The finding of normal %LGLs indicates that the NK cell defect in patients with euthyroid exophthalmos is functional.

REFERENCES

1. Pedersen B.K., Allergy, 40, 547, 1985.
2. Pedersen B.K., Oxholm P., Manthorpe R., Andersen V. Clin. Exp. Immunol. 63, 1, 1986.
3. Burman K.D., Baker J.R. Endocrine Reviews, 6, 183, 1985.

INTERACTION OF PURIFIED GRAVES' IMMUNOGLOBULINS

WITH THE TSH-RECEPTOR

P.G.H. Byfield and Jane Worthington

Endocrinology Research Group
Clinical Research Centre
Harrow, HA1 3UJ, UK

INTRODUCTION

We have previously demonstrated directly, by chromatographic separation, the coexistence of multiple immunoglobulin activities against the TSH-receptor (GIg) in sera from patients with Graves' disease (Worthington et al. 1986). Biological properties of these GIg varied from blocking to stimulating with the mix present in an individual being unpredictable. These components were all detected initially using a radioreceptor assay which employs the inhibition of ^{125}I-TSH from binding to solubilised receptors. We have therefore, examined the interaction of mixtures of TSH and the purified GIg with the TSH-receptor in order to clarify the relationship between structure and function for these antibodies.

METHODS

Chromatography: Ammonium sulphate precipitates from serum were eluted from columns of Remazol yellow GGL-Sepharose 4B using gradients of pH (5.0-7.4) and sodium chloride (0-0.3M).
Radioreceptor assay: Solubilised porcine TSH-receptors were used as a binding reagent (Southgate et al., 1984) with reduction in ^{125}I-bTSH (RSR Ltd) binding as the response due to active ligands.
Biological assay: Stimulation of uptake, or inhibition of TSH-stimulated uptake, of iodide-125 by FRTL5 cells was used to characterise stimulating or blocking Graves' immunoglobulins respectively.

RESULTS

Several purified GIg were selected for their different characteristics. LC was the single peak of binding activity obtained from an hypothyroid patient. The protein had no stimulating activity in the bioassay. AR1 and AR2 were the two peaks obtained from a thyrotoxic subject (AR); each had a similar, high stimulating potency in the bioassay. DC2 was one of two peaks present in another subject (DC) with Graves' disease, both had a similar stimulating activity but were less potent than those from AR.

Constant amounts of each of these immunoglobulin activities were mixed with increasing amounts of bTSH and assessed for biological activity and for the response in the binding assay. The results are shown in Fig. 1A as the resultant activity in TSH equivalents plotted against TSH added. In all cases, whether the immunoglobulin tested was a blocker or stimulator, the bioactivity of TSH plus immunoglobulin was less than the sum of the two components. As the quantity of TSH rose this effect became more pronounced and at 100 µU/ml added TSH all tested immunoglobulins acted as apparent blockers of TSH stimulation; AR1 and DC2 even appeared more effective than the blocker LC. This, however, may only be an effect of the different (and unknown) mass of antibody used in each case.

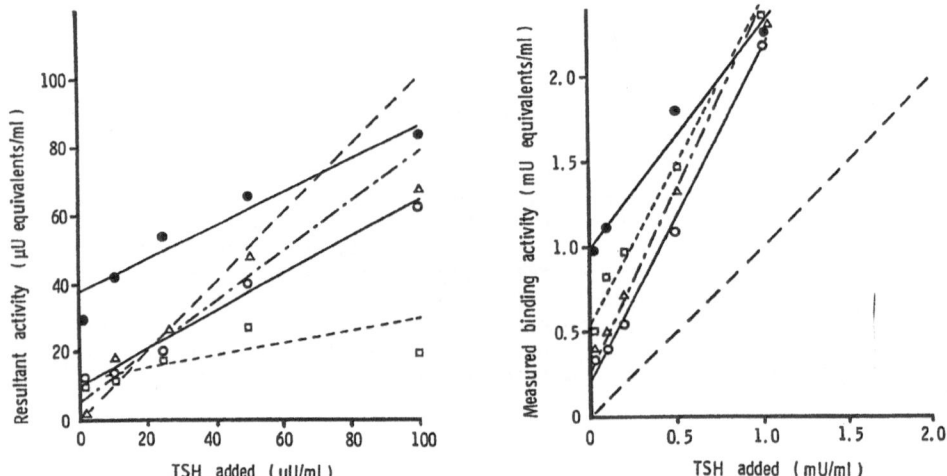

Fig. 1. A. The resultant biological activity of mixtures of bTSH and purified Graves' immunoglobulins. Constant amounts of antibody were mixed with increasing amounts of bTSH.
B. The apparent analyte concentration of mixtures of bTSH and purified Graves' immunoglobulins. Constant amounts of antibody were mixed with increasing amounts of bTSH.
Key. LC △ —·—·— △ ; AR1 ○ ——— ○ ;
AR2 ● ——— ● ; DC2 □ - - - - □ .

These results are consistent with the hypothesis that all the antibodies studied interacted with the receptor at the same site and that this is the TSH binding site. Moreover an increasing mass of TSH does not result in the displacement of GIg that would be expected in a simple equilibrium system and indicates that these antibodies bind irreversibly. Thus the resultant biological activity is the sum of intrinsic (but low or absent) biological activity of GIg plus the activity of TSH acting at a reduced number of binding sites.

These ideas are supported by the results from the radioreceptor assay. In this experiment tracer binding was lower than expected and hence the apparent measured concentration of (TSH + GIg) was greater than the sum of the two components (Fig. 1B) for both the blocker and the stimulators. Again both types of GIg must bind at the TSH binding site. This is probably irreversible and thus restricts TSH and tracer ^{125}I-TSH to fewer binding sites than expected. The consequent lower tracer binding (in a radioreceptor assay) appears to show a high analyte concentration.

CONCLUSION

These results show that both blocking and stimulating immunoglobulin act directly at the TSH binding site. The biological activity of a GIg must therefore be related to its structure and to the precise way in which it binds at the hormone-binding site. Thyroid stimulation in a patient with a mixture of GIg with different properties will be determined by the aggregate activity of the particular mixture.

REFERENCES

Southgate, K., Creagh, F.M., Teece, M, Kingswood, C. and Rees-Smith, B., 1984, A receptor assay for the measurement of TSH-receptor antibodies in unextracted serum. Clin Endocrinol 20:539-543.

Worthington, J., Himsworth, R.L. and Byfield, P.G.H., 1986, Isolation of both agonist and nonagonist Graves' immunoglobulins from the sera of individual patients, in: "The Thyroid and Autoimmunity", H.A. Drexhage and W.M. Wiersinga, eds., Elsevier, Amsterdam.

THYROID STIMULATING IMMUNOGLOBULINS WITHOUT EVIDENCE OF IN VIVO THYROID STIMULATION IN SOME NON-THYROID AUTOIMMUNE DISEASES

K.Bech, U.Feldt-Rasmussen, H.Bliddal, C.Bregengaard, B.Danneskiold-Samsøe, S.Husby, K.Johansen, C.Kirkegaard, T.Friis, K.Siersbæk-Nielsen, and H.Nielsen

Frederiksberg Hosp, Hvidøre Hosp, Gentofte Univ Hosp, Municip Hosp, Steno Memorial Hosp, State Hosp, Odense Univ Hosp, Denmark

INTRODUCTION

Thyroid stimulating immunoglobulins(TSI) are widely accepted to be responsible for the hypersecretion of thyroid hormones in Graves' disease. TSI have also been demonstrated in patients with non-thyroid autoimmune diseases[1]. The aim of the present study was to evaluate if presence of TSI has an influence on thyroid function in vivo in these patients.

MATERIALS AND METHODS

Three different groups of consecutive euthyroid patients were studied. Twenty-five patients (4 men, 21 women) with classical or definite rheumatoid arthritis(RA)(median age: 64 years, range 37-79 years). Rheumatoid factor(RF) was detected in 18 subject. Nineteen of the patients were treated with myocrisine and 2 with penicillamine, whereas none received steroids. Thirty-four patients with insulin dependent diabetes mellitus (IDDM)(19 men, 15 women). Median blood glucose level was 8.9 mmol/l (range 1.8-20.6 mmol/l) and median age 40 years (range 16-72 years). Nine patients with primary biliary cirrhosis(PBC) (2 men, 7 women) aged 65 years (range 52-77 years). Finally, ninety-eight controls (52 men, 46 women) without previous or present evidence of thyroid disease. Median age was 42 years (range 19-83 years). None of them received any medication known to interfere with thyroid function or thyroid hormone assays. Serum TSH levels were measured using an ultrasensitive immunoradiometric assay (sucrosep, Boots Celltech)[2]. TSI were measured both by activation of human thyroid adenylate cyclase(AC) in thyroid membranes (TSAb), and as thyrotropin binding inhibiting immunoglobulins (TBII)[1]. Serum thyroglobulin(Tg) and its autoantibody(TgAb) were quantified as described previously[3], and presence of RF was evidenced by Latex-RF-reagens (BehringWerke). Sera from 3 patients with RA containing both RF and TSAb were fractionated by size chromatography using Sepharose CL6B[3]. The fractions thus obtained were tested for TSAb and RF activity, as well as IgG and IgM by radial immunodifusion. TgAb was

Table 1. Serum TSH, Tg and thyroid autoantibodies in non-thyroid autoimmune disease (medians and ranges).

	N	TSH	Tg	TgAb	TBII >25%	TSAb >108%	level
		mU/l	µg/l	No(%)pos	No(%)pos	No(%)pos	%
RA	25	$\frac{1.3}{(0.2-5.9)}$	$\frac{21}{(11-55)}$	4 (16)	2 (8)	17 (68)	$\frac{121}{(87-196)}$
IDDM	34	$\frac{2.3^*}{(0.4-7.3)}$	$\frac{31^*}{(16-110)}$	8 (24)	3 (9)	8 (24)	$\frac{98}{(72-152)}$
PBC	9	$\frac{1.3}{(0.1-12.7)}$	$\frac{19}{(16-56)}$	3 (30)	0 (0)	4 (44)	$\frac{105}{(100-135)}$
Contr.	98	$\frac{1.3}{(0.5-3.2)}$	$\frac{23}{(7-71)}$	7 (8)	0 (0)	0 (0)	(73-108)

* P < 0.001 compared to normal persons (Mann Whitney)

affinity purified[4] from 3 different sera from patients with Graves' or Hashimoto's diseases, and tested for its ability to stimulate cAMP in thyroid membranes (n=16).

RESULTS

Serum TSH and Tg were not significantly different from controls in RA and PBC, but slightly elevated in IDDM (Table 1), and with a significantly positive association (r=0.69, P < 0.02). Thyroid autoantibodies were present at increased frequency in both RA, IDDM, and PBC (Table 1). There was no significant association between presence of TSAb and sex, age, thyroid function or presence of the other autoantibodies. Serum TSH was not significantly different in patients with or without TSAb (Fig 1). In vitro experiments could not exclude an interference from RF in the TSAb assay as RF and TSAb activities were detected in the same fractions by size chromatography (Fig 2). Purified TgAb did not elicit any AC stimulation in vitro in human thyroid membranes neither when added alone nor together with TSH, TSI or fluoride. On the contrary, in some cases an inhibition of TSH, TSI or fluoride stimulated AC activity was seen by addition of TgAb. However, this inhibition could not account for the lack of in vivo thyroid stimulation by TSAb.

DISCUSSION

The development of ultrasensitive methods for measurement of serum TSH has enabled a complete distinction between hyperthyroid patients and normal control[2]. In the present study TSAb in non-thyroid autoimmune diseases (RA, IDDM, and PBC) was not associated with in vivo thyroid stimulation, assuming that biologically active TSI would release thyroid hormones and Tg, and thereby reduce serum levels of TSH. There was a discrepancy between the frequency of TBII and TSAb in all patient groups. The lack of TBII in RA was in agreement with previous findings[5]. Some of the patients with IDDM showed evidence of incipient thyroid failure despite the presence of

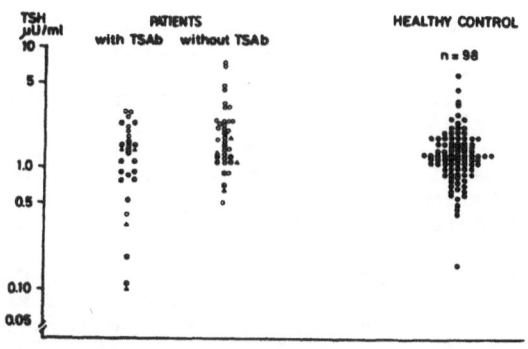

Fig,1 Serum TSH in patients
(RA ●, IDDM o, PBC Δ) with
or without presence of TSAb.
No significant differences
were noted.

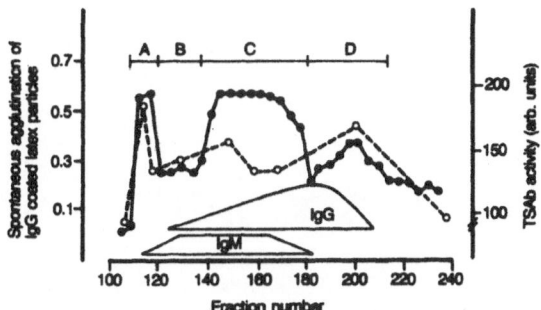

Fig,2 Fractionation of serum
from a patient with RA and both
RF (●) and TSAb (o)(% of buffer).
Similar fractionation of normal
human serum was negative.

TSAb. There was a statistically insignificant tendency towards
a slightly higher TSAb level in RF positive sera, indicating
that RF might stimulate thyroid AC <u>in vitro</u>. This was in agreement with the chromatography studies. The presence of TSAb in
non-thyroid autoimmune disease might thus be an <u>in vitro</u> phenomenon, the reason for which is unclear. Probably TgAb, RF,
or other autoantibodies stimulate the formation of AC through
a pathway which is inaccessible <u>in vivo</u>. This might be due to
the use of disrupted thyroid membranes rather than intact cells.

REFERENCES

1. Bliddal H. and K. Bech, Correlation between TSH receptor
    and adenylate cyclase stimulation assays for thyroid stimu-
    lating immunoglobulins, <u>in</u>: Current Topics in Thyroid Au-
    toimmunity, D.Doniach and H.Schleusener, eds., Georg Thieme
    Verlag, Stuttgart(1984).

2. J. Seth, H.A. Kellet, G. Caldwell, V.M. Sweeting, G.S. Beckett, S.M. Gow and A.D. Toft, A sensitive immunoradiometric assay for serum thyroid stimulating hormone: A replacement the thyrotrophin releasing hormone test? <u>Brit. Med.J.</u> 289:1334(1984).
3. U. Felst-Rasmussen, P.H. Petersen, J. Date and C.M. Madsen, Sequential changes in serum thyroglobulin(Tg) and its auto-antibody(TgAb) following subtotal thyroidectomy of patients with previously detectable TgAb, <u>Clin. Endocrinol.(Oxf.)</u> 12:29(1980).
4. U. Feldt-Rasmussen, S. Husby, O. Blåbjerg, J. Date and H. Nielsen, <u>In vitro</u> characterization of synthesized thyroglobulin <u>immune</u> complexes(IC), <u>Allergy</u> 36:107(1981).
5. C.R. Strakosh, D. Joyner and J.R. Wall, Thyroid Stimulating antibodies in patients with autoimmune disorders, <u>J.Clin. Endocrinol.Metab.</u> 47:361(1978).

THE EFFECT OF THYROID STIMULATING IMMUNOGLOBULINS (TSI) ON THYROID cAMP: COMPARISON WITH TSH ACTIVITY

Sebastiano Filetti, Giuseppe Damante, Daniela Foti, Rosaria Catalfamo and Riccardo Vigneri

Cattedra di Endocrinologia, Università di Catania, Ospedale Garibaldi, USL 34, 95123 Catania, Italy

Thyroid stimulating immunoglobulins (TSI) are believed to act by interacting with TSH receptor as indicated by the ability of TSI to inhibit radiolabeled TSH binding to its receptor.[1] However a good correlation between the inhibition of TSH binding and TSI biological activity is not always demonstrable.[2] Moreover, other antibodies interact with the TSH receptor and block TSH activity but do not have any agonist activity.[3] The possibility remains, therefore, that TSI binds to the TSH receptor on a site different from the TSH-binding site, or alternatively that TSI may influence the TSH receptor via an allosteric mechanism.

The continuous thyrotropin stimulation of thyroid cells induce desensitization of the thyroid adenylate cyclase complex (homologous desensitization). This process is related to an "uncoupling" of the TSH receptor and the stimulatory N protein (Ns).[4]

Little information is available on the desensitization of thyroid tissue by TSI. If TSI primarily interacts with the TSH receptor: 1) it should be able to induce an homologous desensitization in respect to TSH stimulation; 2) thyroid desensitization to TSI stimulation should be similar to that observed for TSH.

The present study compares the thyroid desensitization by TSI and TSH. Since their actions are very similar, these observations provide indirect evidence that both agents are acting at a close related site and with a similar mechanism.

METHODS

Human thyroid cells in monolayer culture were obtained by a collagenase digestion procedure from normal thyroid tissue as previously described.[5] IgGs were purified from sera of Graves' patients by DEAE affy-gel column chromatography. Thyroid cell stimulation was performed as previously described and cellular cAMP was measured by radioimmunoassay.[5]

RESULTS AND DISCUSSION

a) TSH- and TSI-induced desensitization is homologous.

Preexposure of human thyroid cells to TSI for 8 hours reduced the subsequent cAMP response to both TSI and TSH (Figure 1). In parallel

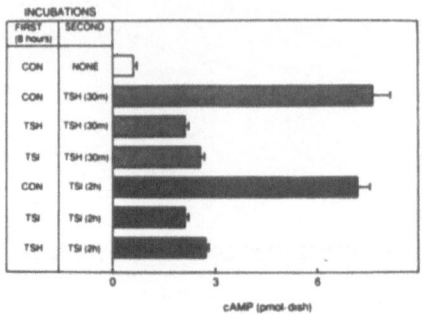

FIG. 1. Desensitization of the thyroid cell cAMP response induced by TSH
and TSI. Human thyroid cells were incubated (8 h) in control
medium or in medium supplemented with TSH (100 μU/ml) or TSI
(10 mg/ml). Then, a second incubation was performed in fresh
medium containing 1 mM MIX plus TSH (100 μU/ml) or TSI (10 mg/ml)
for the indicated times. Cellular cAMP content was then determined
Each bar represents the mean ± SD of values.

experiments, preincubation with TSH for 8 hours was also associated with
a reduced cell response to either stimulators. These results indicate that
TSH and TSI can substitute for each other in inducing an homologous
desensitization. Similarly to human cells, also in FRTL-5 cells, TSH and
TSI cross-desensitized each other.[6] Recovery from desensitization to either
agent occurred at the same rate, suggesting that TSH and TSI induced
desensitization by the same mechanism.

Cholera toxin stimulates cellular cAMP generation by interacting with
a specific cell surface receptor and then permanently activating the
stimulatory (Ns) regulatory protein of adenylate cyclase. Forskolin, on the
contrary, is believed to predominantly activate the adenylate cyclase
catalytic unit. The cAMP response to both these agents was equally effective
in thyroid cells preexposed to TSH or to TSI, confirming the homologous
nature of the desensitization (data not shown).

b) <u>Cycloheximide prevents both TSH- and TSI-induced desensitization</u>

Inhibitors of protein synthesis prevent TSH desensitization in cultured
human, dog and rat thyroid cells.[6,7] Similarly, in human thyroid cells the
presence of cycloheximide (10^{-4} M) for 8 h, together with TSI was able to
prevent the development of TSI-induced desensitization of adenylate cyclase ·
and greatly enhanced the thyroid cAMP response to TSI stimulation (Figure 2).

c) <u>Ni activation inhibits both TSH and TSI cAMP stimulation</u>

When thyroid cells are preexposed to epinephrine in the presence of
propranolol (α_2-adrenergic effect) an inhibition of the cAMP response to
TSH occurs and it is due to the Ni activation.[8] As shown in figure 3, the
activation of Ni also inhibits TSI induced cAMP stimulation, supporting
the idea that TSH and TSI follow similar pathways in stimulating thyroid
adenylate cyclase.

d) <u>Iodide inhibits the cAMP activation by both TSH and TSI</u>

When thyroid tissue is preexposed to iodide a form of desensitization
different from that induced by TSH occurs. The iodide-induced

352

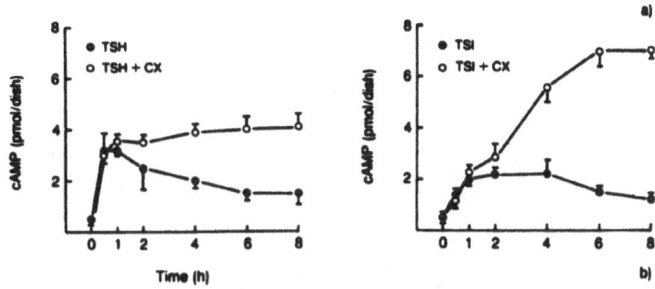

FIG. 2. Cycloheximide prevents TSH and TSI desensitization.
Human thyroid cells were incubated with (o) or without (•)
cycloheximide 10^{-4} M for 30 min. Then TSI (10 mg/ml) (panel a) or
TSH (100 μU/ml) (panel b) were added in the presence of 1 mM MIX.
At the indicated times cAMP content was determined. Each point
represents the mean ± SD of the values obtained in triplicate dishes.

desensitization involves an alteration in the functional activity of the
catalytic subunit of adenylate cyclase.[8] Preexposure of freshly dispersed
human thyroid cells to increasing concentrations of iodide led to a
progressive decline in the cAMP response to both TSH and TSI stimulation
(Figure 4). The dose response for iodide-induced inhibition was almost
superimposable for both TSH and TSI stimulation, once again illustrating
the remarkable similarities between the stimulations by these two agonists.

CONCLUSIONS

In conclusion, our data demonstrate remarkable similarities between
the desensitization induced in human thyroid cells by TSH and TSI. These
similarities provide indirect evidence that TSI interacts with the binding
site of the TSH receptor, and not through an allosteric mechanism.

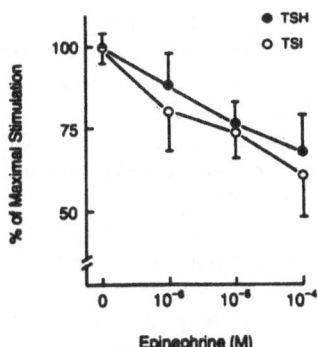

FIG. 3. Effect of Ni activation. Human thyroid cells were incubated in
medium plus propranolol (10^{-4} M) and epinephrine at the indicated
concentrations. Then TSH (100 μU/ml) or TSI (10 mg/ml) were added
in presence of MIX (1 mM). After 30 min (TSH) or 2 hours (TSI) the
cAMP content was determined. Each point represents the mean ± SD
of values obtained in triplicate dishes of cells.

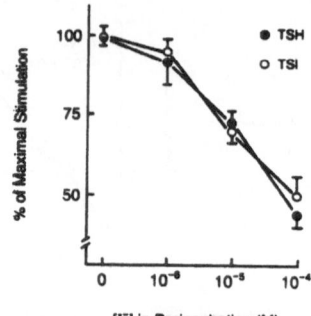

FIG. 4. Iodine effect. Inhibition by iodide of TSH (●) and TSI (o) cAMP
stimulation in cultured human thyroid cells. Thyroid cells were
preincubated for 4 hour in medium containing the indicating
concentrations of iodide. Subsequently, the cells were incubated
with TSH (100 μU/ml, 30 min) or TSI (10 mg/ml, 120 min) in presence
of 1 mM MIX, and the intracellular content of cAMP was then
determined. Each point represents the mean ± SD of values obtained
in triplicate dishes of cells.

REFERENCES

1. A. P. Weetman, A. M. McGregor, Autoimmune thyroid disease: Developments
   in our understanding. Endocr. Rev. 5:309 (1984).
2. E. Macchia, G. Fenzi, F. Monzani, L. Bartalena, F. Lippi, V. Aloisio,
   C. Cupini, L. Baschieri, A. Pinchera, TSH-displacing activity versus
   TSH-binding inhibiting activity of immunoglobulins from patients with
   Graves' disease. J. Endocrinol. Invest. 6:375 (1983)
3. M. Zakarija, J. M. McKenzie, D. S. Munro, Immunoglobulin G inhibitor of
   thyroid-stimulating antibody is a cause of delay in the onset of
   neonatal Graves' disease. J. Clin. Invest. 72:1352 (1983)
4. B. Rapoport, S. Filetti, N. Takai, P. Seto, Studies on the
   desensitization of the cyclic AMP response to thyrotropin in thyroid
   tissue. FEBS letters 146:23 (1982)
5. S. Filetti, M. Vetri, G. Damante, A. Belfiore, Thyroid autoregulation:
   effect of iodine on glucose trasport in cultured thyroid cells.
   Endocrinology 118:1395 (1986)
6. P. Vitti, L. Chiovato, P. Ceccarelli, A. Lombardi, M. Novaes, G. F. Fenzi
   A. Pinchera, Thyroid-stimulating antibody mimics thyrotropin in its
   ability to desensitize the adenosine 3',5'-monophosphate response to
   acute stimulation in continuously cultured rat thyroid cells (FRT-L5).
   J. Clin. Endocrinol. Metab. 63:454 (1986)
7. S. Filetti, B. Rapoport, Inhibitors of specific aminoacyl-tRNA
   synthetases prevent thyrotropin-induced desensitization in cultured
   human thyroid cells. J. Biol. Chem. 257:1342 (1982)
8. S. Filetti, B. Rapoport, Evidence that organic iodine alterates the
   adenosine 3',5'-monophosphate response to thyrotropin stimulation in
   thyroid tissue by an action at or near the adenylate cyclase catalytic
   unit. Endocrinology 113:1608 (1983)

PROLIFERATION IN CULTIVATED FOLLICLES OF GRAVES' THYROIDS:

IMMUNOHISTOCHEMICAL STUDIES WITH ANTIBODY KI-67

Michael Derwahl, Christian Sellschopp,
Heinrich M. Schulte, and Edgar E. Ohnhaus

I. Medizinische Klinik
Christian-Albrechts-Universität
Kiel, W.-Germany

INTRODUCTION

Widely varying growth rates in follicles of human multinodular goiters have been demonstrated (1). It has been suggested that vigorous stimuli such as thyroid growth stimulating immunoglobulins in Graves' disease may bring most of the follicular cells into mitotic cycle. To further investigate this issue, we studied the proliferation rates of cultivated thyroid follicles from tissue of patients with Graves' disease. Growth fractions were determined by immunostaining of tissue with the monoclonal antibody KI-67, which reacts with a human nuclear antigen, present in proliferating cells (G_1,S,G_2 and M phase of cycling cells) and absent in quiescent cells (2).

MATERIAL AND METHODS

Collagenase was obtained from Boehringer Mannheim (W-Germany). Eagle's minimum essential medium (MEM) with Earle's salt was obtained from Gibco Laboratories (Detroit, Michigan, USA) Insulin, bovine TSH and epidermal growth factor were obtained from Sigma Chemical Company (Munich, W-Germany). Fetal calf serum (FCS) was obtained from Seromed (Berlin, Germany).
Monoclonal antibodies were obtained as follow: antibody KI-67 and peroxidase-conjugated rabbit anti-mouse immunoglobulins from Dakopats (Copenhagen, Danmark), peroxidase-conjugated goat anti-rabbit IgG serum from Dianova (Hamburg, W.-Germany).
Tissue specimen were collected at surgery from enlarged thyroids (size II-III/WHO) of patients with Graves' disease (n=3),treated preoperatively with thiamazole, and from patients with multinodular goiters (size III, n=4). Thyroid follicles were prepared by technique of Herzog and Miller (3), using collagenase (10 mg/ml) for enzymatic digestion. Isolated follicular cells were cultivated in MEM supplemented with insulin (10 µg/ml) and 10 % FCS forming closed follicular structures within 24 h. Follicles were then kept in medium with different doses of TSH (0.01, 0.1, 1.0, 10 mU/ml) and/or epidermal growth factor (EGF 5 ng/ml) for further 72 h. Afterwards, cultivated follicles were cytocentrifuged and stained by indirect immunoperoxidase method using KI-67 as primary, peroxidase-conjugated rabbit anti-mouse IgG as secondary and peroxidase-conjugated goat

anti-rabbit IgG as tertiary antibody (6). Peroxidase was visualized by method of Graham and Karnowsky (5). Last, cytocentrifuge slides were counterstained with haemalum and mounted.
Unstimulated follicles incubated in vehicle medium were used as controls. Percentage of KI-67 positive cells were estimated at x 400 magnification by counting 500 cells.

The viability of cultivated follicles were assesed by trypan blue staining.

RESULTS

In unstimulated follicular cells derived from Graves' thyroids less than 10 % of nuclei were stained by KI-67 antibody (Table 1). Widely varying rates of KI-67 positive cells were found in unstimulated follicular cells of multinodular goiters. Incubation of follicles from Graves' thyroids with TSH concentrations (0.1 - 10 mU/ml) resulted in increasing numbers of KI-67 stained cells with a maximum at 1 mU/ml of TSH (Table 1). Adding TSH (1 mU/ml) and EGF (5 ng/ml) to culture dishes further increases of cycling cells were determined in Graves' thyroids (up to 45.1 %) and in follicles of multinodular goiters (up to 55.3 %).

Table 1: KI-67 positive cells in cultivated follicles of
Graves' thyroids and multinodular goiters
(percent of total)

	Graves' thyroids (n = 3)	Multinodular goiters (n = 4)
unstimulated	5.2 - 9.6	0 - 25
TSH 0.01	5.0 - 10.5	
(mU/ml) 0.1	8.3 - 15.8	
1.0	16.2 - 30.8	18.1 - 34.2
10.	11.8 - 17.3	
TSH 1.0 (mU/ml) + EGF 5.0 (ng/ml)	20.2 - 45.1	18.2 - 55.3

DISCUSSION

The monoclonal antibody KI-67 was developed for immunohistological estimation of the growth fractions in malignant tumours (6).
We applied this technique to determine the rates in cultivated follicles of Graves' disease comparing with growth rates in multinodular goiters.

Intense stimuli such as thyroid growth stimulating immunoglobulins were suggested to induce high proliferation rates in Graves' disease. In contrast, we determined low proliferation rates in unstimulated Graves' thyroids.
In multinodular goiters a wide variation of growth fractions were found as it is well known by autoradiographic studies of human goiter transplants (7).
Numbers of KI-67 labelled cells in Graves' disease and multinodular goiters were markedly increased by stimulation with TSH potentiated by addition of EGF. This potentiating effect suggest that both TSH and EGF are stimulators of thyroid cell growth.

The wide variance of growth rates in stimulated and less in unstimulated follicles of Graves' disease were surprising. However, the same phenomenom has been observed in other tissue cultures (8). Further investigations are needed to clarify this issue.

REFERENCES

1. H. Studer and F. Ramelli, Simple goiter and its variants: euthyroid and hyperthyroid multinodular goiters, Endocr. Rev. 3:40 (1982).
2. J. Gerdes, H. Lemke, H. Baisch, H.H. Wacker, U. Schwab and H. Stein, Cell cycle analysis of a cell proliferation-associated human nuclear antigen defined by the monoclonal antibody KI-67, J.Immunol. 133:1710 (1984).
3. V. Herzog and F. Miller, Membrane retrieval in epithelial cells of isolated thyroid follicles, Eur.J.Cell.Biol. 19:203 (1979).
4. J. Gerdes, An immunohistological method for estimating cell growth fractions in rapid histopathological diagnosis during surgery, Int.J.Cancer 35:169 (1985).
5. R. C. Graham and M. J. Karnowsky, The early stages of absorption of injected horseradish peroxidase in the proximal tubes of mouse kidney: ultrastructural cytochemistry by a new technique, J.Histochem.Cytochem. 14:291 (1966).
6. J. Gerdes, U. Schwab, H. Lemke and H. Stein, Production of a mouse monoclonal antibody reactive with a human nuclear antigen associated with cell proliferation, Int.J.Cancer, 31:13 (1983).
7. H.J. Peter, H. Gerber, H. Studer and S. Smeds, Pathogenesis of heterogeneity in human multinodular goiter, J.Clin.Invest., 76:1992 (1985).
8. A. Pardee, W.R. Dubrow, J.L. Hamlin and R.F. Kletzien, Animal cell cycle, Ann.Rev.Biochem., 47:715 (1978).

THE SIGNIFICANCE OF IMMUNOGLOBULINS RELATED TO STIMULATION OF THYROID GROWTH IN PATIENTS WITH ENDEMIC GOITER

Alfredo Halpern and Geraldo Medeiros-Neti

Thyroid Laboratory, Division of Endocrinology
Hospital das Clínicas, Univ São Paulo Medical School
05403. São Paulo, Brazil

The most prevalent and complicated form of thyroid disease is ironically named "simple goiter" and synonyms include euthy' roid goiter, nontoxic, diffuse or multinodular goiter. Most of these goiters are due to absolute or relative iodine deficiency or goitrogens in the diet or water supply. However, even in areas with plenty of iodine, the prevalence of simple or multino' dular goiter still ranges from 5-10%. The etiopatogeny of simple or multinodular goiter is related to stimuli to new follicle ge' neration induced by TSH (Iodine deficiency, inborn errors), local tissue growth factors or a controversial immunogenic growth fac' tor (TGI). Other factors leading to structural or functional he' terogeinity can also induce continuous pathological growth (1). Although thyroid autoimmunity has been studied intensively since 1956, the possibility that simple or endemic goiters may also arise from disturbances in the immunological system (Table 1) was raised only in the past fifteen years (2-14):

TABLE 1. IMMUNOGLOBULINS AFFECTING THYROID GROWTH IN GOITER.

AUTHOR(YEAR)	SOURCE	METHOD	RESULTS (POSITIVE)
BROWN (1978)	Porcine membranes	Inhibit TSH binding	42%
DREXHAGE (1980)	Guinea pig	Cytochemical bioassay	67%
CHIOVATO (1983)	Rat follicles	3-H Thymidine incorp.	30%
SCHATZ (1983)	Porcine follicles	3-H Thymidine incorp.	38%
WIENER (1985)	Guinea pig	Cytochemical bioassay	77%[2]
VAN DER GAAG (1985)	Guinea pig	Cytochemical bioassay	67%[1]
ROTELLA (1985)	FRTL-5	3-H Thymidine uptake	53%[1]
KNOBEL (1986)	Porcine membranes	Inhibit TSH binding	39%
SMYTH (1986)	Guinea pig	G6PD increase	63%
MEDEIROS-NETO (1986)	FRTL-5	3-H Thymidine uptake	63%[1]
SCHATZ (1986)	Porcine follicles	3-H Thymidine uptake	27-38%[1]

[1] Endemic   [2] Plummer

As shown in this Table the diversity of the methods used by different investigators and laboratories made it difficult to as' certain if these results are comparable. Moreover Valente et al (5) could not detect any growth-promoting antibodies in simple goiter (sporadic) nor could find any correlation between goiter

size and "in vitro" TGI activity. Later, Rotella et al(9), how'
ever, was able to demonstrate in a serie of sera obtained from
endemic areas of Tuscany (Italy) that IgG samples from 16 of 30
patients with nontoxic multinodular goiter (53%) and 13 of 21
with nontoxic simple goiter (62%) had growth promoting activity.
More recently Van der Gaag et al (8) studying 62 consecutive ca'
ses of sporadic simple euthyroid goiter (15 as diffuse, 39 as
multinodular and 8 as single nodules) observed that 43 (67%) we'
re positive for TGI by the Feulgen cytochemical assay, using Gui'
nea pig cells in culture. Negative results were obtained in 20
normal subjects. It was claimed that defects in T supressor cell
function in such patients may underlie the exaggerated response
of TGI-specific autoimmune B-cell clones. None of the positive
TGI sera studied showed cAMP stimulation. Some were weakly posi'
tive for TBII (blocking) but the responses failed to correlate
with the presence of TGI. This lack of correlation may imply
that TGIs are either not TSH receptor antibodies or, if they are
recognized antigenic determinants on the receptor differently
from the TSH-binding size, probably with a strong affinity for
the ganglioside receptor component (12).

Smith and co-workers (11) using a different method, in
which TGI was measured by its effect on glucose-6-phosphate dehy'
drogenase (GGPP) and thyroid stimulating antibody is measured by
its effect on lysosomal naphthylamidase (L Nase) activity in Gui'
nea pig thyroid follicular cells, demonstrated that 50% of pati'
ents with Plummer's disease and 62% of subjects with simple goi'
ter had a positive TGI activity. Schatz and co-workers (13)
using the stimulation of ^{3}H thymidine incorporation into isola'
ted porcine thyroid follicles and IgG from goitrous patients li'
ving in an iodine-deficient region indicated that the sera of 20
out of 72 patients (27%) with euthyroid goiter and of 10 out of
26 patients (38%) with recurrent euthyroid goiter contained IgGs
stimulating thyroid growth (TGI). There was no correlation of
TGI with other thyroid antibodies (TSAb or TBII).No clear-cut re'
lationship could be demonstrated between TGI and goiter size.

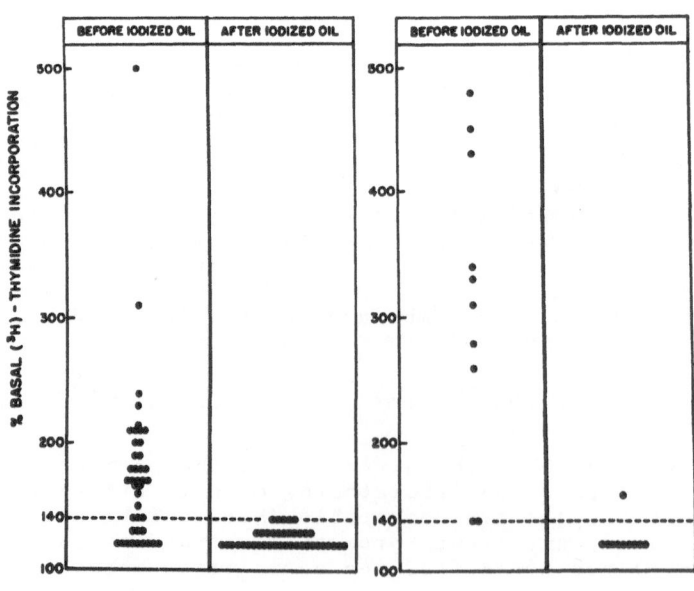

Finally Medeiros-Neto et al (14) using FRTL-5 system and
3-H thymidine uptake were able to demonstrate that 63% of the en'
demic multinodular goitrous patients living in iodine deficiency
areas had a positive test for TGI. Only four of the positive TGI
patients had a concomitant increase in cAMP following introduc'
tion of IgG. All patients, except 1 had no IgG stimulation
(<120%) of growth promoting activity 1 year after an im injec'
tion of iodized oil, that also induced a remarkable shrinkage of
the glands.

There was a significant positive correlation between thyroid
growth promoting activity and serum Tg concentration (r= .58,
p<0.01). It was concluded that growth promoting IgGs lacking
ability to stimulate cAMP production may play a role in the lar'
ge multinodular goiter due to chronic iodine deficiency. In or'
der to test that the growth promoting activity was present in
the IgG fraction, anti-human, anti-rat, and anti-goat immunoglo'
bulins coupled with sepharose were incubated with IgG prepara'
tions from patients from endemic goiter areas (14).

Only with anti-human IgG there was a significant reduction
in the growth promoting activity, not obtained with anti-rat or
anti-goat. Similarly anti-human TSH was unable to block the
growth promoting ability of the IgG preparations for these pa'
tients. Thus the activity could not be explained by TSH contami'
nation. The increase in thymidine uptake was confirmed by stu'
dies measuring cell number, in culture, for 14 days. The IgGs
from endemic goiter patients were able to increase the cell num'
ber in a fashion similar of IgG's from patients with Graves' di'
sease.

In general, in all the studies that were mentioned here, TGI
in sporadic and simple goiter was approximately 10 times less po'
tent than that in goitrous hyperthyroid Graves' disease. As the
thyroid gland is composed of follicular cells which differ in
their ability to synthetize thyroid hormones, to respond to TSH
and to replicate, it is possible that a mild stimuli as brought
by TGI will act upon a normal heterogeneous gland and cause en'
largement with both hyperthrophy and hyperplasia. Within this
same concept growth promoting activity, arising from disorders
of immune regulation, could increase the size and nodularity of
the goiter in patients already under chronic iodine deficiency.
Further studies are needed, however, to support this concept.

References

1. H.Studer & F.Ramelli, Endocrine Rev 3:40-61 (1982).
2. R.S.Brown, I.M.D.Jackson, S.C.Pohl & S.Reichlin, Lancet i:
   904-906 (1978).
3. H.A.Drexhage, G.F.Botazzo, D.Doniach, Bitensky & J.Chayen,
   Lancet i:287-292 (1980).
4. L.Chiovato, L.J.Hammond, T.Hanafusa, R.Pujol-Borrel, D.Do'
   niach & G.F.Botazzo, Clin Endocrinol 19:581-590 (1983).
5. W.A.Valente, P.Vitti, C.M.Rotella, M.M.Vaughan, S.M.Aloj,
   E.F.Grollman, F.S.H.Ambesi-Impiombato & L.D.Kohn, N Engl J
   Med 309:1028-1034 (1983).
6. H.Schatz, F.H.Beckman & M.Floren, Horm Metab Res 15:627-628
   (1983).
7. J.D.Wiener & R.D.Van der Gaag, Clin Endocr (Oxf) 23:635-642
   (1986).

8. R.D.Van der Gaag, H.A.Drexhage, W.M.Wiersinga, R.S.Brown, R. Dolter, G.F.Botazzo & D.Doniach, J Clin Endocr Metab 60:972 979 (1985).
9. C.M.Rotella, R.Toccafondi, W.Hoffman, W.A.Valente, G.A.Medei' ros-Neto & L.D.Kohn, American Thyroid Association, New York, Abstract nº 17 (1984).
10. M.Knobel & G.A.Medeiros-Neto, IRCS Med Sci (Endocrine) 14: 366-367 (1986).
11. P.P.A.Smith, Giubeck-Loebeinstem & N.M.McMullan, In: Medeiros -Neto GA & Gaitan E(eds) "Frontiers in THyroidology". Plenum Press. New York (1986).
12. S.M.Aloj, G.Mariocci, M.De Luca, S.Shifrin, E.Grollman, W. Valente & L.A.Kohn, In: Peptide Hormones, Biomembranes and Cell Growth, L.Bolis, E.Verna, L.Frati (eds), Plenum Press, New York, 169-195 (1984).
13. H.Schatz, K.Pschierer-Berg, J.A.Nickel, R.Bar, F.Muller, R. G.Bretzel, H.Muller & H.Stracke, Acta Endocrinol 112:523- 530 (1986).
14. G.A.Medeiros-Neto, A.Halpern, Z.S.Cozzi, N.Lima & L.D.Kohn, J Clin Endocrinol Metab 63:644-650 (1986).

REGULATION OF GROWTH OF THYROID CELLS IN CULTURE BY TSH RECEPTOR ANTIBODIES AND OTHER HUMORAL FACTORS

Donatella Tramontano, Gary W. Cushing, Masanobu Mine,
Alan C. Moses, Francesco Beguinot and Sidney H. Ingbar

Beth Israel Hospital and Joslin Diabetes Center
Harvard Medical School, Boston, MA, USA

Highly differentiated target endocrine epithelia provide a valuable model for studies of cell replication, since their growth is regulated by their specific trophic hormone and since they may possibly respond as well to those growth factors that interact with a variety of cell types. Hence, studies of the independent and conjoint effects of trophic hormones and growth factors in target endocrine cells have the potential to elucidate both general mechanisms for the regulation of cell growth and abnormalities in endocrine cell growth that occur in disease.

As a part of studies on the regulation of thyroid cell growth, both normally and in disease states, we have examined growth regulation in FRTL5 cells, a line of non-transformed rat thyroid follicular cells, that over many years in culture have retained most of the differentiated functions of thyroid tissue (1). Most importantly, growth of FRTL5 cells is largely dependent on the presence of TSH. Even in the presence of high concentration of serum, FRTL5 cell remain quiescent and fail to grow in the absence of TSH, but resume their growth upon the readdition of the hormone (2,3). This effect of TSH is mimicked by TSH receptor antibodies (TRAb) of Graves' disease, which, like TSH, promptly stimulate adenylate-cyclase activity in FRTL5 cells (4). The growth promoting activity of TSH and TRAb is mimicked by various agents which increase intracellular levels cAMP in FRTL5 cells, suggesting that the mitogenic effect of TSH receptor agonists is, at least in part, cAMP mediated.

The particular objective in these studies has been to examine the effects on the growth of FRTL5 cells of well known classical growth factors, whose effects are not tissue specific, and their possible interaction with specific thyroid growth-stimulating factors, such as TSH and TRAb. Our attention has focused mainly on the effects of insulin-like growth factor I (IGF-I) and interleukin-1 (IL-1). IGF-I has been shown to stimulate growth and metabolic functions in various tissues, principally those of mesenchimal origin. IL-1, on the other hand has been thought to stimulate proliferation only of lymphocytes and some cells of mesenchymal origin.

Contrary to the expectation that growth of FRTL5 cells is absolutely dependent on the action of TSH receptor agonists, our results show that both IGF-I (5) and IL-1 alone can stimulate growth of FRTL5 cells. When added to quiescent FRTL5 cells, IGF-I and IL-1 produced a dose-dependent stimulation of ^{3}H-thymidine incorporation into DNA. In some system growth factors do not promote cell replication although they stimulate DNA synthesis (6); therefore to ascertain that DNA synthesis stimulated

Table 1. Independent effects of growth factors on FRTL5 cells

Functions	TSH	TRAb	IGF-I	IL 1
DNA synthesis	++	++	++	+
Increase in cell number	++	++	+	+

by IGF-I and IL-1 reflected actual cell proliferation, we have examined growth curves on cells treated with each growth factor. As expected quiescent FRTL5, in the absence of TSH failed to grow, while those treated with IGF-I or IL-1 showed a significant increase in cell number (Table 1).

Of greatest interest is the finding that, with respect to DNA synthesis, IGF-I and IL-1 strongly potentiate the mitogenic effects of TSH receptor agonists. When quiescent FRTL5 were treated with IGF-I or IL-1 in the presence of TSH or TRAb, a dramatic enhacement of ^{3}H-thymidine incorporation into DNA was observed. The extent of these effects was dependent upon the concentration of each agent and it was far greater than the sum of ^{3}H-thymidine incorporation stimulated in the presence of each agent alone. When cell numbers were measured in the same condition an additive, rather than synergistic effect, was observed (Table 2).

The mechanism through which IGF-I and IL 1 stimulate cell proliferation is not clear, but it is apparently not cAMP mediated, since the two peptides have failed to stimulate adenylate-cyclase in many systems of cells in culture. As expected, when tested in FRTL5 cells, IGF-I and IL 1 neither increased adenylate-cyclase activity directly nor increased the stimulation thereof produced by TSH and TRAb (Table 2). Thus, there exist in FRTL5 cells at least two separate pathways for growth stimulation: one cAMP-dependent, that is stimulated by TSH receptor agonists, and one (or more) cAMP-independent that can be stimulated by IGF-I and IL-1. When these pathways are concomitantly activated their interaction results in a pronounced enhancement of growth.

The interaction of IGF-I and IL-1 with Graves'-IgG mimics almost perfectly their interaction with TSH, suggesting that the diverse effects of Graves'-IgG in FRTL5 cells, including their ability to stimulate thyroid cell growth, are mediated at the same receptor and by the same mechanism as those which mediate the response to TSH.

The results obtained with cell in cultures should be extrapolated to

Table 2. Modification of TSH and TRAb effects

	DNA synthesis	Cell number	cAMP generation
IGF-I	potentiates	additive	no effect
IL 1	potentiates	additive	no effect

Table 3. Factors that influence thyroid cell growth and their interactions.

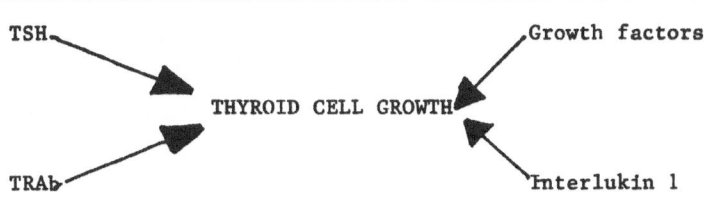

the _in vivo_ situation only with great caution. Nontheless, the independent stimulatory effect of IGF-I on thyroid cell growth may relate to the inordinate frequency of goiter in patients with acromegaly. In addition, the effect of IL-1 on FRTL5 cells raises the possibility that IL-1 generated locally in the thyroid beset by autoimmune diseases can act directly on the thyroid by a short-loop mechanism, both to stimulate follicular cell growth and to synergize the goitrogenic effects of TSH and TRAb.

The findings that we have described are summarized in Table 3. The schema indicates that control of thyroid cell replication is the result of complex interactions among various hormones, nutrients and growth factors. In FRTL5 cells, factors other than TSH receptor agonists are capable of stimulating growth, in some cases, as with IGF-I and IL 1, acting through pathways that differ from those utilized by the trophic hormone. As shown by the connecting arrows, these pathways may interact with one another to produce an amplified growth response.

Despite its complexity, this schema undoubtedly represents a gross oversimplification of the mechanism of regulation of thyroid cell growth. Other interactions between these classes of growth regulators have not yet been studied and remain possible. Surely, the pursuit of a full understanding of the regulation of thyroid cell growth will diffi- cult and time consuming, but will be worth the effort for the under- standing, not only of thyroid growth in health and disease, but also for the regulation of cell growth in general.

REFERENCES

1. Ambesi-Impiombato FS, Picone R, Tramontano D, 1982 In: Sirbasku DA, Sato GH, Pardee A (eds) Cold Spring Harbor Conference on Cell Proli- feration. Cold Spring Harbor Laboratory. vol 9:483
2. Valente WA, Vitti P, Kohn LD, Brandi ML, Rotella CM, Toccafondi R, Tramontano D, Aloj SM, Ambesi-Impiombato FS, 1983 Endocrinology 112:71
3. Tramontano D, Chin WW, Moses AC, Ingbar SH, 1986 J. Biol. Chem. 261:3919
4. Valente WA, Vitti P, Rotella CM, Vaughan MM, Aloj SM, Grollman EF, Ambesi-Impiombato FS, Kohn LD, 1983 New Engl. J. Med. 309:1028
5. Tramontano D, Cushing GW, Moses AC, Ingbar SH, 1986 Endocrinology 119:940
6. Moses AC, Cohen KL, Johnsonbaugh R, Nissley SP, 1976 J. Clin. Endo. Metab. 46:9

POLYAMINE MODULATION OF RESPONSES TO

GRAVES'IgG IN GUINEA PIG AND HUMAN THYROID

P.P.A. Smyth and A.E. Corcoran

Department of Medicine
University College, Dublin, Ireland

INTRODUCTION

The ubiquitous naturally occurring polyamines have been implicated as intracellular messengers in a variety of tissues. An early consequence of TSH stimulation of thyroid follicular cells is the induction of ornithine decarboxylase(ODC)activity leading to increased production of polyamines. It is the aim of this study to investigate if Graves' IgG exert their stimulatory action on the thyroid via the polyamine pathway both in the established guinea pig thyroid system used in cytochemical bioassay(CBA) for thyroid stimulators or in organ cultures of human thyroid.

MATERIALS AND METHODS

Segments of guinea pig thyroid or blocks of human tissue from surgical specimens with a histologically demonstrated rich supply of follicles were incubated for 5 hours with test substances. The tissues were snap frozen and changes in glucose-6-phospate dehydrogenase (G6PD) activity within thyroid follicular cells from frozen sections of tissue were studied cytochemically. The ODC inhibitor difluoromethylornithine (DFMO) was a gift from Merrell Dow, Strasbourg, France.

RESULTS

As shown in Fig.1 incubation of guinea pig or human thyroid with individual polyamines spermidine (10^{-8} - 10^{-3} M) or putrescine (10^{-7} - 10^{-3} M) resulted in the increases in G6PD activity over control values in both tissue types. The responses to both polyamines were greater in human than in guinea pig thyroid thissue.

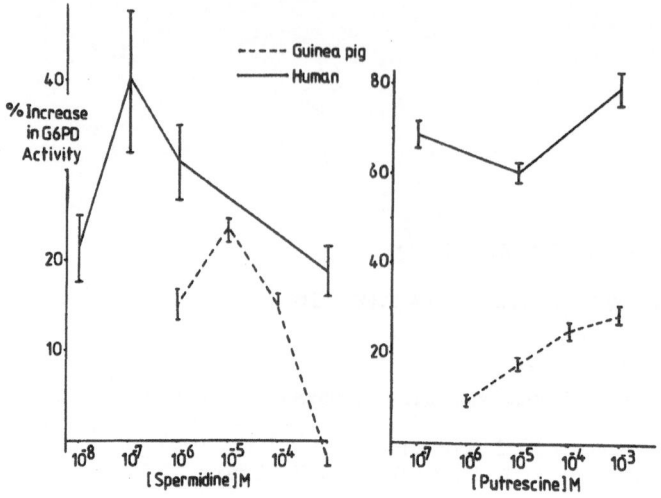

Fig.1 In vitro effects of individual polyamines on G6PD activity in
guinea pig or human thyroid.

Incubating segments of human thyroid for 5 hrs with bovine TSH(5mu/1)
or Graves'IgG(100ug/ml)produced significant increases in G6PD activity in
thyroid follicular cells as shown in Fig,2. Inclusion in the incubation
medium of the ODC inhibitor DFMO which inhibits polyamine production resulted in highly significant reductions of both TSH and Graves' IgG
stimulated G6PD activity.

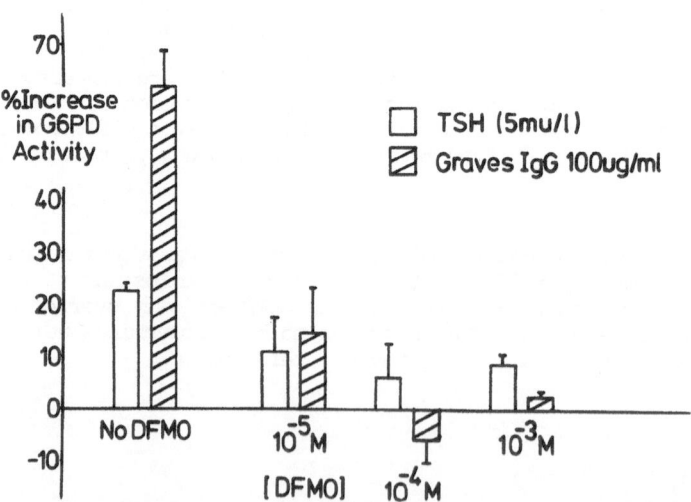

Fig.2 inhibitory effects of DFMO on TSH and Graves' IgG stimulated G6PD
activity in human thyroid.

Fig.3 shows the effect on G6PD activity of incubating thyroid tissue from another patient with Graves' IgG. Addition of DFMO (10^{-3} M) to the incubation medium significantly inhibited the increase in G6PD activity although in this case did not remove it. However, inclusion of the polyamines spermidine (10^{-6} M) or putrescine (10^{-3} M)restored the initial stimulatory response observed with Graves' IgG alone.

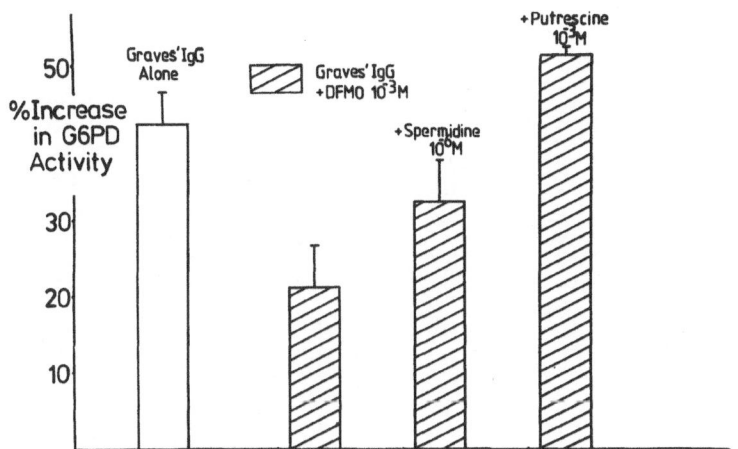

Fig.3 Reversal by polyamines of DFMO inhibited Graves' IgG induced G6PD activity in human thyroid.

DISCUSSION

The results suggest that Graves'IgG in vitro exert their trophic action on guinea pig or human thyroid via ODC induced polyamine biosynthesis. The findings while demonstrating a critical role for polyamines in mediating thyroid stimulation also support the concept of common trophic pathway for TSH and Graves' IgG.

1. E. Pegg,Biochem J 234: 249(1986)

2. W. I. Combest and D. H. Russell, Mol. Pharmacol 23: 641 (1983)

3. P.P.A. Smyth, N.M. McMullan, B.Grubeck Loebenstein and D. K. O'Donovan. Acta Endocr. iii: 321 (1986)

Fig. 3.

EVIDENCE FOR INTRATHYROIDAL PRODUCTION OF

THYROID GROWTH-STIMULATING IMMUNOGLOBULINS

H. Schatz, I. Ludwig, F. Wiss and P.E. Goretzki[+]

Center of Internal Medicine, University of Giessen and
[+]Surgical Department, University of Düsseldorf

INTRODUCTION

Thyroid stimulating antibodies appear to be produced predominantly by intrathyroidal lymphocytes (1). In this study it should be tested whether thyroid growth-stimulating immunoglobulins (TGI) are also mainly produced within the thyroid gland.

PATIENTS AND METHODS

During thyroid surgery blood was drawn simultaneously from a thyroid vein (vena thyreoidea media) and from a peripheral vessel (the arteria brachialis in Graves' disease having been hyperthyroid prior to preoperative treatment, n=1o , or a cubital vein in goitrous Graves' disease being euthyroid since longer time, n=3 , and in nontoxic goitre, n=7) in a first series of altogether 2o patients. The immunoglobulins were fractionated by ammonium sulphate precipitation followed by dialysis and all antibody determinations were carried out with these fractionated immunoglobulins. TGI were estimated by measuring H-3-thymidine incorporation into FRTL-5-cells (2) kindly donated by Dr. L. Kohn, Bethesda, and thyrotropin binding inhibiting antibodies (TBIAb) by a commercial kit (TRAK-Assay, Henning). Antibodies against thyroglobulin and thyroid microsomes were also determined (Thymune T and M, Wellcome).

In a second series of patients mostly operated for nontoxic goitre total thyroxine and total triiodothyronine were estimated in serum samples of thyroid venous and peripheral blood using a coated tube - assay commercially avaible from Diagnostic Products Corporation. (The antibody determinations will also be performed for this second series within the next time).

RESULTS

From figure 1 it can be seen that TGI were , altogether, higher in venous blood compared to peripheral blood. Similar data were obtained for TBIAb (figure 1, right part) whereas there was not much difference for anti-thyroglobulin and anti-microsomal antibodies (figure 2).

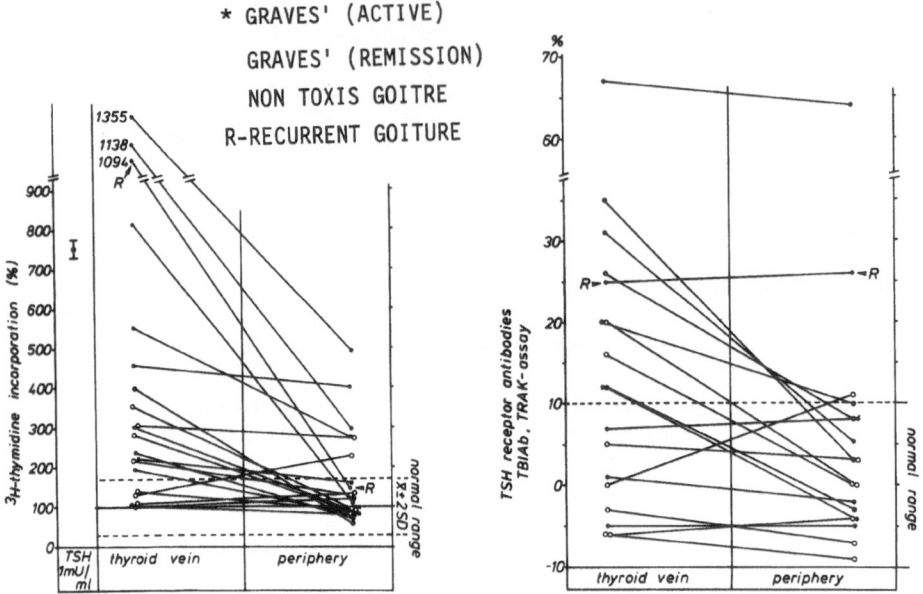

Fig. 1. Thyroid growth-stimulating immunoglobulins (TGI, left part), and
TSH-binding inhibiting antibodies (TBIAb, right part) in thyroid
venous and peripheral blood taken simultaneously during thyroid
surgery.

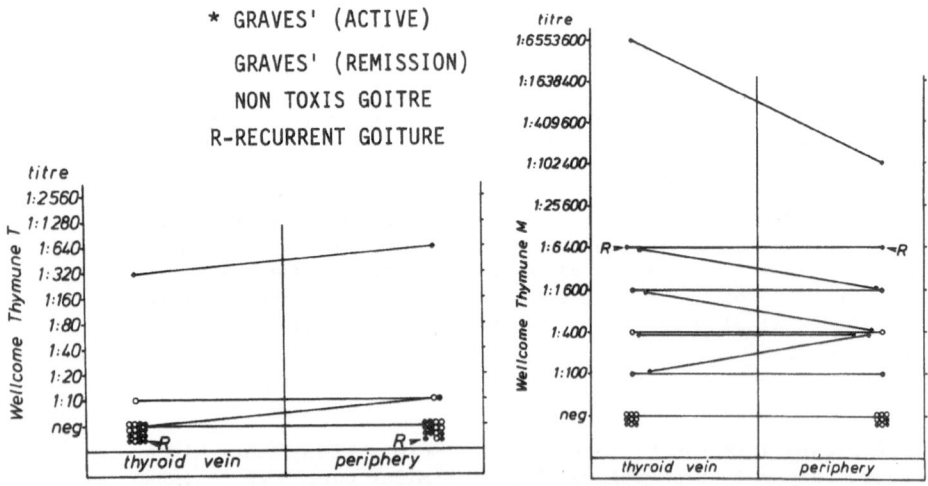

Fig. 2; Antibodies against thyroglobulin (Thymune T) and thyroid microsomes (Thymune M) in thyroid venous and peripheral blood (see
legend to fig. 1).

In the second series of (mostly euthyroid) patients triiodothyronine was significantly higher in the thyroid vein compared to peripheral blood whereas thyroxine showed hardly any difference (table 1).

Table 1. Triiodothyronine and thyroxine levels in serum simultaneously drawn from thyroid venous and peripheral blood during surgery of 25 patients with mostly euthyroid goitre. MEAN $\pm$ SEM

	thyroid vein	periphery
triiodothyronine ng/dl	131 $\pm$ 9.8 p o.o5	lo5 $\pm$ 7.96
thyroxine µg/dl	11.2 $\pm$ o.76 n.s.	lo.7 $\pm$ o.59

DISCUSSION

TGI appear to be produced mainly within the thyroid gland thus resembling TBIAb(1). The highest (thyroid venous) TGI and TBIAb levels were observed in goitrous patients with Graves' disease as it was to expect from the literature. In nontoxic goitre, TGI were much lower or negative, and TBIAb values in thyroid venous blood were only in the low positive range in 2 out of 7 cases,and in peripheral blood borderline positive in 1 case. The findings for TGI aggree with previous reports about a lower incidence of TGI in iodine-deficient areas with endemic goitre compared to sporadic goitre regions (cf.4). In the second series of (mostly euthyroid) patients triiodothyronine levels were significantly higher in the thyroid vein compared to peripheral blood, however not too much. No significant difference was calculated for thyroxine. Considering the relatively long halflife of immunoglobulins one is wondering why the differences for TGI and TBIAb were numerically so high. This may be explained by the test systems for TGI and TBIAb giving non-arithmetically distributed results. It may also be speculated that both TGI and TBIAb are bound (and degraded) on peripheral receptor sites too, e.g.on fat cells. A preferential production within the thyroid gland of antibodies against thyroglobulin and thyroid microsomes is not apparent from our study.

REFERENCES

1. P. Kendall-Taylor, A.J. Knox, N.R. Steel, S. Atkinson, Evidence that thyroid-stimulating antibody is produced in the thyroid gland, Lancet 2 : 654 (1984).

2. H. Schatz, I. Ludwig, F. Wiss, P.E. Goretzki, Pathophysiological and clinical implications of thyroid growth stimulating immunoglobulins, in: "Advances in Thyroidology", B. Wenzel, P.C. Scriba and D. Beysel eds., Acta endocrinol. (Kbh), Suppl., in press.

3. H. Schatz, K. Pschierer-Berg, J.-A. Nickel, R. Bär, F. Müller, R.G. Bretzel, H. Müller and H. Stracke, Assay$_3$for thyroid growth stimulating immunoglobulins: stimulation of ^{3}H-thymidine incorporation into isolated thyroid follicles by TSH, EGF, and immunoglobulins from goitrous patients in an iodine-deficient region, Acta endocrinol. (Kbh) 112 : 523 (1986).

4. H.A. Drexhage and R. van der Gaag, Thyroid growth stimulating immunoglobulins (TGI) and goitre, in:"The Thyroid and Autoimmunity", H.A. Drexhage and W.M. Wiersinga , eds., Excerpta Medica, ICS 711 Amsterdam - New York - Oxford (1986).

PRESENCE OF THYROID GROWTH PROMOTING ANTIBODY IN PATIENTS WITH GRAVES' DISEASE IN REMISSION: MEDICAL versus SURGICAL THERAPY

Carlo M. Rotella, Carmelo Mavilia, Enrico Vallin[*], Andrea
Lopponi and Roberto Toccafondi

Clinica Medica III   Surgery Section[*]
Universita' di Firenze   I.N.R.C.A., Sede di Firenze
Firenze, Italy

INTRODUCTION

FRTL-5 rat thyroid cells are a stable line of cultured rat thyroid cells whose growth and function exhibit a requirement for TSH in the culture medium (1). We have already reported on the value of these cells for detecting thyroid stimulating antibody (TSAb) in Graves' patients by measuring the effect on cAMP levels (2). We have also reported on the ability of these cells to measure thyroid growth promoting antibody (TGPAb) using (3H)-thymidine incorporation into DNA as an assay tool (3). When these systems were used, the incidence of TSAb and TGPAb in untreated Graves' disease patients is very high (95% and 83% respectively) and a good correlation between the two assays esixts (3). It has already been demonstrated that Graves' disease patients in remission maintain detectable TSAb values in a limited number of cases (0-20%)(4-6), but no data are available about the persistence of TGPAb after therapy. In the present report we have studied the presence of both TSAb and TGPAb in 85 patients previously affected by Graves' disease, but at present in phase of remission after surgical (40 patients) or pharmacological (45 patients) treatment.

PATIENTS AND METHODS

The diagnosis of hyperthyroidism due to Graves' disease was based on clinical findings, including diffuse goiter, elevated serum levels of thyroid hormones, and absent response to TRH, high thyroid radioiodide uptake values and diffuse isotope uptake on thyroid scan. 40 of these patients underwent subtotal thyroidectomy when first diagnosed, while the other 45 were treated with methymazole (MMI). The group of 40 surgically treated patients ranged in age from 19 to 75 years, 36 of them were women. Surgical treatment was undertaken at the utmost after two months the diagnosis of Graves' disease was placed; surgery, as a treatment of choice, was determined by the dimension of goiter, or the presence of compression symptoms. All patients were euthyroid at the time of the present study, but six of them were treated with thyroxine (150–200 μg/day). The phase of remission lasted 12 to 141 months. The 45 patients treated with MMI had an age ranging from 12 to 74 years, 35 of them were women. The pharmacological treatment lasted 10 to 18 months, in order to obtain a complete remission; at the time of the present study all patients were euthyroid in the absence of any therapy, except two, who were treated with thyroxine (150 μg/day). Time elapsed from the remission of Graves' disease and this study varied from 6 to 12 months. The functional state of 85 Graves' patients in remission was evaluated on the basis of the clinical findings, of serum levels of thyroid hormones and of the normality of TSH response to TRH stimulation.

The immunoglobulins obtained from sera of patients with HT were tested using the FRTL–5 thyroid cell system to detect both TSAb and TGPAb. TSAb activity was measured by cAMP cellular levels in 24 well plastic plates, after two hour incubation with the IgG preparations (2). The intracellular cAMP was measured by a protein binding assay and the amount of cAMP was corrected by the DNA content of each well, as assesed by the ethidium bromide fluorescence method. The TGPAb activity was evaluated by measuring the tritiated thymidine incorporation into FRTL–5 cell DNA, measured by the diphenylamine method (3).

RESULTS AND CONCLUSIONS

We have compared TSAb, measured cAMP accumulation in FRTL–5 cells, and TGPAb, measured as tritiated thymidine incorporation in FRTL–5 cell DNA, in 40 Graves' patients in remmission after surgical therapy. When the responsiveness in the individual tests was considered, 8 patients (20%) were TSAb(+)ve and 27 patients (67.5%) were TGPAb(+)ve. When combined assays were considered in the 40 surgically treated patients, the following results were obtained: 12 (30%) were TSAb(−)ve/TGPAb(−)ve; 1 (2.5%) was TSAb(+)ve/TGPAb(−)ve; 20 (50%) were TSAb(−)ve/TGPAb(+)ve; and 7 (17.5%) were TSAb(+)ve /TGPAb(+)ve.

We have also compared TSAb, measured as cAMP accumulation in FRTL–5 cells, and TGPAb, measured as tritiated thymidine incorporation in FRTL–5 cell DNA, in 45 Graves' patients in remmission after therapy with MMI. When the responsiveness in the individual tests was considered, 9 patients (20%) were TSAb(+)ve and 18 patients (40%) were TGPAb(+)ve. When combined assays were considered in the 45 MMI treated patients, the following results were obtained: 22 (48.9%) were TSAb(−)ve/TGPAb(−)ve; 5 (11.1%) were TSAb(+)ve/TGPAb(−)ve; 14 (31.1%) were TSAb(−)ve/TGPAb(+)ve; and 4 (8.9%) were TSAb(+)ve/TGPAb(+)ve.

When the incidence of TGPAb in surgically treated Graves' disease patients was correlated to the time elapsed after surgery, no correlation between the number of months elapsed after surgery and the percent (3H)–thymidine incorporation in the growth assay exists. On the other hand, if the patients studied between 12 and 36 months alone were considered, the incidence of TGPAb(+)ve cases is 10 out of 12 (83.3%), which is similar to that of untreated patients. In the patients studied between 37 and 132 months after surgery, the incidence of TGPAb(+)ve cases is 17 out of 28 (60.7%).

TSAb and TGPAb values of MMI treated Graves' patients were compared to those of same patients studied before the onset of treatment. Mean (+ SD) TSAb value of these patients before therapy was 289.5 + 179.0 % and 111.2 + 84.7 % after therapy (p < 0.01). Mean (+ SD) TGPAb value in the same patients was 260.8 + 135.1 % before therapy and 139.2 + 72.5 % after therapy. TSAb(+)ve Graves' patients were 37 (82.2%) before therapy and 18 (40.0%) after therapy.

Present data indicate that in treated Graves' disease patients there is not such a good correlation between TSAb and TGPAB, as before the onset of therapy; that a considerable number of TGPAb(+)ve /TSAb(-)ve cases appear; and that the incidence of TGPAb is higher than that of TSAb, this incidence being significantly higher in patients treated surgically, with respect to those treated with MMI (67.5 vs. 40.0 %). Considering that treated Graves' patients were in a phase of clinical remission, and that no recurrence of goiter was present in surgically treated patients, we can conclude that the presence of TGPAb is of poor prognostic value in the follow-up of Graves' disease patients.

REFERENCES

1. F. S. Ambesi-Impiombato, R. Picone, and D. Tramontano, Influence of hormones and serum on growth and differentiation of the thyroid cell strain FRTL, in: "Growth of cells in hormonally defined media", Cold Spring Harbor Laboratory, p.483 (1982).
2. P. Vitti, C. M. Rotella, W. A. Valente, J. Cohen, S. M. Aloj, P. Laccetti, F. S. Ambesi-Impiombato, E. F. Grollman, A. Pinchera, R. Toccafondi, and L. D. Kohn, Characterization of the optimal stimulatory effects of Graves' monoclonal and serum immuno-globulin G on adenosine 3', 5' monophosphate production in FRTL-5 thyroid cells: a potential clinical assay, J. Clin. Endocrinol. Metab. 57:782 (1983).
3. W. A. Valente, P. Vitti, C. M. Rotella, M. M. Vaughan, S. M. Aloj, E. F. Grollman, F. S. Ambesi-Impiombato, and L. D. Kohn, Antibodies that promote thyroid growth: a distinct population of thyroid promoting antibodies. New Engl. J. Med. 309:1028 (1983).
4. F. A. Karlsson, and P. A. Dahlberg, Thyroid stimulating antibodies (TSAb) in patients with Graves' disease undergoing antithyroid drug treatment: indicators of activity of disease, Clin. Endocrinol. 14:579 (1981).
5. K. Bech, U. Feldt-Rasmussen, H. Bliddal, J. Date, and M. Blichert--Toft, The acute changes in thyroid stimulating immunoglobulins, thyroglobulin and thyroglobulin antibodies following subtotal thyroidectomy, Clin. Endocrinol. 16:235 (1982).
6. H. Bliddal, K. Bech, and C. Kirkegaard, Thyroid stimulating immunoglobulins in patients in long-term remission after Graves' disease, Horm. metab. Res. 16:602 (1984).

THYROTROPHIN AND GROWTH PROMOTING IMMUNOGLOBULIN(TGI) OF FRTL-5 CELLS HAVE NO GROWTH STIMULATING ACTIVITY ON HUMAN THYROID EPITHELIAL CELL CULTURES

B.E. Wenzel, M. Dwenger, T. Mansky, U. Engel*, V. Bay*, and P.C. Scriba

Klinik für Innere Medizin, Med. Universität zu Lübeck;D-2400 Lübeck,FRG and * Chirugische Klinik, Allg. Krankenhaus, Hamburg-Harburg, FRG

INTRODUCTION

When growth promoting activity on thyroid cells was dis-covered in immunoglobulin fractions (TGI) from patients with goitrous Graves' disease (GD), an intriguing concept to ex-plain goitre formation was created (1). Indeed, TGI-like activity subsequently was described in patients with non-toxic (NTG) or recurrent goitres (2,3,4). Recently however, some doubts were cast on this concept for goitre formation, since TGI activity could not be found in highly purified IgG fractions and growth promoting activity in IgG fractions prepared by ammonsulfate precipitation was attributed to contaminations with epidermal growth factor (EGF) (5). More-over, TGI has not yet been convincingly detected with assay systems using human thyroid epithial cells (TEC).

Our own interest to reassess TGI activities was triggered by the inability to find TGI in serum from patients with euthyroid or recurrent goitres (not shown). We therefore investigated the growth promoting activities of TGI samples, TSH and EGF on human TEC and on rat FRTL-5 cells. In both assay systems tritriated thymidin (^{3}HTdR) uptake, glucose-6-phosphate dehydrogenase (G-6-PD) and adenylcyclase (cAMP) were measured.

METHODS

TECs were established from thyroid tissue obtained at operation of patients with GD or NTG. After separating TECs from debris and erythrocytes by density centrifugarion cells were plated in Iscove medium supplemented with insulin, transferrin, hydrocortisone, somastatin, and gly-his-lys tripeptide in 0.5% FCS (5H medium) (6). 20 x 10^3 cells 1 per well of 96 well Microtiter flat bottom plates were growing in semi follicle-like structures (domes) displaying "right side out" polarity. The differentiated function of TECs in cultures was verified by their ability to secrete thyroglobulin and to express microsomal(M) antigen on TSH stimulation.

The rat FRTL-5 cells were grown in Coon's 5H medium plus 1 mU bTSH/ml. Before these cells were used for TGI assays TSH was withdrawn for 5 days. Both TECs and FRTL-5 cells were used for ^{3}HTdR uptake in 96 well plates after cultures reached 2/3 confluency. The supernatants of cultures were used for measuring cAMP stimulation (7) of cells. Cell cultures were preincubated for 48 h with IgGs (0.1mg/ml),TSH $(10-10^4\mu U/ml)$ or EGF (0.1- 5 ng/ml). In order to measure the 24h ^{3}HTdR uptake cells were washed, detached from plastic bottoms by trypsin digestion and harvested on cellulose acetate filter with a cell harvester using 10% tri- chlor-acetic acid, and 96% cold ethanol. Results were calculated as stimulation indices(8). The G-6-PD was measured kinetically (9) using cells grown and preincubated in 16 well Costar plates. The G-6-PD activity was expressed as % over control cultures. Three IgGs from patients with GD were used for the study. They were positive for thyroid stimulating antibodies (TSab) and showed growth promoting activity in the ^{3}HTdR uptake assay of FRTL-5 cells. As a normal control a pool of IgGs from healthy individuals of the laboratory staff was used. All IgGs were prepared from serum by ionexchangechromotographie on Affi-Gel- Blue and concentrated by Minicon- ultrafiltration chambers. All IgG samples were adjusted to 1mg/ml and stored in liquid nitrogen until use.

MATERIALS

Collagenase (Dispase II) was from Boehringer, Mannheim, FRG. Fetal calf serum (FCS), Iscove medium and additives were from Biochrom, West Berlin. Coon's modified medium was from GIBCO, Europe, Karlsruhe, FRG. TSH (Thyrostimulin) was from Organon, Munich, FRG. EGF and all hormone additives were from Sigma Chemie, Deisenhofen, FRG. Tritiated thymidin and the cAMP binding-protein assay were from NEN, Dreieich, FRG. Affi-Gel- Blue was from BioRad Lab., Munich, FRG. The FRTL-5 rat cells were kindly provided by Dr. L. Kohn, Bethesda, USA.

RESULTS

By stimulating FRTL-5 rat cells with TSH (Fig.1a) the growth promoting activity is apparently mediated by adenylcyclase activation. In addition, the ^{3}HTdR uptake is paralleled by the activation of G-6-PD. Human TECs display a different pattern of TSH stimulation (Fig.1b). Although TSH is stimulating the adenyl-cyclase, HTdR uptake as well as G-6-PD stay flat.

A similar result is obtained with IgG preparations from GD-patients (n=3): With FRTL-5 cells the ^{3}HTdR uptake increases by 2.8 - 5.9 times accompanied by an cAMP increase of 200-600% (Fig. 2). In contrast, human TECs after incubation with IgGs (GD) do not incorporate significantly more thymidin than control IgGs, although cAMP increases by 120-400% compared to pooled normal IgG.EGF served as a control for the proliferation assay with human TECs. Thymidin uptake was increased by 2.5-7.1 fold (n=4), while FRTL-5 cells of course could not be stimulated by EGF.

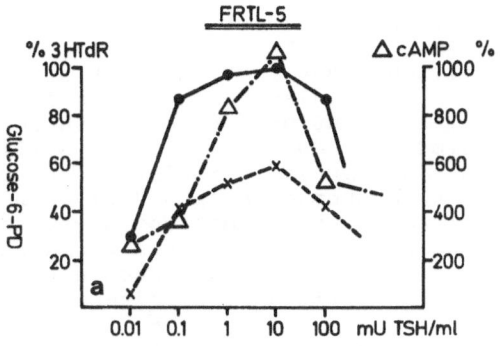

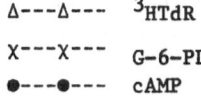

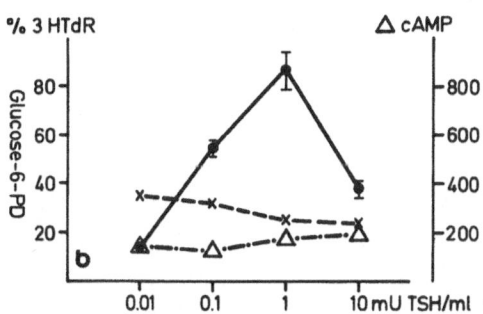

FIGURE 1.

Growth and cAMP
stimulation by bTSH

DISCUSSION

Various experimental assay systems (1,2,3,4) using thyroid cells from different species (1,3,4) have been employed to demonstrate thyroid growth stimulators in IgG preparations from patients with auto-immune and non-immune goitrous thyroid disorders (1,2,4). Both, the assay systems and the origin of thyroid cells have rather contributed to confusion than to clarify thyroid cell growth in vitro and goitre formation in vivo. This is particularly true for the human thyroid, where the mechanisms of proliferation control are not yet understood.

While TSH mediates growth stimulation through a cAMP signal in dog and rat cells (10,11), no such effect is observed in pig and sheep thyroid cells (12,13). We here confirm that TSH does not induce proliferation in human TECs, although it activates adenylcyclase (Fig. 1b)(14,15,16). In contrast, FRTL5 cells stimulated with TSH showed increased cAMP thymidine uptake and G-6-PD activation, which is indirectly linked to DNA-synthesis (Fig.1a) (17). Since in FRTL-5 cells growth is mediated by adenyl cyclase activation , it makes FRTL-5 cells a dubious tool to measure TGI activities from hyperthyroid GD-patients. Characteristically, these patients mostly have cAMP stimulating Tsab. Thus,with TSab positive GD-IgGs, the FRTL-5 cell system should always detect growth stimulation. But even the FRTL-5 cell system has been reported to detect selectively TGI in IgGs of goitrous GD-patients (3).This might be due to the insensitivity of assay systems employed. It does , however, still allow an adenyl-cyclase independent growth stimulator acting on FRTL-5 cells.

These growth promoting IgGs derive from humans and sup-posedly stimulate goitre formation in vivo. One should there-fore assume that these stimulators would promote growth of human TECs in vitro, if they do react directly on the thyroid cells and if TECs still have differentiated characteristics in vitro. TECs in our hands, were almost free of fibroblasts (5H medium). They displayed M-antigen on TSH and TSab stimu-lation and they synthesized thyroglobulin. With our, admittedly, small number of IgGs from goitrous, hyperthyroid GD-patients, we could not detect growth promoting activity (Fig. 2), although the same IgGs stimulated [3]HTdR uptake in FRTL-5 cells.

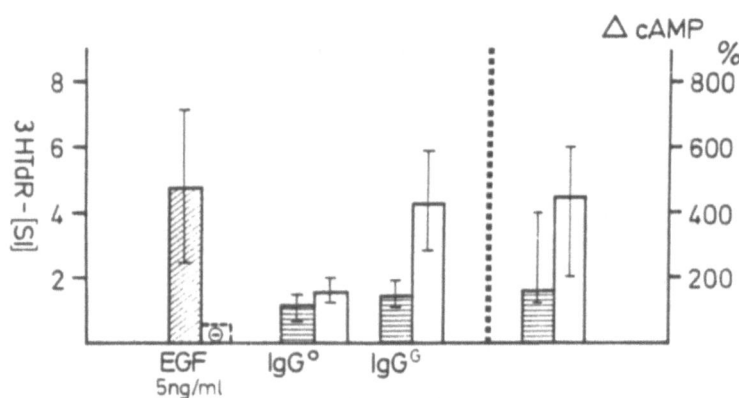

FIGURE 2.

Growth promoting and stimulating activities of IgG from GD-patients(IgG[G]),IgG from normals(IgG[∅]) and of EGF.

☐-- FRTL-5 cells   ▨-- Human TECs

The situation in euthyroid and recurrent goiters appears even more conflicting, since growth promoting activity in IgG prepared by ammoniumsulfate precipitation was attributed to EGF contaminations. We were not able so far to demonstrate stimulation of cell growth with IgGs prepared by ionexchange-chromatography using the HdR uptake of human TECs.

In conclusion, future work on growth promoting activi-ties in human IgGs , should not only define better the acting agent but also the mechanism by which cell proliferation is modulated.

ACKNOWLEDGEMENTS

The expert technical assistance of Ms. S. Grammerstorf and the help of Ms. A. Bullasch is gratefully acknowledged. This work was supported by "Deutsche Forschungsgemeinschaft", SFB 232/C4.

REFERENCES

1. Drexhage HA, Bottazzo GF, Doniach D, Bitensky L, Chayen Evidence for thyroid-growth-stimulating immunoglobulins in some goitrous thyroid diseases. Lancet II: 287-292.(1980)

2. Valente WA, Vitti P, Rotella CM, Vaughan MM, Aloj SM, Grollman EF, Ambesi-Impiombato FS, Kohn LD, Antibodies that promote thyroid growth: a distinct population of thyroid stimulating autoantibodies. N Eng J Med 309: 1028 (1983)

3. McMullan NM, Smyth PPA ,In vitro generation of NADPH as a index of thyroid stimulating immunoglobulins (TGI) in goitrous disease. Clin Endocrinol (Oxf) 20:269 (1984)

4. Schatz H, Pschierer-Berg K, Nickel JA, Bär R, Müller F, Bretzel RG, Müller H, Stracke H, Assay for thyroid growth stimulating immunoglobulins: stimulation of ^{3}H-thymidine incorporation into isolated thyroid follicles by TSH, EGF, and immunoglobulins from goitrous patients in an iodine-deficient region. Acta Endocrinol (Kbh) 112: 523-530 (1986)

5. Gärtner R, Greil W, Tzavella A, What is Thyroid Growth Promoting Activity, in "The Thyroid and autoimmunity", H.A.Drexhage :and W.M. Wiersinga, eds.,Elsvier Science Pub, 1986, p. 191.

6. Ambesi-Impiombato FS, Picone R, Tramontano D : Influence of hormones and serum on growth and differentiation of thyroid cell strain FRTL, in:Sirbasku A et al. (eds.) "Growth of cells in hormonally defined media," vol 9: 483-492. Cold Spring Harbour Laboratories New York. (1982)

7. Schleusener H, Kinke R, Kotulla P, Wenzel K.W.,Meinhold H, Roedle H.D., Determination of thyroid stimulating immunoglobulins (TSI) during the course of Graves' disease. A reliable indicator for remission and persistence of this disease ?,J. Endocrinol. Invest. 2:155, (1978).

8. Wenzel B, Averdunk R, Differentiation between various effects of cytoxic fractions of lymphocyte culture medium,Z Immun Forsch vol 153,pp.380-394 (1977).

9. Bishop C, Assay of glucose-6-phosphate dehydrogenase in red cells, J Lab & Clin Med 68:149, (1966).

10. Roger PP, Servais P, Dumont JE, Stimulation by thyrotropin and cyclic AMP of the proliferation of quiescent canine thyroid cells cultured in a defined medium containing insulin, FEBS Lett 157:323-329 (1983),

11. Chiovato L, Hammond LJ, Hanafusa T, Pujol-Borell B, Doniach D, Bottazzo GF, Detection of thyroid growth immunoglobulins (TGI) by 3H-thymidine incorporation in cultured rat thyroid follicles, Clin Endocrinol (Oxf.) 19:581-590,(1983).

12. Gärtner R, Greil W, Demharter R, Horn K, Involvement of cyclic AMP, iodide and metabolites of arachidonic acid in regulation of cell proliferation of isolated porcine thyroid follicles, Mol Cell Endocrinol 42:146-152 (1985b).

13. Eggo MC, Bachrach LK, Fayet G, Errick J, Cohen MF, Kudlow JE, Burrow GN, Effect of grwoth factors and serum on DNA synthesis and differentiation in thyroid cells in culture, Mol. Cell. Endo. 38:141-150, (1984).

14. Errick JE, Ing K, Eggo MC, Burrow GN, Growth and TSH-mediated differentiation in cultured human thyroid cells, In Vitro. 22:28-36, (1986).

15. Watanabe Y, Amino N, Tamaki H, Iwatani Y, Miyai K, Bovine thyrotropin inhibits DNA synthesis inversely with stimulation of cyclic AMP production in cultured porcine thyroid follicles, Endocrinol Japon, 32:81-88, (1985).

16. Westermark B, Karlsson FA, Walinder O, Thyrotropin is not a growth factor for thyroid cells in culture, Proc Natl Acad Sci, 76:2022-2026, (1979).

17. Coulton LA, Temporal relationship between Glucose-6-phosphate Dehydrogenase activity and DNA- Synthesis, Histochemistry, 50:207-215, (1977).

AUTOANTIBODIES STIMULATING THYROID GROWTH AND ADENYLATE CYCLASE
CANNOT BE SEPARATED IN IgGs FROM PATIENTS WITH ACTIVE GRAVES'
DISEASE

Claudio Marcocci, Paolo Vitti, Guadalupe Lopez, Claudia
Mammoli, Luca Chiovato, Gianfranco Fenzi, and
Aldo Pinchera

Cattedra di Endocrinologia e Medicina Costituzionale,
Università di Pisa, Viale del Tirreno 64, 56018
Tirrenia (Pisa), Italy

INTRODUCTION

Previous studies have shown that immunoglobulin G (IgG) able to
stimulate thyroid adenylate cyclase (TSAb) or growth (TGSAb) are
present in sera of patients with active Graves' disease. The
question of whether these two effects are produced by the same or
different IgG is still under investigation. Valente et al. (1)
reported that the stimulation of adenylate cyclase and growth were
two separate bioeffects of TSH, and that TGSAb and TSAb could be
independently found in patients with thyroid autoimmune disorders
(2). Moreover, in patients with nontoxic goiter, other authors
reported that TGSAb could be detected by a cytochemical assay in the
absence of any adenylate cyclase stimulatory activity (3).It is
worth noting that in all these studies TGSAb and TSAb were measured
in separate assays, under different assay conditions.

To further investigate the relationship between TSAb and TGSAb
we have developed an assay for simultaneous measure of TSAb and
TGSAb using FRTL-5 cells.TSAb were detected by their ability to
stimulate I^- uptake, a direct consequence of cAMP stimulation; TGSAb
were measured by a ^3H-thymidine incorporation assay.In the present
study we report the results obtained in patients with active Graves'
disease.

MATERIALS AND METHODS

Cells. FRTL-5 cells were cultured in 96-well plates under standard
conditions in 6H medium and deprived of TSH (5H medium) for 7 days
before use (4).

IgG. IgG was prepared by the DEAE-Sephadex method from sera of 34
patients with active Graves' disease and from 10 normal subjects.

Simultaneous assay of I^- uptake and ^3H-thymidine incorporation. The
procedure was a modification of the I^- uptake assay previouslly
described (5). Experiments were initiated by adding to cells 100 μl
of 5H medium containing 5 μM IBMX, 0.2 μCi ^3H-thymidine, and either

TSH or IgG (1 mg/ml). After 48-60 h the medium was removed and washed cells were pulsed with $^{125}I^-$ for 40 min at 37C. Incubations were terminated by aspirating the medium and washing the cells with ice-cold buffer. TCA (5%) was added and the supernatant, containing the $^{125}I^-$ released, was collected and counted. Cells were then solubilized with the dyphenylamine reagent for 12-18 h and aliquots were counted for ^3H-thymidine. Results were expressed as % of control (incubations without TSH or IgG).

RESULTS AND DISCUSSION

The results of I^- uptake and ^3H-thymidine incorporation assays simultaneously performed in the same well were not significantly different from those obtained when the two assays were performed separately (data not shown).

IgG from 10 normal subjects slightly affected basal activities in both assays: 104±12 % and 101±19 % (mean ± SD) for I^- uptake and ^3H-thymidine incorporation assays, respectively. Results were considered positive when higher than the mean + 2SD of those of normal subjects.

As shown in Fig. 1, 24/34 (71%) patients were positive in the I^- uptake assay and 20/34 (59%) in the ^3H-thymidine incorporation assay. The analysis of individual data showed that the results of the two assays were generally concordant. However few IgGs had different potency in the two assays.

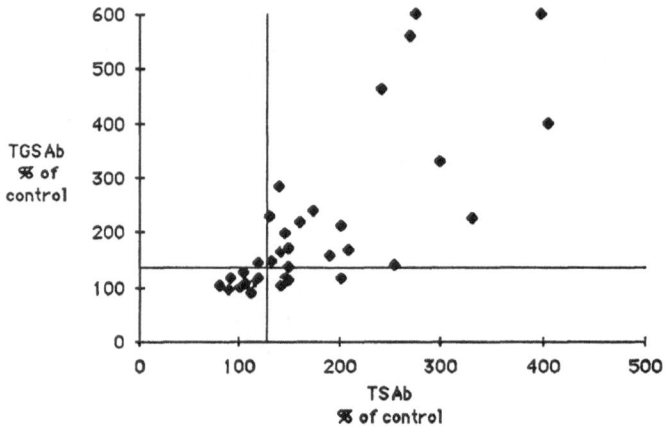

Fig. 1. Correlation between the results of TGSAb and TSAb (measured by stimulation of I^- uptake) in 34 patients with active Graves' disease. The vertical and horizontal lines represent the upper limit of normal range.

Recent studies have shown that TSH stimulation of FRTL-5 cell growth is largely (6), but not completely (7), mediated by the adenylate cyclase-cAMP system. Therefore it can be hypothesized that in Graves' patients a single IgG able to stimulate the adenylate cyclase can also promote cell replication. The finding of IgG with different potency in the two assays may be explained by the fact that the two activities measured, i.e. I⁻ uptake and ^{3}H-thymidine incorporation, although initiated by the same mechanism, represent the end result of a complex series of events that are highly regulated in an independent way.

Two IgGs were clearly TGSAb+ve, but showed only borderline positive results in the TSAb assay. In these cases it can be hypothesized that, as for TSH, other pathways of growth stimulation, in addition to the adenylate cyclase-cAMP system, are also operating (7). The finding of four TSAb+ve and TGSAb-ve IgGs may be attributed to the lower sensitivity of the growth assay.

CONCLUSIONS

The results of the present study indicate that in patients with Graves' disease TGSAbs are generally detected only in TSAb+ve IgGs. This finding is consistent with the observation that the adenylate cyclase-cAMP system mediates cell replication in FRTL-5 cells. However, since additional pathways are involved in the growth of these cells, it cannot be excluded that in other thyroid autoimmune disorders TGSAb+ve but TSAb-ve IgGs can occur.

REFERENCES

1. W.A. Valente, P. Vitti, L.D.Kohn, M.L. Brandi, C.M. Rotella, R. Toccafondi, D. Tramontano, S.M. Aloj, and F.S. Ambesi Impiombato, The relationship of growth and adenylate cyclase activity in cultured thyroid cells: separate bioeffects of thyrotropin, Endocrinology 112:71 (1983).
2. W.A. Valente, P. Vitti, C.M. Rotella, M.M. Vaughan, S.M. Aloj, E.F. Grollman, F.S. Ambesi-Impiombato, and L.D. Kohn, Antibodies that promote thyroid growth. A distinct population of thyroid stimulating antibodies, N. Engl. J. Med. 3098:1028 (1983).
3. P.P.A. Smyth, N.M. McMullan, B. Grubeck-Loebenstein, and D.K. O'Donovan, Thyroid growth-stimulating immunoglobulins in goitrous disease: relationship to thyroid-stimulating immunoglobulins, Acta Endocrinol. (Kbh) 111:321 (1986).
4. F.S. Ambesi-Impiombato, L.A.M. Parks, and H.G. Coon, Culture of hormone-dependent epithelial cells from rat thyroids, Proc. Natl. Acad. Sci USA 77:3455 (1980).
5. C. Marcocci, W.A. Valente, A. Pinchera, S.M. Aloj, L.D. Kohn, and E.F. Grollman, Graves' IgG stimulation of iodide uptake in FRTL-5 rat thyroid cells: a clinical assay complementing FRTL-5 assays measuring adenylate cyclase and growth promoting antibodies in autoimmune thyroid disease, J. Endocrinol. Invest. 6:463 (1983).
6. S. Jin, F.J. Hornicek, D. neylan, M. Zakarijia, and J.M.McKenzie, Evidence that adenosine 3',5'-monophosphate mediates stimulation of thyroid growth in FRTL-5 cells, Endocrinology 119:802 (1986).
7. C. Marcocci, D. Gianchecchi, I. Masini, and E.F. Grollman, TSH stimulation of thyroid cell proliferation: role of the adenylate cyclase-cAMP system. Ann. Endocrinol. (Paris) 47A:50 (1986).

ANTIIDIOTYPIC BLOCKING OF GRAVES' DISEASE BIOLOGIC ACTIVITY WITH AUTOLOGOUS SERA BUT NOT CONSISTENTLY WITH HOMOLOGOUS SERA: EVIDENCE FOR POLYCLONALITY OF THYROID RECEPTOR ANTIBODIES (TRAb)

R. Paschke, J. Teuber, U. Schwedes, and K.H. Usadel
II. Medical Dept., Klinikum Mannheim der Universität
Heidelberg, Theodor-Kutzer-Ufer, 6800 Mannheim 1, FRG

INTRODUCTION

Although there is multiple evidence for the functional heterogeneity and polyclonality of TRAb (1 - 3) both statements are questioned by some investigators (4, 5). Furthermore there is growing evidence for an idiotypic-antiidiotypic regulation of Graves disease and other autoimmune diseases (6, 7).

The nude mouse bioassay permits to study the behaviour of intact human thyroid tissue and the simultaneous determination of several biologic parameters. This way the biologic profile of a patients TRAb (determined by radio ligand assay) can be analysed. Therefore we tried to further elucidate the question of TRAb clonality and functional heterogeneity by the use of the nude mouse bioassay.

MATERIAL AND METHODS

Thyroid tissue of 3 patients with Graves disease undergoing subtotal thyroidectomy was transplanted to 28 thymus-dysplastic nude mice. Each animal received 2 transplants. 4 weeks after transplantation the animals received an injection of 0.5 ml serum intraperitonally. The serum samples which were used for the autologous experiments were obtained from 2 patients with Graves disease during active disease and during remission. In these patients disease activity and TRAb values happened to correlate (i.e. high titer = active disease, low titer = remission or low activity).

For the autologous experiments 2 groups of animals received serum samples of patient 1 with TRAb 197 mU/ml, TRAb 48 mU/ml and the 1:1 mixture of these serum samples. Controls received TRAb negative serum (Fig. 1). This experiment was repeated by using serum samples from patient 2 with TRAb 700 mU/ml, TRAb 279 mU/ml and the 1:1 mixture of these sera. Again controls received TRAb negative serum (Fig. 1).

For the study of the homologous serum samples, serum samples of 3 different Graves' disease patients with different TRAb values were used. 2 of these patients had goiter class I - II (TRAb 5.0 mU/ml = patient 3 and 16.3 mU/ml = patient 4). The serum sample with TRAb 17.3 mU/ml was obtained from a 79 year old thyrotoxic patient without thyroid enlargement (= patient 5). Groups of nude mice were injected with these serum samples and their 1:1 mixtures. Controls received TRAb negative serum.

4 days after injection the animals received 20 µCi of ^{3}H-thymidine intraperitonally and were killed in anaesthesia 1 hr later. The transplants were fixed in Boins' solution and embedded in parafine. Nuclear volume was determined histometrically ($V = \frac{\pi}{6} \times ab^2$) for 100 nuclei of epithelial cells. The fraction of ^{3}H-thymidine labeled cells (FLC) was determined for 1 000 thyroid epithelial cells in 2 sections per transplant.

RESULTS

The results are shown in figure 1 and 2. Controls showed the following data: autologous experiments, serum donor 1 :

Autologous Serum Samples

Serum donor	Goitre size	T R A b (mU/ml)	biologic potency: nuclear volume (μm^3)	biologic potency: ^{3}H-thymidine incorporation (%)	biol. potency related to TRAb: ^{3}H-thymidine / T R A b	biol. potency related to TRAb: nuclear volume / T R A b	
1	II	48	71			1,48	
1	II	197	86			0,44	
		4,1	1,2			0,29	increase of parameters
		48/197	54 (78,5)				
2	I-II	279	67	1o,3	0,036	0,23	
2	I-II	700	86	16,7	0,024	o,12	
		2,5	1,2	1,6	0,66	0,52	increase of parameters
		279/700	69 (76,5)	8,7 (13,5)	0,02	0,16	

( ) = calculated mean value of biolog. parameters

FIG.1

Homologous Serum Samples

Serum donor	Goitre size	T R A b (mU/ml)	biologic potency: nuclear volume (μm^3)	biologic potency: ^{3}H-thymidine incorporation (%)	biologic potency rel. to TRAb: ^{3}H-thymidine / T R A b	biologic potency rel. to TRAb: nuclear volume / T R A b
3	I-II	5,0	62,9	18,2	3,6	12,5
4	I-II	16,3	75,3	31,7	1,9	4,6
5	no thyr. enlargm.	17,3	68,2	20,4	1,2	3,9
3/4		5,o/16,3	61,2 (1,12)	13,4 (1,86)		
3/5		5,0/17,3	79,2 (0,82)	14,5 (1,33)		
4/5		16,3/17,3	74,5 (0,96)	13,0 (2,0)		

( ) = calculated mean value of biol.pram. / detected mean value of serum samples

FIG.2

nuclear volume 58 μm³, serum donor 2: nuclear volume 39 μm³, FLC 9.4%. Homologous experiment, serum donor 3 - 5 : nuclear volume 64.9 μm³, FLC 9.4%.

DISCUSSION

Different autologous thyroid receptor antibody (TRAb) titers determined by radioligand assay (RLA) show a corresponding but not proportional increase of ³H-thymidine incorporation and likewise nuclear volume of transplants. Homologous serum samples with different TRAb titers and with different patient characteristics (i.e. goiter size) do not show a consistent relation between TRAb titers determined by RLA and the biologic parameters ³H-thymidine incorporation and nuclear volume.

The biologic parameters ³H-thymidine incorporation and nuclear volume may not neccessarily represent or discriminate between stimulation of thyroid growth (TGI) or thyroid function (TSI) but they do seem to represent different qualities of stimulation. The corresponding relation of TRAb and both biologic parameters in the autologous comparison together with the lack of correlation between TRAb titer combined with clinical characteristics and biologic parameters in the comparison of homologous serum samples are evidence for polyclonality of TRAb.

This hypothesis is further substantiated by the results of the blocking studies. Mixture of autologous sera shows blocking of both biologic parameters (i.e. nuclear volume and FLC) when compared with the calculated mean values of the biologic parameters. This kind of antiidiotypic response in the homologous system, taylored to the individual polyclonality of TRAb could not be expected in the homologous system. Since patient 1 and 2 both had progressive growth of their thyroids and hence probably a prominent clone of thyroid growth stimulating immunoglobulins (TGI) the antiidiotypic blocking response can be demonstrated best by the blocking of the FLC. This theory is confirmed by the "protective" antiidiotypic antibodies of patient No 5 without thyroid enlargement which shows a prominent blocking of the FLC but not nuclear volume. This antigen specific blocking effect presupposes a polyclonal TRAb which produces a corresponding antiidiotypic response.

REFERENCES

1. S.H. Ingbar (1986) The role of antibodies and other humoral factors in the pathogenesis of Graves disease In: the thyroid and autoimmunity, H.A. Drexhage, W.M. Wiersinga ed, Excerpta MEDICA

2. C.R. Strakosch, B.E. Wenzel, V.V. Row, R.Volpé (1982) Immunology of autoimmune thyroid disease. New Engl. J. Med. 307: 1499

3. J. Worthington, R.L. Himsworth, P.G.H. Byfield (1986) Isolation of both agonist and nonagonist Graves immunoglobulins from the sera of individual patients. In the thyroid and autoimmunity. H.A. Drexhage, W.M. Wiersinga ed, Excerpta MEDICA

4. M. Zakarija, S.Jin, J.M. McKenzie(1986)
   Support for the identity of thyroid stimulating
   antibody (TSAb) and thyroid growth stimulating IgG
   (TGI) in Graves' disease. 61st meeting of the American Thyroid Association, Sept 11-13, Abstract 34.

5. B.S. Hawe, N.R. Farid(1986)
   An antiidiotypic antibody against Graves' IgG
   Advances in thyroidology, International Symposium,
   Lübeck, Germany, Oct 2 - 4th, Abstract 16.

6. M.Zanetti, P.E. Bigazzi(1981)
   Antiidiotypic immunity and autoimmunity. In vitro
   and in vivo effects of antiidiotypic antibodies to
   spontaneously occuring autoantibodies to rat thyroglobulin. Eur. J. Immunol. 11: 187.

7. K.B. Raines, J.R. Baker, Y.G.Lukes, L. Wartofsky,
   K.D. Burman(1985)
   Antithyrotropin antibodies in the sera of Graves' di-
   sease patients. J. C. Endocr. Metab. 61: 217

AUTOANTIBODIES BLOCKING THE TSH-INDUCED ADENYLATE CYCLASE STIMULATION IN IDIOPATHIC MYXEDEMA AND HASHIMOTO'S THYROIDITIS

Vitti P., Chiovato L., Lombardi A., Lopez G., Santini F., Ceccarelli P., Mammoli C., Giusti L.F., Battiato S., Fenzi G.F., and Pinchera A.

Cattedra di Endocrinologia, University of Pisa, Italy

INTRODUCTION

Adult idiopathic myxedema (IM) is believed to be the end stage of a lymphocytic thyroiditis in which humoral and cellular autoimmune processes lead to failure of the thyroid function (1). Recent data indicate that this disease may be associated with the presence of autoantibodies which block the effect of TSH on thyroid adenylate cyclase (2, 3) and cell growth (4). In the present report we describe a new method for the detection of blocking autoantibodies (TBkAb) by determining their blocking effect on the TSH-induced thyroid cAMP accumulation in FRTL-5 cells (5, 6).

MATERIALS AND METHODS

FRTL-5 cells was cultured as previously described (5, 6) and maintained for 4 days in medium without TSH before the assay.

IgGs were prepared by DEAE Sephadex separation from sera of 38 consecutive patients with IM (23 untreated, and 15 already under l-thyroxine when first observed), from 44 patients with Hashimoto's thyroiditis (23 hypothyroid and 21 euthyroid). Sera from 33 normal subjects matched for sex and age, and from 10 patients with nonautoimmune untreated hypothyroidism following total thyroidectomy for thyroid carcinoma were used as controls.

FRTL-5 cells were incubated for 1 h at 37 C with TSH (40 μU/ml), IgG (1 mg/ml), or IgG plus TSH. All assays were performed in NaCl-free medium containing 0.5 mM isobutyl-methyl-xantine (IBMX) and the production of cAMP was measured in the extracellular medium by RIA. Results were calculated according to the following formula:

1 - $\dfrac{\text{cAMP (TSH+sample IgG) - cAMP (sample IgG)}}{\text{cAMP (TSH) - cAMP (control buffer)}}$ X 100

For the preabsorption experiment human thyroid membrane or rat testis membrane were prepared by differential ultracentrifugation.

RESULTS AND DISCUSSION

None of the IgG preparations obtained from patients and controls was found to significantly alter basal cAMP production (i.e. in the absence of TSH). Normal IgGs did not significantly modify the stimulation of adenylate cyclase produced by TSH (mean ± SD = -2±16). Fifteen out of 23 (65%) IgGs from patients with untreated IM elicited a significant inhibition of the TSH-stimulated cAMP production (> 2 SD of the mean of normal IgG). Only a minority (2/15) of IgG preparations from patients with IM under treatment were positive for TBkAb. In the group of Hashimoto's thyroiditis, antibodies blocking the TSH-induced adenylate cyclase stimulation were found in 10/23 (43%) hypothyroid patients and only in 2/21 (9%) untreated euthyroid cases. No IgG from patients with nonautoimmune hypothyroidism caused any significant effect. It is interesting to note that only a minority of patients with long standing and treated idiopathic myxedema gave positive results for TBkAb. This phenomenon could be ascribed to a spontaneous disappearance of these autoantibodies during the natural course of the disease or to an effect of I-thyroxine therapy (7). Longitudinal studies are needed to clarify this point. To exclude the possibility that the inhibition of the TSH-stimulated adenylate cyclase was due to anti-TSH antibodies, a preabsorption experiment was performed incubating IM IgG (30 μg) with human thyroid or rat testis membranes (3 mg) for 3 h at 37 C. After preabsorption with human thyroid membrane the inhibiting activity of IM IgG was reduced by 50% with respect to control (Fig. 1).

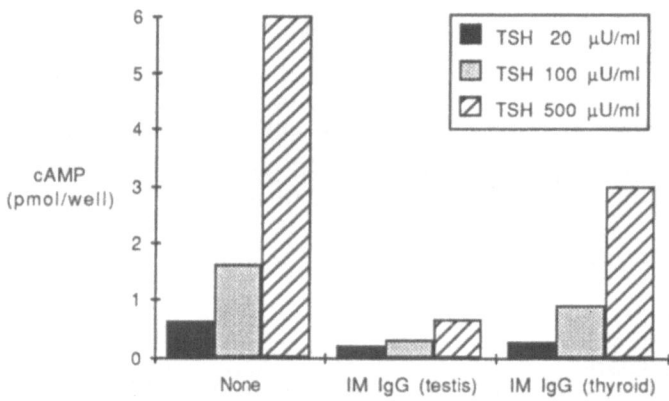

Fig. 1. Effect of preabsorption with thyroid tissue on the adenylate cyclase inhibiting activity of an IM IgG. On the ordinate is reported the cAMP produced per each well of FRTL-5 cells under the stimulation of TSH. The three sets of columns represent the results obtained adding to the assay mixture the preabsorbed IM IgG. None = preabsorption buffer. IM IgG (testis) = IM IgG preabsorbed on rat testis. IM IgG (thyroid) = IM IgG preabsorbed on thyroid membrane.

In conclusion, the results of our study indicate that: i) using FRTL-5 cells autoantibodies blocking the stimulating effect of TSH on thyroid adenylate cyclase can be found in 65% of patients with untreated idiopathic myxedema, in 43% of patients with hypothyroid Hashimoto's thyroiditis and are undetectable in patients with nonautoimmune hypothyroid following total thyroidectomy; ii) positive results for inhibiting antibodies were found only in a small minority of patients with euthyroid Hashimoto's thyroiditis; iii) these antibodies are directed to thyroid membrane components, possibly the TSH receptor, and could play a role in the pathogenesis of thyroid failure in autoimmune thyroiditis.

REFERENCES

1. Pinchera A., Fenzi G.F., Vitti P., Chiovato L., Bartalena L., Macchia E. & Mariotti S. (1985) Significance of thyroid autoantibodies in thyroid autoimmune diseases. In: Autoimmunity and the Thyroid (Eds. P.G. Walfish J.R. Wall & R. Volpé) pp. 139-151, Academic Press, Toronto.

2. Matsuura N., Yamada Y., Nohara Y., Konishi J., Kasagi K., Endo K., Kojima H. & Wataya K. (1980) Familial neonatal transient hypothyroidism due to maternal TSH binding inhibiting immunoglobulins. New England Journal of Medicine, 303, 738-741.

3. Konishi J., Iida Y., Kasagi K., Misaki T., Nakashima T., Endo K., Mori T., Shinpo S., Nohara Y., Matsuura N. & Torizuka K. (1985) Primary myxedema with thyrotropin-binding inhibiting immunoglobulins. Annals of Internal Medicine, 103, 26-31.

4. Drexhage H.A., Bottazzo G.F., Bitensky L., Chayen J. & Doniach D. (1981) Thyroid growth blocking antibodies in primary myxedema. Nature, 289, 594-596.

5. Vitti P., Valente W.A., Ambesi-Impiombato F.S., Fenzi G.F., Pinchera A. & Kohn L.D. (1982) Graves' IgG stimulation of continuously cultured rat thyroid cells: a sensitive and potentially useful clinical assay. Journal of Endocrinological Investigation, 5, 179-182.

6. Vitti P., Rotella C.M., Valente W.A., Cohen J., Aloj S.M., Laccetti P., Ambesi-Impiombato F.S., Grollman E.F., Pinchera A., Toccafondi R. & Kohn L.D. (1983) Characterization of the optimal stimulatory effects of Graves' monoclonal and serum immunoglobulin G on adenosine 3'5' monophosphate production in FRTL-5 thyroid cells: a potential clinical assay. Journal of Clinical Endocrinology and Metabolism, 57, 782-791.

7. Chiovato L., Marcocci C., Mariotti S., Mori A. & Pinchera A. (1986) L-thyroxine therapy induces a fall of thyroid microsomal and thyroglobulin antibody in idiopathic myxedema and in hypothyroid but not in euthyroid Hashimoto's thyroiditis. Journal of Endocrinological Investigation, 9, 299-305.

RELEVANCE OF MATERNAL THYROID AUTOANTIBODIES ON THE DEVELOPMENT OF

CONGENITAL HYPOTHYROIDISM

Lia   Giusti,   Claudio   Marcocci,   Luca   Chiovato,
Mariella Ciampi, Ferruccio Santini, Paolo Vitti, Nunzio
Formica, and Gianfranco Fenzi

Cattedra di Enocrinologia e Medicina Costituzionale,
Università di Pisa, Viale del Tirreno 64, 56018
Tirrenia (Pisa)

INTRODUCTION

Previous studies have suggested a potential role of maternal thyroid
autoantibodies in the prediction and the development of congenital
hypothyroidsm. Maternal antibodies able to inhibit thyroid adenylate
cyclase[1] or cell growth[2] have been described in selected cases of
congenital hypothyroidism. More recently it has been suggested that
the presence of immmunoglobulin G (IgG) capable to increase
TSH-stimulated I^- uptake in FRTL-5 rat thyroid cells could predict
the occurrence of congenital hypothyroidism[3]. To investigate this
problem we have studied the effect of IgGs from mothers of children
with congenital hypothyroidism (MHC) on several biological function
of FRTL-5 cells.

MATERIALS AND METHODS

Sera. Sera were obtained from 16 MHC detected during a screening
program. Sera from 7 mothers of newborns with normal thyroid
function (MNC) were used as controls. Circulating thyroglobulin
(TgAb) and thyroid microsomal (MAb) autoantibodies were found in 4
MHC, with titers ranging between 1: 6,400 and > 1: 102,400. One MHC
had hypothyroid Hashimoto' thyroiditis and was under 1-thyroxine
replacement therapy at delivery. IgG was prepared by the
DEAE-Sephadex method and used at concentrations of 0.5-1.0 mg/ml.
The effect of these IgGs on TSH-stimulated cAMP production, I^-
uptake and ^{3}H-thymidime incorporation by FRTL-5 cells was studied.

Cells. FRTL-5 cells were cultured in 24- or 96-well plates under
standard conditions in 6H medium and deprived of TSH (5H medium) for
7 days before use[4].

Simultaneous assay of I^- uptake and ^{3}H-thymidine incorporation.
Experiments were initiated by adding to cells 100 µl 5H medium
containing 5 µM IBMX, 0.2 µCi ^{3}H-thymidine, TSH (1 mU/ml) and IgG
(0.5 mg/ml). After 48-60 h the medium was removed and washed cells
were pulsed with $^{125}I^-$ for 40 min at 37C. Incubation was terminated

by aspirating the medium and cells were rapidly washed with ice-cold HBSS. TCA (5%) was added and $^{125}I^-$ released in the supernatant was counted. Cells were treated with the dyphenylamine reagent for 12-18 h and aliquots were counted for ^{3}H-thymidine. Results were expressed as % of control (incubations without IgG).

cAMP production assay. Cells were incubated for 60 min with IgG alone (1 mg/ml), TSH alone (40 µU/ml) or TSH+IgG. cAMP was measured in the extracellular medium as previously described[5]. Results were expressed as follows:

$$1- \frac{cAMP\ (TSH+IgG)\ -\ cAMP\ (IgG)}{cAMP\ (TSH)\ -\ cAMP\ (control\ buffer)} \times 100$$

RESULTS AND DISCUSSION

IgG from MNC or MHC, without humoral signs of thyroid autoimmunity, did not affect TSH-stimulated cAMP production when compared to normal controls. At contrary, 2 of the 4 IgGs from MHC with circulating thyroid autoantibodies significantly inhibited TSH-stimulated cAMP production (Fig. 1).The more potent IgG was obtained from the MHC with hypothyroid Hashimoto's thyroiditis, who delivered a newborn with transient hypothyroidism.Similar findings have been recently reported by other authors[1].

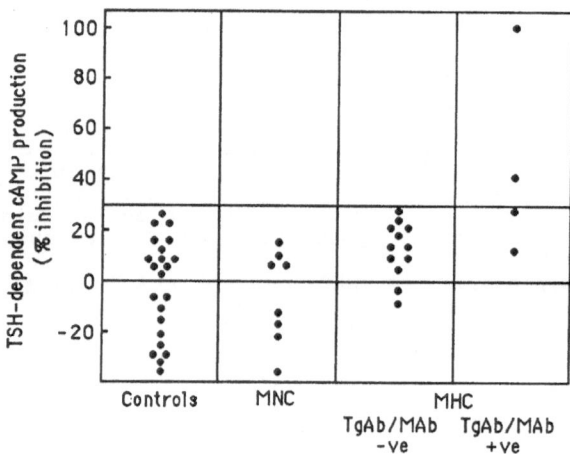

Fig. 1. Effect of IgG preparations on TSH-stimulated cAMP production by FRTL-5 cells.The higher horizontal line represents the upper limit of normal range.

The effects of IgGs on TSH-stimulated I^- uptake and ^{3}H-thymidine incorporation are reported in Figure 2. All but one MHC and all MNC IgGs did not significantly affect these TSH-stimulated activities. The remaining MHC IgG produced a profound inhibition in both assays. This IgG was the same that completely inhibited TSH-stimulated cAMP production (see above).

At variance with the study of Dussault and Bernier[3], we found no evidence that IgG from MHC increase TSH-stimulated I^- uptake in FRTL-5 cells[6]. We have no explanation for such discrepancy. The importance of regional and ethnic differences cannot be excluded. We also failed to confirm the observation of van der Gaag et al.[2] that IgG able to inhibit TSH-induced thyroid growth are present in about half serum samples from MHC

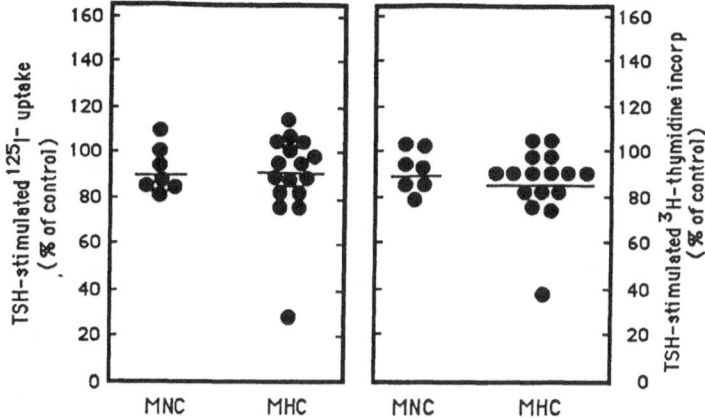

Fig. 2. Effect of IgG preparations on TSH-stimulated I⁻ uptake and ^{3}H-thymidine incorporation by FRTL-5 cells.

CONCLUSIONS

The results of the present study indicate that autoantibodies able to inhibit TSH-stimulated functions in FRTL-5 cells can be detected in MHC only when clinical, or at least humoral signs of thyroid autoimmunity are present. Furthermore, we found that IgG from MHC are not able to increase TSH-stimulated I⁻ uptake by FRTL-5 cells. Therefore this assay cannot be used as a screening to predict the delivery of a hypothyroid baby.

REFERENCES

1. N. Matsuura, Y. Yamada, Y. Nohara, J. Konishi, K. Kasagi, K. Endo, H. Kojima, and K. Wataya, Familial neonatal transient hypothyroidism due to maternal TSH-binding inhibitor immunoglobulins, N. Engl. J. Med. 303:738 (1980)
2. R. D. van der Gaag, H. A. Drexhage, and J. H. Dussault, Role of maternal immunoglobulins blocking TSH-induced thyroid growth in sporadic forms of congenital hypothyroidism, Lancet 1:246 (1985).
3. J. H. Dussault, and D. Bernier, ^{125}I uptake by FRTL-5 cells: a screening test to detect pregnant women at risk of giving birth to hypothyroid infants, Lancet 2:1019, (1985).
4. F. S. Ambesi-Impiombato, L. A. M. Parks, and H. G. Coon, Culture of hormone dependent epithelial cells from rat thyroids, Proc. Natl. Acad. Sci. (USA), 77:3455 (1980).
5. P. Vitti, W. . Walente, F. S. Ambesi-Impiombato, G. F. Fenzi, A. Pinchera, and L. D. Kohn, Graves' IgG stimulation of continuously cultured rat thyroid cells: a sensitive and potentially useful clinical assay, J Endocrinol. Invest. 5:179 (1982).
6. C. Marcocci, L. Giusti, L. Chiovato, M. Ciampi, G. Fenzi, and A. Pinchera, Screening for risk of delivery of a hypothyroid baby, Lancet 2:403 (1986).

ABILITY OF IMMUNOGLOBULINS FROM PATIENTS WITH THYROID DISEASE TO
STIMULATE SKIN FIBROBLASTS

P. Wadeleux and R. Winand

Université de Liège, Institut de Pathologie, C.H.U., B. 23

4000 Sart-Tilman par Liège 1, Belgium.

INTRODUCTION

Thyroid cells in culture are widely used to detect antibodies present
in thyroid disease and particularly the anti-TSH receptor antibodies.
However, TSH also binds specifically to membranes from several extrathyroidal tissues (fat, leukocytes, testis, adrenal tissue, retro orbital tissue).
In this study, we have investigated the action of TSH on fibroblasts from
calf reticular dermis; we have tested these cells as target for the detection of antibodies in sera of patients with simple goitre or with Graves'
disease goitre; we have estimated the possible correlation of the detected
antibodies with other thyroid anti-TSH receptor antibodies.

MATERIALS AND METHODS

Serum samples were obtained from patients on the basis of clinical history and examination. Patients referred to as simple goitre were euthyroid;
they were subdivided as patients with diffuse non toxic goitre and patients
with colloid nodular goitre. Patients with Graves'disease were hyperthyroid.
Ig fractions were precipitated from sera with 1.6 M ammonium sulphate.

Calf skin fibroblasts were isolated from reticular dermis and subcultured as described by Delvoye et al.[1]. Primary cultures of porcine thyroid
cells were prepared as previously described[2]. Cellular cAMP level was
determined after incubating the cells in the presence of TSH or Ig fractions (2 mg/ml)[2]. Incorporation of ($^{35}SO_4$) into glycosaminoglycans was
performed by incubating the cells in the presence of ($^{35}SO_4$)[3]. Collagen
synthesis was measured after labelling with (^{3}H) proline and determination
of the formation of the radioactive hydroxyproline in the medium[3].

Thyroid Growth Stimulating Immunoglobulin (TGI) was determined by (^{3}H)
thymidine incorporation.by porcine thyroid follicles after addition of gamma
globulin[4]. TSH Binding Inhibiting Immunoglobulin (TBII) was tested by using
a commercial kit and porcine thyroid membrane as target. Thyroid Stimulating
Immunoglobulin (TSI) was determined by the stimulation of cellular cAMP on
porcine thyroid cells[2].

RESULTS AND DISCUSSION

A. Action of TSH

When calf fibroblasts were cultured in the presence of increasing amounts of TSH (0.005 to 1 mU/ml), a bell-shaped dose response curve was observed for the cellular cAMP level (Fig. 1). This phenomenon was identical to that obtained with human or porcine thyroid cells (Fig. 1). In this last case, elevation of cAMP level was correlated positively with stimulation by TSH of iodide incorporation[3]. In fibroblasts, TSH (100 μU/ml) also increased the radioactivity associated with the glycosaminoglycans isolated from the culture medium and from the cell layer of the cells incubated in the presence of ($^{35}SO_4$) (Data not illustrated).

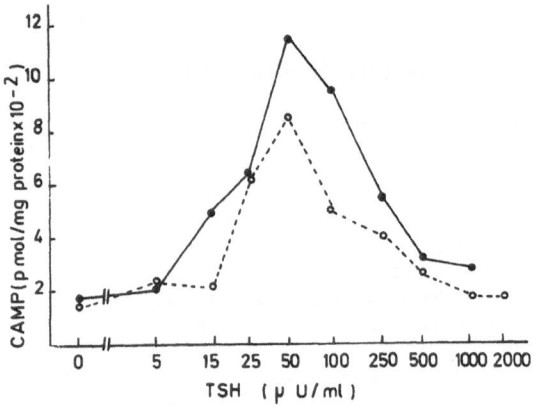

Fig. 1. Action of TSH on the cAMP level of fibroblasts (●————●) or porcine thyroid cells (O-----O). Identical results were obtained with different TSH preparations (0.5 U/mg to 30 U/mg).

B. Action of the gamma globulins

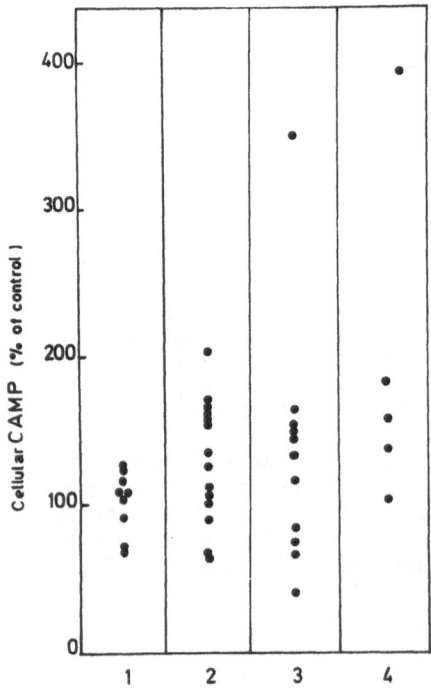

a. Cellular cAMP (Fig. 2)

Fig. 2. Action of gamma-globulins on the cAMP level of fibroblasts. Fibroblasts were cultured for 48 h in the presence of gamma-globulins (2 mg/ml) from control subjects (1) or from patients with diffuse non toxic goitre (2), colloid nodular goitre (3) or Graves'disease (4).

When fibroblasts were incubated with immunoglobulins from patients with Graves'disease, an increase in cAMP level was obtained when compared to immunoglobulins from control subjects; stimulation of the cAMP level was also observed in a significant proportion of immunoglobulins from patients with simple non toxic goitre.

b. Collagen synthesis (Fig.3)

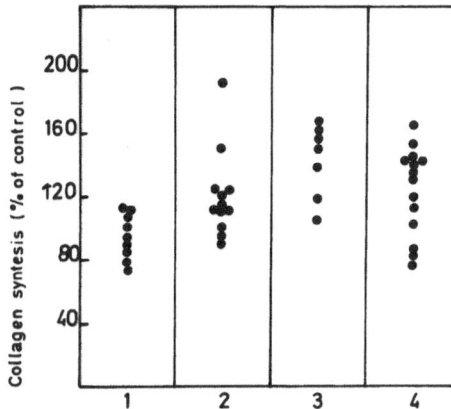

Fig. 3. Action of gamma-globulins on the collagen synthesis by fibroblasts. Fibroblasts were cultured for 24 h in the presence of gamma-globulins (2 mg/ml) from control subjects (1) or from patients with diffuse non toxic goitre (2), colloid nodular goitre (3) or Graves'disease (4). (^{3}H) proline was then added and incubation was continued for 24 h.

Graves'disease immunoglobulins stimulated the collagen synthesis by the skin fibroblasts. An increase in collagen synthesis was also observed in a significant proportion of immunoglobulins from patients with simple non toxic goitre. By contrast, no effect could be obtained by incubating fibroblasts with immunoglobulins from patients with primary hypothyroidism (data not shown).

c. Correlation with other thyroid anti-TSH receptor antibodies

TSI[2], TGI[4] and TBII (data not shown) were evidenced in a high proportion of patients with Graves'disease. In patients with simple non toxic goitre, TGI was present in a significant proportion (16/58)[4] but these patients were negative for TSI[2] and for TBII (data not shown).

REFERENCES

1. P. Delvoye, B. Nusgens, Ch.M. Lapière, The capacity of retracting a collagen matrix is lost by dermatosparatic skin fibroblasts, J. Invest. Derm. 81:267 (1983).
2. J. Etienne-Decerf, R. Winand, A sensitive technique for determination of thyroid-stimulating immunoglobulin (TSI) in unfractionated serum, Clin. Endocrinol. 14:83 (1981).
3. P. Wadeleux, B. Nusgens, J.M. Foidart, Ch.M. Lapière, R. Winand, Synthesis of basement membrane components by differentiated thyroid cells, Biochim. Biophys. Acta 846:257 (1985).
4. P. Wadeleux, R. Winand, Thyroid growth modulating factors in the sera of patients with simple non toxic goitre, Acta Endocr. 112:502 (1986).

SOME EVIDENCES THAT THYROTROPIN AND AUTOANTIBODIES BINDING SITES
ARE LOCATED ON DIFFERENT POLIPEPTIDE CHAINS OF THYROID PLASMA
MEMBRANE PROTEINS

Andrzej Gardas, and Hanna Domek

Biochemistry Department
Medical Center of Postgraduate Education
Marymoncka 99, Warsaw 01-813, Poland

INTRODUCTION

It is generally assumed that autoantibodies present in the sera of
Graves' patients react with thyroid cell plasma membrane at the thyrotropin /TSH/ receptor level /1 - 3/. A structure for the TSH receptor has
been proposed as a protein built from two different subunits linked by
a disulphide bridge /3/. The relative resistance of the TSH binding sites
to disulphide bridges reducing agents is well known and dithiothreitol has
been used to dissociate the TSH binding peptides from thyroid plasma
membranes /3/. We report the high sensitivity of autoantibodies binding
sites to dithiothreitol pretreatment in solubilized thyroid plasma membrane
protein in contrast to relative stability of TSH binding sites. The data
presented suggest a different localization of the TSH and autoantibodies
binding sites and location of the autoantibodies binding sites on two
polipeptide chains linked by a disulfide bridge or bridges.

MATERIAL AND METHODS

Preparation of thyroid plasma membrane, solubilized thyroid plasma
membrane and microsomal membrane antigesn, solubilized TSH binding proteins, ELISA assay of autoantibodies in the sera of Gravesń patients,
and autoantibodies binding to thyroid plasma membrane were estimated as
described previously /4/. The reaction of soluble thyroid plasma membrane
proteins with autoantibodies have been estimated by their ability to inhibit
autoantibodies binding to a solid phase bound thyroid plasma membrane
proteins in the ELISA assay as follows; solubilized thyroid plasma membrane
proteins with or without pretreatment with the designated compound were
incubated with pooled serum obtained from 20 untreated hyperthyroid Graves'
patients at 1:1000 dilution in PBS containing 0.05% Tween 20 and ovoalbu-
min 2 mg/ml to 16 hours at 4°C. The solution was then added in triplicate
to wells of polistyren plates coated with thyroid plasma membrane antigens
and the ELISA carried out as described previously /4/. Thyroid plasma
membrane and solubilized thyroid plasma and microsomal membrane proteins
were treated with dithiothreitol /DIT/ or other designated compound for
60 minutes at 20°C at 2mg/ml protein concentration and after dialysis
to PBS for 18 hours used in inhibition experiments. In some experiments,
solubilized thyroid plasma membrane proteins were treated with 0.1% glutardialdehyde for 30 minutes at 20°C and after dialysis to PBS, used for
further experiments. Dot-immunoblotting experiments with soluble thyroid

Table 1. Effect of disulphide bridges reducing agents and other compounds on autoantibodies and TSH binding of human thyroid plasma membrane antigens.

Compound		Autoantibodies binding capacity /% of control/			TSH binding capacity /% of control/
		Soluble thyroid plasma membrane proteins	polistyrene bound plasma membrane proteins	particulate plasma membrane	soluble thyroid plasma membrane proteins
Dithiothreitol	0.03mM	50	100	100	100
	0.10mM	2	100	100	100
	1.00mM	0	40	100	90
	10.00mM	0	20	100	60
Cystein	25mM	50	90	100	100
Mercaptoethanol	1mM	0	20	80	90
Iodoacetamid	10mM	100	100	100	90
Methimazole	25mM	100	100	100	100
Glutardialdehyde	0.1%	100	100	100	100
Glutardialdehyde and 10mM dithiothreitol	0.1%	100	100	100	100

plasma membrane proteins were carried out as described by Towbin and Gordon /5/.

RESULTS

The reaction of soluble thyroid plasma membrane proteins with auto-antibodies from sera of Graves' patients is abolished by low concentration of dithiothreitol /DIT/, and 50% of inhibition of autoantibodies binding is obtained at 0.03mM. The inactivation curve is steep and complete inactivation achived at 0.1mM DIT. TSH binding to solubilized thyroid plasma membrane proteins was not significantly reduced by 1mM DIT pretreatment. Inactivation of autoantibodies binding sites in soluble preparation of thyroid plasma membrane was not reversed by dialysis to PBS or to alkaline buffer /carbonate-bicarbonate pH 9.6/ or by low concentrations of hydrogen peroxide /0.01%/. Thyroid plasma membrane proteins bound to polistyren plates are 20 times as much resistant to DIT inactivation. The inactivation curve of solid phase bound antigens is shallow, 50% of inactivation is obtained at 0.6mM DIT and even after 10mM DIT pretreatment, 20% of the antibodies binding capacity is still detectable, table 1. Binding of autoantibodies to particulate thyroid plasma membrane before solubilization is not affected by 10mM DIT pretreatment. Other disulphide reducing agents such as cystein and mercaptoethanol have a similar effect to that of DIT, on the binding of antibodies by soluble thyroid plasma membrane proteins. Preincubation of soluble thyroid plasma membrane proteins with 0.1% glutadialdehyde did not affect their ability to bind autoantibodies but protected them from the subsequent inactivation by DIT. Soluble thyroid plasma membrane proteins after 0.1% glutardialdehyde pretreatment retained 100% of the autoantibodies binding capacity even after 10mM DIT incubation for 16 hours at 4°C and they reacted with autoantibodies even in the presence of 10mM DIT.
Soluble thyroid plasma membrane antigens can be easily detected by immunoblotting on nitrocellulose paper and the detection limit is 0.05µg of protein per spot at 20 000 serum dilution. However, after 10mM DIT or mercaptoethanol pretreatment no specific reaction with autoantibodies from Graves' patients can be detected at 1:500 dilution of the same serum.
The ability to bind autoantibodies by soluble microsomal antigens is diminished by 40% by 0.1mM DIT pretreatment, the remaining 60% is not abolished after 1mM of DIT.

DISCUSSION

Thyrotropin binding sites on thyroid plasma membranes are sensitive to disulphide bridges reducing agents /6/ but they can be reactivated by dialysis or oxidation and DIT was used to dissociate the TSH binding peptited from plasma membranes /3/. The high sensitivity of autoantibodies binding sites on soluble thyroid plasma membrane proteins to disulphide bridges reducing compunds show that they are highly conformation dependent and different from the TSH binding sites. The disulphide bridge is not directly involved in the autoantibodies binding site as the glutardialdehyde linked proteins retain their ability to bind antibodies in the presence of DIT. The resistance of glutardialdehyde linked thyroid antigens to DIT in contrast to the soluble preparation point to the localisation of the binding sites on two /or more/ polipeptide chains, kept together in a proper conformation by an -S-S- bridge. The localisation of TSH binding sites on a single polipeptide chain has been demonstrated by Kajita et al /3/. The conformation of autoantibodies binding sites in particulate plasma membrane and in solid phase bound antigens is preserved also by other forces /hydrophobic interactions/ as they are resistant to disulphide bridges reducing compounds. Particulate thyroid plasma membranes bind autoantibodies even in the presence of 10mM DIT. Our data allow us to put forward a hypothesis that the autoantibodies epitopes are made up of two polipeptide chains linked by disulphide bridge and both chains are involved in making of the epitope.

In solution, after reduction of the disulphide bridges the polipeptides chains dissociate and reactivation in a complex protein mixture is improbable. By contrast, when the polipeptide chains can not seperate because they are fixed on polistyren plates or in the plasma membrane, reactivation is easily obtained. The antigenic deterimnants for Graves' autoantibodies can be classified as discontinuous /7/ concisting of residues from different parts of aminoacids sequence, brought together by the folding of the protein molecule. By analogy to antigenic determinants TSH binding sites can be regarded as continuous and composed of residues which are local in the polipeptide sequence.

REFERENCES

1. D.Doniach and J.N.Marshall. Autoantibodies to the thyrotropin receptor on thyroid epithelium and other tissues, in: Autoimmunity, N.Talal, ed., Academic Press, New York /1977/.

2. E.Davies Jones, F.A.Hashim, Kajita, F.M.Creaght, P.R.Buckland, V.B.Petersen, R.D.Howells and B.R.Smith, Interaction of autoantibodies to thyrotropin receptor with a hydrophilic subunit of the thyreotropin receptor with a hydrophilic subunit of the thyreotropin receptor, Biochem.J.228:111 /1985/.

3. Y.Kajita, C.R.Rickards, P.R.Buckland, R.D.Howells and B.R.Smith, A structure for the porcine TSH receptor, FEBS Lett. 181:218 /1985/.

4. A.Gardas, K.Rives, Enzyme-linked immunosorbent assay of autoantibodies reacting with thyroid plasma membrane antigens in sera of patients with autoimmune thyroid diseases, Acta Endocrinol. 113:265 /1986/.

5. H.Towbin and J.Gordon, Immunoblotting and dot immunobloting - current status and outlook, J.Immunol.Methods 72:313 /1984/.

6. J.Ginsberg, B.R.Smith and R.Hall, Evidence that porcine thyrotropin receptor contains an essential disulphide bridge, Mol,Cell.Endocrinol. 26:95 /1982/.

7. D.J.Barlow, M.S.Edwards and J.M.Thornton, Continuous and discontinuous protein antigenic determinants, Nature 322:747 /1986/.

PRESENCE OF THYROID GROWTH PROMOTING ANTIBODY IN PATIENTS WITH HASHIMOTO'S THYROIDITIS: EFFECT OF LONG-TERM THYROXINE TREATMENT

Annalisa Tanini, Carlo M. Rotella, Leonard D. Kohn[*] and
Roberto Toccafondi

Clinica Medica III   N.I.D.D.K.[*]
Universita' di Firenze   National Institutes of Health
Firenze, Italy   Bethesda, MD, U.S.A.

INTRODUCTION

The development of new procedures to detect the presence of circulating autoantibodies capable of promoting thyroid cell growth (TGPAb) has opened new ways to explore the pathogenesis of goitrous diseases (1-6). Methods to detect these autoantibodies include a cytochemical bioassay (CBA) based on DNA cytophotometry or pentose shunt analysis or the (3H)-thymidine incorporation into DNA of thyroid follicles, or thyroid cells in culture. The FRTL-5 thyroid cell thymidine incorporation assay appears to be more simple than the CBA, enables direct interassay comparisons and has an incidence of positive cases not so different from the more sensitive CBA (6); in addition the same cells can be also used to detect the presence of thyroid stimulating antibodies (TSAbs) (7).

The FRTL-5 cell growth assay has been shown to be positive in most patients with Graves' disease and in some with nontoxic goiter (3,6). The aim of the present report was to evaluate if the FRTL-5 tritiated thymidine incorporation assay is able to measure TGPAbs in untreated patients with Hashimoto's thyroiditis, and if it is to correlate their presence with goiter size, and to study the effect of therapy with thyroxine.

PATIENTS AND METHODS

Sera were obtained from 36 patients affected by Hashimoto's thyroiditis (HT), attending the Florence University Clinic. There were 29 women and 7 men, aged 18-77 yrs. The diagnosis of HT was based on: (a) diffuse enlargement of the thyroid gland, (b) clinical and laboratory finding of thyroid disfunction, (c) high titres of circulating antithyroid antibodies. Laboratory measurements included total T3 and T4 levels, as well as TSH measurements in all cases. Among the 36 patients, 25 (19 women and 6 men, ages 26–61 yrs) were studied before the start of any therapy; 12 of these, all TGPAb positive, were also studied after 13–22 months of treatment with thyroxine (150–200 µg/day). The remaining 11 patients were first studied after having been treated with thyroxine (150–200 µg/day) for several months.

Of the 25 untreated patients, 10, all hypothyroid, exhibited a moderate enlargement of thyroid gland. 25 had higher degrees of thyroid enlargement; 12 out of 15 were hypothyroid and 3 were hyperthyroid, i.e. had "Hashitoxicosis". The 12 patients also studied after 13–22 months of therapy with thyroxine were all euthyroid. Five of these had a small goiter, 7 a larger one.

At the time of onset of disease, all the 11 patients (10 women and 1 men, ages 18–77 yrs) affected by HT and treated for 12–22 months with exogenous thyroxine (150–200 µg/day) prior the study presented the same clinical and laboratory characteristics as the untreated patients, but TGPAbs were not studied before the onset of treatment since the test was not operational. At the time of these study all patients were euthyroid; 6 of them had a small goiter and 5 a larger one.

The immunoglobulins obtained (3,7) from sera of patients with HT were tested using the FRTL-5 thyroid cell system to detect both TSAb and TGPAb. TSAb activity (7) was measured by cAMP cellular levels in 24 well plastic plates, after two hour incubation with the IgG preparations. The intracellular cAMP was measured by a radioreceptor assay, correcting cAMP values by the DNA content of each well, as assesed by the ethidium bromide fluorescence method. The TGPAb activity (3) was evaluated by measuring the tritiated thymidine incorporation into FRTL-5 cell DNA, measured by the diphenylamine method.

RESULTS AND CONCLUSIONS

IgG preparations (3,7) did not contain other Ig classes as evaluated by immunoelectrophoresis, and exhibited 88 $\pm$ 10% purity based on differences between IgG RIA analyses and total protein content. The growth activity could be ascribed to the IgG itself since stimulatory activity was lost after preincubation of IgG with rabbit anti-human IgG coupled to Sepharose 4B. IgG preparations from HT patients did not contain TSH, as assessed by IRMA Sucrosep, even if tested at high IgG concentrations.

When the IgG of untreated HT patients were tested in the FRTL-5 growth assay, 17 out of 25 were positive (68.0%). The increase in tritiated thymidine incorporation into FRTL-5 cell DNA of TGPAb positive cases was variable, reaching in some instances 4 to 5 times the basal levels. Out of the 17 TGPAb positive patients only 3 were also TSAb positive in the cAMP assay using FRTL-5 cells; these patients were those affected by "Hashitoxicosis". For that concerns the goiter volume, among the 10 untreated HT patients with a small goiter, only 4 were TGPAb positive (40.0%). Of the 15 patients with larger goiters, 13 were positive in the FRTL-5 growth assay (86.7%).

In 12 of the 17 TGPAb positive patients it was possible to study the growth promoting activity in FRTL–5 cells after 13 to 22 months of treatment with adequate doses of T4. Only in 2 of these patients was TGPAb activity still detectable, and these patients were also the only ones in which therapy failed to reduce the goiter size. When TGPAb was studied in the 11 HT patients, who underwent T4 treatment prior to their TGPAb assay, only one had detectable thyroid growth promoting activity, and was also the only one in which therapy failed to reduce the size of goiter. All 11 treated Hashimoto's patients of this series were TSAb negative.

The TGPAb activity of the IgG of 4 untreated hypothyroid HT patients was also studied with respect to TSH effect on growth. The addition of a fixed amount of TGPAb (2 mg/ml) to increasing amounts of TSH (from 0.01 to 10 nM) in each case resulted in the same value that of TSH alone, in none of the cases studied was there an addictive effect as might be anticipated if the antibodies were modulating a receptor as signal much different from TSH.

In conclusion, also if the existence of TGPAb activity independent from TSAb activity has been questioned (see Zakarija elsewhere in this book), our data bring evidence for the polyvalent antibody production during an autoimmune mechanism, and TGPAb can be considered, along with TSH, as responsible for goiter formation in thyroid disorders.

REFERENCES

1. H. A. Drexhage, G. F. Bottazzo, D. Doniach, L. Bitensky, and J. Chayen, Evidence for Thyroid growth stimulating immunoglobulins in some goitous diseases, Lancet ii:287 (1980).
2. L. Chiovato, L. J. Hammond, T. Hanafusa, B. Pujol-Borel, D. Doniach, and G. F. Bottazzo, Detection of thyroid growth promoting immunoglobulins (TGI) by 3H-thymidine incorporation in cultured rat thyroid follicles, Clin. Endocrinol. 19:581 (1983).
3. W. A. Valente, P. Vitti, C. M. Rotella, M. M. Vaughan, S. M. Aloj, E. F. Grollman, F. S. Ambesi-Impiombato, and L. D. Kohn, Antibodies that promote thyroid growth: a distinct population of thyroid promoting antibodies. N. Engl. J. Med. 309:1028 (1983)
4. N. M. McMullan, and P. P. A. Smyth, "In vitro" generation of NADPH as an index of thyroid stimulating immunoglobulins (TGI) in goitrous disease, Clin. Endocrinol. 20:269 (1984).
5. R. D. van der Gaag, H. A. Drexhage, W. M. Wiersinga, R. S. Brown, R. Docter, G. F. Bottazzo, and D. Doniach, Further studies on thyroid growth stimulating immunoglobulins in euthyroid nonendemic goiter, J. Clin. Endocrinol. Metab. 60:972 (1985).
6. C. M. Rotella, C. Mavilia, L. D. Kohn, and R. Toccafondi, Thyroid growth promoting antibody in patients with non toxic goiter, in: "The thyroid and autoimmunity", H. A. Drexahage and W. M. Wiersinga, eds, Elsevier Science Publisher, Amsterdam, p.198, (1986).
7. P. Vitti, C. M. Rotella, W. A. Valente, J. Cohen, S. M. Aloj, P. Laccetti, F. S. Ambesi-Impiombato, E. F. Grollman, A. Pinchera,

R. Toccafondi, and L. D. Kohn, Characterization of the optimal
stimulatory effects of Graves' monoclonal and serum immunoglobulin G on adenosine 3', 5' monophosphate production in
FRTL-5 thyroid cells: a potential clinical assay, J. Clin.
Endocrinol. Metab. 57:782 (1983).

LIMITED CLINICAL VALUE OF TBII AND TSAB FOR PREDICTION OF THE OUTCOME OF PATIENTS WITH GRAVES' DISEASE

R. Hörmann, B. Saller, and K. Mann

Medical Department II, Klinikum Grosshadern
University of Munich
Munich, FRG

INTRODUCTION

According to the interim results of a German multicenter study the clinical value of TSH binding inhibiting immunoglobulin (TBII) determinations as a prognostic parameter in Graves' disease is questionable. Usually employed radioreceptorassays are measuring a heterogeneous population of functionally different antibodies, such as stimulating, binding and even inhibiting antibodies. Currently, the significance of stimulating antibodies is not well defined.
The aim of the present study was to compare the results of a radioreceptorassay with that obtained by a bioassay determining the stimulation of T3 release from porcine thyroid slices and to evaluate the clinical and prognostic implications of both assay systems.

PATIENTS

The study group consisted of 70 patients with active untreated GD (46 ± 14 years mean age). Diagnosis was confirmed by clinical observation, 99m technetium scintigraphy, hormone analysis and presence of signs of endocrine orbitopathy (stage III-IV) and/or elevated titres for microsomal and/or thyroglobulin antibodies.
25 patients were selected for a longitudinal study according to the following criteria: positive TSAb and TBII titres before therapy, standardized drug treatment (12 months, thiamazole: 10-30mg/day according to serum hormone levels), antibody determinations at 1-3 month intervals during therapy and a minimum time of 24 months of surveillance after drug withdrawal).

METHODS

TSH binding inhibiting immunoglobulins (TBII) were determined by a radioreceptorassay (TRAK-Assay, Fa. Henning,

Berlin). TBII activities >15% were regarded as positive (1).
Thyroid stimulating antibodies (TSAb) were evaluated by an
in vitro bioassay which determines the T3 release from
porcine thyroid slices (2). The assay procedure has been
described in detail previously (3). Briefly, thyroid slices
(0.5x1x1 mm) were incubated with 100ul of serum (5h, 37 ° C,
95% O_2 /5% CO_2) in the upper part of a bipartite teflon pot
with a dialysis membrane. After equilibrium dialysis (24h,
30°C, shaking water bath) free T3 was determined by a
sensitive RIA in aliquots of the lower compartment
containing 5ml of buffer. TSAb activities >30% were regarded
as positive.

RESULTS

The incidence of TBII / TSAb in 70 patients with untreated,
active GD was 90% / 91%. There was no correlation between
TSAb and TBII activities in these patients (r=0.20, p=n.s.).
41 (59%) showed signs of endocrine orbitopathy (stage
III-IV), 49 (70%) had elevated titres of microsomal and 21
(30%) of thyroglobulin antibodies. Neither TBII nor TSAb
activities were correlated to the titres of microsomal or
thyroglobulin antibodies or the presence of endocrine
orbitopathy.
During antithyroid treatment TBII decreased into the normal
range in 14 out of 25 selected patients, TSAb in 19
patients. Relapse after drug withdrawal (13/25 patients) was
seen in 5/5 patients with positive TSAb activities at the
end of therapy and in 8/20 TSAb negative patients. Out of
the patients with positive TBII titres 7/11, with negative
TBII 6/14 patients relapsed. Relapsing disease was always
associated with reappearance of TSAb and TBII.
Thus, TSAb determination with the T3 bioassay at the end of
therapy showed a higher specificity for prediction of
relapse after antithyroid drug treatment than TBII
radioreceptorassay. However, the sensitivity and predictive
value were poor for both methods (table 1).

Table 1. Sensitivity, specificity and predictive value of
TBII radioreceptorassay and TSAb bioassay for relapse or
remission of Graves' hyperthyroidism after 12 months of
antithyroid drug treatment.

	RRA (TBII)	Bioassay (TSAb)
sensitivity	54 %	38 %
specificity	67 %	100 %
predictive value for remission	60 %	57 %

CONCLUSION

Our results show a high and comparable incidence of TSAb and TBII in patients with untreated hyperthyroid Graves' disease. Persistence of TSAb during antithyroid drug treatment could specifically indicate an early relapse of hyperthyroidism after drug withdrawal. However, TSAb bioassay as well as TBII radioreceptorassay lack sufficient sensitivity and predictive value for relapse or remission after antithyroid drug treatment to have a decisive impact on therapeutic considerations.

REFERENCES

1. Hörmann R, Saller B, Müller R, Hobelsberger A, Moser E, Mann K: Methodische Probleme und klinische Wertigkeit der Bestimmung von TSH-Rezeptor-Antikörper mit einem kommerziellen Kit. Lab Med 9 (1985),208-213
2. Atkinson S, Kendall-Taylor P: The stimulation of thyroid hormone secretion in vitro by thyroid-stimulating antibodies. J Clin Endocrinol Metab 53 (1981),1263-1266
3. Mann K, Schneider N, Hörmann R: Thyrotropic activity of acidic isoelectric variants of human chorionic gonadotropin from trophoblastic tumors. Endocrinology 118 (1986), 1558-1566

TSH RECEPTOR ANTIBODIES IN NEONATAL HYPERTHYROIDISM

P.M. Hale, M. Liebert, N.J. Hopwood and J.C. Sisson

Departments of Pediatrics and Internal Medicine
The University of Michigan
Ann Arbor, Michigan, USA

Introduction

The hyperthyroidism in Graves' disease is caused by circulating autoantibodies which stimulate the thyroid gland (Burman and Baker, 1985). If these antibodies are present in a pregnant woman, they may cross the placenta and cause transient neonatal hyperthyroidism (Munro et al., 1978). Delays in treatment or failure to detect neonatal hyperthyroidism may lead to chronic complications such as mental impairment or craniosynostosis (Daneman and Howard, 1980). A method to predict and diagnose neonatal hyperthyroidism would be valuable. Historically, methods to detect Graves' autoantibodies involved laborious and difficult bioassay (Hensen et al., 1984). We report here the use of a simple, commercially available radioimmunoassay to detect Graves' autoantibodies in four cases of neonatal hyperthyroidism.

Materials and Methods

Thyroxine (T4) levels were determined using a standard competitive radioimmunoassay. Antibodies to the thyroid stimulating hormone (TSH) receptor were detected by the ability of the patient's serum to block the binding of radioiodinated TSH to solubilized TSH receptors from porcine thyroids. This activity is called TSH binding inhibiton (TBI). The TSH receptor antibody assay kit was obtained from Clinetics Corporation (Tustin, CA, USA), and was performed as previously described by Southgate et al., 1984. The TSH binding inhibition index (TBII) was calculated using this formula.

TBII=

$$\left(1 - \frac{\% \text{ receptor bound I-125 TSH is patient assay}}{\% \text{ receptor bound I-125 TSH in negative control}} \right) \times 100$$

The mean TBII observed in 18 normal individuals was 3.4% and the upper limit of normal was 15%.

Results

In maternal infant pair 1, a 20 year woman with a history of Graves' disease gave birth to a 2.33 kg infant at 35 weeks gestation. A diagnosis of neonatal Graves' disease was made at 6 days of age after the baby presented with irritability, tachycardia, vomiting, and increased stooling. As shown in the table, both mother and infant had TBII elevated above the normal range.

Maternal infant pair 2 represents a 30 year old woman who was diagnosed with Graves' disease during the 2nd trimester of her pregnancy. She was treated with PTU and delivered a 3.15 kg infant at term. The baby was diagnosed with Graves' disease at 12 days of age after presenting with diarrhea and hyperalertness. The table shows the presence of TBI in the mother and infant. TBI gradually disappeared in the infant over time.

In maternal infant pair 3, a 21 year old woman was diagnosed with Graves' disease during the third trimester of her pregnancy. She was treated with PTU and a beta blocker, and gave birth to a 2.96 kg infant at term. The baby was diagnosed with Graves' disease at 15 days of age after presenting with a possible apneic episode. TBII measurements were made in the mother before, on the day of, and after delivery (see Table) and were consistently elevated. The infant showed an elevated TBII which diminished over time and was undetectable by 85 days of age.

Maternal infant pair 4 represents a 26 year old woman who was diagnosed with Graves' disease and treated with radioactive iodine and PTU. Shortly afterward she became pregnant and delivered a 3.35 kg infant at term. The baby was diagnosed with Graves' disease at 6 days of age after presenting with diarrhea. The table demonstrates elevated maternal and infant TBII.

TBII[a] in Maternal Infant Pairs

| | Mothers | | Infants | |
	time (days)	TBII (%)	time (days of age)	TBII (%)
Pair 1	31 posp.[b]	67.8	25	26.7
			29	20.5
Pair 2	13 postp.	60.6	13	49.5
			18	44.9
			68	27.0
			103	18
Pair 3			1	61.9
	48 prep[c]	72	7	54.4
			21	25.0
	day of			
	delivery	70.7	29	20.3
	113 postp.	52.1	85	0
Pair 4	1 postp.	85	1	77
			6	86

[a] TSH binding inhibition index; upper limit of normal = 15%
[b] post partum
[c] pre partum

Conclusions

TBII was shown to be elevated in each of the four mothers studied and in their offspring. The TBII decreased over time in two infants in which serial samples were taken over several months.

Our results suggest that this commercially available test is of value in the diagnosis of neonatal hyperthyroidism and may be useful in identifying mothers at risk of delivering affected infants.

References

Burman, K.D., and Baker, J.R., Jr., 1985, Immune mechanism in Graves' disease, Endo. Rev. 58: 980.

Daneman, D., and Howard, N.J., 1980, Neonatal thyrotoxicosis: Intellectual impairment and craniosynostosis in later years, J. Peds. 97: 257.

Hensen, J., Kotulla, P., Finke, R., Bogner, U., Badenhoop, K., Meinhold, H., and Schleusener, H., 1984, Methodological apsects and clinical results of an assay for thyroid-stimulating antibodies: Correlation with thyrotropin binding-inhibiting antibodies, J. Clin. Endo. Metab., 58: 980.

Munro, D.S., Dirmikis, S.M., Humphries, H., Smith, T., and Broadhead, G.D., 1978, The role of thyroid stimulating immunoglobulins of Graves' disease in neonatal thyrotoxicosis, Brit. J. Obs. Gyn., 85: 837.

Southgate, K., Creagh, F., Teece, M., Kingswood, C., and Smith, B.R., 1984, A receptor assay for the measurement of TSH receptor antibodies in unextracted serum, Clin. Endo., 20: 539.

THYROID AUTOIMMUNITY AS A MAJOR CAUSE FOR CONGENITAL HYPOTHYROIDISM

U. Bogner, A. Grueters*, H. Peters, G. Holl, R. Finke and H. Schleusener

Endocrine Departments of the Medical and *Pediatric Clinics of the Free University of Berlin, FRG

INTRODUCTION

A causal relationship between maternal autoimmune thyroid disease and congenital hypothyroidism (CH) of the infant has been suggested as early as 1960.[1,2] Subsequent observations in single families with maternal autoimmune thyroid disease and repeated occurrence of congenital hypothyroidism in the children were reported.[3] With the establishment of a TSH-screening program for CH a large number of newborns with CH were tested for microsomal (Mab) and thyroglobulin (Tab) antibodies in the neonatal period, which did not show an increased frequency of these antibodies in affected children compared to normal newborns.[4] However, since during the last years, other types of antibodies than Mab and Tab could be measured in those newborns, increasing evidence for supporting the hypothesis of maternal autoimmune thyroid disease as a pathogenetic mechanism of CH was raised.[5,6] Therefore we determined the frequency of different types of thyroid antibodies in newborns with CH and their mothers in correlation to the type of congenital hypothyroidism.

PATIENTS AND METHODS

In 46 newborns with permanent CH and 8 newborns with transient CH, detected by the newborn TSH-screening program in Berlin, and in 15 of their mothers, the following types of antibodies were determined: 1) Microsomal (Mab) and thyroglobulin (Tab) antibodies were measured by passive hemagglutination using a commercial kit. 2) TSH-binding inhibitory-immunoglobulins (TBII) were determined by a radioreceptor binding assay using membrane fractions.[7] 3) Antibody-dependent cell-mediated cytotoxicity (ADCC) was measured using a ^{51}chromium-release assay against human thyroid cells.[8] 4) Thyroid-growth-blocking-antibodies (TGBAb) were measured by the inhibition of the TSH-induced ^{3}H-thymidine uptake into human thyroid cells by serum of affected infants and their mothers.[9]

This work was supported by Deutsche Forschungsgemeinschaft

Table 1. Clinical data of newborns with CH (median and range)

	n	TSH mU/ml	T$_4$ /ug/dl	Tg ng/ml	Scan Results n
Athyreosis	18	200 (150-380)	2.6 (1.8-7.3)	0 (0-1.8)	8
Dysgenesis	28	120 (50-200)	7.2 (2.5-10.1)	78 (25-400)	15
transient CH	8	50 (40-200)	7.7 (2.5-10.5)	113 (80-250)	-

RESULTS

Table 1 gives the clinical data of the newborns with CH. The diagnosis of athyreosis was made by a negative ^{123}I-thyroid scan at the age of two years or by absent thyroglobulin (Tg) levels at the time of diagnosis. Ectopic or hypoplastic glands (dysgenesis) were detected by ^{123}I-thyroid scan or the diagnosis was based on normal thyroglobulin levels in the newborn period. Transient hypothyroidism normalized within four weeks without replacement therapy. The three groups of patients differed also in the levels of TSH and thyroxin (T$_4$) at the time of diagnosis, with those newborns with athyreosis presenting significantly higher TSH and lower T$_4$ levels.

A significant percentage of positive antibodies could be found in newborns with permanent CH but they were absent in transient hypothyroidism (Tab. 2). The highest frequency was observed for TGBAb. In five cases, positive TGBAb and ADCC were accompanied by positive TBII.

Fig. 1 shows the corresponding values of positive thyroid antibodies (TBII, TGBAb, ADCC) in infants and their mothers. All mothers positive for TGBAb and TBII transmitted their antibodies to their infants.

Table 2. Incidence of positive thyroid autoantibodies in newborns with permanent CH and their mothers

Type of Ab	n	pos. infants (%)	n	pos. mothers (%)
Mab	46	9	12	8
Mab	46	4	12	8
TBII	43	9	12	33
ADCC	24	20	9	11
TGBAb	14	57	9	55

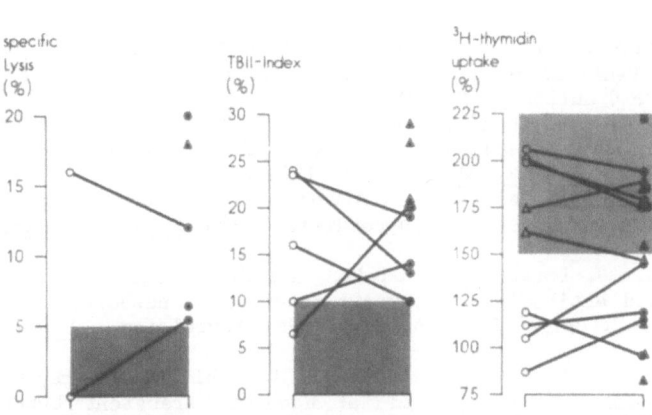

Fig. 1.   TBII, ADCC and TGBAb in infants with athyreosis (O), dysgenesis
(▲) and transient hypothyroidism (■) and their mothers
(o △). Normal values of TBII (52 infants with permanent or
transient CH and 12 mothers) and ADCC (19 infants and 8 mothers)
are included in the shaded area, which indicates the normal range.

DISCUSSION

     The high frequency of TGBAb we found in newborns with congenital
hypothyroidism and their mothers is in keeping with results presented by
van der Gaag et al.[6]   Additionally, we were able to demonstrate
TSH-binding inhibiting and cytotoxic antibodies in the sera of some of
these children, but Tab and Mab only in a low frequency.   Although TBII
and TGBAb did not show a positive correlation and seem to be antibodies
with different properties, they are both directed against structures of
the TSH-receptor or binding sites closely related to the receptor, whereas
cytotoxic antibodies are thought to bind to a different antigen on the
cell surface, i.e. to the microsomal antigen.   Altogether, our data show
that various types of antibodies are present in sera of infants with CH
and their mothers, supporting the hypothesis that autoimmune reaction
might be responsible for the inhibition of the regular development of the
fetal gland and subsequently permanent congenital hypothyroidism.

     Since it is possible to measure TBII, TGBAb and cytotoxic antibodies
in small amounts of serum, in the future, large series will probably
clarify the pathogenetic role of maternal autoimmune thyroid disease for
congenital hypothyroidism.   Additionally, the determination of these
antibodies might be helpful in the genetic counseling of mothers with
autoimmune thyroid disease.

REFERENCES

1. J.M. Sutherland, V.M. Esselborn, R.L. Burket, T.B. Skillman, and J.T. Benson, Familial nongoitrous cretinism apparently due to maternal antithyroid antibody, N Engl J Med 263: 336 (1960).
2. R.M. Blizzard, R.W. Chandler, B.H. Landing, M.O. Pettit, and C.D. West, Maternal autoimmunization as a probable cause of athyrotic cretinism, N Engl J Med 263: 327 (1960).
3. E.M. Ritzén, H. Mahler, and A. Alveryd, Transitory congenital hypothyroidism and maternal thyroiditis, Acta Paediatr Scand 70: 765 (1981).
4. J. Dussault, J. Letarte, H. Guyda, and C. Leberge, Lack of influence of thyroid antibodies on thyroid function in newborns and on a mass screening program for congenital hypothyroidism, J Ped 96: 385 (1980).
5. N. Matsuura, Y. Yamada, Y. Nohara, J. Konishi, K. Kasagi, K. Endo, H. Kojima, and K. Wataya, Familial neonatal transient hypothyroidism due to maternal TSH-binding inhibitor immunoglobulins, N Engl J Med 303: 738 (1980).
6. R.D. van der Gaag, H.A. Drexhage, and J.H. Dussault, Role of maternal immunoglobulins blocking TSH-induced thyroid growth in sporadic forms of congenital hypothyroidism, Lancet 1: 246 (1985).
7. H. Schleusener, P. Kotulla, R. Finke, H. Sörje, H. Meinhold, F. Adlkofer, and K.W. Wenzel, Relationship between thyroid status and Graves' disease specific immunoglobulins, J Clin Endocrinol Metab 47: 379 (1978).
8. U. Bogner, H. Schleusener, and J.R. Wall, Antibody-dependent cell-mediated cytotoxicity against human thyroid cells in Hashimoto's thyroiditis but not Graves' disease, J Clin Endocrinol Metab 59: 734 (1984).
9. H. Peters, U. Bogner, G. Holl, A. Grueters, R. Finke, and H. Schleusener, Thyroid growth blocking antibodies in congenital hypothyroidism, in: "Thyroid autoimmunity 30th anniversary: memories and perspectives," A. Pinchera, ed., Plenum Publishing Corp., London (1986).

THYROID GROWTH BLOCKING ANTIBODIES IN CONGENITAL HYPOTHYROIDISM

H. Peters, U. Bogner, G. Holl, A. Grueters*, R. Finke, and
H. Schleusener

Endocrine Departments of the Medical and *Pediatric Clinics
of the Free University of Berlin, FRG

INTRODUCTION

The causes of transient and permanent congenital hypothyroidism (CH) have not been entirely clarified, although there is increasing evidence that these diseases might be the result of an immunological disorder. Thyroid growth blocking antibodies (TGBAb), detected in the sera of affected infants and their mothers, might suggest that the development and maturation of the fetal thyroid gland might be suppressed by these antibodies. Recently, Drexhage et al.[1] described TGBAb in patients with primary myxedema. Applying the same technique, van der Gaag et al.[2] detected thyroid growth blocking antibodies in about 50% of infants with congenital hypothyroidism.

In order to evaluate the frequency of thyroid growth blocking antibodies in newborns, found to be hypothyroid in the Berlin TSH-screening program, we developed a new method of measuring the inhibition of TSH-induced ^{3}H-thymidine incorporation into human thyroid cells in serum instead of IgG fractions from affected infants.

METHOD

Human thyroid tissue, obtained by surgery, was minced and digested by collagenase and cultured in Iscove's medium. The medium contained 0.5% FCS, 5 /ug/ml transferrin, 10 /ug/ml somatostatin, 10^{-8}mol/l hydrocortisone, 10 /ug/ml insulin and 10 /ug/ml iodide. After 2 days of incubation at 37°C in 5% CO_2 in air, the cells were transferred in suspension by trypsinization. 10^4 cells/well were incubated in microtiter plates with increasing concentrations of TSH (0 - 100 mU/ml), 100 /ul 1:10 diluted serum, and 1 /uCi ^{3}H-methyl-thymidine. After 2 days of incubation, the supernatant was decanted and each well washed twice. Thyroid cells were detached from the plastic wall by addition of 150 /ul trypsin-EDTA solution (0.5%/0.2%) and precipitated by addition of 50 /ul trichloroacetic acid solution (20%). The precipitate was then harvested by a cell harvester and the radioactivity was determined in a ß-counter. The basal thymidine uptake in the absence of TSH was called the 100% value.

This work was supported by Deutsche Forschungsgemeinschaft

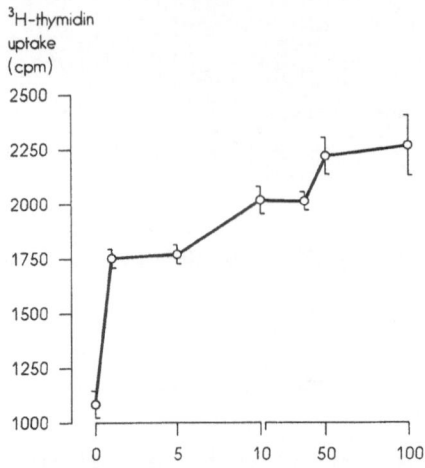

Fig. 1. Dose response curve of increasing concentrations of TSH and
^{3}H-thymidine uptake into human thyroid cells.

RESULTS

^{3}H-thymidine uptake was stimulated by increasing concentrations of
TSH (0 - 100 mU/ml) (Fig. 1). Addition of 1 mU/ml TSH resulted in a steep
increase of thymidine incorporation, whereas no further increase could be
seen at TSH values of 50 - 100 mU/ml. The thymidine uptake blocking
activity of sera was measured at a TSH concentration of 10 mU/ml.

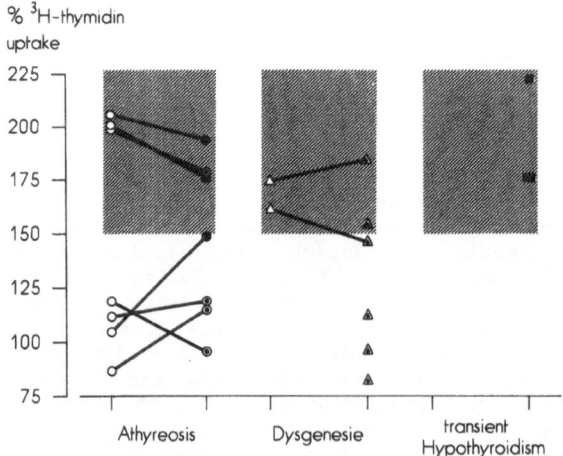

Fig. 2. TBGAb in infants and their mothers in permanent (athyreosis,
dysgenesis) and transient congenital hypothyroidism. Shaded area
indicates the normal range. Light symbols = mothers, dark symbols
= infants.

426

The thymidine uptake was 185 + 15% in the presence of serum from normal infants (n = 8). Sera exhibiting blocking activity were called positive when being below the mean value - 2 SD (<150%) of normal sera. Thirteen infants with permanent CH (athyreosis and dysgenesis), 9 of their mothers and 3 infants with transient CH were investigated. In 8 infants and 4 of their mothers, TGBAb was positive. TGBAb could be detected in 4 children with athyreosis as well as in 4 children with dysgenesis (ectopic or hypoplastic gland), whereas in transient hypothyroidism blocking activity was always negative (Fig. 2).

DISCUSSION

In several case reports[3-5], the influence of maternal autoimmune thyroid disease on the development of the fetal thyroid gland were described. Antibodies directed against the TSH-receptor seem to be of more importance in inducing fetal hypothyroidism than thyroglobulin and microsomal antibodies.[5] TSH-binding inhibiting antibodies as well as antibodies, which inhibit TSH-induced cAMP increase in thyroid cells, were reported to be increased in infants with CH and their mothers.[6] Very recently, van der Gaag et al.[2]described thyroid growth blocking antibodies in about 50% of newborns with CH, a finding confirmed by our results applying a different technique. Our assay system has the advantage of measuring TGBAb in human thyroid cells, excluding any problems of species specificity. Furthermore, the use of serum instead of IgG makes the assay suitable for determination of TGBAb in newborns from whom, in general, only limited amounts of serum are available.

REFERENCES

1. H.A. Drexhage, G.F. Bottazzo, L. Bitensky, J. Chayen, and D. Doniach, Thyroid growth-blocking antibodies in primary myxoedema, Nature 289: 594 (1981).
2. R.D. van der Gaag, H.A. Drexhage, and J.H. Dussault, Role of maternal immunoglobulins blocking TSH-induced thyroid growth in sporadic forms of congenital hypothyroidism, Lancet 1: 246 (1985).
3. J.M. Sutherland, V.M. Esselborn, R.L. Burket, T.B. Skillman, and J.T. Benson, Familial nongoitrous cretinism apparently due to maternal antithyroid antibody, N Engl J Med 263: 336 (1960).
4. R.M. Blizzard, R.W. Chandler, B.H. Landing, M.O. Pettit, and C.D. West, Maternal autoimmunization as a probable cause of athyrotic cretinism. N Engl J Med 263: 327 (1960).
5. N. Matsuura, Y. Yamada, Y. Nohara, J. Konishi, K. Kasagi, K. Endo, H. Kojima, and K. Wataya, Familial neonatal transient hypothyroidism due to maternal TSH-binding inhibitor immunoglobulins, N Engl J Med 303: 738 (1980).
6. N. Takasu, M. Naka, T. Mori, and T. Yamada, Two types of thyroid function-blocking antibodies in autoimmune atrophic thyroiditis and transient neonatal hypothyroidism due to maternal IgG, Clin Endocrinol 21: 345 (1984).

INCIDENCE OF TSH RECEPTOR ANTIBODIES IN PATIENTS WITH TOXIC DIFFUSE GOITER

Enrico Macchia, Roberto Concetti, Giovanni Carone, Lucia Gasperini, Flavia Borgoni, Gianfranco Fenzi, and Aldo Pinchera

Cattedra di Endocrinologia e Medicina Costituzionale, Università di Pisa; Pisa, Italy

INTRODUCTION

Graves' disease is considered to be an autoimmune disorder characterized by hyperfunction and diffuse enlargement of the thyroid gland, frequently associated with ophthalmopathy and sometimes with pretibial myxedema. The hyperthyroidism of Graves' disease is attributed to the stimulation of the thyrotropin receptor by an antibody directed against this structure (1-3). Moreover changes in the number and the function of T-lynphocytes has been observed in patients with Graves' disease (4). The TSH receptor antibodies are detected by two different systems: a truly stimulatory assay and a binding assay. The autoantibodies detected by the former assay are commonly known as "thyroid stimulating antibodies"(TSAb), those detected by the latter "thyrotropin-binding inhibiting antibodies" (TBIAb). A variety of other autoantibodies directed towards different constituents of the thyroid cell, such as thyroglobulin antibody (TgAb) and thyroid microsomal antibody (MAb), have been detected in patients with autoimmune thyroid diseases. TgAb and MAb are widely used in the diagnosis of Graves' disease as an index of humoral autoimmunity. However, some patients with toxic diffuse goiter do not show circulating TgAb or MAb, or other clinical signs of thyroid autoimmunity, such as ophthalmopathy or pretibial myxedema.

The aim of this study was to evaluate the prevalence of TSH receptor antibodies (TRAb) in patients with toxic diffuse goiter without humoral features of autoimmunity and in those patients with active ophthalmopathy or pretibial myxedema.

MATERIALS AND METHODS

Patients : the study group included 128 hyperthyroid patients with Graves' disease of whom 99 untreated and 29 relapsed after withdrawal of antithyroid drug therapy. The presence of active ophthalmopathy, pretibial myxedema, TgAb , MAb and TSH receptor antibodies was evaluated.

Preparation of IgG: IgG fraction was prepared by a modification (5) of the Baumstark method. Protein concentration was determined by the Lowry method (6). In the adenylate cyclase (AC) stimulation assay the IgG were used at a final concentration of 1 mg/ml.

Preparation of human thyroid plasma membranes for AC assay: thyroid tissue from patients with non toxic goiter was obtained at surgery and immediately processed at 4°C. Human thyroid homogenate was centrifuged at 300xg; the 30,000xg pellet of the supernatant was resuspended in an isotonic medium and stored in liquid nitrogen until used.

Adenylate cyclase activity assay: the crude thyroid plasma membrane preparation (60 µg/tube) was incubated with normal or Graves' immunoglobulins. The incubation took place at

34°C in 50 mM Tris HCl buffer, pH 7.9, O.1% BSA, with 1 mM ATP, 4 mM Mg^{++}, a phosphodiesterase inhibitor and an ATP regenerating system, and was stopped after 60 min. by the addition of a cold methanol/ethanol mixture. A 50 µl aliquot of the supernatant was dried and its cAMP content was measured by a specific radioimmunoassay.

TSH-binding inhibition assay: TBIAb was measured by a radioreceptor assay. Briefly, solubilized porcine thyroid plasma membranes were incubated for 20 min. at 22°C with ^{125}I-TSH and normal serum or patient serum. The inhibitory effect of patients' sera on the binding of ^{125}I-TSH to porcine thyroid plasma membranes was expressed as TBIAb index:

$$TBIAb = (1 - \frac{cpm\ unknown\ sample}{cpm\ normal\ serum}) \times 100$$

Values exceeding 2 SD from the mean value obtained with normal patients' sera were considered positive.

Miscellaneous: serum TgAb and MAb were measured by the standard haemagglutination technique.

RESULTS

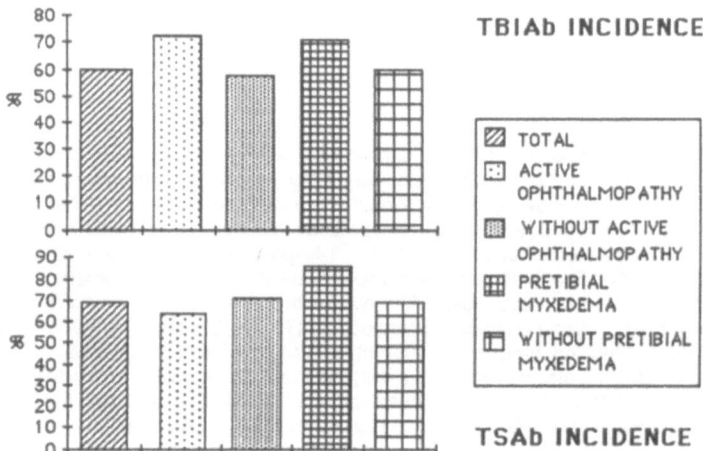

Fig. 1: TBIAb and TSAb incidence in the various groups of patients.

Active ophthalmopathy was present in 22/128 patients and pretibial myxedema in 7/128. 54/128 patients had no sign of Graves' ophthalmopathy. TBIAb was positive in 60.1% and TSAb in 68.7% of patients. TBIAb and TSAb were found positive in 72.7% and 63.6%, respectively, of patients with active Graves' ophthalmopathy and in 57.4% and 70.4%, respectively, of patients without ophthalmopathy. Subjects with pretibial myxedema showed a TBIAb and TSAb prevalence of 71.4% and 85.7%, respectively, compared with 59.5% and 67.8% in the patients without this clinical sign. The χ^2 analysis of these results did not show any significant difference in the incidence of TSH receptor antibodies in the various groups of patients. In patients with toxic diffuse goiter 15/128 did not have circulating TgAb and MAb. None of them had pretibial myxedema and only 3 had active ophthalmopathy; TBIAb and/or TSAb were positive in 13 of these subjects. No correlation was observed between TBIAb and TSAb activities.

DISCUSSION

Several authors have demonstrated the presence of TBIAb and/or TSAb in the majority of patients with active Graves' disease (1; 7-9). Schleusener et al. (10) found a higher prevalence of TBIAb in patients with ophthalmopathy, compared with those without this symptom. Our study confirmed this observation, although the difference between the two groups of patients did not reach the level of statistical significance. As far as TSAb is concerned, we did not see any noticeable difference.

We extended our investigation to study the prevalence of TSH receptor antibodies in another typical, even though infrequent, sign of Graves' disease, i.e. pretibial myxedema. An elevated incidence of TBIAb and TSAb was observed, but, again,the difference in prevalence compared to those subjects without this symptom was not significant.

A minority of patients with toxic diffuse goiter do not present either TgAb and/or MAb in their sera or clear clinical signs of thyroid autoimmunity, so that the autoimmune origin of the disease could be challenged. In order to understand the problem better, we looked for thyroid receptor antibodies in those patients without humoral and clinical stigmata of thyroid autoimmunity: only 2 out of 15 subjects did not show the presence of TBIAb and/or TSAb in their sera. This observation supported the concept that the presence of thyroid receptor antibodies is the most specific marker of Graves' disease; MAb, even if present in the majority of cases and sometimes correlated with TRAb (5), can be considered merely as an index of an autoimmune attack to the thyroid gland, but not as having any pathogenetic role in the hyperthyroidism of Graves' disease, which is actually due to antibodies directed against the TSH-receptor and able to stimulate thyroid function.

REFERENCES

1-J. Orgiazzi, D. E. Williams, I. J. Chopra, D. H. Solomon: Human thyroid adenyl cyclase-stmulating activity in immunoglobulin G of patients with Graves' disease. J. Clin. Endocrinol. Metab. 42: 341 (1976).

2-B.R. Smith, R. Hall: The interactions of Graves' immunoglobulins with the TSH receptors. In: Thyroid Research (Stcking J. R. and Nagataki S., eds.) Australian Acad. Sci., Camberra, vol. 8, pp. 715-716 (1980).

3-A. Pinchera, G. F. Fenzi, E. Macchia, L. Bartalena, S. Mariotti, F. Monzani: Thyroid stimulating immunoglobulins. Horm. Res. 16: 317 (1982).

4-R. Volpé: Autoimmune thyroid disease. A perspective. Mol. Biol. Med. 3: 25 (1986).

5-G. F. Fenzi, E. Macchia, L. Bartalena, F. Mazzanti, L. Baschieri, L. J. De Groot: Radioreceptor assay of TSH: its use to detect thyroid stimulating immunoglobulins. J. Endocrinol. Invest. 1: 17 (1978).

6-H. Lowry, N. J. Rosenbrough, A. L. Farr, N. J. Randall: Protein measurement with the folin phenol reagent. J. Biol. Chem. 193: 265 (1951).

7-B. R. Smith, R. Hall: Measurement of thyrotropin receptor antibodies. Method in Enzymology 74: part C 405-420 (1981).

8-J. M. Mc Kenzie, M. Zakarija: A reconsideration of thyroid stimulating immunoglobulin as the cause of hyperthyroidism in Graves' disease. J. Clin. Endocrinol. Metab. 42: 778 (1976).

9-E. Macchia, P. Carayon, G. F. Fenzi, S. Lissitzky, A. Pinchera: A sensitive method for assaying thyroid stimulating immunoglobulins of Graves' disease: use of the guanyl nucleotide-amplified thyroid adenylate cyclase assay. Acta Endocrinol (Kbh.) 103: 345 (1983).

10-J. Hensen, P. Kotulla, R. Finke, K. Badenhoop, K. Koppenhagen, H. Meinhold, H; Schleusener: 10 years experience with consecutive measurement of thyrotropin binding inhibiting antibodies (TBIAb). J. Endocrinol. Invest. 7: 215 (1984).

BLOCKING-ANTIBODIES APPARENTLY WITHOUT ANY STIMULATORY ACTIVITY ARE PRESENT IN SERA OF PATIENTS WITH GRAVES' DISEASE

Enrico Macchia, Roberto Concetti, Giovanni Carone, Flavia Borgoni, Gianfranco Fenzi, and Aldo Pinchera

Cattedra di Endocrinologia e Medicina Costituzionale, Università di Pisa; Pisa, Italy

INTRODUCTION

Over the last ten years a radioreceptor assay for thyrotropin has been developed to detect immunoglobulins able to inhibit the binding of TSH to its receptor in patients with Graves' disease (1). These immunoglobulins were originally called thyroid stimulating immunoglobulins (2), but later on they were more appropriately termed TSH-binding inhibiting antibodies (TBIAb). In fact subsequent methods directly measuring the thyroid stimulating activity of Graves' IgG, have not shown any clear correlation with TBIAb, whereas the existence of TBIAb without any stimulatory activity was demonstrated(3, 4). Immunoglobulins able to inhibit TSH binding to its receptor were also found in other autoimmune thyroid diseases such as Hashimoto's thyroiditis and idiapathic myxedema (5). TBIAb, which not only lacked thyroid stimulating activity but also blocked the action of TSH in vitro, were found in several patients with idiopathic myxedema and hypothyroid Hashimoto's thyroiditis (6). Blocking antibodies have also been reported in some patients with Graves' disease after treatment (7).

In this study we investigated the presence of these blocking antobodies in the sera of patients with active Graves' disease. We then compared this blocking activity with that of an IgG preparation, showing a potent blocking activity, from an idiopathic myxedema patient.

MATERIALS AND METHODS

Patients: Blood samples were obtained from 135 hyperthyroid Graves' patients and from 1 patient with idiopathic myxedema. The thyroid stimulating and TSH-binding inhibiting activities were evaluated.

Preparation of immunoglobulins: 3 ml of patients' serum were submitted to ion-exchange chromatography with DEAE-Sephadex A-50. Immunoglobulins were then precipitated with ammonium sulphate and extensively dialyzed against 10 mM Tris HCl buffer, pH 7.4 (8). The final concentration of IgG in the adenylate cyclase activity assay was 1 mg/ml.

Preparation of human thyroid plasma membranes for adenylate cyclase assay: thyroid tissue from patients with non-toxic goiter was obtained at surgery and immediately processed at 4°C. Human thyroid homogenate was centrifuged at 300xg; the 30,000xg pellet of the supernatant was resuspended in an isotonic medium and stored in liquid nitrogen until used.

Adenylate cyclase activity assay: the crude thyroid plasma membrane preparation (60 µg/tube)was incubated with normal or Graves' immunoglobulins. The incubation took place at 34°C in 50 mM Tris HCl buffer, pH 7.9, O.1% BSA, with 1 mM ATP, 4 mM Mg^{++}, a phosphodiesterase inhibitor and an ATP regenerating system, and was stopped after 60 min. by the addition of a cold methanol/ethanol mixture. A 50 µl aliquot of the supernatant was dried and its cAMP content was measured by a specific radioimmunoassay.

When the IgG blocking activity was evaluated, the thyroid membrane preparation was incubated with b-TSH or with a potent TSAb in the absence, or in the presence, of different concentrations of Graves' or I.M. immunoglobulins.

TSH-binding inhibition assay: TSH-binding inhibiting antibodies were measured by a radioreceptor assay. Briefly, solubilized porcine plasma membranes were incubated for 20 min. at 22°C with ^{125}I-TSH and normal immunoglobulins or patients' immunoglobulins. The inhibitory effect of patients' immunoglobulins on the binding of ^{125}I-TSH to porcine thyroid plasma membranes was expressed as TBIAb index:

TBIAb = (1-cpm unknown sample/cpm normal immunoglobulin) x 100

Values exceeding 2 SD from the mean value obtained with normal patients' immunoglobulins were considered positive.

RESULTS

Nineteen out of 135 Graves' patients were found positive for TBIAb assay and negative for TSAb assay. The IgG of 15 of these patients inhibited significantly (> 20%) TSH-stimulated adenylate cyclase activity. In this latter group 2 IgG preparations were strong inhibitors of the adenylate cyclase activity stimulated by TSH. In conditions of submaximal adenylate cyclase stimulation by TSH (6.6 mU/ml), the two Graves' TBIAb produced a dose-dependent inhibition of TSH-stimulated adenylate cyclase activity up to 75% and 82% respectively; the IgG from I.M. showed a similar effect up to 79%. The adenylate cyclase stimulation produced by a potent TSAb preparation with weak TBIAb activity was also inhibited in a dose-dependent way by the two Graves' TBIAb up to 77% and 90% respectively, and by I.M. TBIAb up to 89%.

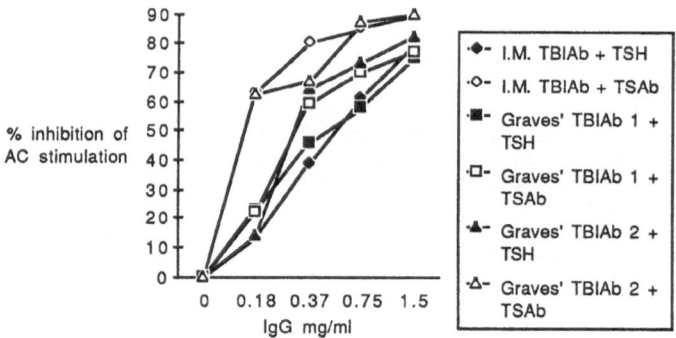

Fig. 1. inhibition of TSH- or TSAb-stimulated AC activity by I.M. and Graves' IgG with TBIAb activity.

DISCUSSION

In this study we examined the IgG preparations from a group of 135 patients with active Graves' disease and observed a significant inhibition of the thyroid adenylate cyclase activity stimulated by TSH in 15 out of 19 patients positive for TBIAb but lacking thyroid stimulating activity. Of these 15 IgG preparations 2 showed a strong inhibitory effect on TSH binding and greatly inhibited the adenylate cyclase activity stimulated by a submaximal dose of b-TSH and by a potent TSAb in a dose-dependent way. The effect of these 2 IgG was similar to that observed with an IgG derived from a patient with idiopathic myxedema. Several studies demontrated the presence of blocking antibodies directed against the thyrotropin receptor in patients with idiopathic myxedema and hypothyroid Hashimoto's thyroiditis (6). These antibodies were able to inhibit TSH binding to its receptor and also to inhibit TSH-stimulated adenylate cyclase activity. Blocking antibodies have also been reported in some patients with Graves' disease after radioiodine administration (7).

Our finding of blocking antibodies in 15 patients with hyperthyroid Graves' disease, both untreated and relapsed, apparently without any thyroid stimulating activity, is rather surprising. However the the existence of at least two types of TSH receptor antibodies in the sera of patients with Graves' disease has been suggested by the lack of correlation between TSH -binding inhibiting and thyroid stimulating activities (3). Thus, it should not seem such a paradox that the sera from some Graves' patients appear to contain blocking activity only. At least two hypotheses can be made to explain the thyroid hyperfunction in these patients: the first one is that the possible stimulating effect of these Graves' immunoglobulins is present at concentrations higher than those we can use with our method. The second one is that the sera of these 15 Graves' patients do in fact contain thyroid stimulating antibodies, but their action is masked _in vitro_ by the blocking immunoglobulins, which bind with high affinity to our membrane system, while these stimulators can exert their action on the patients' thyroid.

In conclusion we can postulate that the activity of the Graves' immunoglobulins on, the TSH receptor-adenylate cyclase system could be attributed to different antibodies varying with regard to their concentration, binding affinity and intrinsic biological activity.

REFERENCES

1- A. Pinchera, G.F. Fenzi, E. Macchia, L. Bartalena, S. Mariotti, F. Monzani: Thyroid-stimulating immunoglobulins. Horm. Res. 16: 317 (1982).
2 - B.R. Smith, R. Hall: Thyroid-stimulating immunoglobulins in Graves' disease. Lancet 2: 427 (1974).
3 - E. Macchia, G.F. Fenzi, F. Monzani, F. Lippi, P. Vitti, L. Grasso, L. Bartalena, L. Baschieri, A. Pinchera: Comparison between thyroid stimulating and TSH binding inhibiting immunoglobulins of Graves' disease. Clin. Endocrinol. (Oxf.) 15: 175 (1981).
4 - A. Sugenoya, A. Kidd, V.V. Row, R. Volpé: Correlation between thyrotropin-displacing activity and human thyroid-stimulating activity by immunoglobulins from patients with Graves' disease and other thyroid disorders. J. Clin. Endocrinol. Metab. 48: 398 (1979).
5 - K. Endo, K. Kasagi, J. Konishi, K. Ikekubo, T. Okuno, Y. Takeda, T. Mori, K. Torizuka: Detection and properties of TSH binding inhibitor immunoglobulins in patients with Graves' disease and Hashimoto thyroiditis. J. Clin. Endocrinol. Metab. 46: 734 (1978).
6 - J. Konishi, Y. Iida, K. Kasagi, T. Misaki, T. Nakashima, K. Endo, T. Mori, S. Shinpo, Y. Nohara, N. Matsuura, K. Torizuka: Primary myxedema with thyrotropin-binding inhibitor immunoglobulins. Ann. Intern. Med. 103: 26 (1985).
7 - K. Bech, H. Bliddal, K. Siersbaek-Nielsen, T. Friis: Production of non-stimulating immunoglobulins that inhibit TSH binding in Graves' disease after radioiodine administration. Clin. Endocrinol. (Oxf.) 17: 395 (1982).
8 - G.F. Fenzi, E. Macchia, L. Bartalena, F. Mazzanti, L. Baschieri, L.J. DeGroot: Radio-receptor assay of TSH: its use to detect thyroid-stimulating immunoglobulins. J. Endocrinol. Invest. 1: 17 (1978).

INCREASED FREQUENCY OF HLA-DR5 IN METRO TORONTO PATIENTS WITH GOITROUS

AUTOIMMUNE THYROIDITIS AND POST-PARTUM THYROIDITIS

Paul G. Walfish, Maria T. Vargas, and Daphne Gladman

Depts. of Medicine, Mount Sinai, Wellesley and Women's College
Hospitals, University of Toronto, and Thyroid Lab. Mount Sinai
Hospital Research Insititute,
Toronto, Ontario, Canada

INTRODUCTION

Previous human leukocyte antigen (HLA) typing studies of Caucasian
patients with goitrous autoimmune thyroiditis (GAT) had demonstrated
an increased association with DR5 (1,2) or Dw5 (3) while no significant
associations were noted in another study (4); whereas, studies of Caucasian
patients with post-partum thyroiditis (PPT) from Canada had observed an
increased association with DR5 (5) while a study from Sweden reported an
increase in DR4 but not DR5 (6) and that from the United States had no
significant HLA associations (7). However, subsequent studies from
Newfoundland, Canada have reported the association of both GAT and PPT with
DR4 (8,9). In order to further assess the possibility that the differences
in HLA association between these various studies were related to variations
in antisera, and/or patient selection, we performed repeat studies in
Toronto, Canada using a new series of patients in comparison to regional
control subjects and utilized new antisera which had been standardized
according to the 9th International W.H.O. Workshop.

MATERIAL AND METHODS

HLA typing results for 98 Caucasian control subjects in our region were
compared to 60 Caucasian females with GAT diagnosed by the presence of a
palpable goiter with hypothyroidism and a positive antimicrosomal
antithyroid antibody (AMA) titre equal or greater than 1:400 and/or
cyto/histopathology compatible with chronic lymphocytic thyroiditis, as well
as 38 Caucasian females with PPT, all of whom had transient hyperthyroidism
with low (< 2%) ^{131}I thyroid uptake results and/or subsequent
hypothyroidism. HLA typing was performed using Canadian Red Cross trays
standardized according to the 9th International W.H.O. Workshop for: 44-A,
B, C, and 10-DR antigens as well as DQw1,2,3 and DRw52,53 antigens, using
routine microdroplet cytotoxicity tests. Chi-square tests (x^2) with
appropriate corrections for the number of antigens tested as well as Yates'
correction for continuity (x^2correct) were used to analyze the frequency
of HLA associations. Relative risk was calculated using Woolf's method
(10). Fisher's exact and x^2correct tests were used for comparison between
groups when appropriate. Two tailed P values < 0.05 were considered to be
significant.

RESULTS

In comparison to our regional control subjects, no significant associations were obtained within A,B,C antigens. The results of DR typing are illustrated in Table 1. Note that DR5 occurred in 12/98 controls: vs. 22/60 GAT (x^2correct = 11; P = < 0.001; Pc = < 0.01) with a relative risk (RR) = 4.2: vs. 11/38 PPT, (x^2correct = 4.5, P = < 0.05) with a RR = 2.9. Also, the mean frequency of DR4 and DRw53 (data not shown) were increased in both GAT and PPT compared to controls but these increases did not reach statistical significance.

Table 1. Summary of HLA-DR Typing Results for Patients with PPT and GAT in Comparison to 98 Regional Caucasian Controls.

HLA-DR Antigen	Controls (n = 98)	PPT (n = 38)	RR Values	GAT (n = 60)	RR Values
1	19 (19.3%)	4 (10.5%)	0.49	9 (15.0%)	0.73
2	19 (19.3%)	7 (18.4%)	0.94	13 (21.6%)	1.2
3	22 (22.4%)	4 (10.5%)	0.29	12 (20.0%)	1.6
4	28 (28.1%)	16 (42.1%)	1.8	22 (36.6%)	1.4
5	12 (12.2%)	11 (28.9%)	2.9 *	22 (36.6%)	4.2 **
6	9 (9.1%)	2 (5.2%)	0.55	8 (13.3%)	1.5
7	30 (30.6%)	12 (31.5%)	1.1	14 (23.3%)	0.69
8	5 (5.1%)	2 (5.2%)	1.0	5 (8.3%)	1.6
10	2 (2.0%)	2 (5.2%)	2.6	2 (3.3%)	1.7

* x^2c = 4.5;   P = < 0.05
** x^2c = 11.0;   P = < 0.001; Pc = < 0.01

Additional HLA typing studies also revealed that DQw3 antigen positivity occurred in 53% of PPT (RR = 1.8) and 57% of GAT (RR = 1.9), representing mean percentage increases in comparison to the 38% prevalence in controls, but these increases did not reach statistical significance (P = > 0.05). Also, there was an interesting reduction in the percentage of positivity for the occurrence of DQw1 in PPT and GAT with values of 42% (RR = 0.55) and 36% (RR = 0.4) respectively compared to 56% in controls, but these changes also did not reach statistical significance. Although AMA positivity occurred in 100% of DR5 PPT subjects vs. 75% of non-DR5 PPT, no significant association (P = > 0.05) was observed in PPT patients between AMA positivity and any DR antigen.

DISCUSSION

Our HLA results confirm previous reports (1-3) of a strong association for GAT with DR5 or Dw5, and the RR value of 4.2, (P_c = < 0.01) represent one of the highest associations reported to date. Also, the present report has again confirmed the association of PPT with DR5 for patients studied within our Toronto, Canada region using local Caucasian control subjects and W.H.O. HLA-antisera standardized according to the 9th International Workshop. The previous HLA study of PPT from Toronto had been performed using regional controls and additional PPT patients from Newfoundland, Canada (5). In the present study, the association of DR5 with PPT at an RR = 2.9 (P = < 0.05) is weaker than its association with GAT RR = 4.2, (P_c = < 0.01). In comparison to our results, the report from Sweden which observed a DR4 association (6), had possible differences in diagnostic clinical criteria for PPT by selecting hypothyroid patients with milder increases in serum TSH and not routinely confirming the occurrence of a prior transient thyrotoxic phase in all PPT patients. Also, there were possible differences in the HLA-DR4 antisera used and the prevalence of DR5 in controls had to be estimated (6). Workers in Newfoundland, Canada who recently reported an increased association of DR4 for GAT and PPT also observed a reciprocal reduction in the frequency of DR5 in these patients (8,9). However, the increase in DR5 in our GAT and PPT patients was accompanied by an increase rather than a reduction in DR4 prevalence relative to controls, but this change did not reach statistical significance. Such observations were further supported by a parallel mean percentage increase of DQw3 (which frequently correlates with the presence of HLA-DR4,5,8,9 antigen positivity) in both GAT and PPT without reaching statistical significance. Hence, our observations are entirely consistent with an increased association of DR5 and possibly DR4 with both GAT and PPT. Since DR4 and DR5 remain less well-defined HLA antigens, distinguishing between these two antigens could depend upon the antisera employed as well as typing differences in regional control groups and other local environmental factors such as dietary iodine which may mediate the clinical expression of PPT and GAT and could thereby account for the variations of HLA associations reported. Nevertheless, our overall results for DR and DQ typing are consistent with an increased DR5 and possibly DR4 prevalence in GAT as well as PPT. The relative decrease of association for DQw1 in both GAT and PPT is of interest and suggests that its presence may have a protective role, which resembles its postulated influence on the occurrence of certain complications within Type I diabetes mellitus patients (11).

In summary, using a new series of patients and regional controls, we have documented in our region a strong HLA association of DR5 with GAT and demonstrated again a significant but lesser association of DR5 with PPT. The association of DR5 with GAT as well as PPT, is in agreement with the current evidence favouring the view that PPT is likely a subclinical variant of GAT (12) which becomes activated post-partum by autoimmune pathogenic mechanisms in those mothers with the appropriate immunogenetic predisposition (13).

ACKNOWLEDGMENTS

Funded in part by grants from the physicians of Ontario by the Physicians Services Incorporated Foundation and the Mount Sinai Hospital Department of Medicine Research Fund (PGW) as well as the Women's College Hospital Research Fund (DG). MTV was a Research Fellow supported by an award from the Mount Sinai Hospital Department of Medicine Research Fund. The technical assistance of K. Anhorn and C. Williams in the performance of HLA typing is also gratefully acknowledged.

REFERENCES

1. M. Weissel, R. Hofer, H. Zasmeta and W. R. Mayr, HLA-DR and Hashimoto's Thyroiditis. Tissue Antigens, 16:256, (1980).
2. N. R. Farid, L. Sampson, H. Moens, J. M. Barnard, The Association of Goitrous Autoimmune Thyroiditis with HLA-DR5, Tissue Antigens, 17:265 (1981).
3. M. Thomsen, L. P. Ryder, K. Bech, H. Bliddal, U. Feldt-Rasmussen, J. Molholm, E. Kappelgaard, H. Neilsen, A. Svejgaard, HLA-D in Hashimoto's Thyroiditis, Tissue Antigens, 21:173 (1983).
4. H. G. Fein, S. Metz, T. F. Nikolai, A. H. Johnson, R. C. Smallridge, Goitrous Hashimoto's Thyroiditis: Lack of Association with HLA Antigens, Mol. Biol. Med., 3:195 (1986).
5. N. R. Farid, B. S. Hawe and P. G. Walfish, Increased Frequency of HLA-DR3 and DR5 in the Syndrome of Painless Thyroiditis with Transient Thyrotoxicosis; Evidence for an Autoimmune Etiology, Clin. Endocrinol. (Oxf.), 19:699 (1983).

6. R. Jansson, J. Safwenberg, P. A. Dahlberg, Influence of the HLA-DR4 antigen and Iodine Status on the Development of Autoimmune Post-partum Thyroiditis, J. Clin. Endocrinol. & Metab.,60:168 (1985).
7. H. G. Fein, S. Metz, T. F. Nikolai, A. H. Johnson, R. C. Smallridge, HLA Antigens: Difference Between Silent and Post-partum Lymphocytic Forms and Comparisons with Subacute and Goitrous Autoimmune Thyroiditis, in: "Autoimmunity and The Thyroid" P.G. Walfish, J.R. Wall and R. Volpe , eds., Academic Press, Orlando, Florida, pp. 373 (1985).
8. C. Thompson, N. R. Farid, Post-partum Thyroiditis and Goitrous (Hashimoto's) thyroiditis are associated with HLA-DR4, Immunology Letters, 11:301 (1985).
9. N. R. Farid, C. Thompson, HLA and Autoimmune Endocrine Diseases, Mol Biol Med, 3:85 (1986).
10. B. Woolf, Estimating the Relationship between Blood Group and Disease, Ann. Hum. Genet., 19:251 (1955).
11. D. Gladman, S. Sukenik, E. Gertner, C. Bombardier, A. Hanna, Skin Thickening and Joint Contractures in Adults with Insulin Dependent and Non-Insulin Dependent Diabetes: Relationships to Microvascular Diabetic Complications and HLA Antigens, in: "Program 1st I.U.I.S. Conference of Clinical Immunology", Toronto, Canada, Abstract #P9.11, pp. 67, (1986).
12. P. G. Walfish, J. Y. C. Chan, Post-partum Hyperthyroidism, Clinics in Endocrinolology and Metabolism, 14:417 (1985).
13. P. G. Walfish, N. R. Farid, The Immunogenetic Basis of Autoimmune Thyroid Disease, in: "Autoimmunity and the Thyroid" P.G. Walfish, J.R. Wall, and R. Volpe , eds., Academic Press, Orlando, Florida, pp. 9 (1985).

POST-PARTUM THYROID DYSFUNCTION AND HLA STATUS

Münire Koloğlu[1], Hedy Fung[1], C. Darke[2], C.J. Richards[3],
R. Hall[1] and A.M. McGregor[1]

Department of Medicine, University of Wales College of
Medicine, Heath Park, Cardiff CF4 4XN[1], Tissue Typing Lab.
Blood Transfusion Centre, Rhydlafar, Cardiff CF5 6XF[2] and
Department of Obstetrics and Gynaecology, Caerphilly District
Miners Hospital, Caerphilly CF8 2WW[3]

INTRODUCTION

Syndromes of post-partum thyroid dysfunction (P-PTD) have been described
in women not previously recognised as having thyroid disease[1,2,3,4]. The
classical syndrome has been defined as transient (or permanent) hypothyroidism, which is sometimes preceded by transient hyperthyroidism, occurring
8-12 weeks after delivery and resolving spontaneously at 6-8 months post-
partum. The severity of thyroid dysfunction has been reported to be
associated with the presence of high anti-microsomal antibodies (AMA) during
the first trimester of pregnancy[4].

Previous studies have reported an increased frequency of HLA-DR3 and
DR5[5] and DR4[6] in groups of 25 and 13 women respectively with P-PTD. A
further study of a group of 50 women with positive AMA has also reported an
increased frequency of HLA-DR4[7]. This study, without being biased by retrospective definition of patient groups, prospectively examines the relationship between P-PTD and HLA antigens in an unselected large group of Caucasian
women with no known previous history of autoimmune thyroid disease (AITD).

PATIENTS AND METHODS

Nine hundred and one women, at around the 16th week of pregnancy, were
screened for the presence of anti-thyroglobulin antibodies (ATGA) and AMA by
ELISA. FT3, FT4 and TSH were assessed using commercially available kits.
P-PTD was defined as abnormal thyroid function (the normal range for
pregnancy and the post-partum period (P-PP) was established in 120 normal
anti-thyroid antibody negative pregnant women) on at least 2 occasions during
the P-PP. Three hundred women were selected for the study. Sixty-eight
were lost to follow-up, 7 were excluded from analysis (4 = known AITD,
3 = non-Caucasian) and the remaining women were followed up throughout
pregnancy and for at least 12 months post-partum.

Two hundred and twenty-one women were HLA typed, 113 being anti-thyroid
antibody negative (AB-ve) and 108 being anti-thyroid antibody positive
(AB+ve) during pregnancy or the P-PP. HLA typing for 12 HLA-A and 19 HLA-B

antigens was performed using the standard lymphocytotoxicity test and 8 HLA-DR antigens, HLA-DQw1 and DQw3 were typed using the 7th Histocompatibility Workshop technique. HLA-DQw2 was not included in typing.

HLA antigen frequencies were compared with 600 local Caucasoid subjects for HLA-A and B antigens and with 382 of these subjects for HLA-DR antigen. Statistical analysis was based on x^2 test with Yates' correction. Correction for the number of antigens being compared was performed using the method of Edwards. The distribution of p values for the frequency comparisons of the antigens at each locus was performed by summing the x^2 values being described as "multiplex analysis".

RESULTS

Of the 221 women (Table 1) that were HLA typed, 113 were AB-ve and 108 were AB+ve at some time during pregnancy or·during the P-PP. Of 108 women, 79 had anti-thyroid antibodies at screening whereas 29 women developed AMA and/or ATGA during pregnancy or in the P-PP.

When all 45 women developing P-PTD, irrespective of the presence of anti-thyroid antibodies were analysed, there was an increase in the frequency of HLA-A1 antigen (55.6%; $p < 0.02$) and HLA-B8 antigen (48.9%; $p < 0.01$) compared with the controls (36.0% and 30.2% respectively). However, the p values were not significant after correction. An increase in the frequency of HLA-DR3 (46.7%; $p < 0.01$) and a decrease in the frequency of HLA-DR2 (6.7%; $p < 0.01$) was found when compared with the control population (27.5% and 27.7% respectively). These differences were not significant after correction but multiplex analysis of the DR antigen comparisons showed x^2 = 19.3, $p < 0.02$. No association of HLA-DR4 antigen with the development of P-PTD was observed.

Since there is strong linkage disequilibrium between the HLA-B8 and DR3 alleles, we further analysed our study group. Compared with the normal population (22.5%) the HLA-B8, DR3 combination was significantly increased in women with P-PTD without antibodies (55.6%; $p < 0.05$) and in women with P-PTD irrespective of the presence of antibodies (40.0%; $p < 0.02$). Analysis of the HLA-A1, B8, DR3 combination compared with normals (18.6%) again showed a significant increase in women with P-PTD without antibodies (55.6%; $p < 0.02$) and in women with P-PTD irrespective of the presence of antibodies (35.6%; $p < 0.01$).

When the HLA-DQw3 antigen frequency was compared between the AB+ve group (52.8%) and AB-ve group (33.6%), the difference was found to be significant by multiplex analysis ($p < 0.02$).

DISCUSSION

Within the total group (n = 221) 45 women, 36 in the AB+ve group and 9 in the AB-ve group developed P-PTD. The combinations HLA-B8, DR3 and HLA-A1, B8, DR3 were both significantly more frequently observed in those women developing P-PTD (irrespective of their anti-thyroid antibody status) as was HLA-DR3 alone when compared with a large local control population. We could show no significant association between HLA-DR4 and either the presence of antibody activity or the development of P-PTD in contrast to other authors[6,7].

The well recognised association of HLA-A1, B8, DR3 haplotype with other organ-specific autoimmune diseases provides further support for autoimmune events being implicated in the development of P-PTD.

Table 1. The occurrence of anti-thyroid antibodies
and P-PTD in the 221 pregnant women

Group	Number with anti-thyroid antibodies		Number developing P-PTD
AB+ve (n=108)	AMA	38 (35.2%)	4 (3.7%)
	ATGA	15 (13.9%)	3 (2.8%)
	AMA and ATGA	55 (50.9%)	29 (26.9%)
AB−ve (n=113)		−	9 (7.9%)

REFERENCES

1. J. Ginsberg and P.G. Walfish, Post-partum transient thyrotoxicosis
    with painless thyroiditis, Lancet i:1125 (1977).
2. N. Amino, R. Kuro, O. Tanizawa, F. Tanaka, C. Hayashi, K. Kotani,
    M. Kawashima, K. Miyai and Y. Kumahara, Changes of serum anti-
    thyroid antibodies during and after pregnancy in autoimmune thyroid
    diseases, Clin. Exp. Immunol. 31:30 (1978).
3. P.A. Dahlberg and R. Jansson, Different aetiologies in post-partum
    thyroiditis? Acta Endocrinol. 104:195 (1983).
4. R. Jansson, S. Bernander, A. Karlsson, K. Levin and G. Nilsson, Auto-
    immune thyroid dysfunction in the post-partum period, J. Clin.
    Endocrinol. Metab. 58:681 (1984).
5. N.R. Farid, B.S. Hawe and P.G. Walfish, Increased frequency of HLA-DR3
    and 5 in the syndromes of painless thyroiditis with transient
    thyrotoxicosis. Evidence for an autoimmune aetiology, Clin.
    Endocrinol. 19:699 (1983).
6. H.H. Lervang, O. Pryds, H.P.O. Kristensen, B.K. Jacobsen and A.
    Svejgaard, Post-partum autoimmune thyroid disorder associated with
    HLA-DR4? Tissue Antigens 23:250 (1984).
7. R. Jansson, J. Safwenberg and P.A. Dahlberg, Influence of the HLA-DR4
    antigen and iodine status on the development of autoimmune post-
    partum thyroiditis, J. Clin. Endocrinol. Metab. 60:168 (1985).

METHIMAZOLE, γ - INTERFERON AND GRAVES' DISEASE

M. Bagnasco, D. Venuti, M. Caria
G. Pizzorno, O. Ferrini, and G.W. Canonica

Endocrinologia & Semeiotica Medica III
I.S.M.I. Genoa University V.le Benedetto
XV N. 6 - 16132 Genova, Italy

The ability of antithyroid (namely, thionamide) therapy to directly influence the immunological course of Graves' disease (GD) has been stressed on the basis of a number of "in vitro" and "in vivo" experimental
evidence. However such evidences are mainly concerning the effect of methimazole (MMI) on the function of B cells and or accessory cells:
only a few data are available about possible effect(s) of MMI on T cell
function. In the present study we evaluated 1) the effect of MMI on T
cell proliferation in bulk culture induced through different activation
pathways (namely by PHA-acting on T3 T cell receptor complex, and by a
stimulatory combination of different anti-CD2 Mabs) 2) the effect of MMI
on mitogen induced lymphokine release (namely IL-2 and γ IFN) by mass
cultures of PMNC 3) the effect of the drug on the proliferation and
lymphokine production of T cell clones. The modification of some of these
parameters during MMI therapy were also evaluated in patients with
Graves' disease. The results obtained showed that MMI does not affect T
cell proliferation, but seems to be able to modulate the release of γ IFN.
Materials and Methods: Previously described methods have been used for
isolation for peripheral mononuclear cells and evaluations of proliferative response of T cells to different stimulation. The following
T11$^{(CD2)}$ mabs were used: CD2.1 and CD2.9 (kindly provided by Dr. D. Oli-
ve. INSERM, Marseille).
IL-2 and γ IFN were evaluated on 24 h supernatants of 1% PHA-stimulated
cultures as previously described (1). For the former, the method of Gillis et al. (2) based on the IL-2 dependent CTLL cell line proliferation,
was employed: for the latter a specific immunoradiometric assay (IMRX
Centocor Medical System Italy) was used. T cell clones were raised from
the peripheral blood of normal subjects and Graves' disease patients
using the method of Moretta A. et al. (3). Clonal microcultures were
maintained in U bottomed microwells in culture medium (RPMI 1640 + 10%
FCS) containing the appropriate amount of IL-2-enriched supernatants, or
recombinant IL-2. For evaluating γ IFN and IL-2 production, the microcultures were washed several times, then resuspended at approx.25.000 cells/

well in culture medium and stimulated with 1% PHA (or Ca-ionoph.-TPA) for 24 h. Then the supernatants were collected and IL-2 and γIFN concentration measured as described above.

Results and discussion: The addition of MMI even at high concentrations (up to 100 u Mol) had no detectable effect on T cell proliferation in our systems (see table 1). Similarly no effect of the drug was apparent on IL-2 release in mass culture after mitogen stimulation (see table I). Due to the well-known effect of γ-IFN on "aberrant" MHC class II antigen espression on thyroid cells (hypothesized as a crucial step in the development of autoimmune injury (4), our attention was expecially focused on the possible influence of MMI on γ-IFN release. Surprisingly, MMI increased in a dose-dependent manner PHA-stimulated γ-IFN release by PMNC isolated from 6 out of 7 normal subjects, as well as 6 out of 7 GD patients (P 0.02 by the Wilcoxon test at 100 u Mol MMI concentration). After 15 day MMI treatment (30 mg daily) a slight decrease of PHA-induced "in vitro" γ-IFN release was observed: moreover, no significant "enhancing" effect was observed by adding MMI. In 3 patients, after 35 further months of therapy (15 mg daily), MMI did inhibit (30 to 70%) PHA-stimulated γIFN release (Table II). These experimental evidences, obtained in bulk culture experiments, prompted us to directly evaluate the effect of MMI on lymphokine production by cloned T cells. Preliminary results obtained using 9 clones allowed us to confirm that MMI has no effect both on IL-2 production, and on T cell proliferation (in response to exogeneous IL-2) (not shown). As far as γIFN is concerned, MMI (30 u Mol) inhibited γIFN release by T cell clones.(Table III).
Thus, MMI "in vitro" may modulate γIFN production: it seems to exert an inhibitory action at the T cell level, although the mechanism and the site(s) of action are probably multiple (as shown by the initial "enhancing" effect in mass culture). Moreover, the "in vitro" effect of MMI on γIFN release is different under MMI treatment: thus, it is likely that such a therapy may affect γIFN production. Although the phenomenon requires further investigation, it is of potential interest the fact that MMI may affect a fundamental step in the pathogenesis of autoimmune thyroid disease.

TABLE I . Effect of MMI (100 u Mol concentr.) on T cell proliferation induced by PHA and T11 mabs, and, on IL-2 production induced by PHA. The data, herein reported deal with 5 normal individuals (M + SE). Similar results were obtained in patients with GD (not shown).

	PHA ind. prolif. (ç)	T11 ind. prolif (ç)	PHA ind. IL-2 release (˜)
without MMI	$12.3 \cdot 10^{-3} + 1$	$11 \cdot 10^{-3} + 1.2$	1%
with MMI	$12.3 \cdot 10^{-3} + 0.8$	$10.8 \cdot 10^{-3} + 1.4$	1.2%

ç = CPM ^{3}H-Tdr
˜ = % maximal CTLL prolif.

TABLE II. Effect of MMI on PHA-stimulated γIFN release by PMNC in 7 normal subjects and patients with Graves' disease before and during MMI treatment. For more details see text.

	0	γIFN U/ml (M ± SEM) PHA 1%	MMI 0.1 mM	PHA 1%+МЫII 0.1 mM
Normal subjects	0.5	19.6±6.9	0.5	37.3±12.4
Untreated GD	0.5	15.3±7.5	0.5	24.4±11.6
15-day treatment	0.5	11.0±5.0	0.5	13.7±5.6
3.5-month treatment ^	0.5	12.1±2.1	0.5	5.0±1.8

^ = 3 patients only

Table III. Effect of MMI on -IFN production of PHA stimulated T lymphocyte clones.

		γ IFN U/ml	
Clone	PHA	PHA 1% + MMI 30u Mol	
1	8 U	−	n. detect
2	5 U	−	"
3	7 U	−	"

References

1) Bagnasco M. et al., Inv. Arch. Allergy Appl. Immunol. 1986 in press.
2) Gillis et al. J. Immunol. 1978, 120, 2097.
3) Moretta A. et al. J. Exp. Med. 1983, 158, 571.
4) Bottazzo G.F. et al., Lancet, 1983, 2, 1115.

THE PROGNOSTIC VALUE OF COMBINED MEASUREMENT OF THYROID-STIMULATING
ANTIBODY AND SERUM THYROGLOBULIN LEVELS DURING GRAVES' DISEASE LONG
TERM THIONAMIDE TREATMENT

J.H. Romaldini, R.S. Werner, N. Bromberg, I.D. Pereira,
R.P. Dall'Antonia Jr. and C.S. Farah

Department Endocrinology HSPE-IAMSPE, Sao Paulo, Brasil

INTRODUCTION

Several authors reports a decrease of thyroid-stimulating antibody
(TSAb) and serum thyroglobulin (Tg) levels during thionamide therapy (1,
2) and used them as index of outcome of Graves'disease (3,4). However,
their significance remains a matter of controversy (5,6). The aim of the
present study was to compare the TSAb activity and serum Tg concentration
as prognostic indexes of outcome of thionamide drug therapy in Graves'
disease patients.

MATERIAL AND METHODS

We evaluated the clinical results of 80 Graves'hyperthyroid patients
without autoantibodies to Tg. The mean age was 42 yr (range: 18 to 56 yr).
Forty-four patients received high doses of either methimazole (40 to 90
mg daily) or propylthiouracil (500 to 800 mg daily) and 36 patients were
treated with conventional doses regimen (5 to 20 mg and 100 to 300 mg
daily, respectively of methimazole and propylthiouracil). T_3 (50 to 75
ug daily) was administered to the high doses and some of the conventional
doses patients.
Remission group comprised 40 patients treated for 15 to 30 months who
remained euthyroid for 15 to 96 months (mean + S.D. : 45 + 28). Relapsed
group consisted of 40 patients treated for 15 to 25 months and relapsed
after a euthyroid period of 2 to 96 months (12 + 6).
TSAb activity was determined as cyclic AMP increase in human thyroid
slices as previously described (7). Serum Tg was measured by an IRMA
method (Cis-Sorin). The sensitivity of the assay was 1.25 ng/ml and in
normal subjects the range was: 3 to 30 ng/ml. The data were analyzed by
Student't-test,Spearman correlation and chi-square test.

RESULTS

Serum Tg values in remission (66 + 120 ng/ml) were lower (P < 0.001)
than in relapsed patients (272 + 301 ng/ml)(Fig. 1).
The table 1 summarizes the findings obtained in this study.
We observed a correlation between TSAb activity and serum Tg levels
before treatment (r = 0.45, P < 0.01).However this relationship was not
found at the end of thionamide drug therapy (Fig. 2).

Table 1. Remission-rate of Graves'disease patients:correlation
with TSAb activity and serum Tg concentration

Parameters	Remission (No)	Relapse (No)
Positive-TSAb	7 (27%)	19 (57.5%)
Negative-TSAb	19 (73%)	14 (42.5%)*
Elevated Tg§	17 (42.5%)	34 (85%)
Normal Tg	23 (57.5%)	6 (15%)**
Positive-TSAb and Elevated Tg	4 (19%)	11 (84.6%)
Negative-TSAb and Normal Tg	17 (81%)	2 (15.4%)**

§, Serum Tg levels higher than the upper normal value (30 ng/ml)
*, P < 0.05 ; **, P < 0.001

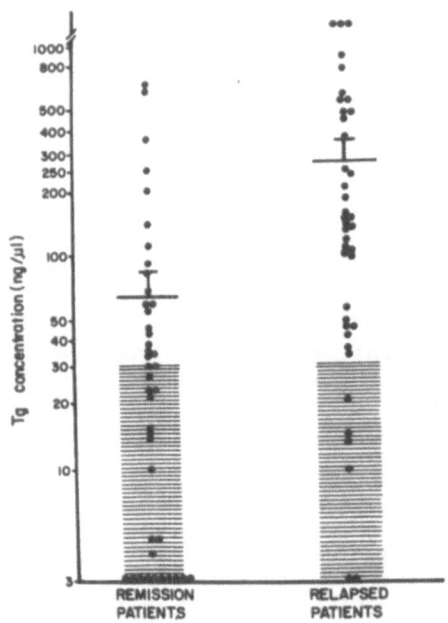

Fig. 1. Serum Tg values at the
end of thionamide therapy.

DISCUSSION

Our findings confirm previous data that correlate the presence of
TSAb with relapse (1,5). Patients negative for TSAb activity did not allow
us to predict the individual remission of Graves'disease (5,8).

The normalization of serum Tg concentration at the end of treatment was
associated with remission of the disease (4). However, elevated serum Tg

concentration did not predict the clinical course of Graves'disease
after thionamide drug therapy.

The combined use of TSAb and Tg levels appears to be more accurate
as predictive value compared with the measurement of either parameter alone.

The high concentration of serum Tg observed in relapsed patients (Fig.
1) may be thought to be an effect of the presence of TSAb stimulation. As
clearly shown in Fig. 2 serum Tg values correlated with TSAb activity at
the beginning but not at the end of thionamide drug therapy. These data
indicate that thionamide drugs interfere with Tg secretion, which provokes
the decrease in the iodine content of Tg (6). Another possible explanation
is that Tg secretion became normal following the thyroidal and immunological homeostasis.

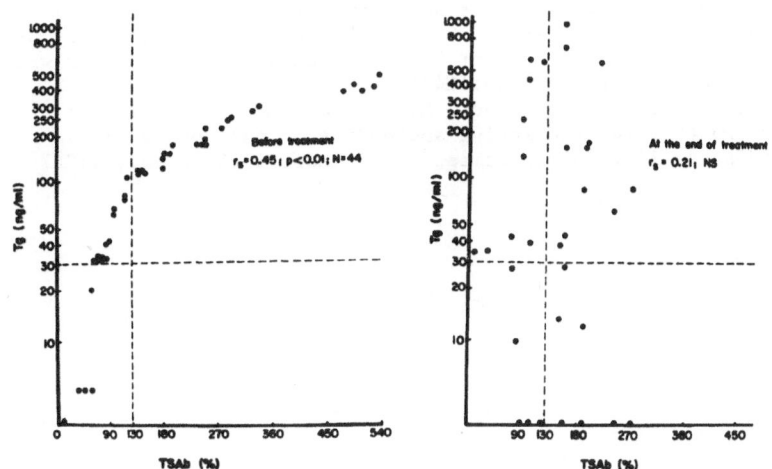

Fig. 2 Correlation of serum Tg and TSAb
values in Graves'disease patients
before (r=0,45, P   0.01) and at
end of thionamide tratment.

REFERENCES

1. M.Zakarija, J.M.McKenzie and K.Banovac, Clinical significance of assay of thyroid-stimulating antibody in Graves'disease, Ann Intern Med, 93:28(1980).
2. R.P.Uller and A.J.Van Herle, Effect of therapy on serum thyroglobulin levels in patients with Graves'disease, J Clin Endocrinol Metab, 46:747(1978).
3. D.F.Gardner, J.Rothman and R.D.Utiger, Serum thyroglobulin in normal subjects and patients with hyperthyroidism due to Graves'disease: effect of T_3, iodide, 131-I and antithyroid drugs, Clin Endocrinol (Oxf), 11:585(1979).
4. S.Kawamura, B.Kishino, K.Tajima, K.Mashita and S.Tarui, Serum thyroglobulin changes in patients with Graves'disease treated with long term antithyroid drug therapy, J Clin Endocrinol Metab, 56: 507(1983).
5. A.M.Madec, M.C.Laurent, Y.Lorcy, A.M.Le Guerrier, A.Rostgnat-Stefanutti, J.Orgiazzi and H.Allanic, Thyroid stimulating antibodies: an aid to the strategy of treatment of Graves'disease ?, Clin Endocrinol (Oxf), 21:247(1984).
6. U.Feldt-Rasmussen, K.Bech, J.Date, P.H.Petersen and K.Johansen, A prospective study of the differential changes in serum thyroglobulin and its autoantibodies during propylthiouracil or radioiodine therapy of patients with Graves'disease, Acta Endocrinol, 99:379(1982).
7. L.M.Tanaka-Matsuura, R.S.Werner, C.S.Farah and J.H.Romaldini, Cryopreserved human thyroid tissue for TSAb determination: comparison with fresh tissue, Hormone Res, 20:124(1984).
8. M.Bagnasco, E.Macchia, G.Ciprandi, M.Caria and G.F.Fenzi, T cell subsets and thyroid-stimulating antibodies in patients with Graves'disease in clinical remission, J Endocrinol Invest, 9:217 (1986).

SERUM THYROID AUTOANTIBODIES IN A LONG-TERM STUDY OF

THYROSTATIC TREATMENT OF GRAVES' DISEASE

Wieland Meng, Sabine Meng, Rainer Hampel,
Manfred Ventz, and Ewald Männchen

Klinik für Innere Medizin
University of Greifswald, Greifswald, GDR

INTRODUCTION

Graves' disease is an autoimmune thyropathy. Therefore, assessment of the course of the disease and recognition of a remission should essentially be based on immunological phenomena. In a prospective study we dealt with the following questions:
- Are antibody titres indicative for the course of the disease?
- Which relations exist between the thyroid suppressibility, the height of antibody titres and the relapse rates?
- Is a highly dosed methimazole treatment more effective than a low dosed therapy?

MATERIAL AND METHODS

In patients with Graves' disease thyroglobulin antibodies (TAb), microsomal antibodies (MAb) and TSH-receptor antibodies (TBIAb) were determined during a methimazole (MMI) therapy for 1 - 2 years. We used the test kits Thymune T, Thymune M (Wellcome corp.) and TRAK-assay[R] (Henning). The thyroid suppression test was performed at the end of the therapy period (80 - 100 µg T3/day, 10 days, positive: 24-h-uptake <35 %). The patients were followed-up for a period of 2 - 5 years(1).

18 patients were treated with 40 mg (initial 60 mg) MMI/day and 19 patients with 5 - 10 mg (initial 20 - 30 mg) MMI/day for one year. After 3 / 6 and 12 months we examined MAb and the thyroid suppressibility. Furthermore we measured MAb 4 - 6 weeks after withdrawal of MMI. Up to now the patients of this group were followed-up only for 6 - 36 months(2).

Table 1. TAb and MAb at the end of treatment and
          relapse rates

TAb	Patients (n)	Relapses (%)	MAb	Patients (n)	Relapses (%)
Negative	134	38.1	Negative	41	24.4
Positive	70	61.4	Positive	83	61.5
≥ 1:250	30	83.3	≥ 1:1600	56	76.8
≥ 1:2500	20	90.0	≥ 1:6400	37	83.8
Total	204	46.1	Total	124	49.2

Table 2. Frequency of positive thyroid autoantibody
          findings (%) in Graves' disease before and after
          treatment of at least 1 year

Graves' disease	n	TBIAb	MAb	TAb
Untreated	50	96	86	32
Unproblematic course	24	17	29	25
Problematic course	30	60	70	27

Valuation: TBIAb >10 U/l, MAb > 1:400, TAb >1:20

Table 3. Preliminary results of highly (n = 18) and
          low dosed (n = 19) methimazole treatment

	Months	Methimazole high	low
Suppression test positive (%)	3	16.7	15.8
	6	55.5	26.3
	12	55.5	42.1
MAb negative (%)	3	50.0	10.5
	6	55.6	47.4
	12	50.0	31.6
	1 (post th.)	50.0	0.0
MAb lowering (%)	3	66.7	31.6
	6	88.9	52.6
	12	66.7	42.1
increasing (%)	1 (post th.)	16.7	57.9
Relapses (%)	6 - 36	38.9	63.2

% of patients

RESULTS

    Antibody titres before therapy were not indicative of
the posttherapeutic course of disease. But at the end of the
treatment the antibody titres showed a significantly positive
correlation with the persistence and relapse rates of
hyperthyroidism (Table 1, Fig. 1). MAb allow a better
prognostic statement than TAb but only by reason of their
higher sensibility and frequency. But if TAb are measurable,
then the predictive value appears to be not lesser (Fig. 1).
There exists a significantly negative correlation between
the intensity of thyroid suppressibility and the height of
antibody titres (t-test: $p < 0.001$).

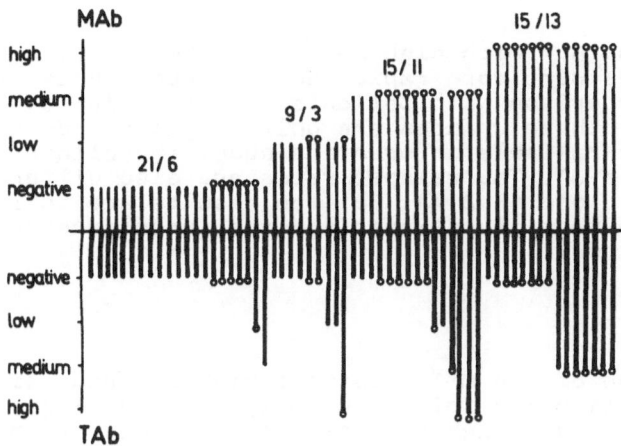

Fig. 1. Microsomal (MAb) and thyroglobulin antibodies (TAb) at the end of treatment in 60 patients and relapse rates (n/n relapses)

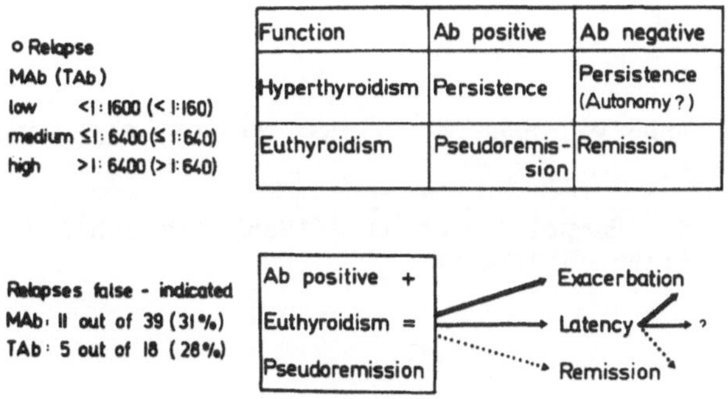

○ Relapse
MAb (TAb)
low   <1:1600 (< 1:160)
medium ≤1:6400 (≤ 1:640)
high   >1:6400 (> 1:640)

Function	Ab positive	Ab negative
Hyperthyroidism	Persistence	Persistence (Autonomy?)
Euthyroidism	Pseudoremis-sion	Remission

Relapses false - indicated
MAb: 11 out of 39 (31%)
TAb: 5 out of 18 (28%)

Ab positive   +
Euthyroidism =
Pseudoremission

→ Exacerbation
→ Latency ← ?
⋯→ Remission

Fig. 2. Possible situations after MMI treatment of Graves' disease

Whereas patients with complicated course of disease (prolonged, persistence, early and repeated relapse) at the end of therapy showed high TBIAb-titres still in 60 %, titres in patients with uncomplicated course (good remission tendency, remissions) were in the positive range with 17 % only. There is a correlation between MAb and TBIAb. But TBIAb can not be substituted by MAb because of their low sensibility (Table 2).

During therapy with high MMI doses the decrease of antibody titres were more rapid and more continuous after therapy in comparison with patients who had a low dose treatment. But these changes are only slight and do not give permission for reliable information about the clinical behavior (Table 3). The relapse rates are also different (high: 39.9 %; low: 63.2 %). But the results are influenced by the small number of patients and the inhomogeneous follow-up periods.

CONCLUSIONS

At the end of the MMI treatment high antibody titres indicate a continuation of the underlying immunological processes and thus a high risk of a persistence or an early relapse of hyperthyroidism (Ab titres high + euthyroidism = "pseudoremission"). By reason of the pathogenetical and pathophysiological processes it can not be expected that antibody findings give absolutly sure prognostic indications. But antibodies are helpful for giving a short time prognosis (Fig. 2).
There exists a close correlation between results of suppression test and antibody titres.
Up to now our results do not offer safe clinical advantages of a highly dosed drug treatment.

REFERENCES

1. Hampel R., Männchen E., Meng W., et al. (1986), Klin. Wochenschr. (in press)

2. Meng W., Meng S., Hampel R. et al. (1986), In Schilddrüse 1985, George Thieme Verlag, Stuttgart.

THE EFFECT OF HIGH DOSES OF CARBIMAZOLE IN PATIENTS WITH GRAVES'DISEASE

AND IN SUBJECTS WITH THYROID ANTIBODIES

P. Tanzi, M. Vitillo, M. Mancuso, V. Fiore, P. Pozzilli, and
U. Di Mario, D.Andreani

Clinica Medica 2(Endocrinologia 1)
Policlinico Umberto I, University of Rome "La Sapienza"
00161 Roma Italy

INTRODUCTION

Several studies have pointed out that Carbimazole (CBZ) may have both
in vivo and in vitro an immunosoppressive effect on the immune response
towards the thyroid (1-4). In this study we have evaluated the immunological change induced by therapy with high doses of CBZ on two different groups
of patients: Group A= patients with Graves' disease; Group B= patients with
normal T3, T4, TSH values but with antithyroid antibodies.

PATIENTS AND METHODS

Patients

Group A. Thirty-three newly diagnosed Graves' patients, age range
14-73 years, were studied at diagnosis. All patients were treated with 60
mg CBZ for 45 days and with 20 mg CBZ and 100-150 µg L-thyroxine for 13.5
months.

Twelve of these patients were followed at regular distances thereafter
(0.5, 1, 3, 6, 9, 12 and 15 months).

Two groups of age comparable control subjects were used: 35 for the
study of TSH-receptors antibodies (TRAb), 26 for the study of the T-cells
subsets.

Group B. Seventeen patients, age range 20-60 years, with normal T3,T4
and TSH, but showing anti-thyroglobulin (TGHA) and anti-thyroid microsomal
(MCHA) antibodies and presenting a palpable thyroid, were followed up for
one year.

Eleven of these patients were treated with high doses of CBZ (60 mg
daily initially; 20 mg daily maintaining dose for one year + L-thyroxine
according to individual need).

Six of these patients acted as controls for the study of humoral immunity, were treated with L-thyroxine only.

Blood samples were taken at diagnosis and 1, 3, 6 and 12 months following CBZ therapy.

Methods

TSH-receptors antibodies (TRAb) were evaluated using a RIA-kit (RIA Ltd., Tyne and Wear UK) based on the capacity of TRAb to inhibit the binding of I-125-labelled TSH to solubilized TSH-receptors. The results of the assay are expressed as a TSH binding inhibitory index (TRAb index);values of TRAb higher than 10 were considered positive.

TGHA were studied using a radio-immune assay; MCHA were assessed using an indirect immunofluorescence technique on thyroid sections.

Total T-cell subpopulations, helper/inducer and suppressor/cytotoxic T-cell subsets were studied with an indirect immunofluorescence technique using mAb OKT3, OKT4, OKT8 (Ortho Diagnostic) respectively .

K/NK cells and activated T-cell subsets were determinated using an indirect immunofluorescence technique with mAb H366.

RESULTS

Group A

91% of these patients showed high values of TRAb at diagnosis versus normal controls with a high statistical significance (p<0.001). The percentage of positivity in the follow up were 100, 89, 82, 80, 66, 60 and 55% after 0.5, 1, 3, 6, 9, 12 and 15 months of treatment respectively.

A significant decrease in the suppressor/cytotoxic T-cell subset in Graves' patients was observed at diagnosis (p<0.02 vs normal controls). On the contrary, the decrease of total T-cells did not reach statistical significance.

29% of Graves' patients at diagnosis were found to have increased levels of K and NK cells.

No correlation was found between the proportion of CD8 positive cells and TRAb values at diagnosis and in the follow up.

Finally, the incidence of relapse within 6 months of therapy with high doses of CBZ was 42%.

Group B

After one year of therapy with high doses of CBZ no differences in T-cell subsets were observed. Activated T-cell subsets were decreased after CBZ therapy (5.0 ± 2.0 before, compared to 0.4 ± 0.3 after treatment.

Disappearance of MCHA and TGHA was observed in 86% of patients treated with CBZ+ L-thyroxine compared to 25% of patients who received L-thyroxine only.

DISCUSSION

The results of this study suggest that CBZ at high doses can be used in the therapy of autoimmune thyroid disease as it can modify the parameters of immune activation which are recognized to play an important role in the pathogenesis of this condition.

Thus, as far as data obtained in group A, both the percentage of Graves' patients who showed high levels of TRAb at the end of treatment and the incidence of relapse within six months of therapy were low compared to data reported elsewhere (5,6).

In group B, patients with thyroid autoantibodies but without hyperthyroidism showed a reduction of the humoral immune resposne towards the thyroid which may have clinical implications in the management of this disorder.

Therefore, treatment with high doses of CBZ could be a useful tool in two different clinical autoimmune thyroid diseases: a) Graves'disease, characterized by immune activation and high T3 and T4 values and b) patients with T3,T4 and TSH within the normal range but with the presence of TGHA and MCHA antibodies.

However, it is still unclear whether the effect of CBZ is due to a direct immunosuppressive action on lymphocytes infiltrating the thyroid or to a reuced thyroid antigen availability to the immune system induced by this therapy (7).

REFERENCES

1. A.P.Weetman, and A.M.McGregor, Autoimmune thyroid disease: developments in our understanding, Endocrine Reviews, 5:309 (1984).
2. B.Hallegren,A.Forsgren,and A.Melander, Effects of anti-thyroid drugs on lymphocyte function in vitro, J.Clin.Endocrinol.Metab., 51:298 (1980).
3. P.Pozzilli,M.Sensi,and D.Andreani, Inhibition of killer cell cytotoxicity induced by carbimazole in vitro, J.Endocrinol.Invest., 5:149 (1982).
4. M.McLachlan,C.Pagg,M.C.Atherton,S.M.Middleton,E.T.Young,F.Clark, and B.R.Smith, The effect of carbimazole on thyroid autoantibody synthesis by thyroid lymphocytes, J.Clin.Endocrinol.Metab., 60:1237 (1985).
5. A.R.Gossage,J.C.W.Crawley,S.Copping,D.Hinge,and R.L.Himsworth, Thyroid function and immunological activity during and after medical treatment of Graves' disease, Clin.Endocrinol., 19:87, (1983).
6. H.Allanic,R.Fauchet,Y.Lorcy,M.Gueguen,M.Le Guerrier,and B.Genetet, Prospective study of the relationship between relapse hyperthyroid Graves' disease after anti-thyroid drugs and HLA haplotype, J.Clin.Endocrinol. Metab., 57:719 (1983).
7. L.Chiovato,C.Marcocci,S.Mariotti,A.Mori,and S.Pinchera, L-thyroxine therapy induces a fall of thyroid microsomal and thyroglobulin antibodies in idiopathic myxoedema and in hypothyroid, but not in euthyroid Hashimoto's thyroiditis, J.Endocrinol.Invest., 9:299 (1986).

THYMULIN DEFICIENCY AND LOW T3 SYNDROME IN INFANTS WITH LOW-BIRTH-WEIGHT

SYNDROMES

E. Mocchegiani*, N. Fabris*, S. Mariotti***, G. Caramia**,
T. Braccili**, F. Pacini*** and A. Pinchera***

*Ctr. Immuno. Res. Dept. INRCA, Ancona, Italy
**Div. Pediatr., Salesi Hosp., Ancona, Italy
***Ctr. Endocrinol. Univ. Pisa, Pisa, Italy

INTRODUCTION

Several immunological abnormalities have been reported during the first week of life in premature and/or low-weight newborns. Impaired thymic function and particularly reduced capacity of the thymus to produce thymic hormones might be implicated in this immunodeficiency [1]. Experimental and clinical data suggest that thymic endocrine activity is regulated by the neuroendocrine system [2], in particular by the thyroid status[3,4]. We have previously reported that in human adults the circulating level of one of the most known thymic hormones, i.e. thymulin[4,5], is decreased in hypothyroidism and increased in hyperthyroidism and these changes are reversed by restoration of the euthyroid state with appropriate therapy. Premature or SGA infants have reduced serum thyroid hormone concentrations during the first post-natal weeks[6]. In order to investigate whether impaired thymic endocrine activity and thyroid function abnormalities are related, we carried out several and parallel measurements of thymulin, T3 and T4 during the first weeks of life in full-term and in preterm newborns with various conditions.

PATIENTS AND METHODS

Subjects. The study was carried out in 131 newborns including: 26 healthy full-term, 23 full-term small for gestational age (SGA), 30 preterm appropriate for gestational age (AGA) and 22 preterm SGA and 30 with respiratory distress syndrome (RDS) of whom 15 were full-term and 15 preterm AGA. Blood samples were obtained 3, 5, 10, 20 and 40 days after delivery.

Thymulin Determination. Plasma thymulin activity was measured by the method of Bach et al. , with minor modification, as previously described[4]

Thyroid Hormone Assay. Serum T4 and T3 concetration were determined by radioimmunoassay using comercial kits (T4 RIA and T3 RIA kits, ARIA II, Becton Dickinson, Spa, Milan, Italy).

461

Table I. Plasma thymulin activity, T3 and T4 concentrations in all
groups of newborns at the tenth day after birth

Groups of newborns	Healtly full-term	AGA pret.	SGA pret.	SGA full-term	AGA pret. + RDS	Full-term + RDS
Thymulin activity (log)	4.20±0.12	2.83±0.3*	2.77±0.2*	2.25±0.16*	1.41±0.17*	1.61±0.2*
T3 (ng/dl)	167±6.64	127.6±6.43	131±17	142±14	73±3.27*	109.27±4.7**
T4 (µg/dl)	9.80±2.7	9.52±1.11	9.0±0.9	9.27±1.48	7.95±1.65	8.63±0.48

*p<0.01 and **p<0.05 when compared to healthy full-term newborns
a:Mean±SEM

RESULTS

    In healthy full-term newborns circulating thymulin concentrations
were low during the first days of life and subsequently increased
reaching normal values for children aged 1-12 months[7] by the tenth day
after birth. Persistently low circulating thymulin and T3 were observed in
the majority of newborns with pathological conditions, the lowest values
of both hormones being observed in infants with RDS. (Table I)
    A highly significant positive correlation was present in all groups
of newborns between mean circulating thymulin and T3 (r=0,80, p<0.001)
but not T4 (r=0,29, p=n.s.). Short-term T3 administration in 6 selected
additional preterm AGA newborns caused a significant increase of plasma
thymulin titers when compared with 6 untreated controls.

DISCUSSION

    The results of the present investigation provide the first evidence
that plasma thymulin levels are low during the first days of life and
reach the normal values reported for children aged 1-12 months[7] about
ten days after birth. Furthermore, our data indicate that in full-term
and preterm SGA, preterm AGA and full-term or preterm AGA newborns with
RDS, plasma thymulin titers remain persistently lower than those of
healthy full-term infants from birth to 40 days of life. These findings
confirm the previous observation of reduced plasma thymulin in full-term
SGA newborns and show that this also occurs in preterm newborns. In
agreement with previous report[6], low circulating T3 and, to a lesser
degree, T4 concentrations were also observed during the first weeks of
life in all the pathological conditions, the lowest values being observed
in preterm SGA and in RDS affected infants. Although the precise
mechanism(s) responsable for thymulin deficiency observed by us in
premature newborns is (are) still unknown the observation of a highly
significant positive correlation between plasma thymulin and T3

concentrations in all groups of our newborns strongly suggests that abnormal thyroid function might play a role in this phenomenon. This concept is in keeping with several adult studies carried out both in animals and in humans showing a direct relationship of thymic endocrine activity and thyroid status [3,4].

Furthermore, the relevance of thyroid hormone in modulating plasma thymulin in sick newborns was further stressed by the observation that short-term T3 administration increased plasma thymulin activity in a small group of preterm AGA newborns. The mechanism by which thyroid hormones influence thymic endocrine activity is still unknown. Although other explanation are possible, the concept that thyroid hormones affect thymic secretion is in agreement with previous experimental data showing that T3 increases either the number or the secretory activity of thymic epithelial cells, which are believed to produce thymulin[8]. In conclusion, the data of the present investigation provide evidence that circulating thymulin is decreased in premature newborns with low T3 syndrome and that this abnormality may be reversed by administration of T3. These findings indicate that thymic endocrine activity is modulated by thyroid function in the early post-natal life.

AKNOWLEDGMENTS

This work was supported by the National Research Council (Rome, Italy), Special Project Preventive Medicine and Rehabilitation Grants N. 83.02625.56, 84.02306.56, 85.00555.56 to N.F. and N. 83.02464.56, 85.00711.56 to A.P.

REFERENCES

1. R. H. Chandra, Serum thymic hormone activity and cell mediated immunity in healthy neonates, preterm infants, and small-for-gestational age infants, Pediatrics 76:407 (1981).
2. N. Fabris and E. Mocchegiani, Endocrine control o f serum thymic factor in young-adult and old mice, Cell Immunol 91:325 (1985).
3. N. Fabris, M. Muzzioli and E. Mocchegiani, Recovery of age-dependent immunological deterioration in Balb/c mice by short-term treatment with L-thyroxine, Mech Ageing Develop 18:327 (1982).
4. N. Fabris, E. Mocchegiani, S. Mariotti, F. Pacini and A. Pinchera, Thyroid function modulates thymus endocrine activity, J Clin Endocrinol Metab 62:474 (1986).
5. J. F. Bach, M. Dardenne, M. Papiernik, A. Barois, P. Lavasseur and H. Le Brigand, Lancet ii:1056 (1972).
6. D. A. Fisher and A.H. Klein, Thyroid development and disorders of thyroid function in the newborn, N Eng J Med 304:702 (1981).
7. N. Fabris, E. Mocchegiani, L. Amadio, M. Zannotti, F. Licastro and C. Franceschi, Thymic hormone deficiency in normal ageing and Down's syndrome: is there a primary failure of the thymus?, Lancet i:983 (1984).
8. W. Savino, B. Worf, S. Aratan-Spire and M. Dardenne, Fluctuations in the thyroid hormone levels "in vivo" can modulate the secretion of thymulin by the epithelial cells of young mouse thymus, Clin Exp Immunol 55:629 (1984).

CONSTITUTIVE EXPRESSION OF HLA CLASS II MOLECULES IN HUMAN THYROID CELLS

TRANSFECTED WITH SV-40

A. Belfiore, T.Mauerhoff, R.Pujol-Borrell, R.Mirakian, and
G.F. Bottazzo
Department of Immunology
The Middlesex Hospital Medical School
40-50 Tottenham Street, London W1

INTRODUCTION

HLA Class II molecules are not constitutively expressed in epithelial
cells but they have been found to be 'inappropriately' expressed in human
thyrocytes (1) and in other epithelia affected by autoimmune diseases (2).
Thus it has been postulated that Class II positive thyrocytes could present
autoantigens and trigger and/or maintain the autoimmune process (3).
The disappearance of Class II positivity when thyrocytes are kept in culture,
suggests the possibility that this inappropriate in vivo expression is induced
and/or maintained by soluble factors (i.e. lymphokines)(4, 5). In fact these
substances are able to induce expression of Class II molecules by human
thyrocytes (6) and other epithelial cells in vitro. However, the little
knowledge about the real mechanism(s) operating in vivo prompted us to explore
the possibility that an oncogenic virus (SV-40) could modulate HLA molecule
expression in human thyrocytes.

MATERIALS AND METHODS

Cell culture and transfection procedure

Thyroid cell monolayers were obtained from a thyroid of a patient
operated from Graves' disease by collagenase digestion (Wortinghton, type IV).
Cells plated in 90 mm Petri dishes were transfected with a modified PBR 322
vector containing the SV-40 early region (6) using the calcium phospate
precipitation technique (7). Culture medium was changed once a week and the
cells were periodically checked for the emergence of colonies. Cell colonies
were detached by a fine bored Pasteur and cultured separately.

Cell characterization and HLA expression

Indirect immunofluorescence technique (IFL) was employed to check the
effectiveness of the transfection, to identify the transfected cells and to
detect HLA product expression. Cells were cultured on glass coverslips and
stained with monoclonal antibodies (moAbs) prior or after fixation with 50%
v/v methanol/acetone for the detection of membrane and cytoplasmic antigens.
The moAb 3C3 anti SV-40 Large T antigen (Dr. D. Lane) was used to detect the
presence of Large T antigen in the nuclei of the transfected cells and moAb
LE-61 (Dr. B. Lane) to stain the cytokeratin network (characteristic of
epithelial cells (8). Class I antigens were detected by moAb W6/32 (Drs. J.

and W. Bodmer) and Class II antigens by moAbs MID$_3$ (Drs. G. Guarnotta and P; Lydyard) and RFDR 1 (Prof. G. Janossy).

RESULTS

Six weeks after the transfection, numerous foci were detected in the transfected monolayer and were individually cultured. The bulk culture was also subcultured. At 16 weeks fast growth of both colonies and bulk culture was observed. At 4 and 6 months cells from the bulk culture were cloned by limiting dilution and 34 clones were obtained.

Cell characterization

All the transfected cells showed a nuclear IFL staining with the moAb anti SV-40 Large T antigen and a cytoplasmic network of cytokeratin. When examined by electron microscope, the transfected cells showed microvilli and junctions reminescent of "tight junctions" providing evidence to be thyrocytes. Thyroglobulin (up to 400 ng/10^6 cells) was detected by radioimmunoassay (Sorin) in the cytosol preparation of most cell population.

HLA molecules expression

HLA Class I and Class II molecules have been periodically determined by IFL. Class I staining was more intense in the transfected cells than in the non transfected parental culture. Surprisingly, Class II products, undetectable in the non transfected cells,started to be expressed at 4 months from the transfection in 5-10% of the cells from the bulk culture. At the same time a similar percentage of cells was also positive in 4 out of 17 colonies examined. This was concomitant with the acquisition of a faster cell growth probably indicating a stable integration of the viral DNA into the host genome. In addition, when clones derived from the bulk culture were analyzed 2 out of 34 were Class II positive in a higher percentage of cells (30-40%), whereas 14 expressed Class II at a lower level and 18 were consistently negative. Individual clones maintained the same percentage of Class II positive cells over a period of several months in culture. The supernatants of Class II positive clones were unable to induce any change in HLA product expression either in negative clones or in normal thyroid cells.

DISCUSSION

SV-40 virus has been extensively used to immortalize cultured mammalian cells (9). Although the mechanism involved is unclear this function is dependent by the presence of the Large T antigen, a protein able to bind the DNA of the host cell and to regulate gene transcription (10). After SV-40 transfection, human thyroid monolayers acquired an extended life span and, interestingly, were found to express "spontaneously" HLA Class II molecules. The fact that the conditioned medium from these cells is unable to induce Class II expression by normal thyrocytes suggests that this characteristic is constitutive to the transfected cells (probaby virus induced) and not mediated by soluble mediators. Thus the possibility exists that a similar mechanism could be responsible for the "aberrant" HLA Class II expression observed in vivo.

REFERENCES

1. T. Hanafusa, R. Pujol-Borrell, L. Chiovato, D. Doniach, G.F. Bottazzo, Aberrant expression of HLA-DR antigen on thyrocytes in Grave's disease: rilevance for autoimmunity, Lancet ii: 1111 (1983)
2. G.F. Bottazzo, I. Todd, R. Mirakian, A. Belfiore, R. Pujol-Borrell, Organ specific autoimmunity: a 1986 overwiew, Immunol. Rev.in press
3. G.F. Bottazzo, R. Pujol-Borrell, T. Hanafusa, M. Feldman, Role of aberrant HLA-DR expression and antigen presentation induction

of endocrine autoimmunity, <u>Lancet</u> ii:1115 (1983)

4. Y. Iwatani, H.G. Gerstein, M. Iitaka, V.V. Row, R. Volpé, Thyrocyte HLA-DR expression and interferon-gamma production in autoimmune thyroid disease, <u>J.Clin. Endocrinol. Metab.</u> 63:695 (1986)

5. A.P. Weetman, D.J. Volkman, K.D. Burman, T.L. Gerrard, A.S. Fauci, The in vitro regulation of human thyrocytes HLA-DR antigen expression, <u>J. Clin. Endocrinol. Metab.</u> 61:817 (1985)

6. I. Todd, R. Pujol-Borrell, L.J. Hammond, G.F. Bottazzo, M. Feldmann, Interferon-gamma induces HLA-DR expression by thyroid epithelium, <u>Clin. Exp. Immunol.</u> 61:265 (1985)

7. M. From, P. Berg, Deletion mapping of DNA regions required for SV-40 early region promoter function in vivo, <u>J. Mol. Appl. Gen.</u> 1: 457 (1982)

8. E.B. Lane, Monoclonal antibodies provide specific intramolecular markers for the study of epithelial tonofilament organization, <u>J. Cell Biol.</u> 92:665 (1982)

9. S.E. Chang, In vitro transformation of human epithelial cells, <u>Bioch. Bioph. Acta</u> 823:161 (1986)

10. P.W. Rigby, D.R. Lane, Structure and function of Simian virus 40 Large T antigen, <u>in</u>: Advances in Viral Oncology, vol 3, G.Klein Ed. New York, Raven Press pp31-58 (1983)

SPECIFIC DNA POLYMORPHISMS IN THE DQ ALPHA REGION OF PATIENTS WITH GRAVES' DISEASE AND HASHIMOTO'S THYROIDITIS

K.Badenhoop, V.Lewis, V.Drummond, V.Algar, G.Schwarz, and G.F.Bottazzo

St.Bartholomews and Middlesex Hospitals
London, UK

INTRODUCTION

Amongst other organ-specific autoimmune diseases Graves' disease and Hashimoto's thyroiditis are generally associated with certain serological HLA DR specificities (DR3 and DR4 and/or 5 respectively). However the associations shown so far have not been as clear as with other autoimmune diseases and the relative risks have been calculated to be around 3-4. Therefore the actual disease susceptibility gene(s) are thought to be in linkage disequilibrium with genes in the HLA D region and might lie in the DQ subregion on the short arm of chromosome 6. To investigate this association further at the genomic level we studied the structure of the HLA class II genes in patients with Graves' disease and Hashimoto's thyroiditis using RFLP (restriction fragment length polymorphism) analysis. Patients and controls were also studied with serological methods.

METHODS

High molecular weight DNA from patients with Graves' disease (G), Hashimoto's thyroiditis (H), and controls (C) was extracted and digested with the restriction endonucleases PvuII(24G,21H,15C), PstI(17G,7H,15C) and TaqI(21G,23H,11C). DNA was size separated on 0.8% agarose gels and transferred to Nylon filters. Filters were then hybridised to a cDNA probe of the DQ alpha chain (provided by Dr.J.Trowsdale, ICRF, London), which had been labelled to a specific activity of 10^9 cpm/ug by oligonucleotide labelling. After stringent washes the filters were subjected to autoradiography for 2 to 10 days. Bands were compared to serology and to recently published polymorphisms in homozygous typing cell lines (1,4).

RESULTS

Amongst the 28 Graves'disease patients no DR3 excess was found. However the 23 Hashimoto's thyroiditis had an increased DR4 (11,48%), giving a weak RR=1.81(NS). RFLP analysis with PvuII showed a 4.8+0.2kb band in 42% of Graves, 33% of Hashimoto's but 6.7% of controls. The difference between the Graves' and the controls reached a level of significance of p<0.05.

PstI digestion resulted in a 4.4+0.2kb band more common in both Graves'(82%) and Hashimoto's (86%) than in controls(47%), although not reaching significant levels. TaqI digestion showed a band of 6+0.2kb in 48% of Graves', 52% of Hashimoto's but 9% of controls.This was significant for the Hashimoto's group (p<0.05).(Table 1).

The DX alpha polymorphism (2.4/2.2kb) was similarly distributed in Graves' and Hashimoto's(52%/65%) but differently in the controls, where 91% had the 2.4kb band and 36.4% the 2.2kb band. As differences in these polymorphisms could be attributed to the differing HLA serology, three groups were examined which recently showed a common DQ alpha RFLP analysis: DR1,2,w6 - DR3,5,8 - DR4,7,9. When corrected for these serological data, differences still occurred in the DR4,7,9 group for the PstI 4.4kb band : 3/5 Graves' vs 5/6 Hashimoto's but 2/8Controls. The TaqI 6kb band was more common in both Graves' and Hashimoto's for all the haplotypes tested: DR1,2,w6: 5/11 Graves' vs 4/8 Hashimoto's vs1/4 Controls ; DR3,5,8: 4/11 Graves', 6/10 Hashimoto's, 0/3 Controls; DR4,7,9: 4/6 Graves', 11/16 Hashimoto's, 0/6 Controls.(Table 2). When looking at DR4 Hashimoto's thyroiditis vs DR4 controls the 6kb band was found in 5/10 Hashimoto's but 0/4 controls. The PvuII 4.8kb polymorphism is present in 5/9 DR4 Hashimoto's patients but 0/4 DR4 controls. (Table 3). We then tested whether the PstI4.4kb and the TaqI6kb bands are related: 7/13G had both,4 only the PstI band, 2 only the TaqI band, none had neither. 5/7H had both bands , 1 the PstI, 1 the TaqI band only, none had neither. In the controls 1/11 had both bands, 4 only the PstI band and 6 had neither. The two bands seem therefore to be related in the disease groups only. (Table 4).

Table 1

	PvuII 4.8+0.2kb	PstI 4.4+0.2kb	TaqI 6+0.2kb
Graves'	10/24 (42%)*	14/17 (82%)	10/21 (48%)
Controls	1/15 (7%)	7/15 (47%)	1/11 (9%)
Hashimoto's	7/21 (33%)	6/ 7 (86%)	12/23 (52%)+

* p<0.05, x^2>3.78(Yates c.)   + p<0.05, x^2>4.17(Yates c.)

Table 2

DQ alpha RFLP - DR serology

	DR1,2,6: TaqI 6+0.2kb	DR3,5,8: TaqI 6+0.2kb	DR4,7,9: TaqI 6+0.2kb
Graves'	5/11 (45%)	4/11(36%)	4/6 (67%)
Controls	1/4 (25%)	0/3	0/6
Hashimoto's	4/8 (50%)	6/10(60%)	11/16(69%)*

*x^2>5.72(Yates c.), p<0.025

Table 3

DR4 only	TaqI 6kb	PvuII 4.8kb
Hashimoto's	5/10 (50%)	5/9 (56%)
Controls	0/4	0/4

Table 4

Combined DQ alpha polymorphisms:

Hashimoto's:	PstI 4.4kb			Controls:	PstI 4.4kb	
	+	−			+	−
TaqI 6kb +	5	1		TaqI 6kb +	1	0
−	1	0		−	4	6

DISCUSSION

Recent data suggest that genetic analysis at the HLA DQ subregion should consider individual alpha and beta polymorphisms (1). This type of analysis will increase our understanding of the existing relationships between serology for DR and DQ. As linkage in both Graves' disease and Hashimoto's thyroiditis with DR serology is not as striking as in e.g. type I diabetes mellitus, disease susceptibility markers might be in the DQ subregion. The DQ alpha polymorphism was recently found to be also in the different lengths of mRNA relating to DQw1, DRw53 and DR3+5 (3).These are specificities, which show the DQ alpha RFLP at the genomic level (1,4). As DRw53 (DR4,7,9) and DRw52 (DR3,5) are DR beta chain related, this seems to be in linkage with the DQ alpha chain. Our findings of the PvuII 4.8kb band in the Graves' patients and the TaqI6kb band in Hashimoto's patients were significant. When corrected for the serological background (by subdividing into DQ alpha RFLP associated haplotype groups) the PstI 4.4kb band was still more common in the DR4,7,9 Hashimoto's compared to controls. The TaqI 6kb polymorphism remained increased in both Graves' and Hashimoto's using the same method. The fact that the two bands seem to be related in the disease groups and that in DR4 Hashimoto's the difference remains compared to DR4 controls indicates that there might be restriction enzyme sites in the DQ alpha non-coding region of Hashimoto's and Graves' patients which differ from controls and others which differ amongst the two disease groups. We have not considered the classical DQ associations, because only DQw1 seems to be correlated with DQ alpha polymorphisms and DQw2 and 3 with DQ beta polymorphisms. Analysis of DQ beta polymorphisms is in progress as well as the enlargement of our patients' and control groups to confirm and extend our preliminary findings.

SUMMARY

RFLP(restriction fragment length polymorphsm) analysis of the DQ alpha subregion with PvuII, PstI and TaqI revealed a PvuII4.8kb, a PstI4.4kb and a TaqI6kb band more common in both Graves' and Hashimoto's patients.These differences persisted when corrected for the HLA serology background and were significant for the PvuII 4.8kb band in the Graves' group and the TaqI 6kb polymorphism in the Hashimoto's group. These observations indicate that markers for the disease susceptibility genes in both Graves' disease and Hashimoto's thyroiditis might lie in the DQ region on the short arm of chromosome 6.

REFERENCES

1) M.Trucco and R.J.Duquesnoy Immunology Today 7, 297, 1986
2) D.A.Hardy, J.I.Bell, E.O.Long et al Nature 323, 453, 1986
3) P.Loiseau, P.Lehn, F.Dautry et al Immunogenetics 23, 111, 1986
4) J.Trowsdale, J.Lee, J.Carey et al PNAS 80, 1972, 1983

SURVEY OF POST-PARTUM THYROID ANTIMICROSOMAL AUTOANTIBODY AS A MARKER FOR THYROID DYSFUNCTION

Paul G. Walfish, Maria T. Vargas, John P. Provias, and
Frederick R. Papsin
Depts. of Medicine and Obstetrics, Mount Sinai Hospital,
University of Toronto, and Thyroid Research Lab., Mount Sinai
Hospital Research Institute
Toronto, Ontario, Canada

INTRODUCTION

The association of post-partum thyroid dysfunction (PPTD) with positive serum antimicrosomal antibody (AMA) has been increasingly recognized (1-5). However, few detailed prospective systematic surveys have been performed on large numbers of patients and controls to determine the precise prevalence of AMA positivity from delivery to one year post-partum (PP) in a series of mothers proven to have developed PPTD compared to those mothers who were also documented to have normal thyroid function (NTF), to evaluate not only the possible utility of a serum AMA test as a marker for the detection of PPTD but also whether such evidence could support an underlying autoimmune etiology for most PPTD patients.

METHODS

261 mothers who were euthyroid at delivery without any previous past history of thyroid dysfunction or nodular goiter were followed at intervals of approximately 2 months from delivery to one year PP to determine the prevalence of positive AMA within those mothers documented to have either PPTD (hyperthyroidism or hypothyroidism) vs. those mothers with normal thyroid function (NTF). Thyroid dysfunction was assessed by routine measurements of serum free thyroxine using a commercial method (Clinical Assays 2-step test, Cambridge, Mass.) and serum total triiodothyronine and pituitary thyroid-stimulating hormone assays as performed by standard double-antibody radioisotopic methods (6). Serum AMA tests were performed using a standard commercial hemagglutination method (Sera-Tek Test, Ames, Division of Miles Laboratory Ltd., Rexdale, Ont.) with a positive titre = > 1:80 (6). Chi square (x^2) and Fisher's exact tests (both with Yates' correction for continuity), i.e. x^2correct, were used for comparison between groups. Relative Risk (RR) was calculated using odd ratios and the validity of the AMA test in its sensitivity and specificity for PPTD was calculated by standard methods. Two tailed P values < 0.05 were considered to be significant.

473

RESULTS

Among the 261 mothers surveyed, the overall prevalence of AMA positive was 15% at delivery; 21% at 2-4 months PP; and 26% at 5-7 months PP. However, a comparison of changes in titer from delivery to 5-7 months PP, revealed that AMA positive NTF mothers had no further increase in mean titer whereas, AMA positive PPTD mothers had a mean 3-fold increase in titer. A retrospective analysis on the of AMA^+ results at delivery in predicting PPTD revealed that it had no significant (P = > 0.05) predictive value for the occurrence of PPTD since AMA^+ at delivery was only 25/55 (43%) for those mothers developed PPTD vs. 15/206 (7%) of those mothers who had NTF. At 2-4 months PP, AMA^+ results were present in 35/46 (76%) of mothers with PPTD vs. 19/215 (9%) for those with NTF, resulting in a x^2correct = 100.5 (p < 0.0001), RR for PPTD = 32.8 with a sensitivity of 0.76, and a specificity of 0.92. At 5-7 months PP, AMA^+ results occurred in 47/55 (86%) for mothers with PPTD vs. 22/206 (11%) for those mothers with NTF resulting in a x^2correct = 121, (P = < 0.0001), RR for PPTD = 49; with a sensitivity 0.86, and a specificity of 0.90.

DISCUSSION

The experimental design employed in our study which assessed not only those mothers who developed PPTD, but also those documented to have NTF has permitted the appropriate calculations of the relative sensitivity and specificity values as well as predictive estimates for AMA positivity as a marker for PPTD. Such studies have demonstrated that patients who developed PPTD had a 3-fold rise in mean AMA positive titer from delivery to 5-7 months PP and that the sensitivity and specificity of AMA positive results was optimal at 5-7 months post-partum at 0.86 and 0.9 respectively, when most patients were in the hypothyroid phase of PPTD. AMA positivity at 2-4 months PP was also a good predictor of PPTD at 0.76 and 0.92 respectively, when most patients were in the thyrotoxic phase of PPTD. Such observations are in agreement with the theory that there is a suppression of immune mechanisms during pregnancy which rebounds post-partum to activate autoimmune diseases, as well as previous studies on a smaller number of patients with PPTD due to painless thyroiditis (1-5, 7-10) which have been reviewed in detail elsewhere (11-13). Serial observations of AMA^+ in the first trimester of pregnancy and post-partum in mothers with known Hashimoto's thyroiditis (11,12) has observed a similar post-partum rebound rise in AMA positive titers. However, the recommendation of a recent report (10) regarding screening for PPTD at delivery is at variance with our observations, since only 43% of those mothers who developed PPTD had a positive AMA titer at delivery, thereby indicating that AMA^+ at delivery had a lesser predictive value for the development of post-partum thyroid dysfunction than AMA^+ at 2-7 months PP when it achieves optimal diagnostic value as a marker for the detection of PPTD.

Moreover, these studies indicate that most PPTD detected in our region likely arises as a result of post-partum activation of anti-thyroidal autoimmune mechanisms and supports recent reviews on the current clinical and experimental evidence favouring post-partum activation of autoimmune mechanisms in the pathogenesis and onset of PPTD from painless thyroiditis (11-13). PPTD occurs at an approximate prevalence of 4-5% for the PP mothers screened in our region (13), being similar to the results of several other surveys (4,5,9,10). While routine screening of post-partum mothers for PPTD is controversial and probably not justified, particularly at delivery, our results indicate that the assessment of thyroid function and autoimmunity should be performed in those mothers who have the post-partum onset of new symptoms, and that a positive AMA titer at 2-7 months PP could be a very useful marker for detecting PPTD.

ACKNOWLEDGMENTS

Supported in part by grants from the physicians of Ontario by the Physicians' Services Incorporated Foundation and the Mount Sinai Hospital Department of Medicine Research Fund. MTV and JPP were Research Fellows supported by awards from the Mount Sinai Hospital Department of Medicine Research Fund. The generous assistance of supplies from Ames, Division of Miles Laboratory Ltd., Rexdale, Ontario and Clinical Assays, Cambridge, Massachusetts and the technical assistance of Mrs. E. Gera, A. Bansil and E. Pike are gratefully acknowledged.

REFERENCES

1. N. Amino, K. Miyai, K., R. Kuro, O. Tanizawa, M. Azukizawa, S. Takai, F. Tanaka, K. Nishi, M. Kawashima, Y. Kumahara, Transient post-partum hypothyroidism: Fourteen cases with autoimmune thyroiditis, Ann. Intern. Med., 87:155 (1977).
2. J. Ginsberg and P. G. Walfish, Post-partum transient thyrotoxicosis with painless thyroiditis, Lancet, 1:1125 (1977).
3. N. Amino, R. Kuro, O. Tanizawa, F. Tanaka, C. Hayashi, K. Kotani, M. Kawashima, K. Miyai and Y. Kumahara, Changes of serum antithyroid antibodies during and after pregnancy in autoimmune thyroid disease, Clin. Exper. Immunol., 31:30 (1978).
4. N. Amino, H. Mori, Y. Iwatani, O. Tanizawa, M. Kawashima, I. Tsuge, K. Ibaragi, Y. Kumahara and K. Miyai, High prevalence of transient postpartum thyrotoxicosis and hypothyroidism, N. Engl. J. Med., 306:846 (1982).
5. R. Jansson, S. Bernander, A. Karlsson, K. Levin and G. Nilsson, Autoimmune thyroid dysfunction in the postpartum period, J. Clin. Endocrinol. Metab., 48:681 (1984).
6. P. G. Walfish, I. S. Gottesman and J. L. Baxter, Graves' Ophthalmopathy and Subclinical Hypothyroidism: Diagnostic Value of the Thyrotropin Releasing Hormone Test, Can. Med. Assoc. J., 127:291 (1982).
7. H. G. Fein, J. M. Goldman, and B. D. Weintraub, Post-partum Lymphocytic Thyroiditis in American women: A spectrum of Thyroid Dysfunction. Am. J. Obstet. Gynec., 138:504 (1980).
8. T. F. Nikolai, G. J. Coombs, and A. K. McKenzie, Lymphocytic Thyroiditis with Spontaneously Resolving Hyperthyroidism and Subacute Thyroiditis, Arch. Intern. Med., 141:1455 (1981).
9. S. Turney, T. F. Nikolai and R. Roberts, The Prevalence in Clinical Course of Post-partum Lymphocytic Thyroiditis, in: "Prog. 64th Ann. Meeting The Endocrine Society", Abst.#557, pp. 219 (1982).
10. C. C. Havslip, H. G. Fein, V. M. O'Donnell, D. S. Friedman, T. A. Klein, R. C. Smallridge, Post-partum Thyroiditis: Should all Patients be Screened at Delivery? in: "Program 61st Annual Meeting American Thyroid Association", Abst.#5, pp.T-3, (1986).
11. N. Amino and K. Miyai, Post-partum Autoimmune Syndromes, in: "Autoimmune Diseases." T. Davies, ed. John Wiley & Sons, New York, pp. 247 (1983).
12. N. Amino, Y. Iwatani, H. Tamaki, H. Mori, M. Aozasa, and K. Miyai, Post-partum Autoimmune Thyroid Syndromes, in: "Autoimmunity and The Thyroid" P.G. Walfish, J.R. Wall, and R. Volpe eds., Academic Press, Orlando, Fl. pp. 289 (1985).
13. P. G. Walfish, J. Y. C. Chan, Post-partum Hyperthyroidism, Clinics in Endocrinology & Metabolism, 14:417 (1985).

HLA REGION GENE INVOLVEMENT IN CONGENITAL HYPOTHYROIDISM

Mariangela Cisternino, Miryam Martinetti*, Renata Lorini,
Angelo Gruppioni, Daniela Larizza, Mariaclara Cuccia Belvede-
re**, Maria Rosaria Romano, and Francesca Severi

Pediatric Clinic 2° Chair, University of Pavia, *Lab. HLA
AVIS, Pavia, **Departments of Genetic and Microbiology, University of Pavia, Italy

INTRODUCTION

Congenital hypothyroidism is commonly due to developmental abnormalities of thyroid resulting in ectopic or hypoplastic thyroid gland as
well as in total thyroid agenesis. The etiology of these abnormalities
has not been yet clarified. Moreover, a less common cause of congenital
hypothyroidism is thyroid dyshormonogenesis,due to several hereditary defects in thyroid hormone synthesis or metabolism[1]. An association among
the human hystocompatibility system and autoimmune thyroid diseases[2] and
non autoimmune endocrine diseases such as congenital adrenal hyperplasia
has been reported[3]. The aim of the present study was to evaluate the HLA
involvement and immune response modulation in congenital hypothyroidism.

MATERIALS AND METHODS

We studied 48 Italian patients with congenital hypothyroidism (9
boys and 39 girls), aged 1.3–24.7 years; 22 patients were affected by
thyroid agenesis, 22 by tnyroid ectopia and/or hypoplasia and 4 by dyshor
monogenesis. The diagnosis was made on the basis of laboratory findings
(including determinations of serum thyroid hormones and TSH) and thyroid
scintigram. All were on appropriate replacement therapy. HLA class I and
II molecules (65 specificities) typing was performed by NIH microlympho-
cytotoxicity test on T and B enriched lymphocyte suspensions from peripheral blood samples. Fisher's exact test was used for comparisons with
a large sample (226) of healthy blood donors from Northern Italy. Autoantibodies (ANA, MA, SMA, RA, LKM, antiribosoma, PCA, IECA, ICA-IgG, CF-ICA,
TgA, MsA, antiadrenal, antigonads) were detected by indirect immunofluorescence or passive haemoagglutination both in 44 patients and in 131 age
and sex-matched normal subjects.

RESULTS

An increased frequency of A31 and DR5 was found in the entire group

477

Table 1. Significant deviations in HLA phenotype frequencies in
patients with congenital hypothyroidism versus controls

HLA antigens	Patients (n=48)		Controls (n=226)		Relative risk
	%	(n)	%	(n)	
A31	12	(6)*	3	(7)*	4.47
DR5	52	(25)**	31	(69)**	2.47

* unc. Fisher's P 0.0110
** "   "   P 0.0077
Values are percentages. Values in parentheses are numbers of subjects

of patients compared to the controls (Tab. 1). When a distinct comparison
was made between various subgroups of thyroid disorders and controls, an
increased frequency of A24, A31, B18, CW6 resulted in the group of patients
with thyroid agenesis; A1 and DR5 frequency was significantly increased
in patients with ectopic and/or hypoplastic thyroid gland (Tab. 2). Comparing HLA phenotypic frequency of patients with thyroid agenesis versus
patients with thyroid ectopia and/or hypoplasia, a significant increase
of A24 and CW6 antigens resulted in athyreotic patients as well as A1 in
patients with ectopia and/or hypoplasia (Tab. 3). HLA phenotype was different in the 4 patients (two of them were siblings) with dysormonogene-
sis. No statistical analysis was performed on these patients. Autoantibodies were present in 35% of the patients and in 24% of the controls (p=
n.s.). No patients had antithyroid antibodies (TgA/MsA). We found no si-
gnificative difference in HLA antigen frequencies in patients positive
and negative for autoantibodies.

Table 2. Differences in HLA frequencies in patients with thyroid
agenesis and with thyroid ectopia and/or hypoplasia compared with controls

HLA antigens	Thyroid agenesis (n=22)		Thyroid ectopia and/or hypoplasia (n=22)		Healthy controls (n=226)		Uncorrected Fisher's P values	Relative risk
	%	(n)	%	(n)	%	(n)		
A1	5	(1)	36*	(8)	19*	(44)	*0.039	2.36
A24	41*	(9)	14	(3)	21*	(48)	*0.026	2.57
A31	14*	(3)	9	(2)	3*	(7)	*0.041	4.94
B18	32*	(7)	18	(4)	16*	(37)	*0.047	2.38
CW6	27*	(6)	0	(0)	12*	(27)	*0.038	2.76
DR5	45	(10)	55*	(12)	31*	(69)	*0.023	2.72

478

Table 3. Statistically different HLA antigen distribution in patients with thyroid agenesis and with thyroid ectopia and/or hypoplasia

HLA antigens	Thyroid agenesis (n=22)		Thyroid ectopia and/or hypoplasia (n=22)		Uncorrected Fisher's P value
	%	(n)	%	(n)	
A1	5	(1)	36	(8)	0.0097
A24	41	(9)	14	(3)	0.0359
CW6	27	(6)	0	(0)	0.0100

DISCUSSION

Our study, involving HLA class I and II molecules, demonstrates a higher frequency of A31 and DR5 antigens in our Italian patients with congenital hypothyroidism. A higher frequency of A24 and CW6 antigens was found in athyreotic patients compared to both controls and patients with ectopia and/or hypoplasia; a higher frequency of A1 was found in patients with ectopia and/or hypoplasia compared to both controls and athyreotic patients. Concerning only HLA class I molecules, Miyai[4] and Cimino[5] suggested an association between congenital hypothyroidism and HLA-A24 in Japanese population and HLA-B18 in white American patients, while Jacobsen[6] didn't find any HLA association in Danish patients. Concerning HLA class II molecules, an involvement of DR5 antigen has been described only in autoimmune thyroid diseases (i.e. Hashimoto's thyroiditis with goitre[7]). On the basis of literature's data and our study, HLA region seems to be probably involved in susceptibility to congenital hypothyroidism.

REFERENCES

1. D. A. Fisher and A. H. Klein, Thyroid development and disorders of thyroid function in the newborn, New Engl. J. Med. 304:702 (1981).
2. A. Svejgaard, N. Morling, P. Platz, HLA and disease associations with special reference to mechanism, Transpl. Proc. 13:913 (1981).
3. L. S. Levine, M. Zachmann, and M. I. New, Genetic mapping of the 21-hydroxylase-deficiency gene within the HLA linkage group, New Engl. J. Med. 299:911 (1978).
4. K. Miyai, H. Mizuta, O. Nose, T. Fukunishi, T. Hirai, S. Matsuda, and T. Tsuruhara, Increased frequency of HLA-Aw24 in congenital hypothyroidism in Japan, New Engl. J. Med. 303:226 (1980).
5. P. Cimino, R. Banks, N. Maclaren, E. Rosembloom, W. Riley, and A. Rosembloom, HLA and congenital hypothyroidism, New Engl. J. Med. 303:1177 (1980).
6. B. B. Jacobsen, N. J. Brandt, and A. Svejgaard, Congenital primary hypothyroidism and HLA, Acta Paediatr. Scand. 71:919 (1982).
7. N. R. Farid, L. Sampson, H. Moens, and J. M. Barnard, The association of goitrous autoimmune thyroiditis with HLA-DR5, Tissue Antigens 17:265 (1981).

PROBABILITY OF A BENEFICIAL, DOSE-DEPENDENT, IMMUNOSUPPRESSIVE ACTION

OF CARBIMAZOLE IN GRAVES' DISEASE

Jacques Duprey, Marie-Françoise Louis*, Maggy Sultan
and Elisabeth Lifchitz

Policlinique and *Laboratoire de Biochimie
Hôpital Ambroise-Paré, 92100 Boulogne, France

INTRODUCTION

It is known that the mean titre of the serum anti-TSH receptor autoantibodies (ATRA) progressively decreases in patients with Graves' disease treated with carbimazole.[1,2] It has been suggested that this decrease may be due to the lowering by carbimazole of thyroid hormones synthesis.[3,4] In order to test whether there is also a direct, dose-dependent, immunosuppressive action of carbimazole, we have compared the evolution of ATRA levels between two groups of patients with Graves' disease at first attack. The patients of the two groups differed by the daily dosage of carbimazole, but were maintained at similar levels of serum T3.

PATIENTS AND METHODS

Patients of group 1 (32 cases) received a "quickly degressive treatment" (QDT): carbimazole 60 mg/day at first, and then rapidly reduced to maintaine an euthyroid state without adding thyroid hormones. Patients of group 2 (32 cases) received a "prolonged high dosage treatment" (PHDT): carbimazole 60 mg/day, maintained during 6 months, and then reduced monthly (50-40-30-20-10-0 mg/day), with adding of substitutive hormonotherapy with L-T3 (25-50 μg/day) to maintain an euthyroid clinical state. Clinical and biological tests were performed before treatment and at different times after starting therapy. Only 23 cases in QDT group and 5 in PHDT group had a survey of 24 months or more. ATRA were measured by the TRAK-Assay (Behring)[5] and expressed as percentages of inhibition of radiolabeled TSH binding to thyroid membranes.

RESULTS

The mean daily dosages of carbimazole in the PHDT group vs the QDT group were respectively, at 0-0.5-1-2-3-4-6-9-12-15-18-21 and 24 months (mean ± sem): 58 ± 1 vs 58 ± 1; 58 ± 1 vs 56 ± 1; 58 ± 1 vs 46 ± 2; 59 ± 1 vs 27 ± 3; 60 ± 0 vs 15 ± 3; 60 ± 0 vs 19 ±4; 59 ± 1 vs 13 ± 2; 35 ± 3 vs 13 ± 3; 10 ± 4 vs 11 ± 2; 5 ± 4 vs 9 ± 2; 4 ± 4 vs 10 ± 3; 0 ± 0 vs 8 ± 3; 0 ± 0 vs 7 ± 3. The differences are highly significant (P< 0.001) from 1 to 9 months (Fig.1).

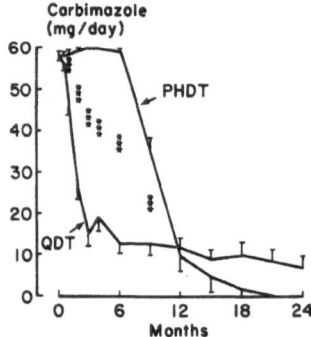

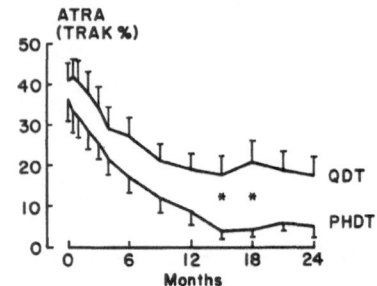

Fig. 1. Carbimazole dosages. QDT: quickly degressive treatment. PHDT: prolonged high dosage treatment. *** P< 0.001

Fig. 2. Titres of anti-TSH receptor antibodies. QDT: quickly degressive treatment. PHDT: prolonged high dosage treatment. * P< 0.05. Anti-TSH receptor antibodies measured by the TRAK-Assay (Behring).

The mean values of serum T3 decreased quickly in the two groups and remained in the normal range from 0.5 to 24 months. They did not differ significantly between the two groups at any time except 3 months.

The mean ATRA levels decreased in the two groups, but more quickly in the PHDT than in the QDT group, respectively (mean ± sem): 36 ± 5 vs 41 ± 4; 33 ± 6 vs 42 ± 5; 32 ± 5 vs 41 ± 5; 29 ± 5 vs 38 ± 5; 26 ± 4 vs 34 ± 5; 22 ± 4 vs 29 ± 5; 17 ± 4 vs 28 ± 4; 12 ± 3 vs 21 ± 4; 9 ± 4 vs 19 ± 4; 4 ± 2 vs 18 ± 5; 4 ± 2 vs 21 ± 5; 6 ± 2 vs 19 ± 5; 5 ± 3 vs 18 ± 4. The differences are statistically significant at 15 and 18 months (P<0.5) (Fig. 2).

We have calculated at every time the ratio R/E, i.e. number of cases relapsing or having relapsed before/number of cases with persistent euthyroid state. R/E in PHDT vs QDT group was: 6 months. 0/27 vs 7/23 (P<0.05); 9 months, 0/22 vs 8/19 (P<0.05); 12 months, 1/19 vs 8/18 (NS); 18 months, 1/13 vs 10/15 (NS); 24 months, 0/5 vs 11/12 (NS) (χ^2 test) (Fig. 3).

The actuarial curves of the cases without relapse, according to the Kaplan-Meïer method, show a high significant difference between the two groups (log rank test: P< 0.01) (Fig. 4).

DISCUSSION

The immunosuppressive effects of antithyroid drugs have been discussed.[3] They might be due to the lowering by these drugs of the thyroid hormones secretion, as these hormones may contribute to the synthesis of the antibodies.[4] Our results, obtained when comparing the action of very different dosages of carbimazole in patients maintained at similar levels of serum T3, seem in favour of a direct, dose-dependent, immunosuppressive action of carbimazole in Graves' disease. They agree with the experimental results of McLachlan.[6] This immunosuppressive action is accompanied by a beneficial, clinical effect : the relapses of thyrotoxicosis are less frequent in patients treated with high dosages than in patients treated with low dosages of antithyroid drugs.[7,8]

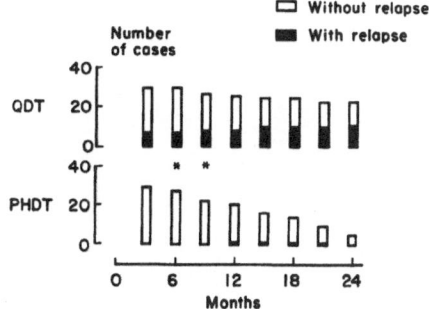

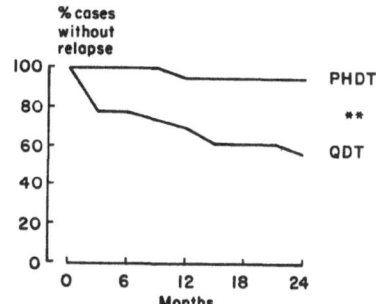

Fig. 3. Numbers of cases with and without relapse. QDT: quickly degressive treatment. PHDT: prolonged high dosage treatment.
* P < 0.05

Fig. 4. Actuarial curves of cases without relapse. QDT: quickly degressive treatment. PHDT: prolonged high dosage treatment. ** P < 0.01

REFERENCES

1. J. Duprey, M. Izembart, G. Vallée, and A. Mossé, Evolution des anticorps antirécepteurs de TSH dans la maladie de Basedow traitée par le carbimazole selon deux modalités thérapeutiques différentes, Ann. Endoc. (Paris) 46:195 (1985).

2. G. Fenzi, K. Hashizume, C. P. Roudebush, and L. J. DeGroot, Changes in thyroid-stimulating immunoglobulins during antithyroid therapy, J. Clin. Endocrinol. Metab. 48:572 (1979).

3. P. Kendall-Taylor, Are antithyroid drugs immunosuppressive? Br. Med. J. [Clin. Res.] 18:509 (1984).

4. S. Ratanachaiyavong, and A. M. McGregor, Immunosuppressive effects of antithyroid drugs, Clinics Endocrinol. Metab. 14:449 (1985).

5. K. Southgate, F. Creagh, M. Teece, C. Kingswood, and B. Rees Smith, A receptor assay for the measurement of TSH receptor antibodies in unextracted serum, Clin. Endocrinol. (Oxf) 20:539 (1984).

6. S. M. McLachlan, C. A. S. Pegg, M. C. Atherton, S. Middleton, E. T. Young, F. Clark, and B. Rees Smith, The effects of carbimazole on thyroid antibody synthesis by thyroid lymphocytes, J. Clin. Endocrinol. Metab. 60:1237 (1985).

7. J. Duprey, B. Ducornet, E. Lifchitz, and M. Sultan, Réduction de l'incidence des rechutes de maladie de Basedow par utilisation de fortes posologies de carbimazole, Ann. Endoc. (Paris) 47:308 (1986).

8. J. H. Romaldini, N. Bromberg, R. S. Werner, L. M. Tanaka, H. F. Rodrigues, M. C. Werner, C. S. Farah, and L. C. F. Reis, Comparison of effects of high and low dosage regimens of antithyroid drugs in the management of Graves' hyperthyroidism, J. Clin. Endocrinol. Metab. 57:563 (1983).

EVIDENCE FOR DR-AG-EXPRESSION BY RHS-CELLS AND NOT BY THYROID EPITHELIAL CELLS

J. Teuber, R. Paschke, U. Schwedes, M. Knoll,
J. Cristophel, and K.H. Usadel

II. Medical Department, Klinikum Mannheim,
University of Heidelberg, Theodor-Kutzer-Ufer
6800 Mannheim, FRG

INTRODUCTION

The class II or MHC II antigens (Ag) play an essential role for the Ag-recognition by macrophages and the interaction between immunologic regulatory- and effectorsystems.

The susceptibility to diseases and the strength of the immune response to certain Ag are genetically controlled by these HLA-DR-Ag and are varying depending on the individual pattern of these MHC II-Ag. DR-Ag expressed on B-lymphocytes (Ly) and activated T-Ly as well as on cells of RHS. Hanafusa et al. (1) demonstrated the occurence of these Ag on thyroid membranes first in native tissue in patients with autoimmune thyroid diseases. They could also induce DR-Ag in cultivated thyrocytes which are cocultivated with lectins. Later Bottazzo et al. (2) described DR-Ag on islet cells in the pancreas of a newly detected diabetes type I. The authors suppose that the membrane expression of DR-Ag is important for the induction of the autoimmune process. In contrast to this asumption Weetman et al. (3) as well as our group (4) could demonstrate that DR expression on thyroid cells does not have any effect as trigger mechanism for the T-cells. We interpreted the appearance of DR-Ag on thyroid epithelial cell membranes as an epiphenomenon caused by lymphokinins which are released during the immune reactions. Up to now IL-1 or IL-2 production by epithelial cells could not be shown. Since on the other hand interleukins are necessary for mediating the immune process we looked for other cell types which would be able to produce these substances.

MATERIAL AND METHODS

Tissue sections of thyroids from patients undergoing subtotal thyroidectomy were screened for the occurrence of DR-Ag, fibronectin, dentritic cells and specific Ag of endothelial cells. Patients were suffering from Graves disease (GD,n=3) and thyroid carcinoma (TC,n=6). The immunohistochemical investigations were performed by indirect immunofluorescence (FITC and rhodamine) and immunoperoxidase-technique using

highly specific monoclonal antibodies as follows:
BMA 020, anti human fibronectin, BMA 340, BMA 120.

RESULTS

DR-Ag staining was found in all tissue sections with different intensity. In TC DR-Ag expression was confined to histologically identify malignant cell areas. In GD DR molecules were distributed over the whole section. The staining was found to be homogeneous. There was a week local prevalence in regions where lymphatic infiltration was present.

The percentage of DR-Ag positive malignant cells varied over a broad range in the different specimens . In the same areas in which DR-Ag was expressed a positive staining could also be detected for fibronectin, reticulum cells and endothelial cells. Routine HE staining could only demonstrate thyroid epithelial cells. in the corresponding areas. By low power magnification it was not possible to discriminate whether DR-staining was localised on cell membranes or between the cells as it can be shown by higher magnification.

DISCUSSION

The occurence of DR-Ag in Graves' disease tissue is well documented. In TC the appearance of these molecules is not jet sufficiently investigated whereas this phenomenon is well known in other malignant neoplasias. Their localisation in areas with malignantly altered cells is discussed as a prognostic marker.

The simultaneous detection of DR-Ag combined with antigens of RHS like fibronectin, dendritic antigen and endothelium in identical areas suggests that characterization of these cells as RHS cells is more likely than epithelial cells. The common occurence of all these antigens for RHS in the same areas makes this assumption more probable.

Since RHS cells are antigen presenting cells (APC) they are able to produce interleukines and other mediators. This capability is a necessary condition for the induction and perpetuation of immune processes. In case of this adequate antigen presentation autoimmune reactions against thyroid epithelial cells in Graves' disease as well as a possible protective effect in TC may be well explained.

During the course of immunologic interactions mediators like interferones and interleukines are released. So far secretion of these substances by epithelial cells has not been described. But earlier investigations (5) could well document the induction of DR-Ag on thyroid epithelial cells by these kinins. In this context an eventual DR-Ag expression on thyroid epithelial cell membranes is a secondary phenomenon induced by an ongoing local autoimmune reaction. We belive that this phenomenon initiated in this way is very unlikely to be of any functional immunological significance.

REFERENCES

1. Hanafusa T, Pujol-Borell R, Chiovato L, Russel RLA, Doniach D, Bottazzo GF (1983) Aberrant expression of HLA-
   DR-Ag on thyrocytes in Graves disease: relevance for autoimmunity. Lancet II, 1111

2. Bottazzo, GF, Dean BM, McNally JM, McKay EH, Swift PGF,
   Gamble DR (1985) In situ characterization of autoimmune
   phenomena and expression of HLA molecules in the pancreas
   in diabetic insulitis. New Engl. J. Med. 313: 353

3. Weetmann AP, Volkmann DJ, Burmann KD, Gerrad TC, Fauci AS
   (1985) The in vitro regulation of human thyrocyte HLA-DR
   expression. J. Clin. Endocrin. Metab. 61: 817

4. Teuber J, Paschke R, Schwedes U, Usadel KH (1986) The role
   of DR expression on thyrocytes for the autoimmunity of
   the thyroid. in: The thyroid and autoimmunity, HA Drexhage
   WM Wiersinga (ed) Excerpta Medica

5. Davies TF Cocultures of human thyroid monolayer cells and
   autologous T cells: Impact of HLA class II antigen expression (1985) J. Clin. Endocrinol. Metab. 61: 418

HLA-DR-β GENE ANALYSIS IN PATIENTS WITH GRAVES' DISEASE

Bernhard O. Boehm, Ekkehard Schifferdecker,
Peter Kuehnl,Christoph Rosak, and Karl Schöffling
University Hospital of Frankfurt Medical School
Center of Internal Medicine,Dept. of Endocrino-
logy, and Institute of Immunehematology,
Frankfurt am Main, Fed.Rep. of Germany

INTRODUCTION

Graves' disease is a HLA-linked autoimmune disease associated with certain HLA antigens, mainly with the HLA class
II antigen HLA-DR 3 (7). Aberrant expression of HLA class II
antigens on thyroidal cells was reported recently and was
suggested to mediate the autoimmune response by presentation
of autoantigens (2). The aim of our study was to determine
HLA-DRβ genes in HLA matched patients suffering from Graves'
disease and Type I (insulin-dependent) diabetics and in
addition in non HLA typed normal controls.

MATERIAL AND METHODS

Subjects. All subjects studied were unrelated Caucasians
selected from the same local area. Graves' and Type I patients were all HLA-DR3 positive. Two HLA-DR3 homozygous typing lymphoblastoid cell lines were kindly donated by Dr.K.
Welte, New York. Controls (free of personal and family history of autoimmune diseases) were age and sex matched to the
patients. We studied 20 Graves' and 20 Type I patients as
well as 45 normal controls.
HLA typing was performed according to standard techniques.
DNA-preparation, DNA digests, electrophoresis, Southern-
transfer. All these techniques were performed according to
standard protocols (5).
DRβ-probe. The DRβ specific recombinant was kindly provided by Dr. E.O.Long, Bethesda (4). An insert spanning the
two extracellular domains, the transmembrane region and the
cytoplasmatic tail, was labelled to a very high specific
activity (1).
DNA-DNA-hybridisation. Filters were hybridised with the
32P labelled insert for 48 hrs at 65°C. Final wash included
0.2xSSC-0.1% SDS at 65°C for 1 hr. Filters were then exposed
to Kodak XAR-5 film with intensifying screens for 2 to 3 days
at -80°C.

RESULTS

Hybridisation of genomic DNA restricted with Taq1 revealed about 6 to 8 restriction fragments per individual blot
as well as several faint hybridisation signals (Fig. 1). The
restriction pattern observed with Taq1 restricted genomic DNA
was closely related to serologically defined HLA-DR types. A
restriction fragment of 10.0kb was markedly increased in Graves' patients (14 out of 20) and Type I diabetics (12 out of
20). This fragment was found to correlate with the HLA-
A1,B8,DR3 haplotype. A restriction fragment of 8.0kb not observed on the blots of the two HLA-DR3 homozygous typing lymphoblastoid cell lines was increased in Graves' patients (positive in 75%) and markedly reduced in the HLA-DR3 positive
Type I diabetics (only 15% positive). In the control group,
this band was detected in 9 out of 45 individuals studied
(20%). A doublet of 10.0 kb and 14.5 kb was indicative in
Type I diabetics of HLA-DR3/HLA-DR4 heterozygosity (Fig. 1).

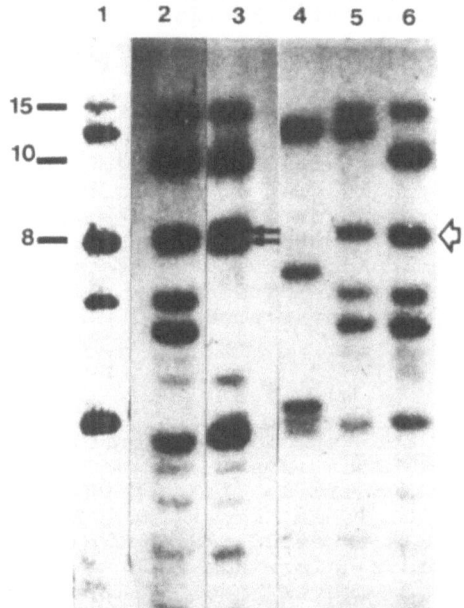

Fig.1. Hybridisation of DRβ cDNA probe to Taq1 restricted genomic DNA.Lane 1:normal control, positive for the 8.0
kb fragment.Lane 2:Type I diabetic. 14.5 and 10.0kb
doublet and the 8.0kb restriction fragment are visible, also several faint hybridisation signals, illustrating the complexity of the hybridisation pattern
obtained with the DRβ full length cDNA probe. Lane 3:
HLA-DR3/-DR4 heterozygous Type I diabetic with a doublet at 8.0 and 7.7kb (arrows). Lane 4: HLA-DR3 positive Graves' patient lacking the 8.0kb fragment. Lane 5:
HLA-B18,DR3 positive Graves' patient with a 12.0kb
fragment indicative for the HLA-B18,DR3 haplotype and
the 8.0kb fragment. Lane 6: HLA-DR3/-DR6 positive Graves' patient with the 8.0kb fragment. At the the left
margin molecular weights in kb. Arrow at the right
margin marks the 8.0 kb fragments.

DISCUSSION

Over the past decade the ability to analyze MHC genes by use of molecular genetics has expanded greatly (6). It was shown that the polymorphism of HLA-DR genes and their products resides almost exclusively in the β-chain of the membrane spanning heterodimer (6). Since Graves' disease is linked to HLA-DR3, we wanted to study by use of a DRβ specific cDNA probe HLA genotypes in two HLA-DR3 matched groups – Graves' patients and Type I diabetics- in comparison with normal controls.

Data from TaqI restricted genomic DNA reveal a pattern closely related to the DR types defined by standard HLA-typing (3). This is illustrated by the high prevalence of the 10.0kb Taq1 fragments which is associated with the HLA-A1,B8,DR3 haplotype, as well as the 10.0kb and 14.5kb doublet in HLA-DR3/DR4 heterozygous individuals.

Data concerning the 8.0kb Taq1 fragment show a different prevalence in the two HLA-DR3 matched populations. This fragment was not found to correlate to another DR specificity suggested to be more prevalent in Graves' disease or Type I diabetes. Recently it has been reported that a 7.7kb and a 8.0kb TaqI fragment correspond to a DRβ a2 and a DRβa1 chain, respectively. These bands describe therefore a split of the HLA-DR3 haplotype (8).

It remains to be clarified on an extended HLA-matched population if there is any difference in the prevalence of HLA-DRβa1 and DRβ a2 chain in the HLA-DR3 haplotype in different disease groups.

Acknowledgement. Work was supported by a grant from Riese Foundation and from Deutsche Forschungsgemeinschaft BO 829/1-1.

LITERATURE

1. Feinberg,A.P. and B.Vogelstein, Addendum: a technique for radiolabelling DNA restriction endonuclease fragments to high specific activity, Anal. Biochem. 137:266(1982)
2. Hanafusa,T., R.Pujol-Borrell, L.Chiovato et al., Aberrant expression of HLA-DR antigen on thyrocytes in Graves' disease: relevance for autoimmunity, Lancet 2:1111(1983)
3. Kohonen-Corish, M.R.J. and S.W.Serjeantson, HLA-DR gene DNA polymorphisms revealed by Taq1 correlate with HLA-DR specifities, Hum.Immunol. 15:263(1986)
4. Long,E.O., C.T.Wake, J.Gorski, B.Mach, Complete sequence of an HLA-DR chain deduced from a cDNA clone and identification of multiple non-allelic DR chain genes, EMBO J. 2:389(1983)
5. Maniatis,T., E.F.Fritsch, J.Sambrook, "Molecular cloning", Cold Spring Harbor Laboratory, Cold Spring Harbor (1982)
6. Shackelford,D.A., J.F.Kaufman, W.J.Korman, J.Strominger, Structure, separation of subpopulations, gene cloning and function, Immunol.Rev. 66:133(1982)
7. Tiwari, J.L. and P.I. Terasaki, "HLA and disease associations",Springer, New York-Berlin-Heidelberg-Tokyo (1985)
8. Bontrop,R., M.Tilanus, M.Mikulski, M. van Eggermond, A. Termijtelen, M.Giphart, Polymorphisms within the HLA-DR3 haplotypes. I.HLA-DR polymorphisms detected at the protein and DNA levels are reflected by T-cell recognition, Immunogenet. 23:401 (1986)

IMMUNE SIGNALS FAIL TO ELICT ENDOCRINE RESPONSES IN THE OBESE STRAIN (OS)

OF CHICKENS WITH HASHIMOTO-LIKE AUTOIMMUNE THYROIDITIS

R. Faessler, K. Schauenstein, G. Kroemer, and G. Wick

Institute for General and Experimental Pathology
University of Innsbruck, Medical School
Fritz-Pregl-Strasse 3, A-6020 Innsbruck, Austria

Much evidence has accumulated proving that the endocrine system can effectively modulate immune functions. Recently, we described a disturbed glucocorticoid hormone tonus in the Obese strain (OS) of chickens[1], which is afflicted with a Hashimoto-like autoimmune disease (spontaneous autoimmune thyroiditis, SAT)[2]. OS chickens exhibit normal serum levels of total corticosterone (CN) (Table 1), but significantly elevated serum concentrations of corticosteroid binding globulin (CBG) as compared to normal controls, indicating that free, hormonally active CN is deficient in this strain. Furthermore, in vivo substitution of OS animals with hydrocortisone led to both normalization of the in vitro T-cell hyperfunction (ConA-hyperreactivity, IL-2 hypersecretion)[3] and prevention of SAT.

In the present study, we examined the influence of immune stimuli on the glucocorticoid system: Recent findings have demonstrated the existence of a pathway in which the immune system controls neuroendocrine functions. It has been shown by several groups[4,5] that antigenic challenge or injection of conditioned medium (CM) from ConA activated lymphocytes lead to a transient increase of glucocorticoid serum levels, which, in turn, regulate the immune response in qualitative terms.

Five month old OS and normal white Leghorn (NWL) chickens were either immunized with a single dose of sheep red blood cells (SRBC) or injected intravenously (i.v.) with different doses of CM from ConA stimulated spleen lymphocytes of NWL chickens, and the CN serum levels were monitored radioimmunologically. NWL chickens showed a transient increase of CN blood levels following immunization with SRBC (Schauenstein et al., submitted for publication) as well as i.v. application of CM (Table 1). OS chickens, however, displayed a significantly diminished CN response against these immune stimuli. CM derived from ConA stimulated lymphocytes from OS and NWL chickens were equally effective in inducing an elevation of CN in NWL animals (Fig.1), clearly excluding an abnormal production of this "corticosterone increasing factor (CIF)" by OS lymphocytes. In a further experiment we could show that the adrenal glands, i.e. the CN secreting organ, respond with a similar CN increase to i.v. ACTH in both OS and control chickens. This normal "CIF" production by OS lymphocytes as well as the unaltered responsiveness of the adrenal gland in OS chickens suggest that the defect underlying the diminished CN response is located in the hypothalamo-hypophyseal system. The discrepancy between normal

Table 1.   CN blood levels and ConA response of PBL after i.v.   injection
of CM from ConA activated NWL lymphocytes [a]

| | CN plasma levels (ug/l; $\bar{x} \pm$ SEM) | | % suppression of the ConA response ($\bar{x} \pm$ SEM) [b] |
	naive	2 hours after "CIF"	
OS (n=4)	2.1 ± 0.2	6.6 ± 0.5 [c]	48 ± 9.0 [c]
CB (n=4)	2.0 ± 0.3	12.8 ± 0.9	77 ± 6.5

[a] Four month old OS and CB (NWL inbred line) chickens were injected with
3 ml of a 10-fold concentrated CM (Amicon membrane filter PM 10, cut
off = 10 kD). CN plasma levels and the ConA response of PBL from both
strains were determined before and two hours after CM administration.

[b] 100% of the ConA response before CM application refer to 6759 ± 1772
cpm ($\bar{x} \pm$ SEM) in CB and 15439 ± 1562 cpm in OS chickens (uptake of 5-
(^{125}J)-2-deoxyuridine), respectively.

[c] Statistically significant different (p<0.01 for the CN increase, p<0.05
for the % suppression of the ConA response) from CB animals as
determined by Student-t-tests.

NWL recipients were injected i.v. with CM from either OS or NWL ConA
activated spleen lymphocytes. CN plasma levels (ug/l; $\bar{x}$ ± SEM) were
determined 2 hours after CM administration (open bars). The IL 2 content
of CM was determined by proliferation assays with IL 2 dependent
lymphoblasts (full bars).

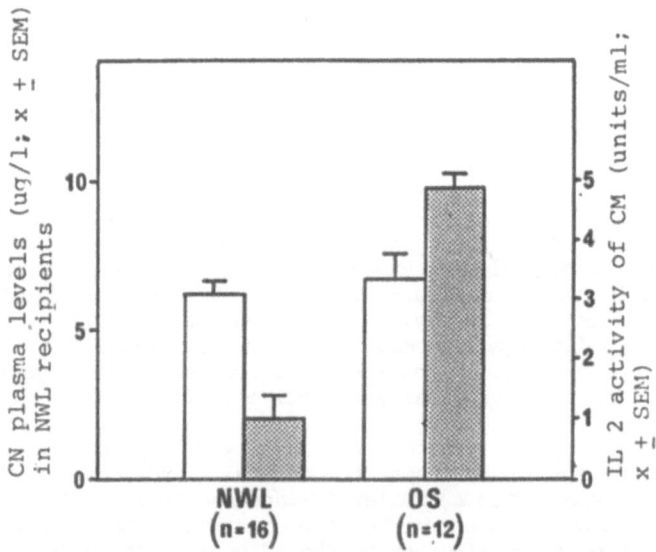

Figure 1.   Comparison of CN inducing capacity and IL 2 content of CM from ·
ConA activated lymphocytes from OS and NWL chickens

"CIF" but constantly enhanced IL-2 production by OS lymphocytes (Fig. 1) clearly indicates that IL-2 is not involved in eliciting a CN response. This defect of the immune-neuroendocrine loop is not of merely theoretical interset but actually has _in vivo_ relevance for the T-cell responsiveness in the OS. Concomitantly with the CN rise in plasma the ConA response of PBL derived from CM treated normal animals is drastically suppressed (Table 1). In contrast, lymphocytes of autoimmune OS chickens are much less inhibited by _in vivo_ administration of "CIF" containing CM.

These data are the first indication that the development of autoimmune disease is not only associated with an intrinsic dysregulation of the immune response[6], but also with a disturbed dialogue between the immune and neuroendocrine system. It was shown by Besedovsky et al.[7] that this immunologically induced CN response plays an important role in the surveillance of the specificity of an immune response against a certain antigen. Since the CN peak occurs several days after immunization and glucocorticoids are only able to exert their suppressive effects during the inductive phase of lymphocyte activation, the CN rise seems not to quantitatively influence the immune response to this antigen. Taking into account that autoimmune reactions may be the result of cross-reactoins to external antigens, defects in this immune-neuroendocrine loop could allow for proliferation of "forbidden" lymphocyte clones, when the autologous structures are antigenically related to foreign antigens.

ACKNOWLEDGEMENTS

This work was supported by the Austrian Research Council (project no. S41-05) and the Jubilaeumsfond of the Austrian National Bank (project no. 2784).

REFERENCES

1. R. Faessler, K. Schauenstein, G. Kroemer, S. Schwarz, and G. Wick, Elevation of corticosteroid-binding globulin in Obese Strain (OS) chickens: possible implication for the disturbed immunoregulation and the development of spontaneous autoimmune thyroiditis, J. Immunol. 136:3657 (1986).
2. G. Wick, J. Moest, K. Schauenstein, G. Kroemer, H. Dietrich, A. Ziemiecky, R. Faessler, S. Schwarz, N. Neu, and K. Hala, Spontaneous autoimmune thyroiditis - a bird´s eye view, Immunol. Today 6: 359 (1985).
3. K. Schauenstein, G. Kroemer, R.S. Sundick, and G. Wick, Enhanced response to Con A and production of TCGF by lymphocytes of Obese Strain (OS) chickens with spontaneous autoimmune thyroiditis. J. Immunol. 134:872 (1985).
4. H.O. Besedovsky, E. Sorkin, M. Keller, and I.W. Mueller, Changes in blood hormone levels during the immune response. Proc. Soc. Exp. Biol. Med. 150:466 (1975).
5. J.E. Blalock, Relationship between neuroendocrine hormones and lymphokines. Lymphokines 9:1 (1984).
6. G. Kroemer, K. Schauenstein, N. Neu, K. Stricker, and G. Wick, In vitro T-cell hyperreactivity in Obese strain (OS) chickens due to a defect in nonspecific suppressor mechanism(s), J. Immunol. 135:2458 (1985).
7. H.O. Besedovsky, A. Del Rey, and E. Sorkin, Antigenic competition between horse and sheep red blood cells is a hormone dependent phenomenon, Clin. Exp. Immunol. 49:273 (1979).

INAPPROPRIATE HLA CLASS II EXPRESSION IN A
WIDE VARIETY OF THYROID DISEASES

R. Pujol-Borrell, A. Lucas Martin*, M. Foz*,
I. Todd, and G.F. Bottazzo

Department of Immunology, Middlesex Hospital Medical
School, London W1. *Hospital Germans Trias i Pujol
badalona (Barcelona), Spain

INTRODUCTION

Thyroid follicular cells from glands afflicted by autoimmune disease often express HLA Class II molecules (1-5). The mechanism(s) by which this 'inappropriate' Class II expression arises in vivo and whether it is restricted to thyroid autoimmune disease remains uncertain. To gain insights into this phenomenon we have studied Class II expression in all the thyrodectomy specimens collected during one year from a major teaching hospital (Hospital General Valle de Hebron, Universidad Autonoma de Barcelona, Barcelona, Spain). Class I and Class II expression were correlated with the clinical diagnosis, with lymphocytic infiltration and with thyroid autoantibodies.

PATIENTS AND METHODS

Summary of patient's data and thyroid antibody results

Diagnosis	Age	M/F	no. cases	no. sera	TMAb(%)	TgAb(%)
Multinodular goitre	49+12	3/51	54	50	12(24)	10(20)
Benign nodules:						
Hyperplastic	38+12	3/14	17	15	4(27)	1 (6)
Colloid Cyst	33	0/2	2	1	0	0
Follicular adenoma	37+11	0/13	13	8	2(25)	1(12)
Malignant nodules:						
Papillary	36+15	3/5	8	5	1(20)	1(20)
Follicular	57	2/0	2	2	0	0
Anaplastic	79	0/1	2	2	0	0
Medullary	36	2/1	3	3	0	1
Graves' disease	32+11	2/12	14	13	10(76)	3(23)
Laryngeal Carcinoma	60+ 8	0/12	12	12	2(17)	2(17)
	TOTALS		126	110	19(17)	8(14)

TMABS: thyroid microsomal antibodies, TgAbs: Thyroglobulin antibodies.
Thyroid antibodies detected by indirect hemagglutination (Wellcome).

Immunofluorescence staining

Serial sections were stained with MoAbs to HLA Class I, beta-2-microglobulin, HLA Class II, CD3 or CD5 followed by biotinylated horse anti-mouse Ig and by FITC-avidin. The next two sections were stained for microsomal antigen and Ig deposition respectively. Selected glands were stained for CD4, CD8, B1 and M1 (results not reported here).

Scoring system

The intensity and extension of the staining for HLA Class I and Class II in the thyroid follicular cells and of the lymphocytic infiltration was assessed semiquantitatively and given a score ranging from negative to +++++.

Statistical analysis

Multiple correlations between Class I, Class II, Lymphocytic infiltration and thyroid antibodies were calculated by contingency and regression analysis.

RESULTS

TABLE 1. HLA EXPRESSION AND LYMPHOCYTIC INFILTRATION IN THE DIFFERENT DIAGNOSIS GROUPS

DIAGNOSIS	Thyrocytes		Lymphocytic Infiltration
	Class I	Class II	
Multinodular goitre:	34 (63)	24 (44)	28 (52)
Benign Nodules:			
Hyperplastic nodule	9 (53)	9 (53)	10 (58)
Colloid cyst	2	2	2
Follicular adenoma	7 (54)	2 (15)	4 (31)
Thyroid Carcinoma:			
Papillary	8 (100)	3 (38)	2 (25)
Follicular	1	1	0
Anaplastic	1*	0	1
Medullary	1	1	1
Graves' disease	12 (86)	10 (71)	13 (92)
Laryngeal Carcinoma	2 (17)	2 (17)	3 (25)

% in brackets

* Class I expression was increased in the C cells which constitute medullary carcinomas.

TABLE 2 MULTIPLE ANALYSIS OF CORRELATION AND ASSOCIATION BETWEEN IMMUNE FEATURES IN THE DIFFERENT DIAGNOSIS GROUPS

	Multinodular goitre	Hyperplastic Nodule	Follicular Adenoma	Thyroid carcinoma	Graves' disease	Laryngeal Carcinoma	All diagnosis
Lymph Infiltr / Class I	****/oooo	o**o	**/o	*		****/o	****/oooo
Lymph Infiltr / Class II	****/oooo	**/oo	**			****/o	****/oooo
Lymph Infiltr / TMAb	*						***/ooo
Lymph Infiltr / TgAb	***/ooo						*/oo
Class I / Class II	****/oooo	****/ooo	***	**	*	***/oo	****/oooo
Class I / TMAb							***
Class I / TgAb							
Class II / TMAb							****/oo
Class II / TgAb	**/o						
No of cases studied	54	17	13	14	14	12	126
No of sera tested	50	15	8	11	13	12	110

* p values by regression analysis, ° p values by Chi square

*,° p<0,05 **,°° p<0,02 ***,°°° p<0,01 ****,°°°° p<0,001

CONCLUSIONS

1. Inappropriate Clas II expression and Class I hyperexpression occurs in non—autoimmune thyroid disorders in two conditions: Focal Thyroidits, and Thyroid neoplasia.
2. Inappropriate Class II expression, Class I hyperexpression and Lymphocytic infiltration tend to be related to each other.
3. Lymphocytic infiltration, Class II and Class I expression were all correlated to TMAb but only lymphocytic infiltration was related to TgAb.
4. The weaker correlation and association between lymphocytic infiltration and HLA expression in Graves' disease and thyroid carcinoma may be indicative of different factors inducing HLA expression in these two conditions.

ACKNOWLEDGEMENTS

Dr J Gomez Perez is thanked for providing most of the thyroidectomy specimen.

REFERENCES

1. T. Hanafusa, R. Pujol-Borrell, L. Chiovato, R.C.G. Russell, D. Doniach, G.F. Bottazzo, Aberrant expression of HLA-DR antgen on thyrocytes in Graves' disease: relevance for autoimmunity, Lancet, ii: 1111-1115 (1983).

2. R. Jansson, A. Karlsson, U. Forsum, Intrathyroid HLA-DR expression and T lymphocyte phenotypes in Graves' thyrotoxicosis, Hashimoto's thyroiditis and nodular colloid goitre, Clin exp Immunol, 58: 264-272 (1985).

3. G. Aichinger, H. Fill, G. Wick, In situ immune complexes, lymphocyte subpopulations and HLA-DR positive epithelial cells in Hashimoto thyroditis, Lab invest, 52: 132-140.

4. A.P. Weetman, D.J. Volkman, K.D. Burman, T.L. Gerrard, A.S. Fauci, The in vitro regulation of human thyrocyte HLA-DR antigen expression, J Clin Endocrinol Metab, 61: 817-824 (1985).

5. R.V. Lloyd, T.L. Johnson, M. Blaivas, J.C. Sisson, B.S. Wilson. Detection of HLA-DR antigens in paraffin embedded thyroid epithelial cells with a monoclonal antibody, Am J Pathol, 120: 106-111 (1985).

ADVERSE REACTIONS RELATED TO METHIMAZOLE AND PROPYLTHIOURACIL
DOSES

M.C.Werner, J.H.Romaldini, N.Bromberg, M.T.A.Boesso
and R.S.Werner
Dept. Endocrinology, HSPE-IAMSPE, São Paulo, Brasil

INTRODUCTION

Graves' hyperthyroidism management with thionamide drugs
has been outwarded because of the risk of toxic reactions (1)
that were related to the patients' age and to the administered
daily dosage (2). Thus, we correlated thionamide side effects,
retrospectively, with methimazole (MMI) or propylthiouracil
(PTU) administration, thionamide dosage, patients' age and sex,
their thyroid status and thyroid microsomal autoantibodies serum
titers (MAb) at the onset of toxic reactions in 360 Graves'
hyperthyroid patients.

PATIENTS AND METHODS

Side effects, classified as major (agranulocytosis and
hepatotoxicity) and minor (arthralgia, gastric intolerance and
skin hypersensitivity), were studied in group I patients (n:261)
who received either MMI (60.6 ± 17.1 mg/daily, mean ± SD) or
PTU (706.7 ± 202.7 mg/daily) high dosage and compared with 99
patients in group II, treated with more conventional dosages
(MMI: 17.7 ± 8.4 or PTU: 210.5 ± 68.9 mg/daily). T3, T4 and
TSH were measured by commercial RIA kits and MAb by passive
haemagglutination technique.

RESULTS

The incidence of side effects in both groups are summarized
in table I. Arthralgia (3.6%: 13/360) was related to MMI (n:10)
and to high dosage regimen (n:11). Its onset varied from the 2nd
to the 25th month of therapy, usually after the 1st semester,
and it was more frequent in euthyroid patients. No pattern of
rheumathologic disease was found in those patients.

TABLE I: Thionamide side effects in Graves' disease patients.

	Drug	n	Dose (mean ± SD)	Side effects
GROUP I	MMI	171	60.0 ± 17.2 mg/day	28 (16.7%)
	PTU	90	706.7 ± 202.7 mg/day	16 (17.7%)
GROUP II	MMI	61	17.7 ± 8.4 mg/day	7 (11.5%)
	PTU	38	210.5 ± 68.9 mg/day	2 (5.3%)

Gastric intolerance (3.6%: 13/360) was related to high dose regimen (n:11) but not to MMI or PTU or to the thyroid status. It occurred after the 6th month of treatment in 69.2%.

Urticaria, pruritus and skin rash (4.4%: 16/360) was not related to MMI or PTU, to their dose regimen or to thyroid status. Its onset was usual in the 1st semester of therapy but it varied widely (1st to 32th month).This group of patients presented the highest MAb titers when compared with other side effects (agranulocytosis, gastric intolerance and hepatotoxicity $p < 0.01$; arthralgia $p < 0.05$), as shows figure 1.

Hepatotoxicity occurred in 1.1% (4/360) patients, all of them receiving high PTU doses (600-1500 mg/day) and after the 3rd month of therapy. It was not correlated with thyroid function. Hepatic damage observed were hepatic cholestasis (n:2) and toxic hepatitis (n:2).

Agranulocytosis was observed in 1.7% (6/360) patients, 5 out of them still hyperthyroid, in the early (1st to 3rd) months

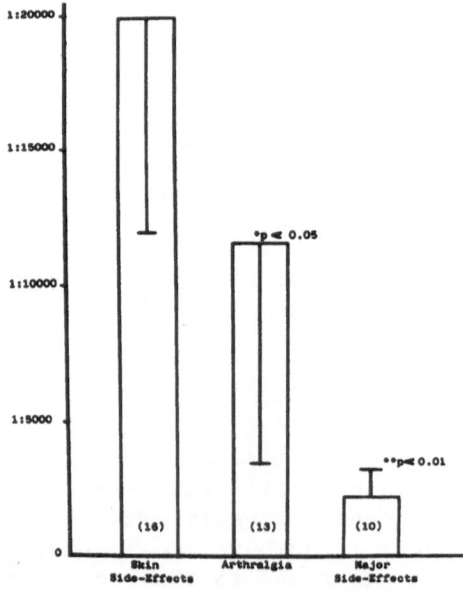

Fig.1 Relationship between MAb and side effects.

of therapy. Patients' age was 35.5 $\pm$ 9.8 yr (25 to 49 yr).It was related to high dose regimen (n:5) and to MMI therapy (n:5).

There was no correlation between patients' age and specific side effects. Minor side effects were restricted to female patients.

DISCUSSION

Our data showed that thionamide side effects were related to high doses. No difference was observed between MMI and PTU. However, the incidence of major side effects (hepatotoxicity, 1.1%; agranulocytosis, 1.7%) was low and no cases of thrombocytopenia and vasculitis were observed (3). Hepatotoxicity was related both to PTU and to the duration of therapy. Recovery following drug withdrawal was observed in 3 out of 4 patients. We found no relationship between hepatic damage and MAb titers or thyroid function.

The relationship between agranulocytosis and hyperthyroidism suggests a facilitating role of thyroid disfunction on the formation of antineutrophilic antibodies (4) induced by drug. The one of our patients who was euthyroid at the onset of agranulocytosis had a previous diagnosis of systemic lupus erythematosus, a condition related to abnormal immunological tolerance. In contrast with Cooper et al (2), there was not a relationship with patients' age. Recovery was achieved in all cases following drug withdrawal.

Minor side effects did not require drug discontinuing. They were related to female patients and did not correlate with thyroid status or patients' age. The relationship between high MAb titers and skin rash/pruritus/urticaria suggests that these patients are prone to cutaneous hypersensibility.

The relatively low risk for major side effects and the high remission rate associated with high dose thionamide therapy (3,5) allow us to indicate this type of treatment for Graves' hyperthyroidism, when carefully managed.

REFERENCES

1. D.S.Cooper, Antithyroid drugs, N Engl J Med, 311:1353(1984).
2. D.S.Cooper, D.Goldminz, A.A.Levin, P.W.Ladeson, G.H.Daniels, M.E.Molitch and E.C.Ridgway, Agranulocytosis associated with antithyroid drugs, Ann Intern Med, 98:26(1983).
3. D.B.Vasily and W.B.Tyler, Propylthiouracil-induced cutaneous vasculitis; case presentation and review of the literature, JAMA, 243:458(1980).
4. S.A.Weitzman, T.P.Stossel, D.C.Harmon, G.Daniels, F.Maloof and E.C.Ridgway, Antineutrophil autoantibodies in Graves' disease, J Clin Invest, 75:119(1985).
5. J.H.Romaldini, N.Bromberg, R.S.Werner, L.M.Tanaka, H.F.Rodrigues, M.C.Werner, C.S.Farah and L.C.F.Reis, Comparison of effects of high and low dosage regimens of antithyroid drugs in the management of Graves' hyperthyroidism, J Clin Endocrinol Metab, 57:563(1983).

THYROID SUPPRESSIBILITY IN GRAVES' DISEASE: RELATIONSHIP WITH THYROID STIMULATING ANTIBODY AND SERUM THYROGLOBULIN LEVELS

R.S. Werner, J.H. Romaldini, N. Bromberg, C.S. Farah,
I.D. Pereira, and R.P. Dall'Antonia Jr.

Department Endocrinology, HSPE-IAMSPE, Sao Paulo, Brasil

INTRODUCTION

The elevated serum thyroid stimulating antibody (TSAb), thyroglobulin (Tg) levels and the T_3 nonsuppressibility of the 24h-radioactive iodine uptake (RAIU) have been used to predict the relapse of antithyroid drug treated Graves'disease patients (1-4). In disagreement with others(3-6), Isozaki et al.,(7) showed a correlation between TSAb and Tg or RAIU during medical treatment. Thus,we studied the correlation among TSAb activity, serum Tg levels, 24h-RAIU, thyroid antimicrosomal antibody (MAb) titers and serum T_4 concentration during the T_3-associated methimazole (MMI) therapy for Graves'disease.

MATERIAL AND METHODS

Graves'disease patients were randomly distributed into two groups: 21 patients using high MMI doses (50 to 80 mg daily) and 19 patients treated with low MMI doses (10 to 20 mg daily) both associated with T_3 (50 to 75 ug daily) during 11 to 18 months (mean $\pm$ S.D.: 15 $\pm$ 4.5). The normal value of T_3 suppressed 24h-RAIU was up to 12%. TSAb activity was measured using the increase of cyclic AMP generation in human thyroid plasma membrane (10,000 g fraction). The thyroid membranes (50 ug) were incubated with either TSH or IgG preparation at 34ºC for 60 min in 30 mM Tris-Hcl-EDTA buffer pH 7.8 containing 2.5 mM ATP, 5 mM $MgCl_2$, 10 mM creatine phosphate, 0.35 mg/ml creatine kinase, 10^{-4} M Gnpp(NH)p, 10 mM theophylline. The sensitivity to bovine TSH was 0.1 mU/ml. Graves' IgG values above 130% of normal IgG were considered positive for TSAb activity. Serum TSH and Tg were determined by IRMA methods (Cis-Sorin) and normal values were 0.08 to 0.6 uU/ml and 3 to 30 ng/ml, respectively. Serum T_4 was measured by RIA. MAb was measured by passive hemagglutination. The data were analyzed by Student't-test and Spearman correlation.

RESULTS

The mean age, sex and thyroid weight did not differ between the two groups. No difference was observed between TSAb activity (157 $\pm$ 59 vs 146 $\pm$ 66%), serum Tg (265 $\pm$ 345 vs 162 $\pm$ 225 ng/ml), T_4 (3.8 $\pm$ 3.4 vs 3.8 $\pm$ 2.6 ug/dl), TSH (1.5 $\pm$ 2.4 vs 1.8 $\pm$ 4.2 uU/ml), MAb titers (1:7720 $\pm$ 9589 vs 1:6382 $\pm$ 9502) and 24h-RAIU (14.8 $\pm$ 17 vs 21.7 $\pm$ 18%) for high and low doses , respectively.

There was a correlation between serum T_4 concentration with either TSAb activity (r= 0.572, P<0.01) or 24h-RAIU (r= 0.513, P<0.01). The relationship between TSAb activity and thyroid suppressibility is shown in Fig. 1 and in Fig. 2. Serum Tg levels were normal in 40% (8/20) nonsuppressible and in 33% (6/18) suppressible patients and also in 29% (5/17) positive TSAb and in 40% (6/15) negative TSAb patients. No relationship was noted neither between MAb titers and others parameters nor serum Tg levels and T_3 suppressed 24h-RAIU.

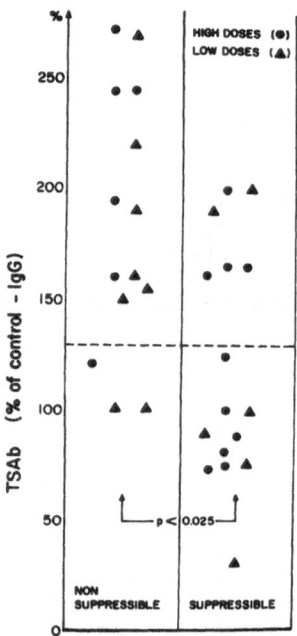

Fig. 1. TSAb activities in Graves' disease patients during MMI therapy.---,The upper limit of IgG from normal subjects.

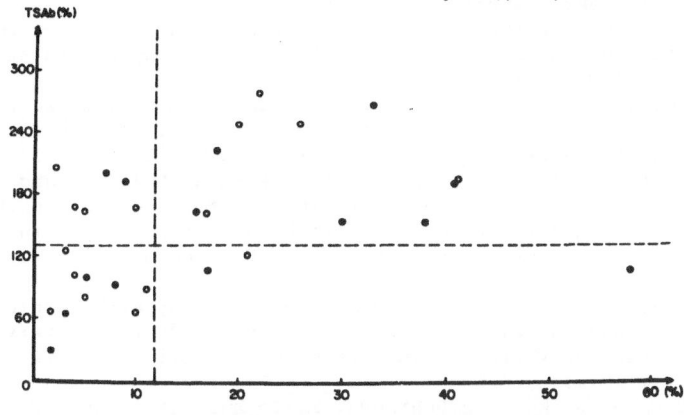

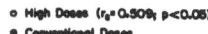

Fig. 2. Correlation between TSAb and T₃ suppressed 24h-RAIU in Graves' disease patients during MMI therapy (r= 0.48, P<0.01; r= 0.51, P<0.05 for high MMI dose group).---,The upper limits in normal subjects.

DISCUSSION

The correlation of thyroid suppressibility with TSAb activity in Graves'disease patients during treatment with MMI was in accordance with Isozaki et al.,(7) but other authors have not noted such association (3-5).

The MMI associated with T_3 throughout therapy regimen utilised in this study or the differences in the sensitivities of the TSAb assays used(5-7) may be accounted for such discrepancies. With this regimen of treatment we are able to obtain both the blocking of thyroid function and a prolonged T_3 suppression test (6,8). In contrast to low MMI dose group the high MMI dose group showed a correlation between TSAb activity and the T_3 suppressed 24h-RAIU.

Our results indicate that 1) Tg secretion, during antithyroid drug treatment, is independent of either thyroid suppressibility or TSAb stimulation (3,4). 2) high MMI doses might decrease the iodine thyroid content and also affect the TSAb levels. 3) the correlation between T_3 suppressed 24h-RAIU and TSAb activity suggest that antithyroid drug associated with T_3 (8) may act both on thyroid gland blocking and on the immunological disturbance.

REFERENCES

1. M.Yamamoto, Y.Totsuka, I,Kojima, N.Yamashita, K.Togawa, N.Sawaki and E.Ogata, Outcome of patients with Graves'disease after long-term medical treatment guided by triiodothyronine(T_3) suppression test, Clin Endocrinol(Oxf), 19:467(1983).
2. A.A.R.Cossage, J.C.W.Crawley, S.Copping, D.Hinge and R.L.Himsworth, Thyroid function and immunological activity during and after medical treatment of Graves'disease, Clin Endocrinol(Oxf), 19:87(1983).
3. T.Yamada, Y.Koizumi, A.Sato, K.Hashizume, T.Aizawa, N.Takasu and H. Nagata, Reappraisal of the triiodothyronine-suppression test in the prediction of long term outcome of antithyroid drug therapy in patients with hyperthyroid Graves'disease, J Clin Endocrinol Metab, 58:676(1984).
4. D.F.Gardner and R.D.Utiger, The natural history of hyperthyroidism due to Graves'disease in remission: sequential studies of pituitary-thyroid regulation and various serum parameters, J Clin Endocrinol Metab, 49:417(1979).
5. N.Kuzua, S.C.Chiu, H.Ikeda, H.Uchimura, K.Ito and S.Nagataki, Correlation between thyroid stimulators and T_3-suppressibility in patients during treatment of hyperthyroidism with thionamide drugs: comparison of assays by thyroid-stimulating and thyrotropin-displacing activities, J Clin Endocrinol Metab, 48:706(1979).
6. J.H.Romaldini, N.Bromberg, R.S.Werner, L.M.Tanaka, H.F.Rodrigues, M.C. Werner, C.S.Farah and L.C.F.Reis, Comparison of effects of high and low dosage regimens of antithyroid drugs in the management of Graves' hyperthyroidism, J Clin Endocrinol Metab, 57:563(1983).
7. O.Isozaki, T.T.Sushima, K.Shizume, M.Saji, Y.Ohba, N.Emoto, K.Sato, Y. Sato and K.Kusakabe, Thyroid-stimulating antibody bioassay using porcine thyroid cells cultured in follicles, J Clin Endocrinol Metab, 61:1105(1985).
8. P.H.Wise, M.Marion and R.Pain, Mode of action of carbimazole in Graves' disease, Clin Endocrinol(Oxf), 10:655(1979).

INFLUENCE OF LYMPHOKINES AND THYROID HORMONES ON NATURAL KILLER ACTIVITY

M. Provinciali, M. Muzzioli, and N. Fabris

Immunology Center, INRCA Research Department

Ancona, Italy

DEVELOPMENT AND FUNCTION OF NK CELLS

Natural Killer (NK) cells are a subpopulation of lymphocytes which have spontaneous cytotoxic activity against tumor cells, virus-infected cells, and some normal cells (Herberman, 1982). NK cells arise from bone marrow and depend on it for their proliferation and/or differentiation. During their maturation to a functionally active form, NK cells acquire the ability to bind to target cells prior to the acquisition of lytic activity. The mechanisms by which NK cells can interact and destroy tumor cells, are largely unknown. Studies have shown that NK cytotoxicity can be resolved into several stages including NK target cell binding, triggering, programming, and killer cell independent lysis. All these stages can be influenced by some humoral factors produced by various lymphoid cells.

LYMPHOKINE-MEDIATED REGULATION OF NK CELLS

The cytotoxicity of NK cells can be strongly augmented by lympho-kines. Interferon (IFN), IFN-inducing agents and Interleukin-2 (IL-2) are the main agents that have been correlated with a stimulating action on NK cells (Djeu et al., 1979; Henney et al., 1981). Interferon affects NK cell activity in several different ways including differentiation of NK precursors, proliferation of mature NK cells and enhancement of NK cyto-toxic activity. IL-2, a lymphokine first described because of its ability to induce proliferation of activated T cells, has been subsequently shown to modulate the functional activity of other cytotoxic lymphocyte popula-tion such as NK cells (Henney et al., 1981). There are at least two mechanisms of IL-2 action: the first one is a direct stimulation of NK cells, the second one is the induction of the synthesis of gamma-IFN from T cells or large granular lymphocytes (LGL) which in turn stimulates NK activity. This assumption is supported by the fact that the simultaneous administration of IFN and IL-2 led to a synergistic effect on NK cytotoxi city (Henney et al., 1981). The basal NK activity in mice is usually low at birth, increases reaching a peak in the 5-8th week of life and finally declines to very low levels during the old age (Muzzioli et al., 1986). With regard to the age-related pattern of IFN or IL-2 stimulation, it has been pointed out that "in vitro" administration of IL-2 causes a relevant increment of NK activity in spleen cells from baby, young-middle aged and old mice, while IFN boosts NK activity only in young-middle aged mice. The additive effect of the combination of IFN plus IL-2 on spleen cells from young-middle aged mice is also present in spleen cells from baby but not in those from old mice (Muzzioli et al., 1986; Muzzioli et al. in preparation). This suggest that IL-2 is able, at least partially, to recover the IFN-insensitivity of spleen cells from baby but not old mice.

NEUROENDOCRINE-MEDIATED REGULATION OF NK CELLS

Much of recent evidence clearly indicates that hormones as well as neuropeptides are able to modulate the expression of NK cell function determining either enhancement or inhibition of NK activity (Table 1) (Fabris, 1986). From a functional point of view, neurohormonal factors such as endorphins, enkephalins and thyroid hormones, may increase whereas others including glucocorticoids, oestrogens and prolactin, depress the NK activity (Table 1). With regard to the mechanisms of action of hormones and neuropeptides, a crucial point is represented by the activation of the cyclic nucleotide messengers (cAMP and cGMP). A second mechanism of action of hormones and neuropeptides on NK activity may involve the activation or inhibition of the synthesis and/or release of those lymphokines which, in turn, modulate NK activity.

THYROXINE-MEDIATED REGULATION OF NK CELLS

Several studies have pointed out that thyroid hormones modulate different immunological functions. The influence of thyroxine is exerted during the whole life-span since thyroxine administration influences the ontogenetic development and maturation of lymphoid cells and reverses many age-related immunological disturbances occuring in old mice.

With regard to the NK cell activity, injection of thyroxine in young-middle aged mice provokes an enhancement of NK spleen cell activity (Sharma et al., 1982).

Experiments performed in our lab. have shown that "in vitro" administration of thyroxine does not directly determine an increase in NK cytotoxicity, but it acts on the NK cell sensitivity to the boosting effect of IFN. Incubation of spleen cells with thyroxine and IFN provokes a very high increase of NK activity when compared with IFN alone. No effect of thyroxine is exerted on the boosting action of IL-2 (Provinciali et al., 1986). This observation suggests that thyroxine exerts his action on specific functional stage of NK cells.

The effect of thyroid hormones on IFN-sensitivity is exerted during the whole life-span of mice. The "in vitro" administration of thyroxine can restore the IFN sensitivity of spleen cells from both baby and old mice (Provinciali et al., in preparation). The reactivation of spleen cell sensitivity to IFN by incubation with thyroid hormone clearly demonstrates that the IFN insensitivity of spleen cells from baby and old

TABLE 1. EFFECT OF NEUROHORMONAL FACTORS ON NK ACTIVITY

Endorphins	↑	Thyroxine	↑
Enkephalins	↑	Glucocorticoids	↓
VIP	↑↓	Oestrogens	↓
GH	↑	Catecholamine	↑↓
PRL	↓		
LH	↓		

↑ : enhancement; ↓ : inhibition; ↑↓ : enhancement or inhibition depending on experimental design.

mice does not rely on the absence of potentially IFN-sensitive cells, but it is the expression of a functional and reversible alteration of "baby" and "old" cells.

ACKNOWLEDGEMENTS

This work was supported by the National Research Council (Rome, Italy), Special Project Preventive Medicine and Rehabilitation, Grant n. 84.02306.56.

REFERENCES

Djeu, J.V., Heinbough, J.A., Holden, H.T., and Herberman, R.B., 1979. Augmentation of mouse natural killer cell activity by interferon and interferon inducers, J. Immunol., 122:175.

Fabris, N., 1986. Hormones and Natural Immunity, in: "Natural Immunity", Academic Press, Australia, in press.

Henney, C.S., Kuribayashi, K.K., Kern, D.E., and Gillis, S., 1981. Interleukin-2 augments natural killer cell activity, Nature, 291:335.

Herberman, R.B., 1982. Immunoregulation and Natural Killer cells, Mol. Immunol., 19(10):1313.

Muzzioli, M., Provinciali, M., and Fabris, N., 1986. Age-dependent modification of Natural Killer activity in mice, in: "New Trends in Aging Research", M. Nijhoff Publ, Copenhagen.

Muzzioli, M., Provinciali, M., and Fabris, N.. Age-dependent modification of basal and lymphokine-induced NK activity, in preparation.

Provinciali, M., Muzzioli, M., and Fabris, N., 1986. Thyroxine-dependent modulation of Natural Killer activity, in: "Immunoactive products in oncology and persistent viral infections", G. Pizza, ed., in press.

Provinciali, M., Muzzioli, M., and Fabris, N. Thyroxine-dependent modulation of NK activity during development and aging, in preparation.

Sharma, S.D., Tsai, V., and Proffitt, M.R., 1982. Enhancement of mouse Natural Killer cell activity by thyroxine, Cell. Immunol., 73:83.

511

RESULTS OF THYROSTATIC DRUG TREATMENT IN HYPERTHYROIDISM

A CLINICAL LONG-TERM STUDY

Wieland Meng, Sabine Meng, Rainer Hampel,
Manfred Ventz, Ewald Männchen, and Bernd Streckenbach[x]

Klinik für Innere Medizin and Radiologische Klinik[x]
University of Greifswald, Greifswald, GDR

INTRODUCTION

In a prospective study we examined:
- The efficiency of therapy with methimazole (n = 400).
- The influence of the duration of the drug treatment on the results (n = 400).
- The value of the thyroid suppression test (n = 344) and the TRH test (n = 152) at the end of drug treatment concerning the detection of remission and the prognosis.
- The relapse rates depending on the type of hyperthyroidism (n = 265).
- The value of the thyroid suppression test and TRH test depending on the type of hyperthyroidism (n = 100).

MATERIAL AND METHODS

Patients: n = 400, Graves' disease 70 %, disseminated autonomy 30 %, goitre class 0 - 2. Drugs: Methimazole, with or without T4-supplementation. Treatment duration: 1 - 5 years. Suppression test: 80 - 100 µg T3/day, 10 days, during methimazole therapy at the end of treatment period, ^{131}I: 24-h-uptake, positive: <35 %, ^{99m}Tc: 20-min-uptake, positive: <10 %. TRH-Test: 200 µg TRH (Berlin Chemie) i.v., 6 weeks after withdrawal of drug treatment, positive ΔTSH >2.0 mU/l. Follow-up: 2 - 10 years(1).

Table 1. Influence of treatment duration on recurrence rates

Treatment duration	Patients n	Relapses (%)		
		Follow-up 1 year	2 years	2-10 years
1 year	151	27.8	32.5	43.1
2 years	163	26.4	30.7	46.0
≥3 years	86	26.7	32.6	47.7

513

Table 2. Regulation tests and relapse rates (%)

Methods	n	Relapses		Test pos.	neg.
Suppression test	344	total		32.5 %	64.5 %
		early		31.3 %	71.9 %
TRH test	152	total		36.7 %	85.1 %
		early		21.4 %	75.0 %

RESULTS AND CONCLUSIONS

We observed a relapse rate of 27.0 % after 1 year, 31.8 % after 2 years and a total relapse rate of 45.3 %. Up to now the treatment results are unsatisfying.

The results of a different treatment duration indicated that relapse rates after 1 and 2 years of follow-up were 26.4 - 27.8 % and 30.7 - 32.6 %, respectively. When patients were followed for 2 - 10 years relapse rates were 43.1 - 47.7 % (Table 1). The time of treatment of more than 1 - 2 years did not decrease the occurence of relapses.

Table 3. Relapse rates dependent on the type of hyperthyroidism

Type	Patients n	Relapses (%)		
		Follow-up 1 year	2 years	5 years
Graves' disease	165	26.7	37.6	54.6
Dissem. autonomy	100	17.0	23.0	37.0

Table 4. Regulation tests and relapse rates (%) in Graves' disease (n = 42) and disseminated autonomy (n = 58)

Test — Relapses	Graves' disease Test pos.	neg.	Dissem. autonomy Test pos.	neg.
Suppression test				
Total relapses	21.4	78.6	25.0	63.6
Early relapses	16.7	63.6	11.1	92.9
TRH test				
Total relapses	16.0	71.4	27.7	70.6
Early relapses	25.0	70.0	20.0	83.3

This fact underlines the importance of methods which are helpful for the detection of remission. For that with good results we used the suppression test as well as the TRH test (Table 2). A disturbed regulation is indicative of a persistence of the disease or an early relapse. In cases with normal regulation the relapse rate is lower and the relapses which occure are mainly late relapses.

The relapse rates after 1 / 2 and 5 years of follow-up were distinctly higher in Graves' disease than in cases with disseminated autonomy (Table 3)(2).

The suppression test and TRH test give the same indications concerning the outcome in cases with Graves' disease and disseminated autonomy (Table 4).

REFERENCES

1. Meng W., Meng S., Hampel R. et al. (1986), In Schilddrüse 1985, George Thieme Verlag, Stuttgart

2. Schicha H. and Emrich D. (1983), Deut. Med. Wochenscr. 108: 6.

PREDICTIVE USE OF TSH-RECEPTOR ANTIBODIES ASSAY AS A PROGNOSTIC INDEX IN GRAVES' PATIENTS TREATED WITH ANTITHYROID DRUGS OR RADIOACTIVE-IODINE

Roberto Concetti, Enrico Macchia, Lucia Gasperini, Giovanni Carone, Flavia Borgoni, Gianfranco Fenzi, and Aldo Pinchera

Cattedra di Endocrinologia e Medicina Costituzionale, Università di Pisa; Pisa, Italy

INTRODUCTION

Thyrotropin receptor antibodies (TRAb) have been implicated in the pathogenesis of Graves' disease and have been found in the majority of patients with active Graves' disease (1). Earlier studies suggested that the disappearance of these antibodies during the course of treatment with antithyroid drugs (ATD) was an index of remission of the underlying autoimmune process (2, 3). More recent reports (4), however, have not confirmed the significance of TRAb measurement as a prognostic index. Methodological differences for the measurement of these antibodies could play an important role, because, on the whole, there is no correlation between the antibody's activity estimated by radioreceptor assay and that tested by a cAMP assay (5, 6). Moreover, it has been postulated that the presence of TSH-binding inhibiting antibodies (TBIAb) in the sera of Graves' patients undergoing radioactive-iodine therapy might be responsible for increasing the therapeutic efficacy of radioactive-iodine (^{131}I), perhaps by directing the ^{131}I towards particularly responsive thyroid cells (7).

In this study we evaluated the usefulness of TSH receptor antibodies, measured either as TSH-binding inhibiting activity or thyroid stimulating activity, as a prognostic index in Graves' disease patients, who were submitted to medical or ^{131}I therapy.

MATERIALS AND METHODS

Patients: we studied 103 patients with hyperthyroid Graves' disease of whom 40 were submitted to long term therapy with ATD (18 months) and 63 were treated with a dose of ^{131}I, calculated on the basis of the estimated weight of the gland and the 24th hour ^{131}I uptake. In all patients TBIAb and thyroid stimulating antibodies (TSAb) were measured before treatment. TSH-receptor antibodies were also measured at the end of treatment in the 40 patients treated with ATD.

Preparation of IgG: IgG fraction was prepared by a modification (8) of the Baumstark method: protein concentration was determined by the Lowry method (9). In the adenylate cyclase stimulation assay the IgG were used at a final concentration of 1 mg/ml.

Preparation of human thyroid plasma membranes for adenylate cyclase assay: thyroid tissue from patients with non-toxic goiter was obtained at surgery and immediately processed at 4°C. Human thyroid homogenate was centrifuged at 300xg; the 30,000xg pellet of the supernatant was resuspended in an isotonic medium and stored in liquid nitrogen until used.

Adenylate cyclase activity assay: the crude thyroid plasma membrane preparation (60 µg/tube) was incubated with normal or Graves' immunoglobulins. The incubation took place at

34°C in 50 mM TRIS HCl buffer, pH 7.9, 0.1 % BSA, with 1 mM ATP, 4 mM Mg^{++}, a phosphodiesterase inhibitor and an ATP regenerating system, and was stopped after 60 min. by the addition of a cold methanol/ethanol mixture. A 50 µl aliquot of the supernatant was dried and its cAMP content was measured by a specific radioimmunoassay.

TSH binding inhibition assay: TSH binding inhibiting antibodies were measured by a radioreceptor assay. Briefly, solubilized porcine thyroid plasma membranes were incubated with normal serum or patient serum and ^{125}I-TSH. Afer centrifugation the precipitate was counted. The inhibitory effect of patients' sera was expressed as TBIAb index: (1- cpm sample/cpm normal serum) x 100. Values exceeding 2 SD from the mean value obtained with normal patients' sera were considered positive.

RESULTS

Before treatment, 80% of the 40 patients treated with ATD were TBIAb positive and 67.5% were TSAb positive; 23 were still in remission one year after drug withdrawal; 17 relapsed. At the end of the medical therapy, none of the patients in remission were positive for TBIAb, while 52.9% of the relapsed patients were found to be positive. TSAb was positive in 21.7% of patients in remission and in 41.1% of those relapsed. The χ^2 analysis of the results showed that, at the end of therapy, TBIAb was significantly more frequent in the relapsed patients than in those still in remission; whereas, TSAb assay had no clear statistical prognostic usefulness. Ten months after ^{131}I therapy, 28.1% of the TBIAb positive patients compared with 19.3% of the TBIAb negative, and 23.7% of the TSAb positive compared with 24% of the TSAb negative, remained hyperthyroid. 28.1% of the TBIAb positive patients compared with 29.0% of the TBIAb negative, and 34.2% of the TSAb positive compared with 20.0% of the TSAb negative, were hypothyroid ten months after ^{131}I therapy; the remaining patients were euthyroid.

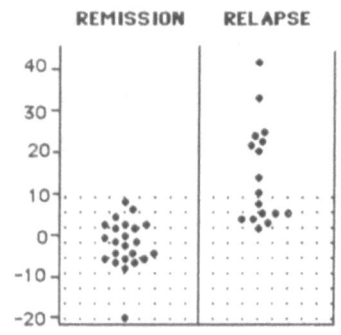

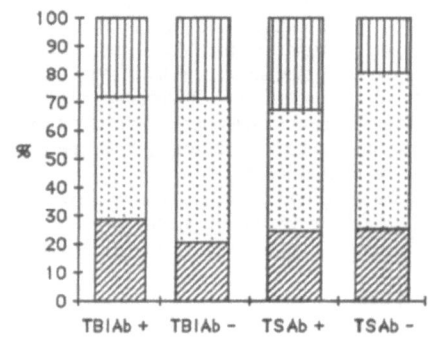

Fig. 1. TBIAb value at the end of therapy with ATD in patients in remission and in those relapsed.

Fig. 2. Thyroid status 10 months after ^{131}I therapy in Graves' patients in relation to the presence or the absence of TRAb: the areas in each column represent hypo-, eu- and hyperthyroid status from top to bottom, respectively.

DISCUSSION

Our results, obtained from a group of 103 patients with hyperthyroid Graves' disease treated with ATD or ^{131}I, highlight the potential prognostic significance of TBIAb and TSAb in this disease. A positive result for the TBIAb assay at the end of ATD treatment preceded, in all cases,

(9/9) a relapse. On the other hand, negative values did not exclude the possibility of a relapse (8/31 TBIAb negative patients relapsed). As far as TSAb was concerned, this assay did not provide a useful tool for predicting post-treatment outcome and only high post-therapy TSAb levels can be considered to precede a relapse. These data confirm previous reports showing that TBIAb assay could be used as a prognostic index for relapse in Graves' patients treated with ATD (10, 11). On the other hand, only high end-treatment TSAb levels may be useful markers of relapse (4). Moreover our data indicate, once again, the lack of correlation between TBIAb and TSAb (5, 6).

Davies et al. (7) measured TBIAb in a series of hyperthyroid Graves' patients prior to the administration of a fixed dose of ^{131}I and concluded that TBIAb could be a predictor of the therapeutic response to ^{131}I. Based on our data, we cannot confirm this observation in fact no significant difference in the subsequent clinical course was found between the patients positive, and those negative, for TBIAb or TSAb. The discrepancy between Davies' results and ours could be due to a difference in the method used to calculate the ^{131}I therapeutic dose. However, our research shows that TRAb do not seem to be relevant in order to predict the therapeutic response to ^{131}I.

REFERENCES

1-A. P. Weetman, A. M. Mc Gregor: Autoimmune thyroid disease: development in our understanding. Endocrine Reviews 5: 309 (1984).

2-A. M. Mc Gregor, B. Rees-Smith, R. Hall, M. M. Petersen, M. Miller, P. J. Dewer: Prediction of relapse in hyprthyroid Graves' disease. Lancet 1: 1101(1980).

3-H. Schleusener, P. Kotulla, R. Finke, H. Sörje, H. Meinhold, F. Adlkofer, K. W. Wenzel: Relationship between thyroid status and Graves' disease-specific immunoglobulins. J. Clin. Endocrinol. Metab. 47: 379 (1978).

4-A. M. Madec, M. C. Laurent, Y. Lorcy, A. M. Le Guerrier, A. Rostagnat-Stefanutti, J. Orgiazzi, H. Allannic: Thyroid stimulating antibodies: an aid to the strategy of treatment of Graves' disease? Clin. Endocrinol. (Oxf.) 21: 247 (1984).

5-E. Macchia, G. F. Fenzi, F. Monzani, F. Lippi, P. Vitti, L. Grasso, L. Bartalena, L. Baschieri, A. Pinchera: Comparison between thyroid stimulating and TSH-binding inhibiting immunoglobulins of Graves' disease. Clin. Endocrinol. (Oxf.) 15: 175 (1981).

6-A. Sugenoya, A. Kidd, V. V. Row, R. Volpé: Correlation between thyrotropin-displacing activity and human thyroid-stimulating activity by immunoglobulins from patients with Graves' disease and other thyroid disorders. J. Clin. Endocrinol. Metab. 48: 398 (1979).

7-T. F. Davies, M. Platzer, N. R. Farid: Prediction of therapeutic response to radioactive iodine in Graves' disease using TSH-receptor antibodies and HLA-status. Clin. Endocrinol. (Oxf.) 16: 183 (1982).

8-G. F. Fenzi, E. Macchia, L. Bartalena, F. Mazzanti, L. Baschieri, L. J. De Groot: Radio-receptor assay of TSH: its use to detect thyroid-stimulating immunoglobulis. J. Endocrinol. Invest. 1: 17 (1978).

9-O. H. Lowry, N. J. Rosenbrough, A. L. Farr, N. J. Randall: Protein measurement with the Folin phenol reagent. Journal of Biological Chemistry. 193: 265 (1951).

10-T. F. Davies, P. P. B. Yeo, D. C. Evered, F. Clark, B. R. Smith, R. Hall: Value of thyroid stimulating antibody determinations in predicting short-term thyrotoxic relapse in Graves' disease. Lancet 1: 1181 (1977).

11-C. S. Teng, R. T. T. Yeung: Changes in thyroid-stimulating anibody activity in Graves' disease treated with antithyroid drug and its relationship relapse: A prospective study. J. Clin. Endocrinol. Metab. 50: 144 (1980).

AFFINITY PURIFICATION OF ORBITAL ANTIGENS USING HUMAN

MONOCLONAL ANTIBODIES IN GRAVES' OPHTHALMOPATHY

M. Salvi and J.R. Wall

McGill University, Montreal General Hospital

Montréal, Québec, Canada

INTRODUCTION

Several authors [1,2,3,4] have reported antibodies against various soluble and membrane eye muscle antigens using different techniques. Although these antibodies may be useful as clinical markers for the disease, only those antibodies directed against eye muscle cell surface or membrane antigens are likely to be pathogenetic. There is good evidence that eye muscle cell surface directed antibodies are cytotoxic, in antibody-dependent cell mediated cytotoxicity[5]. Unfortunately, ELISA assay for the detection of antibodies against crude membrane antigens in the serum of patients with Graves' ophthalmopathy (GO) has proved to be unsuitable[6]. The production of monoclonal antibodies (MCAB) reactive against orbital components and their use to affinity purify membrane autoantigens appear a logical approach for the study of humoral immune mechanisms in GO.

METHODS

Monoclonal Antibodies Production

MCAB were produced by fusion of peripheral blood lymphocytes from 13 GO patients with a human myeloma cell line (GM4572B N1GMS, Camden, NJ) using the method of Köhler and Milstein[7] and previous Epstein-Barr virus infection in order to non-specifically enhance antibody-producing B cells. Twenty out of 312 hybrids were cloned. Twentytwo of the clones showed a high reactivity in ELISA against orbital antigens and have been characterized and used in this study.

Monoclonal Antibodies Characterization

Reactivity. Indirect ELISA has been used to test the various tissue reactivities of the MCAB. Antigens were coated on a 96-well plate and residual sites blocked with 3% BSA. Supernatants from clones were applied and incubated overnight at 4°C. Alkaline phosphatase labelled anti-human IgG+IgM+ IgA was then added and, after a 2 h incubation at 37°C, p-nitrophenol was used as substrate. Tests were read as optical density (OD) at 410 nM.

Ig class determination. "Sandwich" ELISA: fab$\frac{1}{2}$ specific anti-human IgG+

IgM+IgA was coated on the plastic and blocking of sites carried out as before. MCAB were then applied and, after overnight incubation, alkaline phosphatase conjugated goat anti-human IgM or IgG were added. Substrate was p-nitrophenol and reading was performed as before.

Antigen Preparation

Cytosol (soluble), membrane and solubilized membrane fractions of fresh normal human eye muscle (HEM), orbital connective tissue (OCT), thyroid (THY), skeletal muscle (SM) and liver (LIV) were prepared as described previously[6].

Affinity Chromatography

Columns were prepared by binding MCAB-Ig (prepared by DEAE-Sephacell chromatography) to sepharose CNBr and loading with crude antigen fractions. MCAB were chosen according to their reactivity with soluble and CHAPSO or 2% SDS solubilized HEM, OCT and THY membranes. All eluted fractions were tested for reactivity with the same MCAB. Peak fractions were pooled; their protein content was determined and subsequently they were used as antigens in ELISA tests with patients sera.

RESULTS

MCAB reactivity. Reactivities of the 22 MCAB against different crude preparations of orbital and non-orbital antigens are summarized in Table 1.

Ig class determination. All MCAB were tested for their IgG and IgM class. Results are shown in Table 2. Six out of 22 clones proved to be IgM secreting, 3 IgG secreting and 10 showed a positive reaction in both the IgM and IgG assays. Finally, 3 clones seemed not to be secreting either IgM or IgG.

Affinity purification of antigens. We obtained 7 purified antigens from HEM cytosol, 1 from OCT and 2 from THY cytosol, all of which were proteins. Subsequently, we applied solubilized HEM and OCT crude membranes. We obtained

Table 1. Reactivity*of human MCAB against orbital and extra-orbital tissues.

CLONE NO.	EM Cyt	EM Mem	EM Chapso	OCT Cyt	OCT Mem	OCT Chapso	LAC Mem	LAC Chapso	THY Cyt	THY Mem	Tg	SM Mem	SM Chapso	LIV Cyt
39C10B4	+		+											
39C10B5	+		+										+	
39C10B10	+	+	+	+					+			+	+	
39C10B11	+								+			+	+	
39C10F9		+		+	+	+						+		
39C10G4	+						+		+			+		
39G11B8	+		+						+					
39G11B9	+		+						+	+		+	+	
39G11G5	+		+						+			+		
39H6G7		+	+	+	+	+			+				+	
39H11E4		+			+							+	+	
39H11E11		+			+		+							
39H11F10					+									
39H11G5	+				+									
40E2B10		+			+	+		+	+	+				+
40E2B11		+			+	+				+	+	+	+	
40E2C2	+	+		+	+									
40E2C8		+		+	+		+							
40E2D3	+	+	+		+	+				+				
40E2G5		+			+	+								
39H11F10A9		+		+	+	+	+		+	+			+	
39H11F10D11		+		+	+						+			

*Determined using ELISA. (+) indicates a positive test. Negative reactions are not indicated.

Table 2. IgG class of
human MCAB[*]

Monoclonal Ab.	IgG	IgM
39C10B4	−	+
39C10B5	+	+
39C10B10	+	+
39C10B11	−	+
39C10F9	+	+
39C10G4	+	+
39C11B8	+	+
39C11B9	+	+
39G11G5	+	+
39H6G7	+	+
39H11E4	+	−
39H11E11	−	−
39H11F10	−	−
39H11G5	+	−
40E2B10	+	+
40E2B11	+	+
40E2C2	−	+
40E2C8	−	+
40E2D3	−	+
40E2G5	−	+
39H11F10A9	+	−
39H11F10D11	−	−

[*]Measured using
ELISA

Table 3. Characteristics of affinity purified orbital antigens.

ANTIGEN	CRUDE ANTIGEN	PROTEIN CONC (μg/ml)	ELISA ACTIVITY (vs MCAB)
E1-2	HEM Cytosol	30	−
E2-2	OCT "	15	+
E3-1	HEM "	9.5	+
E3-2	HEM "	6.7	+
E3-3A	HEM "	100	−
E3-3B	HEM "	18	−
E4-1	HEM "	4	−
E4-2	HEM "	27	−
E6-1	THY "	7.3	−
E6-2	THY "	22	−
E7-1	HEM CHAPSO-Sol.mem.	2.1	+
E7-2	HEM "	3.2	+
E7-3	HEM "	11.8	−
E8-1	HEM "	3.2	−
E8-2A	HEM "	12.0	n.t.
E8-2B	HEM "	11.0	n.t.
2E7-1	HEM "	−⊛	+
2E7-2	HEM "	6.0	+
2E7-3	HEM "	8.0	+
E5-1	OCT "	−⊛	+
2E9-2	HEM "	n.t.	+
2E9-3	HEM "	n.t.	−
2E9-4	HEM "	n.t.	−
E5-2	OCT "	n.t.	−
E10-1	OCT "	−⊛	+
E10-2	OCT "	9.3	−
E11-1	HEM SDS-Sol.mem.	4.0	−
E11-2	HEM "	4.8	−
E11-3	HEM "	10.3	−
E12-1	HEM "	−⊛	+
E12-2	HEM "	6.5	+

⊛= no detectable protein (non-protein antigen). n.t.= not tested.

523

17 purified antigens from HEM and 4 from OCT. Two OCT and 2 HEM pure antigens were not protein. Concentrations and ELISA reactivity of purified antigens are summarized in Table 3.

DISCUSSION

We have produced and characterized 22 human MCAB from blood lymphocytes of GO patients. The multiple reactivity of such MCAB suggests that cross-reactive antibodies may be one mechanism for the association of organ-specific autoimmune disorder[4].Our preliminary experiments show that purified antigens may be either protein or non-profit and are highly reactive in ELISA with the MCAB used for their preparation and with pooled patients sera, as well. The possibility that, in some cases, putative autoantigens involved in the immune reactions in GO may be other than proteins was already reported[1]. In conclusion, we believe that the use of MCAB-affinity purified antigens is an appropriate approach for the study of the humoral mechanisms associated with GO,since it should allow us to identify relevant autoantigenic targets.

REFERENCES

1. K.Kodama, H.Sikorska, P.Bandy-Dafoe, R.Bayly & J.R.Wall, Lancet ii:1953 (1982).
2. P.Kendall-Taylor, S.Atkinson & M.Holcombe, Brit Med J 288:1183 (1984).
3. M.Faryna, T.Nauman & A.Gardas, Brit Med J 290:191 (1985).
4. M.Mengistu, E.A.Laryea, A.Miller & J.R.Wall, Clin Exp Immunol 65:19 (1986).
5. P.W.Wang, Y.Hiromatsu, E.A.Laryea, J.How & J.R.Wall, J Clin Endocrinol Metab 63:316 (1986)
6. A.Miller, H.Sikorska, M.Salvi & J.R.Wall, Acta Endocrinologica: in press.
7. G.Köhler & C.Milstein, Nature 256:495 (1975).

THE EXOPHTHALMOS-RELATED EYE MUSCLE ANTIGENS ARE NOT RELATED TO THYROID ANTIGENS: LACK OF BINDING INHIBITION USING THYROID MICROSOMES AND THYREOGLOBULIN

Roy Moncayo, Ullrich Bemetz, and Ernst Friedrich Pfeiffer

Department of Internal Medicine, University of Ulm, 7900 Ulm, West Germany

INTRODUCTION

Endocrine exophthalmos with eye muscle involvement is most frequently seen in patients with Graves' hyperthyroidism (1) but also in cases of Hashimoto thyroiditis (2) and even in euthyroid patients. Autoantibodies directed either against thyroid microsomes or thyreoglobulin or both can been found in patients with Graves' disease and Hashimoto thyroiditis The concurrent detection of such autoantibodies in these groups of patients would imply that thyroid antigens could be related in the pathogenesis of eye muscle involvement. In the last years we have succesfully established an Enzyme Linked Immunosorbent Assay (ELISA) for the detection of autoantibodies directed against a soluble eye muscle antigen (3). In this study we have investigated whether a preincubation step with thyroid antigen preparations can lead to a decreased binding of eye muscle specific autoantibodies in our routine ELISA method.

MATERIALS AND METHODS

Thyroid antigen preparations: human thyroids were courteously provided by the Department of Sugery of the University of Ulm. The tissue was subjected to homogenization and centrifugation in order to obtain both the fraction containing thyroid microsomes and that corresponding to thyreoglobulin. Commercially available porcine thyreoglobulin (Sigma) was also used as an inhibitor.

Eye muscle preparations: eye muscle was homogenized in 20mM Tris HCl buffer using a mechanical device (Ultra Turrax). After centrifuging at 500 x g and 50000 x g the final supernant obtained after centrifuging at 80000 x g was used as the soluble antigen. Protein concentration was measured using the Bradford method (4). The ELISA test was done as previously described (3).

Patients: fifteen patients with endocrine ophthalmopathy and three normal controls were investigated. The sera of the patients with exophthalmos had been previously found to be positive in the routine assay for eye muscle antibodies.

Inhibition studies: the sera were pre-incubated with 0, 1, 10 and 100 ug/ml of each inhibitor. For this, microtiter plates (Dynatech M129B) were coated with the corresponding substance: thyroid microsomes, human thyreoglobulin fraction, porcine thyreoglobulin and the soluble eye muscle antigen. Incubation was carried out at room temperature for 1 hour. The pre-absorbed sera were then transferred to the plates with the eye muscle antigen and tested again. Binding of the autoantibodies to eye muscle in the absence of inhibitors was taken as 100%.

RESULTS

Only eye muscle antigen was effective as an inhibitor in this set-up. A 50% inhibition was achieved with an antigen concentration ranging from 8 to 16 ug/ml. Human thyroid microsomes and human thyreoglobulin as well as porcine thyreoglobulin were not effective in inhibiting the binding of eye muscle autoantibodies even at a concentration of 100ug/ml.

DISCUSSION

Although endocrine exphthalmos and thyroid autoimmune disease can coexist in many patients, eye muscle antigens and thyroid antigens do not appear to be related since there was a lack of inhibition when thyroid microsomes and thyreoglobulin were used in pre-absorption assays. Different autoantigens, specific for each organ, seem to be involved.

ACKNOWLEDGEMENTS

This work was supported by the DFG, Project 38/2-1, 1986.

REFERENCES

1. J.M. McKenzie and M. Zakarija, Hyperthyroidism, in: "Endocrinology," DeGroot L.J., Cahill G.F., Potts J.T., Nelson D.H., Steinberger E. and Winegrad A.I., editors, Grune and Stratton, New York (1979).

2. R. Hall and D.C. Evered, Autoimmune Thyroid Disease: Thyroiditis, in: "Endocrinology," DeGroot L.J., Cahill G.F., Potts J.T., Nelson D.H., Steinberger E. and Winegrad A.I., editors, Grune and Stratton, New York (1979).

3. R. Moncayo, W. Scherbaum, U. Bemetz, U. Loos, and F. Seif, ELISA systems for the detection of eye muscle and TSH antibodies in Graves' disease with ophthalmopathy, Acta Endocrinologica 108:85 (1985).

4. M.M. Bradford, A rapid and sensitive method for the quantitation of microgram quantities of protein using the principle of protein dye binding, Anal Biochem 72:248 (1976).

HUMORAL IMMUNITY IN GRAVES OPHTHALMOPATHY

Grazyna Adler, Martha Faryna, Aleksandra Lewartowska
Janusz Nauman, Andrzej Gardas, and Hanna Domek

Department of Biochemistry
Medical Center of Postgraduate Education
Marymoncka 99, Warsaw, Poland

There is a growing evidence that several autoantibodies might be generated in Graves ophthalmopathy (1 - 7) and result in diversiform clinical picture and course of the disease.

To further elucidated this complex humoral immunity we attempted to estimate and to correlate the presence of anti eye muscle plasma membrane autoantibodies /AEMA/, autoantibodies against eye muscle microsomal antigens /AMM/ of both IgG and IgM classes and autoantibodies against thyroid plasma membrane antigens /ATMA/in sera of Graves ohpthalmopathy patients.

MATERIAL AND METHODS

Serum samples were obtained from either untreated or previously treated 58 patients with class II to class VI Graves ophthalmopathy according to ATA classification.

The presence of AEMA was estimated with use of human eye muscle antigen and Protein A-^{125}I as previously described[3] and results expressed as AEMA index. Values of the index above 1.55 were a proof for presence of this type of autoantibodies. AMM were estimated by ELISA[6] with use of pig eye muscle antigen and anti human IgG or anti human IgM antibodies. Optical density index above 1.17 and above 1.29 were proofs for presence of either AMM-IgG or AMM IgM.ATMA were determined by ELISA[8] and results expressed as immunoglobulin titer.

Linear correlation between AEMA,both AMM-IgG,AMM-IgM and ATMA were evaluated at p=0.05 by means of Neptun 2000 computer.

RESULTS

Autoantibodies reacting with eye muscle plasma membrane and microsomal antigens were present in sera of 24 Graves ophthalmopathy patients /41%/ 6 patients have AEMA and AMM of both IgG and IgM classes, 5 patients have AEMA and AMM of IgG class while in 13 cases AEMA and AMM of IgM class were present.Autoantibodies reacting only with plasma membrane antigens were found in 7 patients and autoantibodies selectively reacting with eye muscle microsomal antigens were present in sera of 8 patients.In 19 patients,representing mainly these previously treated, none of autoantibodies investigated were present.

Table 1. The presence of AMM of IgG class,AMM
         of IgM class and AEMA in Graves
         opthalmopathy patients

autoantibody	number of patients	
	present	absent
AMM-IgG,AMM-IgM,AEMA	6	19
AMM-IgG,AEMA	5	4
AMM-IgM,AEMA	13	3
AEMA	7	1

Statistical analysis of the results shown no correlation between AEMA
and AMM of IgG class. Contrary to that, weak but significant correlation
was found between values of AEMA index and values of AMM of IgM class index
/r=0.41 p=0,05/. None of anti eye muscle autoantibodies correlated with
anti thyroid plasma membrane autoantibodies.

DISCUSSION

The present study shown that serum of some patients with Graves ophthalmopathy contain autoantibodies against different component of eye muscle
cells.These findings confirm data presented by others[1]. As our patients
were randomly selected importance of the presence of particular antibody,
two or even all autoantibodies examined for development, clinical picture
and course of the disease can not be at present established. Although we
attempted to correlate presence and titre of different antibodies,results
obtained should be carefully evaluated.It has to be taken into account
that human muscle were used to obtain plasma membrane antigens while porcine
eye muscle served as source of microsomal antigens.In addition the quantity
of antigens used to estimate AEMA and AMM was different.However, we found
rather a high accordance of the presence of anti membrane and anti microsomal
antibodies in patients sera.As in previous study there was no correlation
between ATMA titer and titer of any antibodies directed against eye muscle
cells components.This however, is not a proof that Graves ophthalmopathy
represents a distinct autoimmune disease.

REFERENCES

1.J.R.Wall,Humoral mechanisms in relationship to Graves ophthalmopathy in
  "Autoimmunity and the thyroid"P.Walfish,R.Volpe,J.Wall eds Academic Press
  /1985/.
2.P.Kendal-Taylor,S.Atkinson,M.Holcombe,A specific IgG in Graves ophthalmopathy and its relation to retro-orbital and thyroid autoimmunity,Br.Med.
  J.288:1183 /1984/.
3.M.Faryna,J.Nauman,A.Gardas,Estimation of autoantibodies against human eye
  muscle plasma membranes in Graves ophthalmopathy,Br.Med.J.290:191 /1985/.
4.G.Kahaly,R.Moncayo,U.Bemetz,U.Krause,J.Schresermeir,J.Beyer,E.F.Pfeiffer,
  Spontaneous and therapy induced course of eye muscle antibodies in endocrine ophthalmopathy /EO/in "The thyroid and autoimmunity,H.A.Drexhage,
  W.M.Wiersinga eds,Excerpta Medica,Amsterdam /1986/.
5.T.Kuroki,J.Ruf,L.Whelan,A.Miller,J.R.Wall,Antithyroglobulin monoclonal and
  autoantibodies cross-react with an orbital connective tissue membrane
  antigen:a possible mechanism for the association of ophthalmopathy with
  autoimmune thyroid disorders,Clin.exp.Immunol.62:361 /1985/.
6.G.Adler,A.Lewartowska,A.Gardas,J.Nauman,Autoantibodies of IgM and IgG class
  against eye muscle antigens in patients with Graves ophthalmopathy,this
  volume.

7. U.Feldt-Rasmussen, A.Kemp,K.Bech,S.N.Madsen,J.Date,Serum thyroglobulin, its autoantibody and thyroid stimulating antibodies in the endocrine exophthalmos, Acta Endocrinol.96:192 /1981/.
8. A.Gardas,K.L.Rives,Enzyme linked immunosorbent assay of autoantibodies reacting with thyroid plasma membrane antigens in sera of patients with autoimmune thyroid disease,Acta Endocrinol. 113:255 /1986/.

AUTOANTIBODIES OF IgM AND IgG CLASS AGAINST EYE MUSCLE

ANTIGENS IN PATIENTS WITH GRAVES OPHTHALMOPATHY

Grazyna Adler, Martha Faryna, Aleksandra Lewartowska
Janusz Nauman, Andrzej Gardas, and Hanna Domek

Department of Biochemistry
Medical Center of Postgraduate Education
Marymoncka 99, Warsaw, Poland

The presence of autoantibodies /aab/ reacting with microsomal membrane[1] or plasma membrane /AEMA/[2] eye muscle antigens have been recently reported in Graves ophthalmophathy /GO/.The significance of humoral mediated immunity in GO was further supported by studies in which correlation between presence and development of ophthalmopathy and titer of anti membrane autoantibodies were established[3,4]

The aim of present work was to modify the method of estimation of anti eye muscle antibodies in attempt to increase its sensitivity and to improve its reproductibility. We also have tried to find whether these aab but of IgM class are not more significant than those of IgG class for development and clinical course of GO.

MATERIAL AND METHODS

Serum samples were obtained from 76 untreated or previously treated patients with GO /class II to VI according to ATA/serum samples from 106 healthy individuals matching similar age range served as controls.

Pig eye muscle plasma membranes and microsomes were separated by two steps centrifugations and microsomal membrane proteins were solubilised by 0,2% CHAPSO and sonication. Skeletal muscle and liver microsomes were obtained by the same methods.

ELISA test was performed on polistyrene microtitre plates coated with 6.6 ug/ml of solubilised antigen. Free sites were saturated by 10% pig serum in phosphosaline and the 1 hour reaction at 37° with tested serum at 1:20 to 1:80 dilution were studied.Antibodies of G and M class bound to microsomes were detected with peroxidase conjugated anti human IgG or IgM antibodies /Amersham and Cappel USA/. Optical density /OD/ at 492 mu were read after reaction with o-phenylenediamine. Results are expressed as:

$$OD\ index = \frac{OD\ of\ tested\ serum}{OD\ of\ pool\ normal\ serum}$$

In the above conditions the OD in absence of any serum was up to 10% of value obtained at the presence of normal serum, however the nonspecific absorption of serum was high and only 50% of patients immunoglobulines were displaced by excess of antigen in suspension

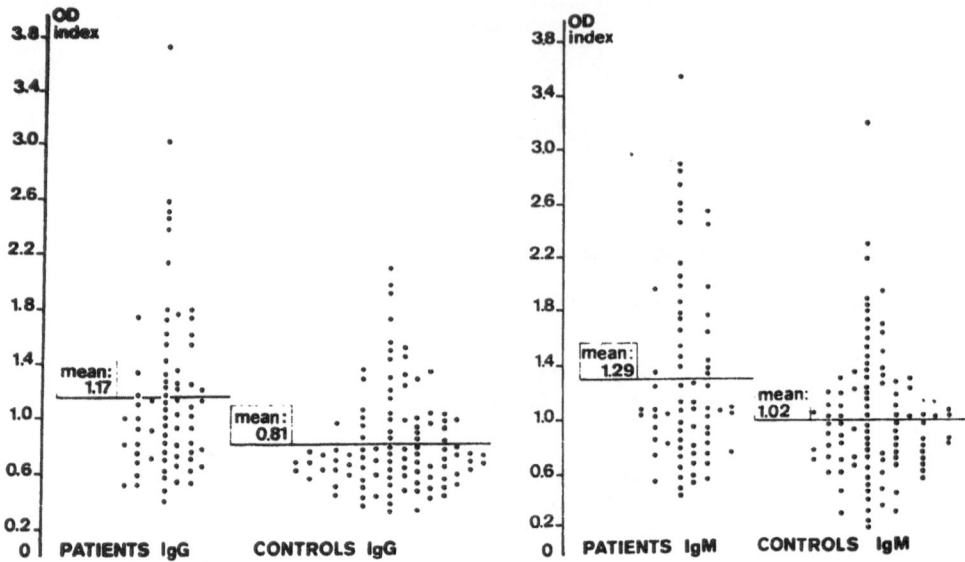

Fig.1. The distribution of autoantibodies against eye
muscle microsomes of IgG and IgM class in sera
of GO patients and in control sera.

RESULTS

The mean OD index in patients with Go was 1.17 $\pm$ 0.63 for IgG class and
1.29 $\pm$ 0.64 for IgM class versus 0.81 $\pm$ 0.35 for IgG and 1.02 $\pm$ 0.49 for
IgM in controls /figure 1/.Both IgG and IgM mean values in GO were
significantly higher then those in controls /p < 0.01/. Values above 1.17
and 1.29 respectively were considered as positive.

Aab reacting with eye muscle microsomal antigens were present in 59%
of GO patients.Among them 17% had both aab 22% only of IgM and 20% only of
IgG class.Falsely positive results for both IgG and/or IgM were seen in
30% of controls.

In randomly selected samples of serum from GO patients and controls
reaction of aab with microsomal antigens from skeletal muscle and liver
were also investigated and presence of respective anti IgG or anti IgM
aab confirmed in some cases /Table 1/.

DISCUSSION

The present results clearly show that aab of both IgG and IgM class are
present in patients with GO. In randomly selected treated and untreated
adult patients both classes of aab appeared with same frequency.Therefore
IgM aab can not be representative for juvenile patients as previously
suggested.[5]
Although ELISA might be expected to be more specific than previously
estimated AEMA, the frequency of falsely positive results found in controls
remain relatively high. The presence of aab reacting with antigens from
skeletal muscle and from liver both in patients in healthy controls
suggest that either similarity of some antigens or crossreactivity of aab
with different antigens remain an obstacle in the investigation of humoral
mediated immunity of Graves ophthalmopathy

Table 1. The presence of anti pig eye muscle /MO/
sceletal muscle /MS/ and liver /L/ microsomal antibodies in representative sera.
Results expressed as OD index.

serum	IgG reaction with:			IgM reaction with:		
	MO	MS	L	MO	MS	L
pool GO	1.6	1.6	1.6	2.1	2.5	2.4
patient no 65	2.2	1.0	0.9	1.4	1.1	0.6
patient no 75	1.2	1.1	0.5	0.5	1.1	0.7
patient no 86	0.6	0.3	0.4	3.1	1.9	1.1
control no 76	1.5	0.9	0.8	1.7	2.5	2.1
control no 80	0.7	1.0	0.8	0.7	0.9	1.0

REFERENCES

1. P.Kendall-Taylor,S.Atkinson,M.Holcome,A specific IgG in Graves
ophthalmopatha and its relation to retro-orbital and thyroid
autoimmunity, Br.Med.J.288:1183 /1984/.
2. M.Faryna,J,Nauman,A.Gardas, Estimation of autoantibodies against human
eye muscle plasma membranes in Graves ophthalmopathy,Br.Med.J.290:191/1985/
3. J.Nauman,M,Faryna,A,Gardas, Humoral immunity in Graves ophthalmopathy in
"The thyroid and Autoimmunity" H.A.Drexhage,W.M.Wiersinga,ed. Excerpta
Medica, Amsterdam /1986/.
4. S.Atkinson,M.Holcome,P.Kendall-Taylor, Ophthalmopathic immunoglobulin
in patients with Graves ophthalmopathy, Lancet ii:374 /1984/.
5. U.Bemetz,R.Moncayo,W.Scherbaum,H.Frisch,K.Badenhoop,G.Hool,H.Schleussener,
E.F. Pfeiffer, Detection of IgG and IgM antibodies directed against eye
and peripheral muscle preparations in juvenile and adult patients with
Graves disease and in patients with hyperhyroidism : "The thyroid and
autoimmunity",H.A.Drexhage W.M.Wiersinga,ed.,Excerpta Medica,Amsterdam
/1986/.

ENDOCRINE EXOPHTHALMOS - NATURAL HISTORY AND RESULTS OF TREATMENT

Ekkehard Schifferdecker, and Karl Schöffling

Department of Endocrinology, Center of Internal
Medicine, University Hospital
Frankfurt am Main, Fed.Rep. of Germany

The appearance of endocrine ophthalmopathy (e.o.) is pathognomonic for Graves' disease, but its outbreak is unpredictable, not correlated with the course and treatment of thyrotoxicosis, and often causing major therapeutic problems. Therefore, history of e.o. and therapeutic efforts in 191 patients suffering from Graves' disease and seen in our outpatient ward were analysed retrospectively.

ASPECTS OF ANALYSIS

1. Manifestation of eye changes in relation to the course of thyrotoxicosis. The beginning of treatment of the first manifestation of thyrotoxicosis was chosen as point of reference.
2. Severity of e.o. according to the classification of the American Thyroid Association (II - soft tissue involvement, III - proptosis, IV - extraocular muscle involvement, usually with diplopia, V - corneal involvement, VI - sight loss (optic nerve involvement)). The highest grade reached by the individual patient was determined.
3. Therapeutic interventions and their efficacy. Only a clearcut improvement was registrated, because retrospective verification of minor changes is difficult (different physicians involved, no standardized documentation). In grade III e.o. a documented persistent improvement of subjective complaints, in grade IV an improvement or disappearance of diplopia were recorded.

RESULTS

1. Table 1 shows the frequency of manifestation of e.o. in different phases of Graves' disease. More than half of the ophthalmopathies appear together with or even before the first manifestation of thyrotoxicosis. Another 25% of e.o. appear during the first six months after starting therapy. Only in 12% of patients the ophthalmopathy followed first manifestation more than two years later.

537

2. Data concerning the severity of e.o. are shown in table 2.
38% of patients reached grade III, 48,1% grade IV and only
1,6% grade V and VI.
3. The results of therapy are also documented in Table 2.
Summarizing the data, an improvement was seen with steroids
alone in 48%, with the combination of steroids and radiation
in 42%, with radiation alone in 17%. Of 94 untreated patients, 17% improved spontaneously.

Table 1. Beginning of symptoms of endocrine ophthalmopathy in
relation to the course of thyrotoxicosis

Beginning of symptoms in relation to initiation of first antithyroid treatment	n	%
< 6 months after initiation	42	24,3
< 12 months after initiation	15	8,7
< 24 months after initiation	7	4,1
> 24 months after initiation	21	12,1
together with initiation	80	46,2
before initiation	8	4,6
total	173	100,0

Table 2. Maximum grade of e.o. reached by 191 patients with
Graves' disease and influence of therapy on clinical pictures

Therapy	Effects	II	II-III	III	III-IV	IV	V	VI	total
no	no change	9	12	44	1	12	-	-	78
therapy	improvement	-	1	7	2	6	-	-	16
steroids,	no change	1	-	10	1	10	-	-	22
1 course	improvement	-	1	4	6	10	-	-	21
steroids,	no change	-	-	1	1	3	-	-	5
>1 course	improvement	-	-	1	-	3	-	-	4
steroids+	no change	-	-	3	1	15	-	-	19
radiation	improvement	-	-	1	1	12	-	-	14
radiation	no change	-	-	-	-	5	-	-	5
alone	improvement	-	-	-	-	1	-	-	1
others		-	-	1	-	2	1	2	6
total		10	14	72	13	79	1	2	191

DISCUSSION

Our data concerning the temporal relation between thyrotoxicosis and ophthalmopathy are in good accordance with the few
reports on this matter in literature (1,6).
Our own experience with severity and course of e.o. confirms
the statement of Gorman (5), that only 2 to 3% of patients
develop severe e.o. (grade V or VI). The impression that e.o.
is a self-limiting disease and burns out in most cases even
without therapy after 3 to 36 months (3) is in agreement with
our data, too. But unfortunately, proptosis and diplopia

often persist in these burned-out cases, in 24% of our patients a grade IV e.o. could not be improved by therapy.
Clinical reports on dramatic improvement of extremely severe
e.o. under steroid therapy are found in the literature (11),
succesfull steroid treatment in 15 patients was performed by
Garber (4), but a critical report on only short-lived beneficial effects appeared early, followed by others (2,7,8).
Experience with more potent immunosuppressive agents like
azathioprine, cyclophosphamide or chlorambucil is negative at
last. Recently, promising results with cyclosporine A were
reported (10), but further studies are necessary to evaluate
this drug.
The bad results of retrobulbar radiation in our patients (improvement in 38% only) may be due to a negative selection,
for radiation was chiefly performed after unsuccesful steroid
therapies. In studies of ophthalmological or radiological
groups better results were achieved with improvement in up to
96% of patients (for ref. see (9)). Only two reports with improvement rates of 44 and 40%, respectively, are comparable
with our observations (for ref. see (9)).
From the reported results it must be concluded that established therapies for e.o. are unsatisfactory and that more
effective therapeutic means with less side effects are
urgently needed, especially under the aspect of earlier
intervention.

LITERATURE

1. Bartels,E.C., M.Irie: in:"Advances in thyroid research",R.
   Pitt-Rivers, ed., Pergamon Press, New York 1961
2. Brain,R.: Cortisone in exophthalmos, Lancet 1:6 (1955)
3. Day,R.M.: Hyperthyroidism: clinical manifestations of eye
   changes, in: "The thyroid: a fundamental and clinical
   text", S.C.Werner, S.H.Ingbar, ed., Harper and Row, New
   York 1978
4. Garber,M.I.: Methylprednisolone in the treatment of exophthalmos, Lancet 1:958 (1966)
5. Gorman,C.A.: The presentation and management of endocrine
   ophthalmopathy, Clin.Endocr.Metab. 7:67 (1978)
6. Gorman,C.A.: Temporal relationship between onset of Graves' ophthalmopathy and diagnosis of thyrotoxicosis,
   Mayo Clin. Proc. 58:515 (1983)
7. Koch,H.-H.: Ergebnisse in der Therapie der endokrinen Ophthalmopathie in den Jahren 1978-1981, in:"Schilddrüse
   1981",P.C.Scriba,K.-H.Rudorff,B.Weinheimer, eds., Thieme
   Stuttgart - New York 1982
8. Schatz,H., S.F.Grebe, U.Schröder, C.Eisenhardt, H.Müller,
   G.-L.Fängewisch: Therapieergebnisse bei 161 Patienten
   mit endokriner Orbitopathie, in:"Schilddrüse 1981",
   P.C.Scriba,K.-H.Rudorff, B.Weinheimer, eds.,Thieme
   Stuttgart - New York 1982
9. Uhlenbrock,D.,H.J.Fischer,R.Rohwerder: Strahlentherapie
   der endokrinen Ophthalmopathie - Auswertung von 56 Fäl-
   len, Strahlentherapie 160:485 (1984)
10.Utech,C., K.G.Wulle, E.U.Bieler, P.Pfannenstiel, N.Panitz,
   H.Kiefer: Treatment of severe Graves' ophthalmopathy
   with cyclosporin A. Acta endocr. 110:493 (1985)
11.Werner,S.C.: Prednisone in emergency treatment of malignant exophthalmos, Lancet 1:1004 (1966)

IMMUNOSUPPRESSIVE TREATMENT OF GRAVES' OPHTHALMOPATHY WITH
OPHTHALMOPATHY WITH CYCLOSPORIN A AND CIAMEXON

Christa Utech, Michael Cordes
Peter Pfannenstiel, and Klaus G. Wulle

Deutsche Klinik für Diagnostik
Fachbereich Nuklearmedizin
6200 Wiesbaden, F.R.G.

INTRODUCTION

Presently Graves' ophthalmopathy is considered to
be an organ specific autoimmune disorder as shown by
Wang et al. (1) and Volpe (2). Since 1983 patients with
severe progressive Graves' disease stage IV to VI
according to the classification by Werner (3) receive
an immunosuppressive treatment with Cyclosporin A (CyA)
in a low dosage alone or in combination with corticosteroids on a short term basis as shown by Wheetman at al.
(4) and Utech et al. (5). We are also examining the efficiency of Ciamexon - a new immunomodulating drug - with
no known side effects.

PATIENTS AND METHODS

23 patients with severe Graves' ophthalmopathy
stage IV to VI who did not respond to corticosteroids
alone and other forms of treatment have been treated
with CyA and corticosteroids over a 6 month period.
Initially a dosage of 4 to 5 mg/kg b.w. was given and
later reduced according to the drug level monitored in
blood 15 to 16 hours after last intake. Corticosteroids
were given in a dosage of 60 mg and reduced weekly by
5 mg.

20 patients with stage III to IV were treated with
Ciamexon in a dosage of 300 mg daily, given as tablets.

Routine laboratory program was performed monthly
and ophthalmological status every 3 months evaluating
vision with subjective and objective refraction, bulbar
motility (Hess chart), measurement of proptosis (Hertel)
and interlid space, tonographic registration of intraocular pressure in straight and upgaze as shown by Draeger
(6) and Wulle et al. (7) visual field test (stat. and
kinet.), slit lamp and ophthalmoscopy.

RESULTS

11 out of 23 patients with Graves' ophthalmopathy
stage IV to VI treated with CyA and corticosteroids over
6 months showed an improvement in all ophthalmological
parameters, 7 remained unchanged and 5 worsened. In 2
patients decompressive surgery was necessary. In 3 patients squint surgery could be done after stabilization
of the status. After 6 months 11 patients were changed
over from CyA to Ciamexon.

Among the 20 patients with Graves' ophthalmopathy
stage III to IV treated with Ciamexon 7 patients improved and 7 patients remained unchanged. In 6 patients
the ophthalmological findings worsened, so that treatment was changed to CyA and corticosteroids in 3 patients,
the other 3 patients received corticosteroids in addition
to Ciamexon over a short term. In severe stages IV to
VI no response was seen with Ciamexon treatment.

SUMMARY

In severe Graves' ophthalmopathy stage IV to VI
combined treatment with CyA plus corticosteroids is more
effective compared to Ciamexon alone. Mostly all the
patients who received Ciamexon after termination of CyA
treatment showed a stabilization of the status over 6
months treatment. After this period a worsening effect
was observed in some patients. A combination with low
dosage of corticosteroids seems to be more effective
in these cases.

Patients with Graves' ophthalmopathy stage III to
IV previously treated ineffectively only with corticosteroids showed an improvement under Ciamexon treatment.
In more severe cases with mainly muscle involvement the
addition of a low dosage of corticosteroids shows better
results.

CONCLUSION

Patients with Graves' ophthalmopathy stage IV to
VI receive CyA plus corticosteroids, changing to Ciamexon
plus a low dosage of corticosteroids after several months.
Our experiences show that the ophthalmological status
then remains stable for 4 to 6 months after changing.
Longterm examinations will show if there is a possibility
to economize CyA with Ciamexon.

In less severe stages III to IV Ciamexon plus a
low dosage corticosteroids are initially administered.

REFERENCES

1. P.W. Wang, Y. Hiromatsu, E. Laryea, L. Wosu, J. How
    and J.R. Wall, J. Clin. Endocrinol. Metab. 63, 316-322
    (1986).
2. R. Volpé, Marcell Dekker, Inc., New York (1985).
3. S.C. Werner, J. Clin. Endocrinol. Metab. 29, 282-284
    (1969).

4. A.P. Weetmann, M. Ludgate, P.V. Mills, A.M. McGregor, L. Beck and J.H. Lazarus, Lancet 2, 486-489 (1983).
5. C. Utech, K.G. Wulle, E.U. Bieler, P. Pfannenstiel, N. Panitz and H. Kiefer, Acta Endocrin. 110, 493-498 (1985).
6. J. Draeger, "Pseudoglaukom" bei endokrinem Exophthalmus, Ber. dtsch. ophthal. Ges. 63: 148-165 (1961).
7. K.G. Wulle, C. Utech, H.L. Christl, Blickrichtungs-tonometrie oder -tonographie bei endokriner Ophthalmo-pathie, Klin. Mbl. Augenheilk., in press.

TREATMENT OF GRAVES' OPHTHALMOPATHY BY RETROBULBAR CORTICOSTEROIDS ASSOCIATED WITH ORBITAL COBALT RADIOTHERAPY

Claudio Marcocci, Luigi Bartalena, Massimo Panicucci, Giuliano Cavallacci*, Claudio Marconcini*, Antonio Lepri*, Michele Laddaga**, Francesco Cartei**, and Aldo Pinchera

Cattedra di Endocrinologia e Medicina Costituzionale *Clinica Oculistica, and **Cattedra di Radioterapia Università di Pisa,Viale del Tirreno 64, 56018 Tirrenia (Pisa), Italy

INTRODUCTION

Combined therapy with systemic corticosteroids and orbital cobalt radiotherapy (RT) has proven an effective method for treatment of severe Graves' ophthalmopathy (1). The use of large doses of systemic corticosteroids is potentially risky. In more than 100 patients treated so far at our Institution with systemic corticosteroids either alone or in combination with radiotherapy, relevant side effects have been observed in 4 cases: one patient had an increase of intraocular tension, one showed depressive psychosis, one developed diabetic syndrome requiring insulin, and one had infective encephalitis within the first month of treatment (2). This prompted us to assess the therapeutic effectiveness of retrobulbar long-acting corticosteroids (RBC) in substitution for systemic corticosteroids in the combined therapy in a group of 44 consecutive patients with active Graves' ophthalmopathy.

MATERIALS AND METHODS

Patients. Forty-four patients (27 F, 17 M, aged 36-78 yr, mean 54 yr) were submitted to RT associated with RBC. The duration of ocular symptoms averaged 29 months, and the follow-up period after the last retrobulbar injection ranged from 12 to 42 months.

Ophthalmopathy Index (OI). The degree of ocular involvement was assessed by the OI (1, 3). Results of treatment at the end of the follow-up period were evaluated both clinically (excellent, good, slight, no response)(1, 3), and by variations of the OI.

Therapeutic protocol. RT, performed as previously detailed (1), was started together with RBC. The latter consisted of 14 bilateral injections of 40 mg methylprednisolone acetate, at 20-30 day intervals.

RESULTS

Before treatment, soft tissue involvement was present in all patients; proptosis in 31 (70%), with a mean Hertel reading of 21.8 mm in the most prominent eye; involvement of extraocular muscles was evident in 42 (95%), with fixation of eye globe in 10 cases; corneal lesions or optic neuropathy were detected in 16 (36%) and 9 (20%), respectively. The ophthalmopathy index ranged from 4 to 10, with a mean value of 5.9 ± 1.8 (± SD).

Table 1. Effects of combined treatment with RT and RBC in 44 patients with active Graves' ophthalmopathy.

| | Before therapy | After therapy | | |
	Abnormality	Regression	Improvement	No change	Worsening
Soft tissue	44	11	24	9	-
Proptosis(≥20 mm)[a]	31	7	5	19	-
Eye muscle	42	7	6	27	2
Corneal lesions	16	8	-	8	-
Optic neuropathy	9	8	1	-	-

[a]Regression indicates a ≥ 2 mm reduction of proptosis and a final reading of < 20 mm; improvement indicates a ≥ 2 mm reduction and a final reading of ≥ 20 mm; no change indicates a < 2 mm reduction.

The effects of treatment on each class of eye changes are reported in Table 1. At the end of the follow-up period, regression or partial improvement was observed in most cases (80%) with soft tissue changes, and in all cases with sight loss due to optic neuropathy. Regression or improvement of proptosis occurred in 12 patients (39%), with a mean final exophthalmometer reading of 20.1 mm, and a decrease of >3 mm in 4 cases. The majority of patients (64%) with extraocular muscle involvement had no beneficial effect from treatment and worsening was observed in 2 cases (5%); only 7 patients (17%) regained normal eye globe motility. Corneal lesions disappeared in 50% of cases, and were not affected by treatment in the remaining 50%. The initial effects of treatment became in general apparent after 2-3 months.

Excellent or good responses were observed in 11 patients (25%), while the majority of patients (n=24, 55%) showed a slight, albeit statistically significant, response to therapy. Ocular conditions did not improve in the remaining 9 patients (20%). The mean final OI was 3.2, with a net change of -2.7.

No side effects of RT and RBC were observed, with the exception of few cases of subconjunctival hemorrhages with no sequelae. No patient had an increase of intraocular tension. Additional therapy was carried out in 7 patients: 3 were given high doses of systemic corticosteroids for persistence or recurrence of ocular symptoms, 4 were submitted to extraocular muscle surgery for persistent distressing diplopia.

DISCUSSION

The results of the present study indicate that combined therapy with RT + RBC was effective on congestive symptoms and optic neuropathy, while proptosis was only partially influenced. Substantially negative results were obtained on ocular motility. This latter finding is in disagreement with the results obtained by Thomas and Hart (4), who using locally injected corticosteroids alone reported satisfactory results in the majority of cases of eye muscle involvement. It is, however, worth noting that about 2/3 of our patients showed a severe restriction of eye movements, with a complete fixation of the globe in 10 cases. Other authors have also been less enthusiastic about the effects of locally administered corticosteroids on extraocular muscle dysfunction (5, see also 6 for review). The different selection of patients may be responsible for these discrepancies. In agreement with previous reports (4, 5), the administration of RBC appeared to be a safe procedure, devoid of any local or systemic major side effects.

In conclusion, on the basis of the present study the association of RT with RBC may be used with advantage in the treatment of severe Graves' ophthalmopathy, but appears to be less effective than the association of RT with systemic corticosteroids (1). This has been recently confirmed in a controlled trial carried out in our Istitution (7). Thus, RBC should be limited to patients with contraindications to the systemic administration of steroids.

REFERENCES

1. L. Bartalena, C. Marcocci, L. Chiovato, M. Laddaga, G. Lepri, D. Andreani, G. Cavallacci, L. Baschieri, and A. Pinchera, Orbital cobalt irradiation combined with systemic corticosteroids for Graves' ophthalmopathy: comparison with systemic corticosteroids alone, J. Clin. Endocrinol. Metab. 56:1139 (1983).
2. A. Pinchera, L. Bartalena, L. Chiovato, and C. Marcocci, Radiotherapy of Graves' ophthalmopathy, in: "The Eye and Orbit in Thyroid Disease", C.A. Gorman, R.R. Waller, and J.A. Dyer, eds., Raves Press, New York, p. 301, (1984).
3. S.S. Donaldson, M.A. Bagshaw, and J.P. Kriss, Supervoltage orbital radiotherapy for Graves' ophthalmopathy, J. Clin. Endocrinol. Metab. 37:276 (1973).
4. I.D. Thomas and J.K.Hart, Retrobulbar repository corticosteroid therapy in thyropid ophthalmopathy, Med. J. Austl. 2:484 (1974).
5. M.I. Garber, Methylprednisolone in the treatment of exophthalmos, Lancet 1:958 (1966).
6. D.H. Jacobson and C.A. Gorman, Endocrine ophthalmopathy: current ideas concerning etiology, pathogenesis and treatment. Endocr. Rev. 5:200 (1984)
7. C. Marcocci, L. Bartalena, M. Panicucci, C. Marconcini, F. Cartei, G. Cavallacci, M. Laddaga, G. Campobasso, L. Baschieri, and A. Pinchera, Orbital cobalt irradiation combined with retrobulbar or systemic corticosteroids for Graves' ophthalmopathy: a comparative study, Clin. Endocrinol.(Oxf) in press

IMMUNOLOGICAL FEATURES OF SIMPLE ENDEMIC GOITRE

A.Costa, C.Ricci[o], V.Benedetto[*], Paola Borelli[o], Emanuela
Fadda[o], Nicoletta Ravarino[**], B. Torchio[**], D. Urbano[**],
P. Fragapane[*], and G. Varvello[*]

[*] 2nd General Surgery Division, Mauriziano Hospital
[**]Pathology Institute, Mauriziano Hospital
[o] Department Clinical Immunology of the University
Turin, Italy

The aim of this research was to study immune aspects of
endemic goiter and throw light on the uncertain boundaries between
autoimmune and non-autoimmune thyroid diseases. For instance the
"European study group of hyperthyroidism" register as "unclassified"
31.3% of the hyperthyroid patients examined[1]. Adult goiter patients from
Piedmont's endemic areas (group E.G.) and "thyroid 0" persons for
control (group C, matched for sex and age) were examined. For the number
of the persons and for methods involved in each research, refer to the
original papers[2,3] . Piedmont's endemic goiter, like that prevalent in
mountain areas, is mostly nodular and poor in iodine (mean value in our
series, I mcg/g 186 ± 200). Toxic multinodular goiters and autonomous
toxic adenomas are the prevailing causes of hyperthyroidism. The
following urine estimates were obtained in adults: I mcg/l 60 ± 14,
thiocyanates mg/l 1.30 ± 0.6, fluorine mcg/l 17.9. A comparison of Ig
G,A,M,C3,C4,k and λ chains in the peripheral blood proved only a IgM
median lower (-21%) in the E.G. group. The incidence of thyroid autoAbs
(T.R.C.) ranged in group E.G. from 7 to 24% with titres up to 1/5120 for
Tg Abs, 1/25.000 for Mi Abs. Higher frequencies and higher titres were
measured in large longstanding goiters. The highest values occurred in
recurrent goiters (43.6%) and in toxic goiters (36.8%). High values of
Mi Abs($\geq$1/6400) were prevalent only in toxic goiters. In toxic adenomas
however, high titres of thyroid Abs were no more frequent than in the C
group. In the E.G. group non thyroid autoAbs were also measured; their
frequency was: Mi Abs 6.7%, Nu Abs 16.9%, Ga Abs 8.5%, Sm Abs 20%. In
the peripheral blood EA,ET lymphocytes, OK and Leu subsets, T DR+ and
NK+ cells (Leu7+/Leu2-, Leu7+/Leu2+) were identified with commercially
available Mo Abs, and enumerated by eye. No significant differences
between the two groups were observed. Lymphocytic infiltration (L.I.)
occurred in 45% of the surgical goiter' specimens, with higher frequency
and intensity in women. There was a direct, though not linear,
correspondence between the L.I. and the incidence and the titres of
thyroid Abs. Lymphocytic germinal centres, plasmacells and oxyphylia
occurred in 8% of simple goiters, and in 30% of toxic ones. In 4 simple

goiters intrathyroidal mononuclear cells were characterized, with the epithelial cells expressing HLA-DR Ag. Using the immunoperoxidase staining method Mo Abs anti-Leu1, anti-Leu3, anti-Leu2b, anti-Leu7 and anti-HLA-DR were employed. Lymphatic follicles, with the germinal centre, and the neighbouring infiltrated areas were stained by HLA-DR Mo Ab. Around the follicles T cells were prevalent, mainly of the T helper phenotype. Leu7+ cells were scattered among the follicles and in both the lymphatic nodes and the germinal centres. HLA-DR+ epithelial cells were more frequent in toxic goiters and easily recognized in the follicles of the less infiltrated areas. In some follicles these cells were scanty, in others nearly all were of this type. Immunohistologic staining by direct and indirect I.F. on serial cryostatic sections showed Ig G,A,M in the follicles of 12 out of 59 simple goiters: in four IgG and C3 were responsible for granular deposits of immunocomplexes (I.C.) at the basal membrane. When L.I. marked by the presence of lymphatic nodules with germinal centres and oxyphylia, I.C. at the follicle basal lamina, occur in endemic goiter, together with high titres of thyroid Abs, we assume the intervention of a lymphatic thyroiditis. Some AA include such cases in Hashimoto's thyroiditis. However, in 5% of our operated endemic goiters not a clear-cut distinction could be drawn between the two forms in the light of the morphologic and immunologic data at our disposal. The above markers of humoral and cell mediated a.i. are more frequent in women, in toxic goiters and in those recurrent after surgery, and appear to proceed with the structural and functional alterations of the gland. "Local abnormality in the gland appears to play an important role in the initiation of thyroid autoimmunity" (Roitt and Doniach)[4]. Because a.i. signs usually are absent in the early stages of the disease, we may conclude that endemic goiter is not of a.i. origin. We are inclined to consider that the a.i. lymphocytic thyroiditis may occur not as a superimposed disease, but rather part of the natural history of the goitrogenic process in immunologically inclined persons. The above observations point to a possible overlapping between true a.i. thyroid disorders and other pathologic thyroid conditions in wich immunological manifestations may follow, overcoming the histological picture and the functional pattern of the primary lesion.

REFERENCES

1. D. Reinwein, G. Benker, M. Koenig, A. Pinchera, H. Schatz and H. Schleusener, Hyperthyroidism in Europe: clinical and laboratory data of a prospective multicentric survey, J.Endocrinol.Invest. 9: suppl.2 (1986).
2. A. Costa, V. De Filippis, A. Balsamo, Nicoletta Ravarino, Ornella Testori, B. Torchio, Piera Valmaggia and G. Zoppetti, Serum autoantibodies and thyroid lymphocytic infiltration in endemic goitre, Clin.Exp.Immunol.56:143 (1984).
3. A. Costa, V. Benedetto, C. Ricci, Paola Borelli, Emanuela Fadda, Nicoletta Ravarino, B. Torchio, D. Urbano, P. Fragapane, G. Varvello and V. De Filippis, Immunological features of endemic goitre, Clin.Immunol.Immunopathol. (in press).
4. I. Roitt and Deborah Doniach, Thyroid Autoimmunity, in: "The Thyroid Gland", British Medical Bulletin 16:152 (1960).

THYROID AUTOIMMUNITY IN FIVE SAMPLES OF GENERAL POPULATION IN ITALY

Giovanni B. Salabè & Helga Lotz (Roma), Alessandro Menotti (Roma), Sergio Muntoni (Cagliari), Giancarlo Descovich (Bologna), Roberto Antonini (Roma), Eduardo Farinaro (Napoli), and Gino Avellone (Palermo)

C.N.R. Special Program on Preventive Medicine "Atherosclerosis Project", Italy

In a previous study carried out in 1978 we have described the prevalence of thyroid autoimmunity and hypothyroidism in a sample of 517 subjects randomly selected from the electoral roll of a quarter of Rome.[1] Thyroid autoimmunity was found in 12.5% of the subjects and latent hypothyroidism in 2.7% (TSH > 5μU/ml, normal T3, T4).

The present article summarizes the results of a collaborative study conducted within the Targeted Programmes on Preventive and Rehabilitative Medicine of C.N.R. Subjects were randomly selected from the electoral roll of the metropolitan area of Bologna and Rome and from three independent municipalities a few km from Cagliari (Capoterra), Palermo (Casteldaria) and Naples (Afragola). Two thousand and eighteen subjects in an age range between 20 and 59 accepted to take part in the study. The enquiry on thyroid autoimmunity was carried out by distributing a questionaire and measuring serum T4, TSH and thyroid antibodies. Thyroid anti-microsomal Abs were measured by tanned red cell haemoagglutination (TRC), anti-thyroglobulin antibodies by TRC and by double antibody technique using 125-I-labelled thyroglobulin (RIA).[2]

The data obtained from the samples of continental Italy have been considered separately from those obtained from the Sardinian sample. The results summarized in Table 1 have shown that:

1) The over-all prevalence of thyroid autoimmunity in continental Italy is 15.8%. In the Sardinian population the prevalence of thyroid autoimmunity is significantly higher than in samples of continental Italy (27.9 vs 15.8%; p < 0.001).

2) In both samples (continental Italy and Sardinian), the prevalence of thyroid autoimmunity is higher in females than in males and increases with age in both sexes.

Table 1. Prevalence of thyroid autoimmunity by sex and age in four
samples of continental Italy and in one Sardinian sample.

Age	20–29	30–39	40–49	50–59	All age groups
Males					
Continental Italy	7.9 (7/88)	7.6 (11/145)	8.2 (17/207)	10.5 (19/181)	8.7 (54/621)
Sardinian sample	9.5 (6/63)	17.1 (13/76)	23.6 (18/76)	16.3 (15/92)	16.9 (52/307)
Females					
Continental Italy	18.4 (21/114)	19.1 (31/162)	16.7 (37/219)	26.5 (58/219)	20.6 (147/714)
Sardinian sample	26.5 (21/79)	33.6 (35/104)	33.7 (30/89)	50.9 (53/104)	37.0 (139/376)

Differences between continental Italy and Sardinian sample by χ^2 were highly significant ($p < 0.001$).

The prevalence of latent and overt hypothyroidism has been found respectively between 0 and 6% and 0 and 1% in the different population samples. The Sardinian population has the highest rate of latent and overt hypothyroidism. Latent and overt hypothyroidism are constantly associated with thyroid autoimmunity.

In summary the average prevalence of thyroid autoimmunity in Italy is comparable to that reported for other European countries.[3] In the Sardinian sample of population, however, a higher prevalence of thyroid autoimmunity, latent and overt hypothyroidism has been found compared with continental Italy.

In recent years geographic differences of thyroid autoimmunity have been reported by us[4] and other AA.[5,6] Several hypothesis can be proposed to explain the geographic differences: iodine intake, low calory diet, viral infections, specific haplotypes of the Major Histocompatibility Complex, breeding of the population sampled and endemic goitre. In one sample of Greece[7] population with endemic goitre, iodine prophylaxis has been able to increase the prevalence of thyroid autoimmunity suggesting a role of iodine in the production of thyroid autoantibodies. This finding however has not been confirmed in another study carried out in Brasil.[8] It is therefore likely that for the expression of thyroid autoimmunity, other environmental and/or genetic factors are essential in addition to iodine intake.

REFERENCES

1. G.B. Salabè, H. Lotz Salabè, G. Urbinati, G. Ricci, A. Fusco, M. Antonucci, A. Beretta Anguissola, A Longitudinal Study of thyroid autoimmunity and subclinical hypothyroidism in a random population of Cen-

tral Italy, in: "Autoimmunity and the Thyroid", P.G. Walfish, J.R. Wall, R. Volpe, ed., Academic Press New York (1985).

2. G.B. Salabè, H. Salabè, R. Dominici, C. Davoli, M. Andreoli, Radioimmunoassay for human antithyroglobulin Antibodies. II Determination of antigen binding capacity, J. Clin. Endocr. Metab. 39: 1125 (1974).

3. W.M.G. Tunbridge, D.C. Evered, R. Hall, D. Appleton, M. Brewis, F. Clark, J. Grimley Evans, E. Young, T. Bird, P.A. Smith, The spectrum of thyroid disease in a community: The Whickam Survey, Clin. Endocrinol. 7: 481 (1977).

4. G.B. Salabè, I. Ilardi, H. Salabè Lotz, C. Petracca, Khalif Bile, Low prevalence of thyroid antibodies in a Somalian population, J. Clin. Lab. Immunol. 9: 55 (1982).

5. I. Mittra, J. Perrin, S. Kumaoka, Thyroid and other autoantibodies in British and Japanese women: an epidemiological of study breast cancer, Brit. Med. J. 1: 257 (1976).

6. A.J. Hedlay, B. Thjodleifsson, D. Donald, J. Swanson Beck, J. Crooks, M.I. Chesters, R. Hall, Thyroid function in normal subjects in Ireland and in Northeast Scotland, Clin. Endocrinol. 7: 377 (1977).

7. M.A. Boukis, Koutras D.A., A. Souvatzoglou, A. Evangelapoulon, M. Vrontakis, S.M. Moulopoulos, THyroid hormone and immunological studies in endemic goiter. J. Clin. Endocrinol. Metab. 57: 856 (1983).

8. M. Knobel, G. Medeiros-Neto, Iodized oil treatment for endemic goiter does not induce the surge of positive serum concentrations of anti-thyroglobulin or anti-microsomal autoantibodies. J. Endocrinol. Invest 9: 321 (1986).

PREVALENCE OF HYPOTHYROIDISM AND HASHIMOTO'S THYROIDITIS IN TWO ELDERLY

POPULATIONS WITH DIFFERENT DIETARY IODINE INTAKE

E. Roti, M. Montermini, G. Robuschi, E. Gardini, D. Salvo[*],
M. Gionet[**],C. Abreau[**],B. Meyers[**], and L.E. Braverman[**]

Cattedra di Endo. dell'Univ. di Parma, Serv. di Med. Nucl.,
Ospedale S.Maria Nuova, Reggio Emilia, Italy[*]; Div. of Endo.
and Metab., Univ. of Massachusetts, Worcester, MA, USA[**]

INTRODUCTION

The prevalence of subclinical and overt primary hypothyroidism in elderly female subjects is variable among different populations, ranging between 1 and 17.5% [1,2]. The etiology of the hypothyroidism is most frequently due to autoimmune or Hashimoto's thyroiditis. Recently, Bastenie et al [3] reported that serum anti-thyroglobulin (Ab-Tg) and anti-microsomal (Ab-M) antibodies are present in a large number of elderly women, reaching approximately 23 percent over age 60 years. A positive relationship between Hashimoto's thyroiditis and iodine intake has been found by some authors[4-6] but not others[7].

In the present study we have determined the prevalence of Hashimoto's thyroiditis, subclinical and overt hypothyroidism, and positive iodine-perchlorate discharge tests among two female populations residing in areas of different iodine intake.

MATERIALS AND METHODS

63 female subjects aged 68 $\pm$ 0.9 years residing in Worcester (USA) and 241 female subjects aged 81 $\pm$ 0.5 years residing in Reggio Emilia (Italy) were studied after informed consent was obtained. Blood samples were obtained from all the subjects.

Serum TSH concentration was measured using commercially available kits. Serum TSH concentrations between 5 and 10 uU/ml and over 10 uU/ml define subclinical and overt hypothyroidism, respectively. The presence of serum Ab-Tg and Ab-M was determined by the tanned red cell technique. Serum Ab-Tg and/or Ab-M titers equal to or greater than 1:400 were considered positive.

Iodine-perchlorate discharge tests were carried out in

the 63 female subjects residing in Worcester and in twenty-seven of those residing in Reggio Emilia. A tracer dose of ^{123}I in Worcester and ^{131}I in Reggio Emilia was administered p.o. with 500 ug of stable iodine at 0 time. Three hours later, radioactive thyroid uptakes were determined and 1 gm potassium perchlorate was then given. An abnormal test was defined as a discharge of radioactive iodine of greater than 15 percent 1 hour after the administration of the potassium perchlorate. Total iodine excretion in the urine was measured by the modified method of Zak[8] and urinary creatinine was determined by autoanalyzer. The iodine:creatinine ratio (micrograms of iodine per g creatinine) was then calculated as an estimate of iodine intake[9].

Data are reported as the mean $\pm$ SE. Statistical analysis was carried out by the Student's t test and by X^2 analysis.

RESULTS

Serum TSH concentrations between 5 and 10 uU/ml occured in 14 percent of the elderly subjecys residing in Worcester and in 0.8 percent of those living in Reggio Emilia (p<0.001). The prevalance of serum TSH concentrations greater than 10 uU/ml was 6.4 percent in Worcester and 0.8 percent in Reggio Emilia (p<0.025).

The prevalence of positive serum Ab-Tg and/or Ab-M titers was 25 percent in Worcester and 0.8 percent in Reggio Emilia (p<0.001).

Urinary iodine/creatinine ratio measured in 51 subjects residing in Worcester was 259 $\pm$ 23 ug/g, a value significantly higher (p<0.01) than that observed in 88 subjects living in Reggio Emilia (84 $\pm$ 4 ug/g).

The prevalence of positive iodine-perchlorate discharge tests was 44.4 percent in Worcester and 3.7 percent in Reggio Emilia (p<0.001). A positive iodine-perchlorate discharge test was the only abnormality in 23 percent of the elderly subjects residing in Worcester.

DISCUSSION

The present study indicates that the prevalence of hypothyroidism and Hashimoto's thyroiditis is far higher in elderly women residing in Worcester than in Reggio Emilia. Furthermore, the prevalence of thyroid iodine organification defects, as measured by the iodine-perchlorate discharge test, is increased in the elderly residing in Worcester. A positive iodine-perchlorate discharge test may be the earliest manifestation of a failing thyroid. It is possible that the increased prevalence of hypothyroidism, Hashimoto's thyroiditis, and positive iodine-perchlorate discharge tests in Worcester is secondary to the marked difference in iodine intake in the 2 populations. Thus, the iodine/creatinine ratio was much higher in Worcester than in Reggio Emilia, an area of mild iodine deficiency. Others have also suggested

that an increased prevalence of Hashimoto's thyroiditis may
be due to increased iodine intake, including the occurence
of autoimmune thyroiditis following iodine supplementation[4-6]. However, more recently Gaitan et al[7] did not
find a correlation between iodine supplementation and
lymphocytic thyroiditis.

REFERENCES

1. E. Nystrom, C. Bengtsson, O. Kindquist, H. Nuppa, G.
Lindstedt, and P.A. Lundberg, Thyroid disease and high
concentration of serum thyrotropin in a population sample of
women. Acta. Med. Scand. 210:39 (1981).
2. W.M.G. Tunbridge, D. Evered, R. Hall, D. Appleton, M.
Brewis, F. Clark, J. Grimley Evans, E. Young, T. Bird, and
P.A. Smith, The spectrum of thyroid disease in a community:
The Whickham survey. Clin. Endocrinol. (Oxf) 7:481 (1977).
3. P.A. Bastenie, M. Bonnyns, and L. Vanhaelst, Natural
history of primary myxedema. Am. J. Med. 79:91 (1985).
4. W.H. Beierwaltes, Iodide and lymphocytic thyroiditis.
Bull. All India Inst. Med. Sci. 3:145 (1969).
5. H.R. Harach, D.A. Escalante, A. Onativia, J.L. Outes,
E.S. Day, and E.D. Williams, Thyroid carcinoma and
thyroiditis in an endemic goiter region before and after
iodine prophylaxis. Acta. Endocrinol. (Kbh) 108:55 (1985).
6. M.A. Boukis, D.A. Koutras, A. Souvatzoglou, A.
Evangelopoulou, M. Vrontakis, and S.D. Moulapoulos, Thyroid
hormone and immunologic studies in endemic goiter. J. Clin.
Endocrinol. Metab. 57:859 (1983).
7. E. Gaitan, R.C. Cooksey, J. Legan, J.M. Montalvo, J.A.
Pino, G.S. Gaitan, N. Guzman, J. Austidillo, R. Guzman, E.
Duque, and H. Gallo, Iodine supplementation and lyumphocytic
autoimmune thyroiditis (AT). 66th Annual Meeting of the
Endocrine Society, Baltimore, MD, 1985, p. 180 (abstract).
8. J. Benotti, and N. Benotti, Total iodine and
butanol-extractable iodine by partial automation. Clin.
Chem. 9:408 (1963).
9. H.M.M. Frey, B. Rosenlund, and J.P. Torgersen, Value of
single urine specimens in estimation of 24 hour urine iodine
excretion. Acta. Endocrinol. (Kbh) 72:287 (1973).

ACKNOWLEDGEMENTS

This work was supported in part by Grant n. 85.005.3304 from
Consiglio Nationale delle Richerche, Roma, Research Grant
AM-19819 from the NIDDK, NIH (Bethesda, MD) and the Dorothy
and Joseph Benotti Iodine Research Fund.

EVIDENCE OF THE INFLUENCE OF IODINE INTAKE ON THE PREVALENCE OF AUTOIMMUNE

FACTORS IN HYPERTHYROID PATIENTS LIVING IN AN ENDEMIC GOITRE AREA

V. De Filippis, A. Balsamo, C. Danni, L. Mongardi, P.A. Merlin,
O. Testori, R. Cerutti, and *R. Garberoglio
Division and Laboratory of Endocrinology
*Ist Division of Medicine, Mauriziano Hospital, Turin, Italy

INTRODUCTION

The influence of iodine on autoimmune thyroid disease is receiving increasing attention. Differences of the prevalence of thyroid autoimmune factors, namely thyroid autoantibodies and/or lymphocitic infiltration, related to iodine intake, in individuals and in animals have been found. The rise of the frequency of Hashimoto thyroiditis after the introduction of iodine prophilaxis and the higher incidence of this disease in areas of high iodine intake compared to iodine deficient countries point to a possible role of iodine in the induction of autoimmune thyroid disease. More recently, conflicting evidences on this problem have been obtained experimentally. Sundick et al., 1986 have demonstrated that high iodine diet in chickens induces thyroid autoantibodies and thyroiditis by increasing the immunogenicity of the Tg molecule. The in vitro experiments of Wenzel et al., 1986 showed that NaJ induces an autoantigen which together with class II antigen stimulates a functional immune response. On the contrary, the recent study of Persson et al. 1986 has demonstrated that HLA-DR expression of the human thyroid can be induced by reducing the iodinating capacity of the gland. We are unaware of studies investigating the role of iodine intake on the prevalence of TSH receptor antibodies. Indirect evidence may be derived by the different frequency of non immune and autoimmune thyroid autonomy associated with deficient or excessive iodine intake respectively (Mc Gregor et al. 1985). The aim of the present work is to investigate in hyperthyroid patients of an iodine deficient area (Piedmont, Italy) on: a) the frequency of thyroid morpho-functional patterns and their association with autoimmune parameters; b) the relationship between urinary iodine excretion/g of creatinine (U.I./g Cr) and the prevalence of thyroid autoantibodies, namely Ab-Tg, MiAb, anti-THS receptor (TRAb). Preliminary data on the fall of TRAb in hyperthyroid patients with different U.I. during a course of methimazole are reported.

MATERIAL AND METHODS

The present work deals with 102 hyperthyroids, in and out-patients of the Mauriziano Hospital, Turin, Italy (age: 49.5 ± 15.4; M/F:1/9). In all patients physical examination (P.E.) and the following laboratory tests were performed: thyroid scintigraphy (SC), ultrasonography (US) Total T_3 and T_4 (Amersham), FT_3, FT_4 (Lepetit), TSH-Irma (Serono), Ab-TG, MiAb (Fuji), TSH-receptor antibody -TRAb- (Bik Goulden). In 87 of 102 patients urinary iodine and creatinine were measured. All patients were hyperthyroid by clinical and laboratory findings; they were examined at the onset of the disease, before treatment was started. On the basis of the results of P.E., SC and US 5 distinct morpho-functional patterns of the thyroid were defined: 14 non enlarged thyroids (NT): thyroid of normal size, diffuse radionuclide uptake and diffuse hypoechogenicity; 36 diffuse goitre (DG): enlarged thyroid, SC and US as in NT; 9 uninodular goitre (UN): thyroid of different size, single, hot nodule at the scan, US characterized by hypoechogenic nodule, sometimes with hemorrhages, fibrosis, calcifications in it; 32 multinodular goitre (MNG): many nodules (P.E.), warm areas interspersed with low uptake areas or nodules (SC), nodules of different size and echogenicity (US). Finally in 11 patients with enlarged thyroid, with or without palpable nodules, the US showed a pattern of low echogenicity with some highly echogenic, variably sized nodules; the scintiscan was not uniform: disomogeneous uptake in thyroids without palpable nodules, scintiscan similar to that of GMN in nodular thyroids. Especially on the basis of US findings we are inclined to consider these thyroids as a separate group, «disomogeneous» (DIS). Work is in progress to better define such thyroids. Autoimmune parameters were measured in all patients with different thyroid morphology and the results are summarized in Table 1. As can be seen, the prevalence of TRAb+, MiAb+, Exophtalmous (Eo) is significantly higher in hyperthyroids with DG, NT, DIS than in those with UN and GMN. The 87 patients in whom urinary iodine was measured were divided according to U.I. in 2 groups: <100 μg/g Cr and > 100 μg/g Cr. The prevalence of autoantibodies was determined in the 2 groups. The results (Table 2) reveal an higher frequency of TRAb+ and of the association TRAb+-MiAb+ in patients with ioduria >100 μg/g Cr. These findings

Table 1. Autoimmune parameters in hyperthyroid patients with different thyroid morphology

	n°	TRAb+(%)	Eo+(%)	MiAb+(%)	TRAb+MiAb+(n°)
DG	36	58	36	58	11
DIS	11	54.5	33	54.5	4
NT	14	57	37.5	43	4
MNG	32	9.4	3	25	2
UN	9	11	–	–	–

$p < 0.001$ p=0.007 $p<0.01$ p=0.015
significancy (DG+DIS+NT) v/s (MNG+UN)

Table 2. Prevalence of autoimmune parameters in hyperthyroid patients with different U.I.

	n°	TRAb+		Eo+		MiAb+TRAb+	
DG	32	1	16	4	9	1	10
DIS	10	–	5	2	–	–	4
NT	14	3	5	2	2	1	3
MNG	26	–	3	–	1	–	2
UN	6	–	1	–	–	–	1

$p = 0.025$ ns $p<0.05$
significancy n° / n°
n° = U.I. <100μg/gCr   n° = U.I. >100μg/gCr

560

Table 3. Rate of disappearance of TRAb in hyperthyroid patients with different
U.I. during Methimazole treatment

U.I. (μg/g Cr)	< 200	> 200	
3rd month	5/11	0/9	p = 0.0198
6th month	4/8	1/8	NS

are more evident in DG, NI, DIS patients. In 2 patients with Amiodarone induced
hyperthyroidism (1 NT, 1 GMN), both TRAb+ with normal eyes at the onset of the
thyrotoxicosis, class 4 ophtalmopathy appeared during the course of the disease
which responded favorably to steroid therapy. We have also examined the rate of
disappearance of TRAb and MiAb in patients with different U.I. during treatment
with Methimazole. The titre of the auto Ab was measured at the onset of the therapy
and at 3 months intervals during treatment. The number of patients in whom TRAb
became undetectable at 3rd and 6th month of treatment in shown in Table 3.

DISCUSSION AND CONCLUSIONS

In our hyperthyroid patients we have tried to correlate the morpho-functional
aspects of the thyroid with the signs of thyroid autoimmunity. By the use of P.E.,
SC and US 5 morpho-functional thyroidal patterns have been defined. Patients with
uninodular or multinodular toxic goitre had significantly lower prevalence of
thyroid autoantibodies and of exophtalmous than patients with other thyroid morphology (DG, NT, DIS). The latter have been classified as having «immunogenic
hyperthyroidism». Hyperthyroids with U.I. > 100 μg/g Cr had significantly higher
prevalence of thyroid autoantibodies than patients with U.I. < 100 μg/g Cr. This
association is particularly evident in patients with immunogenic hyperthyroidism. On the basis of these results we suggest that in patients susceptible to thyroid autoimmune disease high iodine intake facilitates the immune
response. If this suggestion is true, the appearance of the ophtalmopathy in 2
patients with Amiodarone induced hyperthyroidism, both TRAb+, during the course
of the disease is in keeping with the concept of a role of iodine in immune modulation. Furthermore our preliminary results suggest that the iodine intake seems
to influence the fate of the TRAb during antithyroid therapy. It has been
demonstrated that high iodine consumption may be responsible of the resistance
to the effect of antithyroid drugs (ATD) Azizi F., 1985 and that iodine supplementation after discontinuing therapy results in higher recurrence of the disease.
The association of high U.I. with the persistence of TRAb in patients treated
with ATD suggests that iodine influence on TSH receptor could play a role in the
complex relationship between iodine intake, efficacy of ATD and recurrences of
hyperthyroidism.

REFERENCES

1. F. Azizi, Environmental iodine intake affects the response to Methimazole in
   patients with diffuse toxic goiter, J. Clin. Endoc. & Metab. 61:374 (1985).
2. A.M. Mc Gregor, A.P. Weetman, S. Ratanachaiyavong, G.M. Owen, H. Kaye Ibbertson and R. Hall, Iodine: an influence on the development of autoimmune
   thyroid disease?, in «Thyroid disorders associated with iodine deficiency
   and excess, R. Hall and J. Köbberling Edrs. Serono Symposia (1985).
3. P. Persson, S. Smeds, U. Forsum and A. Karlsson, Non immune induction of
   HLA-DR in human thyroid tissue, European Thyroid Association Congress, 1986,
   Proceeding of.
4. R.S. Sundick, D. Herdegen, T.R. Brown and N. Bagchi, Thyroiditis induced
   by dietary iodine may be due to the increased immunogenicity of highly

iodinated thyroglobulin, in «International symposium: Thyroid and autoimmunity, Amsterdam, March 19-21, 1986.

5. B.E. Wenzel, R. Gute Kunst, T. Schultek, P.C. Scriba, In vitro induction of class II and autoantigens expression of human thyroid monolayers stimulates autologous T-lymphocytes in co-cultures, in European Thyroid Association Congress, 1986, Proceeding of.

FURTHER DATA ON IODINE-INDUCED AUTOIMMUNITY

D.A. Koutras, K. Evangelopoulou, K.S. Karaiskos,
M.A. Boukis, G.D. Piperingos, J. Kitsopanides,
D. Makriyannis, J. Mantzos, J. Sfontouris, and
A. Souvatzoglou

Athens University School of Medicine, Department
of Clinical Therapeutics, "ALEXANDRA" Hospital
GR-115 28 Athens/Greece

INTRODUCTION

In a previous study we found that 29 out of 58 goitrous patients
(50 %) injected with 1 ml iodized oil im developed 3 to 6 months later
thyroid autoantibodies against thyroglobulin (TG) and/or the microsomal
antigen (MS)[1]. In the present study we extend previous reports [2,3,4]
that such autoantibodies develop also after small 'physiological' doses
of iodine, and the results are compared with those obtained with iodized
oil [1].

MATERIAL AND METHODS

Four groups of patients with a diffuse or micronodular nontoxic
goitre were studied in our endemic areas. Definitely nodular goitres were
excluded, because of possible autonomy. Before, 3 and 6 months after
treatment, goitre size, serum thyroid hormone levels, the TRH test and
the iodine/creatinine ratio (I/Cr) in spot samples of urine were measured[1].
Antithyroid autoantibodies against TG and the MS antigen were assayed by
passive haemagglutination, using the Thymune-M and Thymune-T kits of Wellcome. Low titres were accepted only after repetition. Group a, 58 patients, were treated with 1 ml of iodized oil (48 % wt/vol), group b, 19
patients, received l-thyroxine, 150 or 200 µg/day, group c, 49 patients,
l-thyroxine 150 µg plus pot. iodide (KI) 150 µg/day, and group d, 25 patients, KI 150 or 300 µg/day.

RESULTS

Table 1.

GROUPS	n	I/Cr ratio in µg/g BEFORE $\bar{x}$	SE	Median	Range	I/Cr ratio in µg/g AFTER $\bar{x}$	SE	Median	Range	DEVELOPED AAB Nr	%
a) Iodized oil	58	42	3	38	10-105	248	19	258	51-829	29	50
b) T4	19	61	17	51	12-165	112	20	84	23-308	2	11
c) T4 + KI	49	81	28	41	7-209	337	58	343	41-595	8	16
d) KI	25	36	5	34	10- 93	237	37	200	27-598	6	24

The I/Cr ratio before treatment was not significantly different
between any two of the 4 treatment groups. After treatment, the I/Cr

ratio rose highly significantly in all groups except group b (treated
with T4), where the rise was of borderline significance (t:1.95, 0.05 <
p < 0.10). After treatment, the I/Cr ratio differed significantly between
group b (T4) and any of the other three groups.

Thyroid autoantibodies against TG and/or the MS antigen developed
after 6 months in 11 to 50 % of the patients in the various groups treated,
with titres ranging from 1:40 to 1:25600 for TG and 1:80 to 1:6400 for MS.
The difference between group a (iodized oil, 50 % AAB) and b (T4, 11 % AAB)
was highly significant (chi-square 9.13, p < 0.005), between a and c (T4 +
KI, 16 % AAB) also highly significant (chi-square 13.19, p < 0.001) and
between a and d (KI, 24 % AAB) just significant (chi-square 4.76, p < 0.05).
The difference between groups b and c, b and d and c and d was statistically not significant.

DISCUSSION

In all groups treated, the I/Cr ratio increased and a sizable number
of patients developed AAB against TG and/or MS. There was no control
group treated with placebo for comparison, but the spontaneous emergence
within 6 months of AAB in 11 (group b) to 50 % (group a) of the patients
seems highly unlikely.

We conclude, therefore, that iodine supplementation, even with modest
'physiological' doses of iodine, leads to the appearance of AAB.

Our results are supported by other evidence found in the literature.
Iodine in vitro enhances the production of IgG by lymphocytes in culture[5].
Histological evidence of autoimmune lymphocytic thyroiditis and/or AAB
are more common in countries with an iodine-rich diet, such as the USA[6,7],
and in patients with iodide goitre[8]. Other authors have also observed the
appearance of thyroiditis and/or AAB after iodine administration and the
correction of iodine deficiency in man[9,10,11,12], in dogs[13] and in chicken[14].
Recent reports point out that dietary iodine increases the immunogenicity
of thyroglobulin[15] and also autoantigen expression in cells from patients
with Graves disease[16]. The mechanism involved is obscure. Large doses
may lead to thyroid tissue necrosis[17] and leakage of thyroid antigen, but
small doses may have a more direct immunogenic effect.

Granted that iodine supplementation facilitates or induces the production of AAB, the possible clinical significance of this phaenomenon
should be considered. It is not known for how long these autoantibodies
persist, or whether they lead to some harm. In group a treated with iodized oil[1], three patients with high AAB titres developed transient hyperthyroidism, but this association may be due to the necrosis which probably
occurred in the thyroid tissue of these patients, resulting in the leakage
of both thyroid hormones and thyroid antigens. In any case, in no way
our results should be taken as evidence against the eradication of iodine
deficiency, whose harmful effects are well known[18].

REFERENCES

1. M.A. Boukis, D.A. Koutras, A. Souvatzoglou, A. Evangelopoulou,
   M. Vrontakis, and S.D. Moulopoulos, Thyroid hormone and immunologic
   studies in endemic goiter, J. clin. Endocr. 57:859 (1983).
2. M.A. Boukis, D.A. Koutras, A. Souvatzoglou, A. Evangelopoulou,
   M. Vrontakis, K.S. Karaiskos, G.D. Piperingos, J. Kitsopanides, and
   S.D. Moulopoulos, Iodine-induced autoimmunity, Serono Symposia
   "Thyroid disorders with iodine deficiency and excess", Freiburg,
   W. Germany, April 24-26 (1984).

3. D.A. Koutras, K.S. Karaiskos, G.D. Piperingos, J. Kitsopanides, M.A. Boukis, D. Makriyannis, A. Souvatzoglou, J. Sfontouris, K. Evangelopoulou, S.D. Moulopoulos, K. Katsouyanni, and D. Trichopoulos, Treatment of endemic goitre with iodine and thyroid hormones, alone or in combination. (Preliminary report), Endocr. exper. 20:57 (1986).

4. D.A. Koutras, K.S. Karaiskos, K. Evangelopoulou, M.A. Boukis, G.D. Piperingos, J. Kitsopanides, D. Makriyannis, J. Mantzos, J. Sfontouris, and A. Souvatzoglou, Thyroid autoantibodies after iodine supplementation, in: "The Thyroid and Autoimmunity," H.A. Drexhage, and W.M. Wersinga, eds., Elsevier Science Publishers B.V. (1986).

5. A.P. Weetman, A.M. McGregor, H. Campbell, J.H. Lazarus, H.K. Ibbertson, and R. Hall, Iodine enhances IgG synthesis by human peripheral blood lymphocytes in vitro, Acta Endocrinol. 103:210 (1983).

6. J.M. Talbot, K.D. Fisher, and J.C. Carr, A review of the significance of untoward reactions to iodine in food, Life Science Research Office, FDA, 71-294, Bethesda Md., (1974).

7. J.M. Talbot, K.D. Fisher, and J.C. Carr, A review of the effects of dietary iodine on certain thyroid disorders, Life Science Research Office, FDA, 223-75-2090, Bethesda Md., (1976).

8. R. Hall, M. Turner-Warwick, and D. Doniach, Autoantibodies in iodine goitre and asthma, Clin. Exper. Immunol. 1:285 (1966).

9. M. Inoue, N. Taketani, T. Sato, and H. Nakajima, High incidence of chronic lymphocytic thyroiditis in apparently healthy school children: epidemiological and clinical study, Endocr. Jap. 22(6): 483 (1975).

10. H.R. Harach, D.A. Escalante, A. Onativia, J. Lederer Outes, H.R. Day, and E.D. Williams, Thyroid carcinoma and thyroiditis in an endemic goitre region before and after iodine prophylaxis, Acta Endocrinol. 108:55 (1985).

11. E. Oechslin, und C. Hedinger, Thyreoiditis Lymphomatosa Hashimoto und Endemische Struma, Schweiz. med. Wochenschr. 115:1182 (1985).

12. C. Hedinger, Geographic pathology of thyroid disease, Path. Res. Pract. 171:285 (1981).

13. T.C. Evans, W.H. Beierwaltes, and R.H. Nishiyama, Experimental canine Hashimoto's thyroiditis, Endocrinology 84:641 (1969).

14. N. Bagchi, T.R. Brown, E. Urdanivia, and R.S. Sundick, Induction of autoimmune thyroiditis in chickens by dietary iodine, Science 230:325 (1985).

15. R.S. Sundick, D.M. Herdegen, T.R. Brown, and N. Bagchi, The incorporation of dietary iodine into thyroglobulin increases its immunogenicity, American Thyroid Association, 61st Meeting, Phoenix-Arizona, Abstr. No 21, September 10-13 (1986).

16. B.E. Wenzel, R. Gutekunst, and P.C. Scriba, Iodine induced autoantigen in human Thyroid Epithelial Cell cultures (TEC) from patients with Graves disease (GD); American Thyroid Association, 61st Meeting Phoenix-Arizona, Abstr. No 32, September 10-13 (1986).

17. B.E. Belshaw, and D.V. Becker, Necrosis of follicular cells and discharge of thyroidal iodine induced by administering iodine to iodine-deficient dogs, J. clin. Endocr. 36:466 (1973).

18. J.T. Dunn, E.A. Pretell, C.H. Daza, and F.E. Viteri, "Towards the Eradication of Endemic Goiter, Cretinism and Iodine Deficiency," Proceedings of the V Meeting of the PAHO/WHO Technical Group on Endemic Goiter, Cretinism and Iodine Deficiency, PAHO Sci. Publ., No 502 (1986).

STUDY OF CLASS I AND CLASS II ANTIGEN EXPRESSION AND LYMPHOCYTIC INFILTRATE ON THYROID TUMORS

C. Betterle, F. Presotto, A. Caretto, B. Pedini, A. Fassina^,
M. R. Pelizzo°, M. E. Girelli and B. Busnardo

Institutes of Semeiotica Medica, ^Pathology and °Semeiotica
Chirurgica
University of Padua, Italy

INTRODUCTION

Class II (HLA-DR) antigens, encoded by genes located in the HLA region, play a key role in antigen presentation and in immunoresponse regulation. The expression of these membrane-associated molecules is normally restricted to B and T-activated lymphocytes, antigen-presenting cells (macrophages, Kupffer, dendritic and Langherans cells, etc.) and capillary endothelium (1). On the contrary, class I (HLA-ABC) antigens are normally present, with different expression, on the membranes of all nucleated tissue cells and platelets (2). The recent observation that in thyroid autoimmune diseases there exists an aberrant epithelial expression of class II and an increased expression of class I molecules by target cells, and the finding that this phenomenon is associated with an infiltration of T lymphocytes (3) permitted new interpretations about the pathogenetic events leading to thyroid autoimmunity and, extensively, to organ-specific autoimmunity (4). Recently it has also been found that paraffin-embedded tissues of different thyroid tumors have an aberrant exhibition of class II molecules and that the lymphocytic infiltration is correlated to HLA expression (5). The aim of this work was to study on unfixed cryostat sections of different thyroid tumors the epithelial expression of class I and class II molecules, the characteristics of the infiltrating cells and the connection between these two events.

MATERIALS AND METHODS

Patients

Surgical thyroid tissues taken from 49 patients with malignant or benign thyroid tumors (24 with papillary carcinoma, 3 with anaplastic carcinoma, 6 with medullary carcinoma and 15 with follicular adenoma) were studied. Normal thyroid tissues obtained from the uninvolved part of 4 thyroid glands affected with benign tumors were used as controls.

Immunofluorescence staining

Thin serial unfixed cryostat sections of each gland were incubated with the following mouse monoclonal antibodies (MoAbs) (Becton-Dickinson), respectively: a) anti-beta2 microglobulin, b) anti-HLA DR (non polymorphic), c) anti-Leu 1 (pan-T lymphocytes), d) anti-Leu 2a (T citotoxic/suppressor), e) anti-Leu 3a (T helper/inducer), anti-Leu 7 (Natural Killer) and g) anti-Leu 10 (cells bearing HLA DQ, equivalent to murine Ia antigens). The sections were then stained with a rabbit biotinylated serum anti-mouse immunoglobulins followed by FITC conjugated Avidin (Sigma Co., St Louis USA). Other sections were directly stained with FITC goat serum anti-human IgG, IgA, IgM and C3 (Wellcome, Beckenham England) to detect immunocomplex deposition.

Serology

In every patient a sample of serum was obtained to detect thyroid autoantibodies (microsomal and thyroglobulin).

RESULTS

Normal thyroids. The cytoplasm of thyrocytes was negative using anti-HLA DR MoAb, while with anti-HLA ABC MoAb only a weak staining was observed. Only a few capillary endothelia were stained. Neither infiltrating cells nor immunocomplexes were seen.

Papillary carcinomas. Nineteen of 24 (79%) revealed the presence of both HLA DR expression and increased expression of HLA ABC. Two other cases (8%) showed only an increased expression of HLA ABC molecules. The remaining 3 cases were negative for these antigens. In general, the fluorescence pattern obtained with MoAb to HLA ABC was diffuse, while with MoAb to HLA DR it was focal. In both cases, the positivity of thyrocytes was slight. A T lymphocytic infiltrate was evident in 11 of the 19 cases expressing both HLA ABC and DR, while it was not demonstrated in the remaining DR- cases. The infiltrate was represented by Leu 1+/10+ cells (T-activated?), however it was moderate and scattered. No NK cells were visible and only 1 tumor had focal granular deposition of IgG and C3 on the follicular basement membrane. Thyroid antibodies were found in 4 of the 19 DR+ and in 1 of the 5 DR- cases.

Anaplastic carcinomas. Two cases (67%) had both HLA DR and ABC antigen expression, and 1 of these showed a small amount of Leu 1+/10+ cells. The third case was negative for both markers and had no infiltrates. Neither NK cells nor immunocomplexes were seen. Thyroid antibodies were found in only one DR+ case.

Medullary carcinomas. Two cases (33%) showed an increased expression of HLA ABC, but none of these tumors expressed HLA DR. Neither infiltrating cells nor immunocomplexes were seen. Thyroid antibodies were not detected.

Follicular adenomas. Four cases (25%) were positive for both HLA ABC and DR, 2 of which showed Leu 1+/10+ cells. A fifth case with increased expression of only HLA ABC was also positive for T infiltrate. Out of the remaining 11 cases which were negative for both HLA markers, 1 showed T infiltrate. In all infiltrated tissues the number of T cells was small. NK cells or immunocomplexes were absent. Thyroid antibodies were detected in 1 of 4 DR+ cases and in 3 of 11 DR- cases.

DISCUSSION

Immunization against an antigen requires both its recognition by lymphocytes and its presentation in an immunogenic form. The presentation of foreign antigens to helper T cells is usually accomplished in the context of the HLA-DR molecules (6). Expression of DR antigens has been observed on cells involved in the immune response, but it has also been described on cells normally not associated with the immune system such as some capillary endothelia and a variety of "barrier" epithelia (7). The presence of DR molecules in these cells has led to the postulate that they can be recruited, under special circumstances, as antigen-presenting cells. The normal endocrine cells are not able to exhibit DR antigens, but in vitro their stimulation with lectins or gamma-interferon induces them to express these antigens (2). Furthermore, during thyroid autoimmune diseases these cells spontaneously express DR antigens (3). This inappropriate DR expression by thyrocytes will result in the efficient presentation of their surface autoantigens to autoreactive T helper cells. Moreover, the increased expression in such diseases of HLA-ABC antigens by these cells could be as efficient signal for the activation of T cytotoxic lymphocytes (4).

The present data reveal that neoplastic thyroid cells in vivo are able to produce class II antigens and to increase the production of those of class I. This phenomenon is less evident compared with that found in thyroid glands affected with autoimmune diseases. In thyroid tumors the lymphocytic infiltrate appears correlated to the expression of DR antigens. Moreover, lymphocytes possess membrane markers of T cells, but are generally few and no NK cells are detectable. This cell infiltration is quantitatively poor with respect to that observed in glands affected with autoimmune processes. The above mentioned data reveal, in addition to the lack of autoantibodies in thyroid tumors, the ineffective involvement of the immune system in these tumors. What induces neoplastic cells to present HLA antigens is not known, but this may be due to a genetic derepression or to environmental stimuli that induce the production of gamma-interferon by local T lymphocytes or by NK cells (2). Why are tumoral DR+ cells not able to engage significant amounts of immunocompetent cells? It might be due to the low concentration of DR antigens on tumoral cells or to the presence of inhibiting factors, as tumoral antigens shedding, immunocomplexes or anti-idiotype antibodies.

REFERENCES

1. A.N. Barclay, D.W. Mason, Graft rejection and Ia antigens - paradox resolved?, Nature 303: 382 (1983).
2. R. Pujol-Borrell, I. Todd, M. Londei, A. Foulis, M. Feldmann, G.F. Bottazzo, Inappropriate major histocompatibility complex class II expression by thyroid follicular cells in thyroid autoimmune disease and by pancreatic beta cells in type I diabetes, Mol Biol Med 3: 159 (1986).
3. T. Hanafusa, R. Pujol-Borrell, L. Chiovato, R.C.G. Russel, D. Doniach, G.F. Bottazzo, Aberrant expression of HLA-DR antigen on thyrocytes in Graves' disease: relevance for autoimmunity, Lancet 2: 1111 (1983).
4. G.F. Bottazzo, R. Pujol-Borrell, T. Hanafusa, Role of aberrant HLA-DR expression and antigen presentation in induction of endocrine auto-immunity, Lancet 2: 1115 (1983).
5. R.V. Lloyd, T. Johnson, M. Blaivas, J. Sisson, B.S. Wilson, Detection of HLA-DR antigens in paraffin-embedded thyroid epithelial cells with a monoclonal antibody, Am J Pathol 120: 106 (1985).
6. E.R. Unanue, Antigen presenting function of the macrophage, Annu Rev Immunol 2: 395 (1984).
7. K. Wiman, B. Kurman, V. Forsum, L. Klareskog, L. Malmas-Tjernlund, L. Rask, L. Tragardh, P.A. Peterson, Occurence of Ia antigens on tissues of non-lymphoid origin, Nature 276: 711 (1978).

INCIDENCE OF ANTI-THYROID AUTOANTIBODIES IN THYROID CANCER PATIENTS

Furio Pacini, Stefano Mariotti, Nunzio Formica, Rossella
Elisei, Stefano Anelli, Enrico Capotorti, Lidio Baschieri*, and
Aldo Pinchera.

Endocrinologia e Medicina Costituzionale and   *Clinica Medica
2, University of Pisa, USL 12, Pisa, Italy

INTRODUCTION

The relationship between thyroid autoimmunity and thyroid cancer is poorly studied. No evidence of increased incidence of anti-thyroid microsomal autoantibodies (MAb) was found by Kornstad[1] in a large series of thyroid cancer patients using the complement fixation technique. Employing the more sensitive passive hemagglutination test, other authors[1-4] reported increased incidence of anti-thyroglobulin (TgAb) and MAb in thyroid malignancies, when compared to the normal population.

In this study we report the incidence of TgAb and MAb in a series of 600 patients with thyroid cancer, with particular regard to the relationship between thyroid antibodies and tumor outcome during 10 years of follow-up.

PATIENTS ·

Serum TgAb and MAb were measured by passive hemagglutination in 600 patients (449 females and 151 males, aging 7-85 years), followed 1-12 years after total thyroidectomy. Subsequent therapy was L-thyroxine in suppressive doses, radioiodine for functioning differentiated cancer and any combination of surgery, radiotherapy or chemotherapy for non-functioning metastases and for anaplastic and medullary tumors. Histology was papillary thyroid carcinoma in 401 patients, follicular in 144, anaplastic in 31 and medullary in 24.

RESULTS

Incidence of thyroid antibodies in relation to sex and histology

As shown in Table 1, positive TgAb and/or MAb were present in 96 (23.9%) patients with papillary, 36 (25%) with follicular, 5 (16.1%) with anaplastic and 1 (4.1%) with medullary thyroid cancer, corresponding to a total incidence of 23% (138 patients). Female to male ratio was 4.3:1 in differentiated and 1.5:1 in anaplastic cancer; only one patient (female) with medullary thyroid cancer had positive antibodies.

Anti-microsomal antibodies alone were found in 92 out of 138 positive cases (66.6%), MAb and TgAb in 43 (31.1%) and TgAb alone in 2 cases (2.2%).

Table 1.   Incidence of positive serum anti-thyroid autoantibodies
in 600 patients with thyroid carcinoma.

Histology	Antibody positive patients	
	no.	%
Papillary (no.=401)	96	23.9
Follicular (no.=144)	36	25.0
Medullary (no.=24)	1	4.1
Anaplastic (no.=31)	5	16.1
Total (no.=600)	138	23.0

Incidence of positive antibodies in relation to age.

The incidence of positive antibodies was not statistically different among the various decades of life, ranging from a minimum of 21.9% (21-40 years group) to a maximum of 27.9% (1-20 years group). On the contrary, the incidence of positive anti-thyroid antibodies in 654 sex-matched normal controls was very low (4%) among young people and increased linearly to reach a maximum of 23% in subjects older than 60 years.

Both in the antibody-positive and in the antibody-negative group of patients the maximal incidence of cancer was found in the 3rd-5th decade of life for papillary and after the 5th decade for follicular carcinoma.

Positive antibodies and tumor outcome.

In 76/138 patients with positive antibody tests the follow-up was long enough to correlate the variations of antibody titers with the outcome of the disease. Successful treatment was achieved in 64 patients, while persistent disease occurred in 12. The behaviour of thyroid antibodies in these two groups was substantially different. As shown in Table 2, in successfully treated patients, thyroid antibodies became undetectable in 54.6%, decreased in 32.8%, did not change in 3.1% and increased in 9.3%. On the contrary, antibody titers became undetectable in 8.3%, decreased in 16.6%, did not change in 25% and increased in 50% of patients with persistent disease.

Table 2.   Changes in antibody titers in relation to the outcome of the
tumor in 76 patients with positive antibodies at the first observation

Antibody titers	Successfully treated		Persistent disease	
	No.	%	No.	%
No longer detectable	35	54.6	1	8.3
Decreased	21	32.8	2	16.6
Unchanged	2	3.3	3	25.1
Increased	6	9.3	6	50.0
Total	64		12	

It should be noted however, that no significant difference in the clinical outcome and the mortality rate was observed in patients with differentiated carcinoma with or without positive serum antibodies at the first observation.

DISCUSSION

The present study carried out in a large series of patients with thyroid carcinoma, confirms and extends previous observations performed in smaller series reporting increased incidence of serum thyroid antibodies by passive hemagglutination in thyroid malignancies[1-4]. Our results show that positive circulating anti-thyroid antibodies are rather frequently observed (23%) in thyroid cancer patients. Positive antibody titers were more frequent in female patients in agreement with the well known higher incidence of thyroid autoimmunity in women[5]. Interestingly the presence of positive antibodies was not age-related, in contrast with the reported age-dependent increase of thyroid autoimmune phenomena observed in apparently normal subjects.

Serum thyroid antibody titers generally decreased or become undetectable after total thyroidectomy in patients succesfully treated while the persistence of metastatic thyroid tissue was usually associated with the persistence or increase of antibody titers.

This finding is in keeping with the concept that metastatic tissue is needed to mantain the antigenic stimulus to autoreactive lymphocyte clones for persistent autoantibody production[6].

Finally, regardless of the mechanism(s) responsible for its perpetuation, humoral thyroid autoimmunity apparently does not affect the clinical outcome of thyroid cancer.

AKNOWLEDGEMENT

This work has been partially supported by the Italian Research Council, Target Project "Preventive Medicine and Rehabilitation" Subproject "Mechanisms of aging", Grant n° 86.01899.56 and Special Project "Oncology", Contract n° 86.00532.44.

REFERENCES

1. L. Kornstad, Organ-specific autoantibodies in thyroid cancer, Acta Path Microbiol Scand (Suppl 248) 1974.
2. N. Aoki, G. Wakisaka, T. Higashi, Y. Akazawa, Clinical studies of thyroidal autoantibodies, Endocrinol Jpn 22:89 1975.
3. N. Amino, S.R. Hagen, S. Refetoff, N. Yamada, Measurement of circulating thyroid microsomal antibodies by tanned red cell hemagglutination technique. Its usefulness in the diagnosis of autoimmune thyroid disease. Clin Endocrinol (Oxf) 5:115, 1976.
4. L.J. DeGroot, K. Hoyek, S. Refetoff, A.J. Van Herle, G.T. Asteris, H. Rochmann, Serum antigens and antibodies in the diagnosis of thyroid cancer, J Clin Endocrinol Metab 45:1220 1977.
5. D. Doniach, Humoral and genetic aspects of thyroid autoimmunity, Clin Endocrinol Metab 4:267 1975.
6. M.C. Atherton, S.M. MacLachlan, C.A.S. Pegs, A. Dickinson, P. Bayles, E.T. Young, S.J. Proctor, B.R. Smith, Thyroid autoantibody synthesis by lymphocytes from different lymphoid organs. Fractionation of B-cells on density gradients, Immunology 55:271 1985.

THYROID AUTOANTIBODIES IN THYROID CANCER

K.Bech, H.Bliddal, U.Andersen, Å.Krogh Rasmussen, H.Sand Hansen, U. Feldt-Rasmussen, and J. Witten Hvidöre Hospital, Med. dept. E, Frederiksberg Hospital, Surg. Dept. R, Rigshospitalet, Finsen Institute Copenhagen, Denmark.

INTRODUCTION

It has previously been shown that thyroid autoantibodies are frequent in patients treated for differentiated thyroid cancer[1,2] Whether these antibodies are due to therapy or are involved in the pathogenesis of the disease has, however, not yet been clarified. We were therefore interested in studying these antibodies in thyroid cancer before and after treatment.

MATERIALS AND METHODS

Two groups of patients were studied. The first group consisted of 10 patients (2 men, 8 women) with newly diagnosed thyroid cancer. Six patients had papillary carcinoma (PC)(median age 47 years, range 19-75) and four follicular carcinoma (FC) (median age 46 years, range 35-50). These patients were observed from diagnosis until 3 months after thyroidectomy and have not been treated with radioiodine or thyroid hormone suppression within this period. The second group consisted of 34 patients (7 men, 27 women). Eighteen had PC (median age 50 years, range 18-83), and 16 FC (median age 65 years, range 33-85). They had been treated for thyroid cancer by surgery and radioiodine and thyroid hormone suppression from 0 to 35 years before (PC: median 4 years, range 1-35) (FC: median 6 years, range 1-17). Two patients in group 1 and 12 patients in group 2 had metastases. The thyroid status was measured by routine assays. The thyroid stimulating immunoglobulins were measured by thyroid adenylate cyclase stimulation (TSAb)[3] and by radioreceptor assay (TBII)[4], thyroglobulin antibodies (TgAb) by radio-coprecipitation assay[5] together with thyroglobulin (Tg) measured by radioimmunoassay[6].

RESULTS

Group 1: Before treatment all patients with FC (n=4) were negative for TBII, TSAb and TgAb, but after operation TSAb became positive in two. TBII remained negative. Four patients with PC (n=6) were positive for TSAb, one for TgAb, while TBII were negative. After 7 days TSAb disappeared in all. The levels

Table. Serum thyroglobulin and thyroid autoantibodies

	N	Tg (ng/ml)	TgAb (No.pos.)	TBII (%)(No.pos.) > 25%		TSAb (%)(No.pos.) > 110%	
Group 2							
PC	18	11.9 (<5.3-370)	4	20 (0-56)	7	98 (88-317)	6
FC	16	164 (6.1-7000)	2	32 (0-60)	12	107 (73-178)	6

of TSAb and TBII were significantly higher in PC than in FC (p<0.01). Tg was very high in one patient with metastases, but ranged in the remaining patients from 21 to 200 µg/l (median 47.5 µg/l). A minor peak was observed within the first post-operative day followed by a rapid decrease.

Group 2: The antibody levels in group 2 appear from the table. Tg was significantly elevated in the patients with meta-stases (p<0.001), but there was no relation between metastases and thyroid autoantibodies, as well as radioiodine therapy or mode of operation.

DISCUSSION

Thyroid autoantibodies have been demonstrated in several thyroid diseases depending on the nature of the autoimmune state of the disease. Thus, in Graves' disease thyroid stimu-lating antibodies are very frequent. Differentiated thyroid carcinoma is not suggested to be an autoimmune disease, and the high frequency of thyroid autoantibodies is therefore surpri-sing. However, the finding, that thyroid autoantibodies are very seldom in thyroid cancer before treatment, leads to the conclusion that their presence is secondary to tissue damage following operation and radioablation.

REFERENCES

1. K. Bech, H. Bliddal, U. Feldt-Rasmussen, J. Witten and H.S. Hansen, Thyroid stimulating immunoglobulins in differenti-ated thyroid cancer. EORTC Meeting Thyroid Study Group Rotterdam (1983).
2. F. Pacini, S. Mariotti, N. Formica, S. Anelli, R. Bechi, R. Elisei and A. Pinchera, Thyroid autoimmunity in thyroid cancer, in: "The thyroid and Autoimmunity", H.A. Drexhage and W.M. Wiersinga, eds., Elsevier Sci. Publ. (1986).
3. K. Bech and S.N. Madsen, Thyroid adenylate cyclase stimu-lating immunoglobulins in Graves' disease. Clin Endocrinol (Oxf) 11:47 (1979).
4. H. Bliddal, A stable, reproducible radioreceptorassay for thyrotrophin binding inhibiting immunoglobulins (TBII). Scand J Clin Lab Invest 41:441 (1981).

5. J. Date, U. Feldt-Rasmussen, P.H. Petersen and K. Bech, An improved co-precipitation assay for determination of thyroglobulin antibodies. Scand J Clin Lab Invest 40:37 (1980).
6. U. Feldt-Rasmussen, P.H. Petersen and J. Date, Sex and age correlated reference values of serum thyroglobulin measured by a modified radioimmunoassay. Acta Endocrinol 90:440 (1979).

SOME ASPECTS OF CELL MEDIATED AUTOIMMUNITY IN ENDEMIC NODULAR GOITRE

A. Balsamo, *F. Botto Micca, P.A. Merlin, V. De Filippis, and *A. Stramignoni

Division and Laboratory of Endocrinology of Mauriziano Hospital Turin
* Department of Pathology of the University, of Turin, Turin, Italy

INTRODUCTION

The diagnosis of autoimmune thyroid disease (ATD), when suspected as a result of clinical, hormonal, instrumental (U.S., scintigraphy), and immunological findings, may be confirmed by conventional hystology or immunochemical stainings also applicable to tissue or simple cells obtained by fine needle biopsy. This has been reported by several authors who investigated lymphoid cell subsets from thyroids of patients with suspected ATD[1,2,3,4]. In this present work, and in previous works, we looked for the presence and possibly the meaning of lymphoid tissue infiltrating the thyroid (LI) of goitrous patients living in an iodine deficient area. In these patients frequently we found high prevalence of antithyroid autoantibodies at low title and histological findings of focal thyroiditis.

MATERIAL AND METHODS

Thyroid specimens from patients who underwent the operation for nodular disease of the thyroid, were obtained during surgery. The average age of the patients was 39.7 ± 9.3 yrs; rate F/M 5/1, lenght of the disease from 3mnths to 20yrs. As controls we used normal thyroids obtained from 4 parathyroidectomised patients. The patients were; 12 multinodular goitre (MNG), 5 multinodular toxic goitre (MNTG), 6 uninodular toxic goitre (UNTG), 1 follicular adenoma. The removed nodular tissue was located in 76% of all the cases at the base of the right lobe. The surgical specimens were firstly examined by conventional hystology, i.e. hematoxilin-eosin stained paraffin sections to demonstrate the hystological features, if any: perivascular lymphoid infiltrates, germinal centres, infiltration of thyroid follicles and fibrosis. Criostatic sections were submitted to commercially available MoABs: Leu4, Leu2a, Leu3a, Leu12(B). Selected MoABs to more restricted T-activated cell membrane antigens were also used: 5/9 (T cells mainly responsible for proliferation to soluble antigens and B differentiation), MLR3 and MLR4 (T blasts and PWM-driven B cell differentiation). We also looked for the expression of MHC antigens using MoABs to monomorphic determinants of HLA-ABC and HLA-DR. Ab-Tg and Mi-Ab were detected in all the cases with TRC and/or with RIA. TSH-receptor antibodies (TRAb) were found only in hyperthyroid patients.

Table 1. Infiltrating lymphocytes sub-classes, activated T cells HLA, ABC and
DR expression in thyroid patients with nodular goitre.
Legend: − = absence, + = few, ++ = numerous, +++ = very numerous, m = masses, s
= spread.

	Leu4	Leu2a	Leu3a	Leu12	ABC	DR
MNG	++/+++m	+m	++/+++m	+/++m	+/++m-s	+/++m-s
	+/+++s	+/+++s	+s			
MNTG	+/++m	+/++m	+/++m	−/++m	+/++m-s	+/++m-s
	+s	+/+++s	+s			
UNTG	+/+++m	+/+++m	+/+++m	+/+++m	+/+++m-s	+/+++m-s
	+/+++s	++/+++s	+/++s			

RESULTS

Significant LI was found in: 6/12 MNG, 2/5 MNTG, 3/6 UNTG. Circulating antithyroid antibodies were present in: 4/6 infiltrates MNG, 2/2 MNTG, 3/3 UNTG.
Moreover, the presence of Ab-T in MNG was associated with more consistent LI,
whose entity in MNTG and UNTG created the environment conditions supporting production of antibodies. In 2/3 UNTG with LI, TRAb was also present. The distribution of Tcell sub-population, B cell (Leu12) and the expression of HLA, ABC and
HLA-DR on lymphocytes and thyrocytes are summarised in Table 1.
Independent of the Leu3a/Leu2a ratio, which is higher in the thyroids with largest
infiltrates, 5/9+ T cells were rare or few. In two cases they were located only
en masse. MLR3+ and MLR4+ showed an almost similar pattern, with the former mainly in clusters. B lymphocytes occurred only in germinal centres. HLA-DR and HLA-
ABC increased expression on thyrocytes is correlated to the entity of LI. In
thyroids with moderate LI only a small number of epithelial cells next to LI are
positive. Many thyrocytes become positive as LI increases, whether they be near
or far from focal thyroiditis. Follicular adenoma and normal thyroids were poorly
infiltrated and there was no expression of MHC antigens on thyrocytes.

CONCLUSIONS

Significant evidence of cellular and humoral autoimmunity is easily found in
endemic goitre. The thyroid infiltration normally has the characteristics of the
focal thyroiditis. Unexpectedly, in 3/6 UMTG we found the hystological pattern
of Graves' disease and circulating TSH receptor antibodies. It is not certain
if limited infiltration and, consequently, limited development of specialised
lymphoid tissue is dependent on the presence of T-suppressor specific antigen
lymphocytes[5]. If and when these lymphocytes became reduced in number and in
function the disease is allowed to emerge. According to this interpretation, our
poorly infiltrated thyroids show a higher number of Leu2a, probably T-suppressor
cells. Epithelial thyroid cells presenting class II antigens (molecules) which
are strictly correlated with autoantigens on their surface, may act as antigen-
presenting cells and can induce the sequence of events which results in lymphoid
infiltration. We do not know what are the possible stimuli able to induce aberrant but limited expression of MHC antigens in goitrous thyroids. Moreover, increased expression of HLA-ABC antygens might facilitate recognition by
autoreactive cytotoxic T-cells, which play a pivotal role in the destruction of
the thyroid tissue[6].

REFERENCES

1. T.H. Totterman, Thyroid infiltrating, immunocompetent cells in human autoimmune thyroid disease: subclass distribution and *in vitro* functions. Academic Dissertation, Helsinki, Finland (1978)
2. E. Witebsky and N.R. Rose, Studies on organ specificity. IV. Production of rabbit thyroid antibodies in the rabbit. J Immunol 76:408 (1956)
3. G. Aichinger, H. Fill and G. Wick, In situ immune complexes, lymphocyte subpopulation and HLA-DR positive epithelial cells in Hashimoto Thyroiditis, Laboratory Investigation, 52, 2:132 (1985)
4. R. Jansson, T.H. Tötterman, J. Sällströn and P.A. Dahlberg, Thyroid-infiltrating T-lymphocyte subsets in Hashimoto's thyroiditis, Journal Clinical Endocrinology and Metabolism, 56:6 (1983)
5. R. Volpé and V. V. Row, Role of antigen specific suppressor T-lymphocytes in the pathogenesis of autoimmune thyroid disease, in: Autoimmunity and the thyroid, P.G. Walfish, ed., Academic Press, Inc., (1985)
6. I. Todd, R. Pujol-Borrell, M. Londei, M. Feldman and G.F. Bottazzo, Inappropriate HLA class II expression on epithelial cells: consolidation and progress, in: The thyroid and autoimmunity, H.A. Drexhage, W.M. Wiersinga, ed., Excerpta Medica, International Congress Series, 711 (1986)

CHRONIC LYMPHOCYTIC THYROIDITIS IN ENDEMIC GOITER: LOCAL Ig PRODUCTION AND DEPOSITION

Huang Gao-sheng and Liu Yan-fang

Department of Pathology, Fourth Military Medical College

Xi' an, People's Republic of China

INTRODUCTION

The local production and deposition of Ig in chronic lymphocytic thyroiditis (CLT) had been noticed long the before (1), and has been studied in detail recently, but mostly restricted to Hashimoto's disease (2).

Our previous studies showed clearly that there is a proportion of CLT in endemic goiter, which has a predilection for the lesions in the tissue surrouding goiter nodules (3). And there is the close correlation between serum autoantibodies and the local lymphocytic infiltration in thyroid tissue. Furthermore some people have reported the increased level of a kind of Ig in endemic goiter (4). So the study on the local production and the position of Ig is directly related to understanding the immunological pathogenesis of CLT in endemic goiter.

MATERIALS AND METHODS

Using trypsinization and immunohistochemical techniques, the local production and deposition of IgG, IgM and IgA in 21 cases of CLT in endemic goiter were investigated serial paraffin sections obtained surgically from patients in an endemic area. The tissue of 5 cases of hypothyroidism were used as control. The sections were stained immunohystochemically by FITC and peroxidase labeled horse antihuman IgG, IgA, IgM and C3 antibodies with the direct method. Slides stained with normal horse FITC labeled Ig, blocking test and bleacking of endogenous enzyme were used as controls.

RESULTS AND DISCUSSION

Plasmacytes and proplasmacyte producing IgG are predominant (Fig. 1), IgM, IgA cells are afew (Table 1).

Most of the Ig-active germinal centers of the lymphofollicle are IgM in nature (Fig. 2), less IgG, and no IgA centers are seen. (Table 2).

Table 1. The no. of Ig-positive cells per mm^2 of tissue

Disease	no. of cases	no. of Ig-cell (X ± SE)	% (X ± SE)		
			IgG	IgM	IgA
CLT in endemic goiter:	21	349±99	96.3±4.2	2.3±2.9	1.4±2.3
Hashimoto's disease	3	965±456	98.7±1.8	-	-
CLT	13	326±88	95.8±4.6	-	-
Focal thyroiditis	5	38±10	96.3±4.4	-	-
Hyperthyroidism	5	71±16	98.3±2.4	1.7±4.2	-

With regard to Ig deposition, the small blood vessels in or around the lymphofollicles were heavily deposited by IgG, perhaps related to pathological changes in vessels (Fig. 3).

Table 2. No. and % of Ig-positive germinal center

Disease in endemic goiter	case no.	case with positive centers	total no. of centers	no. of positive		
				IgM	IgG	IgA
Hashimoto's disease	3	3	117	64 (54.7)	41 (35.0)	0
CLT	13	6	62	23 (37.1)	6 (9.6)	0
Focal thyroiditis	5	0	6	0	0	0
Total	21	9	185	87 (47.0)	47 (25.4)	0 0

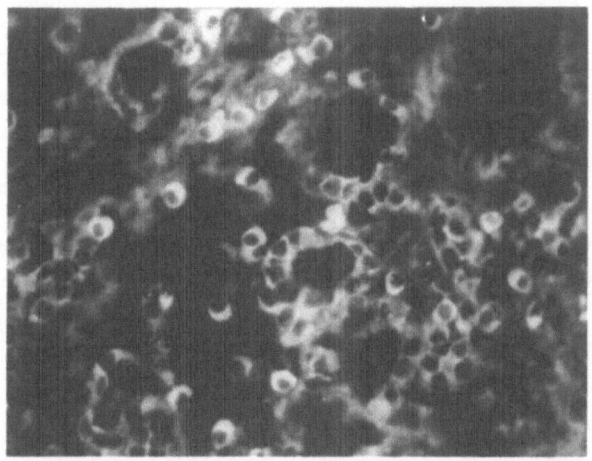

Fig.1 CLT in endemic goiter. Interfollicular IgG-positive
plasma cells and IgG-positive staining of the proliferatiom
acinar cells . x 400

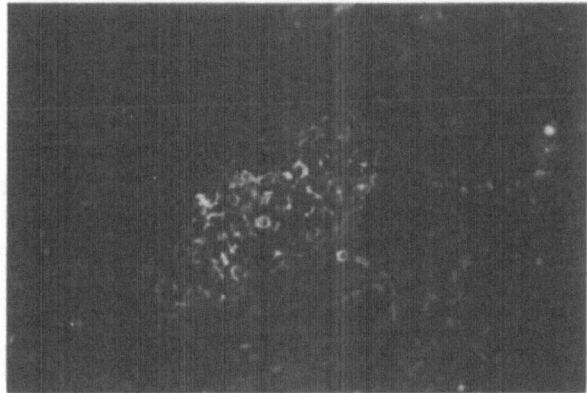

Fig.2 Hashimoto's(or CLT)disease in endemic goiter.
IgM-positive center and a few IgM-positive cells. x400

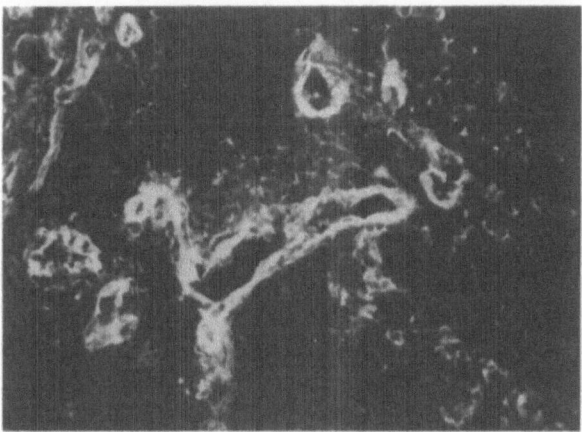

Fig.3 Hashimoto's disease in endemic goiter. IgG-positive
staining of the small blood vessels around the lymphofollicles. X200

From above findings, in spite of a little differences in the number of IgA cells, recent literatures and our present work show marked and rather similar activity of antibody formation in the CLT in general and in endemic goiter. This indicates the inflammation in endemic goiter is also immune or autoimmune in nature.

REFERENCES

1. Robert C. Mellors, Witold J. Brzosko, and Lawrence S. Sonkin, Immunopathology of chronic nonspecific thyroiditis (autoimmune thyroiditis), Am J Pathol. 41:425 (1960).
2. H. Knecht, P. Saremaslani, and Chr. Hedinger, Immunohystological findings in Hashimoto's thyroiditis, focal lymphocytic thyroiditis and thyroiditis De Quevain, Virch Arch Pathol Anat. 393: 215 (1981).
3. Liu Yan-fang, Hu Ming-cin, Niu Shu-miao, and Wu Yan-ling, Chronic lymphocytic thyroiditis in endemic goiter, Chim Med J. 97: 429 (1984).
4. N.G.S. Mota, Y. Kiy, M.T. Rezkallah-Iwasso, and M.T.S. Peracoli, Humoral and cell-mediated immunity in large no-toxic multinodular goiter, Clin Endocrinol 13: 173 (1980).

AUTOIMMUNE THYROID DISEASE IN THE

CITY OF GRAVES

P.P.A. Smyth, T.J. McKenna,
and D.K. O'Donovan

Department of Medicine
University College
Dublin, Ireland

INTRODUCTION

Despite the fact that the disease that bears his name was first des-cribed in 1835 by Dublin physician Robert Graves, the presentation of hyp-erthyroidism in his native city does not always conform to the disease which we now associate with his name. It was the aim of this study to investigate the prevalence and role of IgG thyroid stimulators in the pre-sentation and pathogenesis of hyperthyroidism and euthyroid goitre in an Irish population.

PATIENTS AND METHODS

Patients were classified into hyperthyroid and nontoxic goitrous groups by reference to their charts. The hyperthyroid group included patients with Graves' disease in a diffuse or nodular gland, toxic nodular goitre or those having no palpable goitre. Nontoxic goitre incl-uded those with diffuse or nodular glands.

Thyroid stimulating immunoglobulins (TSI) and thyroid growth stimulating immunoglobulins (TGI), were studied by cytochemical bioassays measuring changes in lysosomal naphthylamidase (LNase)[1] and glucose-6-phosphate dehydrogenase (G6PD)[2] activities in guinea pig thyroid follicular cells.

Table 1. Presentation of newly diagnosed hyperthyroidism.

Table 1 shows that the classical diffuse goitre of Graves' disease was present in only 47.7% of 176 consecutive hyperthyroid patients studied. Also T_3-toxicosis had a high prevalence at 13.6%.

	DIFFUSE GOITRE	NODULAR GOITRE	T3-TOXIC	TOTAL
N	84	92	24	176
%	47.7	52.3	13.6	100

Although TSI was present in all 37 hyperthyroid patients studied as shown in Table 2, TGI was absent in 12 including 8 who had scintigraphically demonstrated toxic nodular goitre and 4 who had no palpable goitre. The findings in nontoxic goitre further support the postulate that 2 separate stimulators were being measured.

	N	TSI	TGI	BOTH
Hyperthyroidism	37	37 (100%)	25 (68%)	25 (68%)
Nontoxic Goitre	53	30 (56%)	34 (64%)	22 (42%)

Table 2. Prevalence of IgG thyroid stimulators measured by cytochemical bioassay.

Tables 3 and 4 show a tendency for TSI and TGI, when present in nontoxic goitre, to occur at lower titres or potencies than in hyperthyroidism.

TSI ESTIMATIONS

	N	TSI TITRE $10^{-2} - 10^{-3}$	TSI TITRE $10^{-4} - 10^{-6}$	MAX.STIMULATION OVER CONTROL%
Hyperthyroidism	60	8	52	30.6 ± 10.9
Nontoxic Goitre	21	16	5	23.3 ± 8.7
				P < 0.005

Table 3. Human plasma TSI titres and maximum stimulation achieved in hyperthyroid and nontoxic goitrous patients.

TGI ESTIMATIONS

	N	MAX.RESPONSE AT IgG 50-100ug/ml	MAX.RESPONSE AT IgG ≥ 500ug/ml
Hyperthyroidism	37	31	2
Nontoxic Goitre	53	12	22

Table 4. IgG concentrations in plasma at which a maximum TGI effect was observed in hyperthyroid and nontoxic goitrous patients.

Although the findings of TGI in both hyperthyroid and nontoxic goitre are consistent with the prevalence of goitre in both conditions, the finding of TSI in nontoxic goitre poses the question as to why such patients do not develop hyperthyroidism.

A difference in properties of TSI between hyperthyroidism and nontoxic goitre are shown in Fig. 1.

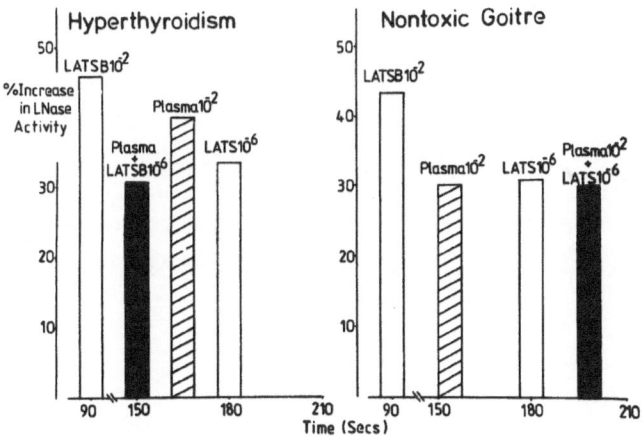

Fig. 1. Effect of incubating patients plasma with LATS-B standard on time of maximum stimulation in the LNase assay

Addition of LATS–B standard to plasma from a hyperthyroid patient caused a shift in the peak of maximum stimulation caused by the plasma from 165 to 150 seconds. This shift in stimulatory peaks is characteristic of enhanced stimulation as shown by the finding of the LATS–B 10^{-2} peak at 90 secs. In contrast, incubation of plasma from a nontoxic goitrous patient with LATS–B standard retarded the plasma induced stimulation peak from 150 to 195 secs.

DISCUSSION

The presentation of hyperthyroidism in Ireland paralleled that encountered in other European countries and is in keeping with a degree of iodine deficiency past or present.[3] The finding of IgG thyroid stimulators in both hyperthyroidism and nontoxic goitre indicate a common (?autoimmune)pathogenesis for both conditions. The apparently greater potency of stimulators found in hyperthyroidism and the possibility of the presence of a circulating TSI blocker in some cases of nontoxic goitre may have a role in determining the natural history of both conditions.

REFERENCES

1.   P.P.A. Smyth, D. Neylan and D.K. O'Donovan.   JCEM 54: 357 (1982)

2.   P.P.A. Smyth, N.M.McMullan, B. Grubeck Loebenstein and D.K. O'Donovan. Acta Endocr. 111: 321 (1986)

3.   Editorial. Lancet ii: 1289 (1985)

A RETROSPECTIVE STUDY OF THYROID AUTOIMMUNITY AND HYPOTHYROI' DISM IN A RANDOM OBESE POPULATION

N. Lima, H. Cavaliere, and G.A. Medeiros-Neto

Thyroid Laboratory, Division of Endocrinology
Hospital das Clínicas, Univ. São Paulo Medical
School, 05403, São Paulo, Brazil

The frequency of autoimmune thyroiditis, that can be iden' tified by the presence of circulating thyroid autoantibodies, has been established in a number of epidemiological studies. Five substantial community surveys have been carried out and these have established that thyroglobulin or thyroid microsomal antibodies are found in 6.5 to 9.5% of the population with a fe' male to male ratio of 4:1 (1-5). There is also evidence that the age-specific prevalence increases with age in the female (4,5). A substantial proportion of subjects with autoimmune thyroiditis have no detectable disturbance of thyroid function, whereas the remainder have varying degrees of thyroid failure. In one commu' nity study approximately 40% of the subjects with autoimmune thy' roid disease have subclinical hypothyroidism (4) broadly similar or higher figures have been published by other workers (6). Fur' thermore it has been recently established that the risk of deve' loping clinical hypothyroidism is approximately 5% per year (6) and a somewhat higher figure has been reported in a highly se' lected population (7). The present report concerns a three-year follow-up of thyroid autoimmunity and subclinical hypothyroidism on a random sample of the obese out-patient population seen at, the University Hospital.

Patients and Methods

The patients were selected from the Obesity out-patient cli' nic in the University Hospital. The cause for their referral was excessive weight and need for nutritional correction. We have examined, consecutively, 1987 patients (1790 females and 197 ma' les) aged 32-69 years, selected from patients seen between 1982- 1986. Clinical examination, routine laboratory tests and a thy' roid function profile (T4, T3, TSH and microsomal antibodies) we' re performed in all patients. Serum thyroid hormones and TSH we' re assayed using commercial kits (Diagnostic Co., USA). The mi' crosomal antibody was assayed using a new technique (Fujirebio, Tokyo, Japan) substituting the tanned red cells usually employed in the hemagglutination method for gelatin particles coated with the antigen, as previously described (8). A standard TSH stimula' tion test, prior to medication, using 200 µg of synthetic TRH (EPM, São Paulo) injected as a iv bolus was performed in 168 sub' jects with a positive microsomal autoantibody test.

Results and Discussion

The results are shown in the Table 1. From the original po'pulation of 1987 patients 314 (15,8%) had a positive microsomal test, indicating the presence of autoantibodies (306 females, 8 males, ratio 7.6) against a cell surface antigen. These patients were subdivided in five groups:

G_1 (n= 34)   Hypothyroid patients (low T4, TSH > 6.0µU/ml)(TRH not performed).

G_2 (n=112)   Euthyroid subjects (normal T4, TSH < 6.0µU/ml)(With'out TRH test).

G_3 (n= 86)   Hypothyroid (low T4, TSH > 6.0µU/ml, exaggerated TSH response to TRH).

G_4 (n= 29)   Subclinical hypothyroidism (T4 N, TSH N but exagge'rated TSH response to TRH).

G_5 (n= 53)   Euthyroid subjects.

Table 1. Thyroid function tests and TRH stimulation test in pa'tients (n= 314) with thyroid autoimmune disease: hypo'thyroidism (G_1 and G_2), low thyroid reserve (G_4) and euthyroidism (G_2 and G_5). Mean ± SEM.

	T4 µg/dl	T3 ng/dl	TSHBasal µU/ml	TSHPeak µU/ml
G_1 (n= 34)	3.1 ± 0.2	95.9 ± 5.0	28.4 ± 4.6	-----
G_2 (n=112)	7.6 ± 0.3	147.0 ± 2.6	2.8 ± 0.1	-----
G_3 (n= 86)	3.2 ± 0.1**	103.1 ± 4.8**	56.5 ± 7.9**	119.5 ± 13.5**
G_4 (n= 29)	6.3 ± 0.4*	130 ± 7.0	3.8 ± 0.2*	48.9 ± 3.3
G_5 (n= 53)	7.7 ± 0.4	143.9 ± 8.5	2.5 ± 0.2	12.3 ± 1.0

**p > .001 as compared with group G4.
 *p > .001 as compared with group G5.

Thus in the total population examined (1987 patients) we we're able to find 120 subjects with "asymptomatic" hypothyroidism, that were never previously treated for their thyroid condition. Furthermore, the TRH test was able to indicate that an additional group of 29 patients had subclinical hypothyroidism, with normal thyroid hormone levels and basal TSH < 6.0µU/ml, but with an exag'gerated TSH peak response to TRH (> 28µU/ml). Twenty of these pa'tients seemed to be in a stable compensated state but 9 patients progressed to symptomatic hypothyroidism in the four years of follow-up. Hypothyroidism was associated with vitiligo in 7 pa'tients and with galactorrhea (with elevated serum prolactin le'vels) in 8 patients. The mean total cholesterol level was signi'ficantly elevated in the hypothyroid group (369 ± 53mg/dl) as compared with the low thyroid reserve group (303 ± 38mg/dl) and the euthyroid subjects (231 ± 18mg/dl).

The significance of thyroid autoimmune disease in an obese population is obviously of great interest. First these subjects are at risk of development of symptomatic hypothyroidism in the near future. Secondly, 16% of these overweight patients have thy'roid failure associated with hypercholesterolemia. Subclinical hypothyroidism has been considered as a risk factor for coronary heart disease. An increase incidence of ischemic heart disease have been described in subjects with autoimmune thyroiditis (9) and obviously obesity would add to that potential risk. Thus re'placement therapy and a nutritional program for reducing the

excessive weight are clearly important in this group of indivi'
duals, mostly because of the long term ill-effects of untreated
thyroid failure.

References

1. K.G.Couchman, R.D.Wigley, M.Prior, J Chronic Dis 23:
   45-53 (1970).
2. A.Gordin, O.P.Hemonen, P.Saarinen, B.A.Lamberg, Lancet
   I:551-554 (1972).
3. B.Hooper,S.Wihingham, J.D.Matthews, Clin Exp Immunol
   12:79-87 (1972).
4. W.M.G.Tunbridge, D.C.Evered, R.Hall, Clin Endocrinol
   (Oxf) 7:495-508 (1977).
5. G.B.Salabè, H.L.Salabè, G.Urbinati, G.Ricci, A.Fusco,
   M.Antonucci, A.B.Anguissola, In: Walfish P, Wall Jr &
   Volpé R (eds) AUTOIMMUNITY AND THE THYROID, Academic
   Press, New York, pp 317-318 (1985).
6. B.R.Hawkins, P.S.Cheah, R.L.Dawkins, Lancet II:1057-
   1059 (1980).
7. A.Gordin & B.A.Lamberg, Lancet II:1234-1238 (1975).
8. M.Knobel & G.Medeiros-Neto, J Endocrinol Invest 10:xxx
   (in press) (1986).
9. M.Tieche, G.A.Lupi, F.Gutzwiller, BR Heart J 46:202-
   206 (1981).

CIRCULATING THYROID AUTOANTIBODIES IN CHILDREN AND YOUNGSTERS WITH INSULIN
DEPENDENT DIABETES MELLITUS (IDDM) ARE NOT PREDICTIVE OF OVERT AUTOIMMUNE
THYROID DISEASE

F.De Luca, S. Bernasconi*, M. Vanelli*, M.F. Siracusano,
L.Di Geronimo°, M.D. Finocchiaro°, and F. Trimarchi°

Istituti di Clinica Pediatrica di Messina e di Parma*
Istituto di Clinica Medica di Messina°
Policlinico Universitario, 98100 Messina, Italy

INTRODUCTION

Several studies unanimously indicate an increased prevalence of circulating
thyroid antibodies in IDDM children,adolescents and young adults[1-6].The clinical significance and the prognostic value of this finding are controversial
in that the risk of overt thyroid disease is high in white North-Americans[1, 3]
and negligible in European patients[2,4-6].Aim of the present study is to evaluate the outcome of IDDM children and adolescents with circulating thyroid
antibodies longitudinally followed during a 5-year period.

PATIENTS AND METHODS

This study covers 99 IDDM subjects(50 males and 49 females),aged between 1.5
and 20.5 years(X 12.7),screened for thyroid microsomal antibodies(MCHA)and
thyroglobulin antibodies(TGHA) by passive haemagglutination methods.Serum
T_4,T_3 and TSH were measured by specific RIAs (Biodata,Milan,Italy).
In 77/99 patients TRH was administered intravenously and serum TSH was measured prior to and after i.v. TRH.Since then all patients were clinically re-
valuated 2-4 times per year.The subjects with circulating MCHA underwent a
second TRH test three years later and are being annually tested for MCHA,
TGHA,T_4,T_3 and TSH.The cases with initially absent MCHA are being annually
screened only for MCHA and TGHA.Control population for MCHA,TGHA,T_4,T_3 and
TSH consisted of 197 healthy children and young adults.TSH response to TRH
was regarded as normal if the peak fell within 3 SD from the mean obtained
for 26 age-matched controls.

RESULTS

The prevalence for MCHA in the serum of our IDDM patients (12.1 %) was significantly higher (X^2=9.5 , p< 0.005) as compared to the one found in the control sera (3%) .TGHA prevalence was also significantly different in both
groups (6.1 vs 0.5 % ;X^2=6.4 ,p< 0.025).MCHA titres persisted substantially
unchanged during the follow-up period in 6/12 patients,whereas they progressively declined through the follow-up period in other five cases.In only one
subject,MCHA were initially absent and became detectable three years later,
with no significant change in thyroid gland size and/or function indices.
No patient of the entire study group shows biochemical evidence of thyroid
dysfunction up to now.On the first sampling,supranormal serum T3 concentra-

tions,not associated with TSH hyporesponsiveness to TRH,were found in two cases(nos.5 and 12 of the Table),but they spontaneously normalized.Enhanced TSH response to TRH (peak > 24 μIU/ml)not associated to subnormal T4 values was initially observed in 4/9 MCHA positive patients (and in 6/68 without MCHA, X^2=8.9 ,p< 0.005)but such finding was not confirmed in two of them at the time of the second TRH test (nos.5 and 10 of the Table).

Table 1. Thyroid function tests in the 12/99 IDDM patients with MCHA at the beginning(A) and at the end (B) of the 5-year follow-up period

Cases	Sex	Titer of MCHA		T4 (μg/dl)		T3 (ng/dl)		TSH (μIU/ml)		TSH peak (μIU/ml)	
		A	B	A	B	A	B	A	B	A	B
1	F	1:1600	1:600	12.7	10.5	155	166	1.0	1.6	–	–
2	F	1:1600	1:1600	11.0	9.8	167	153	2.4	1.7	–	–
3	M	1:100	absent	7.5	10.1	180	187	3.7	1.3	15.4	–
4	F	1:1600	1:6400	7.3	7.2	208	–	3.4	2.5	10.4	14.8
5	F	1:25600	1:1600	6.1	10.3	265	99	3.1	3.0	28.2	19.5
6	F	absent	1:6400	8.0	7.6	195	137	2.4	1.8	–	–
7	F	1:400	1:100	8.8	6.7	136	92	2.9	1.8	16.8	–
8	F	1:100	absent	9.9	7.6	195	104	4.6	3.3	12.7	–
9	M	1:100	absent	9.2	6.5	221	172	5.2	2.2	28.6	29.5
10	M	1:6400	1:400	5.2	8.7	155	179	2.0	2.6	27.2	23.1
11	F	1:1600	1:1600	5.1	7.4	162	150	1.4	2.1	17.5	–
12	F	1:400	1:400	8.2	8.0	250	151	4.5	3.5	26.2	36.0

DISCUSSION

The proportion of diabetic patients carrying thyroid microsomal antibodies, varies widely in the different series, ranging from 6%[4] to 32%[1],but is generally higher in white North-Americans[1,3] than in Europeans[2,4-6]. Other important discrepancies between US reports and the European ones concern the clinical significance and the prognostic value of such humoral finding: the presence of thyroid microsomal antibodies frequently coincides with hypothyroidism (43%) or hyperthyroidism (7%)in US Caucasians[3], whilst the risk of overt thyroid disease appears negligible in European patients with such antibodies[2,4-6].However,whereas hyperthyroidism usually shows itself before or at the onset of diabetes,hypothyroidism tends to arise later[3]. Predictive value of circulating thyroid microsomal antibodies to overt thyroid disease,therefore,may be defined only on the basis of a prolonged follow-up. Our study,based on 5-year follow-up,confirms the increased prevalence of MCHA in the serum of IDDM patients,but indicates that no patient,with such antibodies was hyperthyroid at the moment of the first observation or developed overt or biochemical hypothyroidism during the longitudinal control. US Authors urge that all IDDM patients be screened for thyroid microsomal antibodies and that those with positive results undergo annual thyroid function tests[3]. In the light of our results such protocol is not likewise justified in European patients.

REFERENCES

1. G.M.Bright, R.M.Blizzard, D.L.Kaiser and W.L.Clarke, Organ-specific auto
   antibodies in children with common endocrine diseases,J.Pediatr.100:8(1982).
2. J.Kokkonen, J.Kiuttu, A.Mustonen and O.Räsänen, Organ-specific antibodies in healthy and diabetic children and young adults, Acta Paediatr.
   Scand. 71: 223 (1982).
3. W.Riley,N.Maclaren and A.Rosenbloom,Thyroid disease in young diabetics,
   Lancet ii:489(1982).
4. S.Salardi,A.Fava,A.Cassio,A.Cicognani,P.Tassoni,P.Pirazzoli,E.Frejaville,
   A.Balsamo,E.Cozzuti and E.Cacciari,Thyroid function and prolactin levels
   in insulin-dependent diabetic children and adolescents,Diabetes 33:522
   (1984).
5. F.Trimarchi,F.De Luca,M.Vanelli,S.Benvenga,M.F.Siracusano,C.Volta and S.
   Bernasconi,Circulating thyroid antibodies and thyroid function studies in
   children and adolescents with insulin-dependent diabetes mellitus,Eur.J.Pe-
   diatr.142:253(1984).
6. R.Lorini,D.Larizza,C.Livieri,V.Cammareri,A.Martini,A.Plebani,D.Zanaboni and
   F.Severi,Autoimmunity in children with diabetes mellitus and in their relatives,Eur.J.Pediatr.145:182(1986).

EFFECTS OF CHRONIC AMIODARONE ADMINISTRATION ON HUMORAL THYROID AUTOIMMUNITY

Enio Martino*, Fabrizio Aghini-Lombardi, Stefano Mariotti, Luigi Bartalena, Lucia Grasso and Aldo Pinchera

Cattedra di Endocrinologia, University of Pisa and (*) Cattedra di Endocrinologia, University of Cagliari, Pisa and Cagliari, Italy

INTRODUCTION

Amiodarone, an iodine-rich drug (75 mg/200 mg tablet), is widely used for the treatment of tachyarrhythmias and/or ischaemic heart disease. This drug inihbits the phenolic outer ring deiodination of thyroxine (T4) and 3,3',5'-triodothyronine (rT3) resulting in both decreased production of 3,5,5'-triiodothyronine (T3) from T4, causing a reduction and an elevation of circulating T3 and T4, respectively, and a decreased deiodination of rT3, resulting in an elevated serum rT3 concentration[1].

In addition to the effects on the peripheral metabolism of the thyroid hormones, a major complication of the amiodarone administration is the relatively high frequency of either hyperthyroidism (amiodarone-iodine-induced thyrotoxicosis, AIIT) or hypothyroidism (amiodarone-iodine-induced hypothyroidism, AIIH)[2-4]. The mechanism by which amiodarone induces thyroid dysfunction has not been elucidated; in particular, it is unclear whether amiodarone per se or iodine released from the drug may induce autoimmune reactions responsible for thyroid hyper or hypofunction. In keeping with this concept, recent studies carried out in animals and humans[5-9] suggest that excess iodine may trigger thyroid autoimmunity.

The purpose of this investigation was to evaluate whether and to what extent chronic amiodarone treatment may induce thyroid autoimmune phenomena.

MATERIALS AND METHODS

Retrospective study

To this purpose, the prevalence of anti-thyroblobulin (TgAb) and anti-thyroid microsomal (MAb) antibodies was evaluated in 58 patients with AITT, 28 patients with AIIH and 390 euthyroid subjects chronically treated with amiodarone.

Longitudinal study

In this study, the occurrence of TgAb and/or MAb was assessed in 29 euthyroid subjects before, during and at various time intervals after amiodarone treatment. The follow-up period ranged 1-36 months.

Antibody assays

TgAb and MAb were detected by passive hemagglutination using commercial kits (Fujizoki Pharmaceutical Co., Tokyo, Japan).

RESULTS

Retrospective study

The prevalence of positive TgAb and/or MAb in euthyroid amiodarone-treated subjects was 7%, not significantly different from that previously reported in normal controls[10]. The prevalence of positive TgAb and/or MAb was 24% and 34% in AIIT and in AIIH patients, respectively (Fig.1). However, the large majority of positive antibody tests were confine to patients with independent evidence of Graves' disease (12/14, i.e. 85%) for AIIT and Hashimoto's thyroiditis (9/10, i.e. 90%) for AIIH.

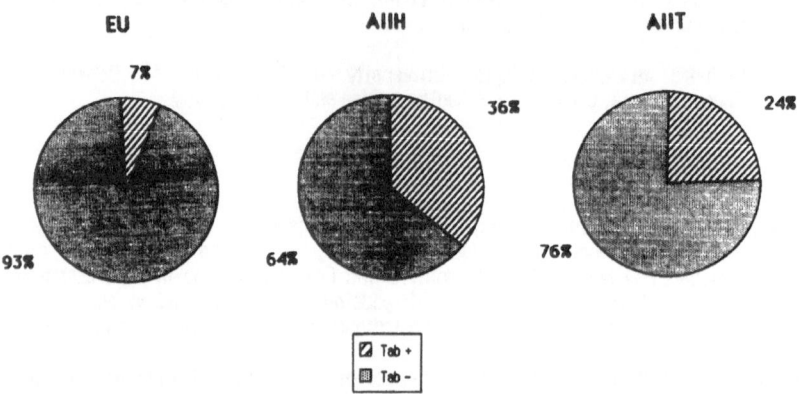

Fig. 1. Incidence of positive (Tab+) and negative (Tab-) thyroid antibody tests in 390 euthyroid subjects under chronic amiodarone treatment (EU), in 28 patients with AIIH and in 58 with AIIT.

Longitudinal study

In the prospective study serum thyroid autoantibodies were undetectable in 28 out 29 subjects before amiodarone treatment and remained negative during administration and after drug withdrawal. Two of these patients developed AIIT and one AIIH. Low titer (1/400) MAb was detected before amiodarone therapy in the remaining euthyroid subject and no change was observed during the follow-up (Table I).

Table 1.   Thyroid autoantibodies and clinical outcome in 29 euthyroid patients during and after chronic amiodarone treatment

	Thyroid autoantibody tests				
	Negative			Positive	
Pretreatment	28			1	
During therapy	28			1	
Final observation	28			1	
Clinical outcome	Eu* 25	AIIT 2	AIIH 1	Eu* 1	

*) Euthyroid

600

CONCLUSIVE REMARKS

The results obatained in the present study indicate that chronic amiodarone administration is not associated with an increased prevalence of circulating thyroid autoantibodies in euthyroid subjects, and that in AIIT and AIIH circulating thyroid autoantibodies are detected only in patients with evidence of coexisting thyroid autoimmune diseases. It is worth noting that in the longitudinal study the amiodarone-treated patients who developed AIIT or AIIH had negative antibody tests at any time interval considered.

Thus, it would appear that amiodarone per se has no relevant effects on humoral thyroid autoimmunity. On the other hand, the excess of iodine released from the drug seems to facilitate the development of thyrotoxicosis or hypothyroidism in subjects with subclinical thyroid autoimmune disorders and circulating thyroid autoantibodies.

AKNOWLEDGEMENTS

This work was partially supported by C.N.R. (Rome, Italy), Target Project "Preventive Medicine and Rehabilitation" Subproject "Mechanisms of aging", Grant n° 86.01899.56.

REFERENCES

1. A. Burger, C., Dinichert, P. Nicod, P. Tenny, T. Lemarchand-Béraud and M.B. Vallotton, Effects of amiodarone on serum triiodothyronine, reverse triiodothyronine, thyroxine and thyrotropin: a drug influencing peripheral metabolism of thyroid hormones, J. Clin. Invest. 58:255 (1976).
2. J. E. Fradkin and J. Wolff, Iodine-induced thyrotoxicosis, Medicine 62:1 (1983).
3. E. Martino, M. Safran, F. Aghini-Lombardi, R. Rajanatanavin, M. Lenziardi, M. Fay, A. Pacchiarotti, N. Aronin, E. Macchia, C. Haffaje, L. Odoguardi, J. Love, A. Bigalli, L. Baschieri, A.Pinchera and L.E.Braverman, Environmental iodine intake and thyroid dysfunction during chronic amiodarone therapy, Ann. Intern. Med. 101:28 (1984).
4. G.C. Hawthorne, N.P.S. Campbell, J.S. Geddes, W.R. Ferguson, W. Postlehwaite, B. Sheridan and A.B. Atkinson, Amiodarone-induced hypothyroidism. A common complication of prolonged therapy: a report of eight cases, Arch. Inten. Med. 145:1016 (1985).
5. E. Martino, E. Macchia, F. Aghini-Lombardi, A. Antonelli, M. Lenziardi, R. Concetti, G.F. Fenzi, L. Baschieri and A. Pinchera, Is humoral autoimmunity relevant in amiodarone iodine-induced thyrotoxicosis (AIIT)? Clin. Endocrinol. (Oxf.) 24: 627 (1986).
6. N. Bagchi, T.R. Brown, E. Urdanivia and R.S. Sundick, Induction of autoimmune thyroiditis in chickens by dietary iodine, Science 230:325 (1985).
7. M.A. Boukis, D.A. Koutras, A. Souvatzoglou, A. Evangelopoulou, M. Vrontakis, K.S. Karaiskos, G.D. Piperingos, J. Kitsopanidis and S.D. Moulopoulos, Iodine-induced autoimmunity. In: Thyroid disorders associated with iodine deficiency and excess, R. Hall, J. Köbberling, eds., Raven Press, New York (1985).
8. A.M. Mc Gregor, A.P. Weetman, S. Ratachaiyavong, G.M. Owen, H.K. Ibberson, R. Hall, Iodine: an influence on the development of autoimmune thyroid disease? In: Thyroid disorders associated with iodine deficiency and excess, R. Hall, J. Köbberling, eds., Raven Press, New York (1985).
9. E. Monteiro, A. Galvao-Teles, M.L. Santos, L. Mourao, M.J. Correia, J. Lopo Tuna and C. Ribeiro, Antithyroid antibodies as an early marker for thyroid disease induced by amiodarone, Br. Med. J. 292:227 (1986).
10. S. Mariotti, A. Pinchera, P. Vitti, L. Chiovato, C. Marcocci, C. Urbano, M. Tosi and L. Baschieri, Comparison of radioassay and haemagglutination methods for anti-thyroid microsomal antibodies, Clin. Exp. Immunol. 34:118 (1978).

SERUM THYROID AUTOANTIBODIES IN PATIENTS WITH BREAST CANCER

U. Feldt-Rasmussen, B. Rasmusson, K. Bech, L. Hegedüs, M. Høier-Madsen, and H. Perrild

Dept of Med E, Frederiksberg Hosp, Dept of Med F
Gentofte Univ Hosp, Dept of Onkol and Endocrinol
Herlev Univ Hosp, and State Serum Inst, Denmark

INTRODUCTION

Previously, an association between Hashimoto's thyroiditis
and breast cancer has been suggested[1]. It is controversial
whether thyroid dysfunction plays a role in the pathogenesis
of breast cancer. The conflicting results may partly be explained by differences in the control groups[2,3,4].The aim of
the present study was to investigate thyroid function and signs
of autoimmune disease in patients with breast cancer, and compare results with those obtained from age-matched controls,
all from the same area without endemic goitre.

MATERIAL AND METHODS

Sixty-two consecutive patients admitted to the Department
of Oncology, Herlev University Hospital after mastectomy for
mammary carcinoma, and 13 patients with recurrent disease more
than 6 months after previous treatment were considered for the
study. Excluded were patients with known past or present thyroid
disease (n=2), interfering medication (n=2), other cancers, impaired renal function or liver disease (n=0) or missed blood
samples (n=12). Thus 58 patients (median age 56 years, range:
27-80 years) were included after informed consent:
Group 1   23 patients recently operated for local mammary car-
           cinoma,
Group 2   23 patients recently operated for mammary carcinoma
           with metastases to axillary lymph nodes,
Group 3   12 patients with disseminated disease treated more
           than 6 months previously with either high voltage,
           irradiation, endocrine- or chemotherapy.
The control group consisted of 75 healthy age-matched women
without a goitre or evidence of previous or present thyroid
disease. None received any medication. Blood was sampled 16-42
days after operation in group 1 and 2. Antithyroglobulin anti-
bodies(TgAb) were measured by radio-coprecipitation technique[5],
and microsomal antibodies(MAb) by immunofluorescence. Thyroid
stimulating antibodies(TSAb) were measured by an adenylate cyclase stimulating assay using human thyroid homogenate[6], and

Table 1. Thyroid autoantibodies in 58 patients with breast cancer.

Antibody	Number positive
TSAb	17
TgAb + MAb	5
TgAb + MAb + TSAb	3
MAb	2
TgAb	1
TgAb + TSAb	1
Total number positive	29 = 50%

serum thyroglobulin(Tg)[7], serum thyroxine(T4), triiodothyronine
(T3), TSH, and T3-uptake test were all measured by radioimmuno-
logical methods.

RESULTS

There was no significant difference in serum concentrations
of T4, T3, TSH or free T4 and T3 indices between patients and
controls. Nor was there any difference between the patient groups
Serum Tg level in patients without TgAb was not different from
that of controls, median: 20.4 ug/l (range: 7.6-185 ug/1), and
22.9 ug/l (range: 2.2-77 ug/1), respectively. Thyroid autoantibodies were present in 29 patients (50%)(Table 1). Ten patients
had TgAb (median: 26 kU/l, range 8-650 kU/1) compared with 3
controls (39 kU/l range 20-1350 kU/1)(P 0.05 by Chi square test)
MAb were found in 1/10-1/160 dilution. A total of 21 patients
(36%9 had TSAb above 108% (median 118%, range 110-156%). The
autoantibodies were equally distributed in the three groups.
There was no relationship between presence of the antibodies
and previous irradiations. No difference in thyroid autoantibodies was noted in relation to thyroid function or serum Tg.
Other serum autoimmune antibodies against salivary gland, adre-
nocortex, parietal cell, smooth muscle tissue, mitochondria, DNA,
extractable nuclear antigen, antinuclear, IgM rheumatoid factor,
granulocyte specific antinuclear were sparsely occurring like in
normal controls (data not shown).

DISCUSSION

In the present study thyroid function was not significantly
different in patients with breast cancer compared to age-matched
controls, in agreement with the study by Abe et al.[8], but in
contrast to others[4,9]. It has not been verified, however, if
the possible changes were due to a specific interrelation between
breast cancer and the thyroid, or to a result of the well-known
influence of non-thyroidal disease on thyroid function[10]. There
was a marked increase in the frequency of thyroid autoantibodies
(both TgAb, MAb, and TSAb) in the patients with breast cancer
compared to the controls, and no evidence of a general autoimmune
activation. This has also been controversial[1,4,11], probably due
to differences in selection of patient and control groups, or to
population differences. In the present study there was no relationship between thyroid antibodies and previous treatment of the

cancer. The levels of the autoantibodies were in all cases low to moderately elevated. The presence of TSAb at low levels without evidence of in vivo thyroid stimulation has been recorded in other diseases of presumable autoimmune origin[12]. Presence of TgAb and MAb without evidence of thyroid dysfunction has been described as asymptomatic autoimmune thyroiditis, which may proceed ultimately to hypothyroidism[13]. Only long-time follow-up may clarify if the antibody positive patients with breast cancer are more exposed to develop overt thyroid dysfunction.

REFERENCES

1. K. Itoh, and N. Maruchi, Breast cancer in patients with Hashimoto's thyroiditis, Lancet ii:1119(1975).
2. C.C. Kapdi, and J.N. Wolfe, Breast cancer. Relationship to thyroid supplements for hypothyroidism, JAMA 236:1124(1976).
3. D.A. Hoffman, W.M. McConahey, L.A. Brinton, and J.F. Fraumeni, Breast cancer in hypothyroid women using thyroid supplements, JAMA 251:616(1984).
4. D.A. Adamopoulos, S. Vassilaros, N. Kapolla, J. Papadiamantis, F. Georgiakodis, and A. Michalakis, Thyroid disease in patients with benign and malignant mastopathy, Cancer 57:125(1986).
5. J. Date, U. Feldt-Rasmussen, P.H. Petersen, and K. Bech, An improved co-precipitation assay for determination of thyroglobulin antibodies, Scand.J.Clin.Lab.Invest.40:37 (1980).
6. K. Bech, Immunological aspects of Graves' disease and importance of thyroid stimulating immunoglobulins, Acta Endocrinol.103, suppl 254:1(1983).
7. U. Feldt-Rasmussen, I. Holten, and H.S. Hansen, Influence of thyroid substitution therapy and thyroid autoantibodies on the value of serum thyroglobulin in recurring thyroid cancer, Cancer 51:2240(1983).
8. R. Abe, A. Hirosaki, and M. Kimura, Pituitary-thyroid function in patients with breast cancer, Tohoku J.Exp.Med. 132:231(1980).
9. D.P. Rose, and T.E. Davis, Plasma thyronine levels in carcino,a of the breast and colon, Arch.Intern.Med. 141:116(1981).
10. I.J. Chopra, J.M. Hershman, W.M. Pardridge, and J.T. Nicoloff, Thyroid function in nonthyroidal illnesses, Ann. Intern.Med. 98:946(1983).
11. I. Mittra, J. Perrin, and S. Kamaoka, Thyroid and other autoantibodies in British and Japanese women: An epidemiological study of breast cancer. Brit.Med.J.1:257(1976).
12. K. Bech, H. Bliddal, and U. Feldt-Rasmussen, Relationship between thyroid stimulating antibodies and other autoantibodies in thyroid diseases, in:"Current Topics in Thyroid Autoimmunity", D. Doniach, H. Schleusener, eds., G. Thieme Verlag, Stuttgart(1984).
13. A. Gordin, and B.-A. Lamberg, Spontaneous hypothyroidism in symptomless autoimmune thyroiditis. A long-term followup study. Clin.Endocrinol.(Oxf)15:537(1981).

COMPLEMENT ACTIVITIES AND CIRCULATING IMMUNE COMPLEXES IN SERA

OF PATIENTS WITH GRAVES' DISEASE AND HASHIMOTO'S THYROIDITIS

K.Kaise, T.Sakurada, N.Kaise, K. Yoshida, T. Nomura,
H.Itagaki, M.Yamamoto, S.Saito, and K.Yoshinaga

2nd Department of Internal Medicine
Tohoku University, School of Medicine
Sendai, Japan

INTRODUCTION

In autoimmune thyroid diseases various immunological abnormalities
were observed. Circulating immune complexes (CIC) have been detected in
sera from patients with Graves' disease(GD) and Hashimoto's thyroiditis
(HT). Intrathyroidal deposition of immune complexes was reported in these
diseases. But the role of CIC in these diseases is not clear. Deposition
of immune complexes induces activation of complement system and leads
cells to lysis. In these process serum complements are consumed and its
activities are reduced in some autoimmune diseases such as systemic lupus
erythematodes and serum sickness. In such diseases serum complement
activities were reported to correlate with the activity of the disease.
In this report we studied about CIC and serum complement activities in
patients with GD and HT to clarify the role of CIC and complement in these
diseases.

MATERIALS AND METHODS

Sera from 20 patients with untreated GD and 28 patients with HT were
subjected to be evaluated serum complement activities and CIC levels.
Blood was kept at room temperature for 1hr and centrifuged at $300 \times g$ for
15 min. Serum samples were stored at $-80°C$ and examined within 4 weeks.
Once thawed, the sera were not stored again.

Circulating Immune Complex

Clq solid phase enzyme immunoassay. The polystylene microtiter plate
coated with purified rabbit Clq was used according to the method of Fukuda
et al. (1985a). Briefly, 100 μl of serum sample diluted 1:12 was added
into the well and incubated at 37°C for 1hr. After washing the well with
PBS-Tween 20, anti-IgG labeled with horseradish peroxidase (HRPO; Sigma
Co.) was added and incubated at 37°C for 1 hr, and the bound HRPO activity
as CIC values developed with O-phenylendiamine was determined by optical
density scanning of the plate at OD492 (Corona E. Co., MTT-12).

Anti-C3 solid phase binding assay. Anti-C3 assay was carried out by
the method of Fukuda et al.(1985b). Briefly, 5% PEG precipitate serum
diluted 1:12 was added into the polystylene microtiter plate coated with

F(ab')2 anti-C3 and incubated at 37°C for 1 hr. After washing with PBS-Tween 20, anti-IgG labeled with HRPO was added, and bound HRPO activity was determined as CIC values as described above.

Complement activity

Total hemolytic activity (CH50) was measured according to Mayer's method. Alternative complement pathway activity (AH50) was measured using rabbit erythrocytes (Platts-Mills and Ishizaka 1974). Serum C3 and C4 concentrations were measured with single radial diffusion using commercially available test kits. Normal ranges of CH50, AH50, and C3 and C4 concentrations were 30 - 45 U/ml, 6 - 12 U/ml, 50 - 100 mg/dl and 15 - 40 mg/dl, respectively.

Other assays

Antithyroglobulin and antimicrosomal antibodies were measured by commercially available hemmaglutination test kits. Serum T4 was measured by radioimmunoassay.

RESULTS

In the present study normal ranges of CIC values measured by C1q binding and anti-C3 assay were below 3 μg AHG/ml and below 2 μg AHG/ml respectively. By C1q binding assay CIC were detected in sera of 2 patients with HT, but not detected in sera of patients with GD. By anti-C3 assay CIC were detected in sera of 7 patients(35%) with GD and 13 patients (50%) with HT. There was no correlation between values measured by C1q binding assay and anti-C3 assay in these patients.

CH50 values were elevated in one and slightly decreased in 3 patients with GD, and were normal in all patients with HT. AH50 were elevated in 8 patients (44%) with GD and 8 patients (33%) with HT. There was no patient with low AH50. Serum C3 concentrations were elevated in 8 patients with GD and 8 patients with HT. In one patient with HT C3 level decreased. Serum C4 concentrations were elevated in 4 patients with GD and 8 patients with HT. There was no patient with low C4 concentrations.

In patients with GD significant negative correlations(p < 0.01) were observed CIC values measured by C1q binding assay with AH50, C3 and C4 concentrations. No correlation was observed between CIC values measured by anti-C3 assay and serum complement activities. In patients with HT there was no correlation between CIC values and serum complement activities. Then we evaluated the relations of serum complement activities and serum T4 concentrations. Positive correlations of serum T4 concentrations with C3 and C4 concentrations were observed in patients with HT but not in patients with GD. Serum T4 levels of patients with HT were 1.2 to 13.0 μg/dl(normal:4.5 - 13). There was no correlaiton of antimicrosomal and antithyroglobulin antibodies with CIC values or serum complement activities.

DISCUSSION

In present study frequencies of elevated levels of CIC in GD and HD were 35% and 50%, respectively, using anti-C3 assay. These results were compatible with those of Calder et al.(1974) (17% in GD and 59% in HT). But using C1q binding assay elevated levels of CIC values were detected in only two patients(7%) with HT. Different frequencies of elevated CIC values, however, have been reported in literatures (Feldt-Rasmussen et

al., 1979 and Mariotti et al., 1979). These discrepancies could be due to
the different methods employed. In this study there was no correlation
between CIC values by Clq binding assay and those by anti-C3 assay. Anti-
C3 assay using PEG precipitated serum is supposed to detect heavy molecular weight CIC. Serum complement activities were elevated in several
patients with GD and HT. AH50 were elevated in 44% of GD and 33% of HT.
C3 and C4 concentrations were also elevated. Serum complement activities
were reported to be elevated in small number of patients with rheumatoid
arthritis(RA). It is speculated that in RA intraarticular inflammation
consumes complements in the synovial fluid but increases the production of
complements in the body. In this study CIC values by Clq binding assay
were correlated with AH50, C3 and C4 levels in GD. These results may be
explained by the fact that alternative pathway of the complement is essential for solubilization of immune complexes (Takahashi et al., 1980).
Serum complements also play a role in the clearance of immune complexes.
So elevated complement activities in GD and HT may work against deposition
of CIC and induction of tissue damage. Correlation of complement levels
with serum T4 in HT may suggest that thyroid function affects the production of complement.

REFERENCE

E.A. Calder, W.J. Penhale, E.W. Barness and W.J. Irvine, 1974, Evidence
        for circulating immune complexes in thyroid disease, Brit Med J.,
        2:30.
U. Feldt-Rasmussen, K. Beck, J. Date, J.H. Larsen and H. Nielsen, 1979,
        Anticomplementary activity in diffuse and nodular goitors, Acta
        Path Microbiol Scand Sect., 87:365.
K. Fukuda, J. Seino, Y. Kinoshita, K. Sudo, I. Horigome, T. Saito, T.
        Furuyama and K. Yoshinaga, 1985a, Circulating immune complex-like
        materials which bind heat inactivated Clq interfere with the Clq
        solid phase assay for immune complexes, Tohoku J Exp Med.,
        146:449.
K. Fukuda, J. Seino, Y. Kinoshita, K. Sudo, I. Horigome, T. Furuyama
        and K. Yoshinaga, 1985b, Modified anti-C_3 immune complex assay
        which avoids inteference by anti-F(ab')$_2$ antibodies, Tohoku J Exp
        Med., 146:337.
S. Mariotti, L.J. DeGroot, D. Scarborough and M.E. Medof, 1979, Study
        of circulating immune complexes in thyroid diseases: comparison
        of Raji cell radioimmunoassay and specific thyroglobulin-
        antithyroglobulin radioassay, J Clin Endocrinol., 49:679.
T.A.E. Platts-Mills and K. Ishizaka, 1974, Activation of the alterna-
        tive pathway of human complement by rabbit cells, J Immunol.,
        113:348.
M. Takahashi, S. Takahashi and S. Hirose, 1980, Solubilization of
        antigen-antibody complexes: a new function of complement as a
        receptor of immune reactions, Prog Allergy., 27:134.

ABNORMALITIES OF THYROID FUNCTION IN SJÖGREN'S SYNDROME

G. Villone, N. Panza, D. Tramontano, B. Merola,
M. Columbo, G. Lombardi, F.S. Ambesi-Impiombato
and G. Marone

Second Medical School, University of Naples
Naples, Italy

INTRODUCTION

Siögren's syndrome is a chronic inflammatory disease, characterized by diminished lacrimal and salivary gland secretion, the "sicca complex", resulting in keratoconjunctivitis and xerostomia. The spectrum of the disease includes a primary form and a secondary form accompanying rheumatoid arthritis or occasionally other diseases of the connective tissue.

Recent observations suggest that the incidence of both primary and secondary forms of Siögren's syndrome is higher than previously reported (1). In addition, Sjögren's syndrome is a disorder in which a benign autoimmune disease can terminate in a malignant lymphoid disorder. Thus, it is a "crossroad" disease that offers potential insight into the mechanism by which B-lymphocytes may become malignant.

The glandular insufficiency in Sjögren's syndrome is secondary to lymphocytic and plasmacell infiltrations. Strand and Talal (2) have recently introduced the term "autoimmune exocrinopathy" for Sjögren's syndrome. Although the involvement of exocrine glands is the hallmark of Sjögren's, abnormalities of thyroid function have been described among these patients (3).

The aim of this study was to estimate the incidence of thyroid function abnormalities in patients with Sjögren's syndrome. Furthermore, in preliminary experiments we examined the ability of sera from these patients to stimulate DNA synthesis in FRTL5 cells.

MATERIALS AND METHODS

Nine outpatients of our Clinical Immunology Department affected with Sjögren's syndrome voluntaired to an evaluation of thyroid functions. The diagnosis of Sjögren's syndrome was established according to standardized criteria (1). All patients were women (age 60.0 ± 3.4 years)). Two of these had an uninodular non-toxic goiter, one had a diffuse non-toxic goiter and another one had been previously submitted to partial thyroidectomy because of a cystic nodule. Serum levels of T_3, T_4, $F-T_3$, $F-T_4$ and basal TSH were determined by radioimmunoassay. Thyroglobulin (Tg), antithyroglobulin and antimicrosomal antibodies were measured by immunoradiometric methods. TSH response to TRH (200 µg i.v.) was calculated by the net increase (Δ-TSH). 38 healthy females in post-menopause were matched as controls. Data were analyzed by Student's test for unpaired data.

FRTL5 cells (4) proliferation was assayed by ^{3}H-thymidine incorporation into DNA.

RESULTS

Mean ($\pm$ SD) of basal hormone levels in Sjögren's patients were as following: T_3: 1.77 $\pm$ 0.4 nM/L; T_4: 98.9 $\pm$ 17.05 nM/L; F-T_3: 6.3 $\pm$ 1.08 pM/L; F-T_4: 14.6 $\pm$ 2.3 pM/L; Tg: 51.9 $\pm$ 38.1 µg/L; TSH: 2.85 $\pm$ 1.2 mU/L. In Sjögren's patients basal serum TSH and Tg levels were significantly higher than in healthy females ($p<0.05$ and $p<0.001$, respectively). The Δ-TSH in Sjögren's patients (11.8 $\pm$ 9.4 mU/L) was not significantly different from that of 38 controls. However, 3 patients had increased TSH response to TRH and 1 had no response to TRH. Serum levels of anti-Tg antibodies were undetectable; circulating levels of antimicrosomal antibodies were found in 3 out of 9 patients.

When tested on quiescent FRTL5 cells, sera from patients affected with Sjögren's syndrome increase ^{3}H-thymidine incorporation into DNA at all concentrations tested (0.5, 1 and 5%/ml), compared to normal serum tested at the same concentrations (Table 1).

DISCUSSION

Consistent with recent data in the literature (5), our results indicate that patients with Sjögren's syndrome have an high incidence of thyroid abnormalities. We have shown that a clear impairment of thyroid functions could be observed in 4 out of 9 patients. In addition, 33% of patients presented in this study show an exaggerated TSH response to TRH stimulation, suggesting the possible coexistence of subclinical hypothyroidism with this disease.

The presence of mild hypothyroidism symptoms, such as dry skin, lethargy and puffyness, may occur in patients with Sjögren's syndrome. We suggest that a complete study of thyroid functions should be part of the routine evaluation of these patients in order to sort out patients with a real thyroid function impairment.

The high frequency of hypothyroidism in patients with Sjögren's syndrome could be caused by idiopathic Hashimoto's thyroiditis. The two syndromes have a common genetic background that can explain the enhanced susceptibility to both deseases (5, 6).

The ability of some sera from Sjögren's patients to stimulate ^{3}H-thymidine incorporation into DNA of FRTL5 cells is suggestive of the

TABLE 1

^{3}H-thymidine incorporation into DNA of the FRTL5 cells *
(data expressed as fold increase over basal)

controls	Sjögren's syndrome
case 1: 23.39	patient 1: 32.48
2: 18.13	2: 29.08
3: 17.42	3: 30.88
Average: 19.64 $\pm$ 2.6	Average : 30.81 $\pm$ 1.3

* treated with 5% serum (either controls or Sjögren's)

presence of a mitogenic activity; it will be of great interest to investigate on the biochemical nature of this factor(s).

ACKNOWLEDGEMENT

G. V. is recipient of a fellowship from the "Associazione Italiana per la Ricerca sul Cancro" (A.I.R.C.).

REFERENCES

1) Whaley K. and Buchanan W.W., 1980, Sjögren's syndrome and associated disease, in: "Clinical Immunology" vol. I, C.W. Parker, ed., W.B. Saunders, Philadelphia.
2) Strand V. and Talal N., 1980, Advances in the diagnosis and concept of Sjögren's syndrome (autoimmune exocrinopathy), Bul. Rheum. Dis, 30:1046.
3) Karsh J., Pavlidis N., Weintaub B.D. and Moutsopoulos H.M., 1980, Thyroid disease in Sjögren's syndrome, Arth. Rheum., 23:1326.
4) Ambesi-Impiombato F.S., Picone R. and Tramontano D., 1982, Influence of hormones and serum on growth and differentiation of thyroid cell strain FRTL, Cold Spring Harbor Conf. Cell Prolif., 9:483.
5) Moens H. and Farid N.R., 1978, Hashimoto's thyroiditis is associated with HLA-DRw3, New Engl. J. Med., 299:133.
6) Moutsopoulos H.M., Mann D.L., Johnson A.H. and Chused T.M., 1979, Genetic differences between primary and secondary sicca syndrome, New Engl. J. Med., 301:761.

THYROID AND RENAL AMYLOIDOSIS IN THYROGLOBULIN IMMUNIZED RABBITS

B. N. Premachandra and H. T. Blumenthal

Veterans Administration Medical Center and
Washington University
St. Louis, Missouri

INTRODUCTION

A variety of forms of immune complex nephritis have been reported in human thyroid disorders of immune origin [1], as well as in animals with an induced lymphocytic thyroiditis [2]. Several types of amyloid also represent expressions of immune system disorders. However, there are no reports of thyroid or renal amyloid associated with human thyroid disorders of immune origin, or in thyroglobulin (Tg) immunized animals. In recent investigations in animals with induced lymphocytic thyroiditis we observed amyloid lesions in thyroid and kidney.

MATERIALS AND METHODS

Six month old New Zealand male albino rabbits were used and were fed Purina lab chow ad libitum. The experimental groups received three weekly intramuscular injections (1 ml) of 1% bovine (n = 36), porcine (n = 22) or human Tg (n = 5) (total of 3 ml per rabbit) in Freund's complete adjuvant. Fifteen rabbits immunized against bovine Tg were also challenged with repeated intravenous doses of antigen (5 mg Tg per animal) for a period of 8 weeks. A control group of 7 rabbits received adjuvant only. A group of untreated rabbits were also maintained. A tanned red cell (TRC) agglutination technique was used to monitor serum Tg antibody levels. Immediately after death all organs were removed and representative blocks were fixed in 10% formalin, embedded in paraffin; sections were stained with haematoxylin-eosin/congo red and were screened for evidence of hyaline deposits. In positive cases, additional sections were subjected to potassium permanganate [3]. Sections of thyroid and kidney were subsequently additionally fixed in Karnovsky solution and stained with lead citrate and uranyl acetate for electron microscopy. Immunological studies for examining immune complex deposits incorporating Tg as the antigen were also carried out.

RESULTS

Characteristics of the Hyaline Lesions

Hyaline lesions were found in the thyroid and kidney of the immunized rabbits, but not in controls. In the thyroid the hyaline was deposited in the interstitial tissues, replacing some thyroid follicles while associated with atrophy of others (Fig. 1). In the renal glomeruli, hyaline was present in a nodular or diffuse form (Fig. 2) or a mixture of the two. The hyaline material was congophilic and exhibited typical green birefringence when examined with polarized light. Electron microscopy of the hyaline substance demonstrated fibrils typical of amyloid (Fig. 3). Following treatment with potassium permanganate most of the congophilic material in the thyroid and glomeruli was removed. Treatment of sections of thyroid with peroxidase tagged anti-rabbit IgG and anti-Tg gave a negative reaction in the hyaline deposits. Tubular casts and periglomerular fluid accumulations (which were negative for amyloid) gave positive reactions, and they were also positive with peroxidase tagged anti-C_3.

Analysis of Thyroid and Renal Lesions

A fairly marked thyroiditis was present in 25% of immunized rabbits with the highest incidence (40%) in the group receiving supplementary Tg injections after the initial immunization series. Amyloid deposits were present in 17% of the immunized rabbits, but all of these were in animals receiving only the initial immunization series. About 44% of the immunized rabbits had normal kidneys, and about another 12% showed only the adjuvant lesion. Diffuse glomerular lesions were present in about 8%, and another 17% showed only nodular glomerular lesions. A mixture of these two forms was found in 19% of the immunized animals. Rabbits which received supplementary injections of Tg showed only nodular glomerular lesions.

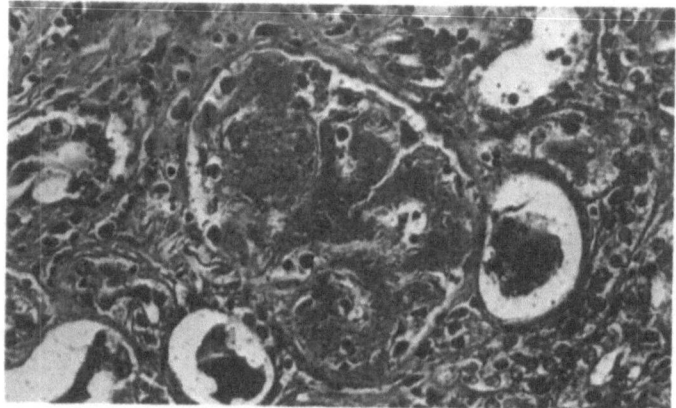

Figure 1.

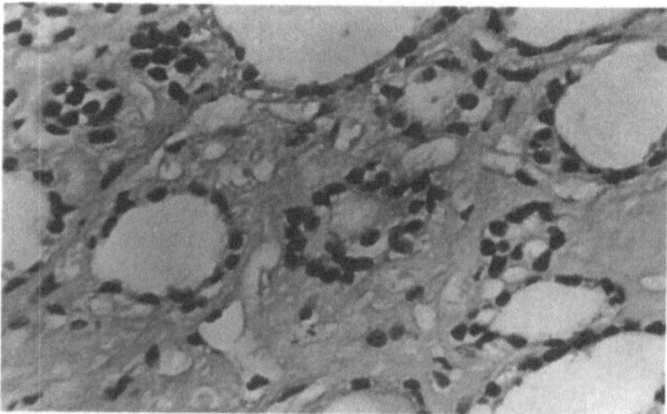

Figure 2.

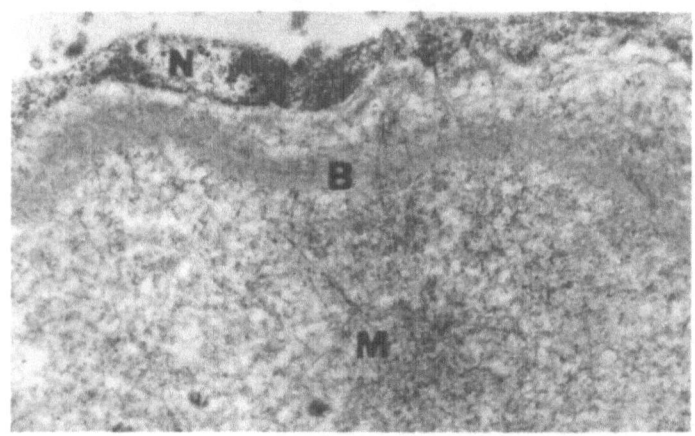

Figure 3.

DISCUSSION

The principal findings in this study are that immunization with Tg in Freund's adjuvant and observation over a period of 6-34 months revealed a moderate lymphocytic thyroidits in about 25% of rabbits, and interstitial amyloid of the thyroid in 17.3%. In the kidney, glomerular and interstitial amyloid deposits were found in about 44% of the immunized animals. Moreover, renal amyloidosis was found in association with lymphocytic thyroiditis as well as with amyloidosis of the thyroid, and there was a small percentage of immunized animals which showed only thyroid lesions or only renal amyloid. The reactions with permanganate indicate a predominance of AA type amyloid. The frequency of thyroid or renal lesions did not correlate with Tg antibody titres. One study in C_3H mice [4] reports systemic amyloidosis with thyroid involvement induced with goitrogens or x-irradiation of the thyroid, procedures which may have induced thyroid immunity.

SUMMARY

The findings noted represent the first report of amyloidosis induced by Tg immunization and are of clinical significance. They suggest that those cases of amyloidosis now classified as idiopathic might have their origin in a thyroid autoimmunity. The studies also indicate that thyroiditis and thyroid amyloidosis may represent mutually exclusive processes. Of further interest is the observation that the variability of amyloid distribution may be related to the method of induction.

REFERENCES

1. Jordan, S.C., Buckingham, B., Sakai, R. and Olson, D. Studies of immune-complex glomerulonephritis mediated by human thyroglobulin. New Eng. J. Med., 304:1212 (1981).
2. Germuth, F.G., Rodriguez, E., Siddiqui, S.Y., Lorelle, C.A., McGee, S., Milano, L.L., and Wise, O. Immune complex disease. VII. Experimental mesangiopathic glomerulonephritis produced by chronic immunization with thyroglobulin. Lab. Invest., 38:404 (1978).
3. Wright, J.R., Calkins, E. and Humphrey, R.L. Potassium permanganate reaction in amyloidosis: A histologic method to assist in differentiating forms of this disease. Lab. Invest., 36:274 (1977).
4. Casas, C.B. and Buso, R. Amyloidosis in C_3H mice treated with goitrogens. Amer. J. Path., 45:645 (1964).

ABSENCE OF THYROGLOBULIN IN KIDNEY OF PATIENTS WITH AUTOIMMUNE

THYROIDITIS AND NEPHROPATHIES

F.X. Thierry, C. Burel, Ph. Caron, I. Vernier,
G.J. Fournie, J.P. Louvet*, and J.J. Conte**

**Service de Néphrologie et d'Hémodialyse
*Service d'Endocrinologie
CHU Purpan, 31059, Tolouse Cedex, France

INTRODUCTION

The possible association of autoimmune thyroid diseases and nephropathies raises the question of a relationship between these two diseases. Only seven cases have been reported in which demonstration of thyroglobulin (Tg) antigen in glomeruli had suggested its responsability in the pathogenesis of nephropathies (1). The aim of our study was to evaluate the frequency of Tg deposits in kidney biopsy of patients with these two diseases.

PATIENTS

37 patients (29 women and 8 men) were studied:
. Renal biopsy was performed in each case for microscopic hematuria (67%), proteinuria (16%), nephrotic syndrome (14%), and chronic renal failure (3%). Hystological studies showed glomerulonephritis (GN) with mesangial deposits in 24 cases (65%), Extracapillary Proliferative GN in 3 cases (8%), Membranous GN in 3 cases (8%), Membranoproliferative GN in 2 cases (5%), Chronic Interstitial Nephritis in 4 cases (11%), Minimal Changes in 1 case (3%).
. Thyroid disease has been diagnosed either before, during or after characterization of nephropathy: Chronic Thyroiditis (Asymptomatic Atrophic Thyroiditis, Hashimoto's Thyroiditis, Primary Myxoedema) was present in 29 cases (78%), Graves' disease in 3 cases (8%), Toxic or Non Toxic Multinodular Goiter and Euthyroid Goiter in 5 cases (14%).
The different association between thyroiditis and nephropathies are showed in table 1.

METHODS

Tg was researched by immunoperoxidase procedure on paraffin section (2). After the paraffination in toluene, sections were incubated during 30 minutes in a methanol-hydrogen peroxide mixture to inhibit endogenous peroxidase. Sections were rinsed with ordinary water. Immunoperoxidase technique required 4 stages:

1. Application of rabbit's polyclonal antibodies during 30 minutes (dilution 1/50)

2. Application of pig's sera anti-rabbit (Dakko-Patts Z126) during 30 minutes (dilution 1/20)
3. Application of pig's sera anti-rabbit's immunoglobulins marked with peroxidase-antiperoxidase (Dakko-Patts Z113 - dilution 1/100)
4. Demonstration of peroxidase with diamine-benzidine.

RESULTS

Tg antigen was not found in any of the 37 biopsies. Tg was absent as well in renal biopsy from 10 patients with various nephropathies but without thyroid diseases. Controls of human thyroid slices were positive, showing Tg in colloid vesicle and thyroid cells.

Table 1. Different associations between thyroid diseases and nephropathies observed in our study

	GN Mes	ECGN	MGN	MPGN	CIN	MC	TOTAL
Chronic Thyroiditis	20	1	2	2	3	1	29
Graves' Disease	1	1	-	-	1	-	3
Toxic Goiter	2	1	-	-	-	-	3
Euthyroid Goiter	1	-	1	-	-	-	2
TOTAL	24	3	3	2	4	1	37

GN = glomerulonephritis. GN Mes = GN with mesangial deposits. ECGN = extracapillary GN. MGN = membranous GN. MPGN = membranoproliferative GN. CIN = chronic interstitial nephritis. MC = minimal changes.

DISCUSSION

In the literature, 9 cases of the association of autoimmune thyroid disease and glomerulonephritis have been reported (3-9). Tg was found in renal biopsy specimens of a total of 7 patients. Thyroid microsomal antigen has been also characterized in 3 cases, but not sought in other patients. Thyroid diseases were Graves' or chronic thyroiditis. Histological kidney studies showed in most of the cases membranous nephropathy.
Thyroid antigenic distribution was in the same pattern as IgG-IgM-C3 5,6,9, IgG-C3 7, IgG 3,4,8 deposits. In one case 6, immunochemical analysis of the circulating immunecomplexes revealed that human Tg was the antigenic component. These observations have suggested development of immune complex GN mediated by thyroid antigens.
Failure of demonstration of Tg in renal biopsy specimens in our study could be in relation with:
. Population study: more than 60% had GN with mesangial deposits and almost 80% chronic thyroiditis.
. Chronological data: whereas nephropathies were characterized before thyroiditis in more 40% of cases, GN was diagnosed, in the literature, at the same time or after thyroid disease.
. Choice of techniques: immunoperoxidase procedure was used in our study whereas other authors employed immunofluorescence technique.
. Possibility of antigenic mask by idiotypic network.
Except for the study of Verger et al. (9), it is never indicated the total number of the renal biopsy studied. Therefore, the frequence of the

association between these two diseases is difficult to evaluate. It is possible that thyroid antigenic factors, other than Tg, could act as prevalent factor in the pathogenesis of the nephropathy. On the other hand, we have never observed a marked improvement in proteinuria, hematuria or renal function after thyroid treatment (Thyroidectomy, Carbimazole, opotherapy). Recently production of human monoclonal antibodies that react with both pancreatic islets and thyroid, is an example of the complex mechanisms involved in autoimmune disease (10).

Whereas association of thyroid diseases and nephropathies seems to be frequent in our study, the frequence of each pathology does not eliminate the possibility of a coincident association. Further studies appear necessary in order to find other thyroid antigenic factors in kidney biopsy and to specify a relationship between these two diseases.

REFERENCES

1. S. O'Regan, M. Smith and K.N. Drummond, Antigens in human immune complex nephritis. Clin. Nephrol. 4: 417 (1976).
2. G. Delsol, T. Al Saati, P. Caveriviere, E. Ancelin and F. Rigal-Huguet, Etude en immunopéroxidase du tissu lymphoide normal et pathologique. Ann. Pathol. 4: 165 (1984).
3. F. Jr. Horvath, P. Teague, E.F. Gaffney, D.R. Mars and T.J. Fuller, Thyroid antigen associated immune complex glomerulonephritis in Graves' disease. Am. J. Med. 67: 901 (1979).
4. T. Iwaoka, T. Umeda, M. Nakayama, T. Shimada, Y. Fujii, F. Miura and T. Sato, A case of membranous nephropathy associated with thyroid antigens, JPN J. Med. 145: 1115 (1982).
5. S.C. Jordan, W.H. Johnston and J.M. Bergstein, Immune complex glomerulonephritis mediated by thyroid antigens. Arch. Pathol. Lab. Med. 102: 530 (1978).
6. S.C. Jordan, B. Buckingham, P. Sakai and D. Olson, Studies of immuno-complex glomerulonephritis mediated by human thyroglobulin. N. Engl. J. Med. 304: 1212 (1981).
7. S. O'Regan, J.S.C. Fong, B.S. Kaplan, J.P. De Chadarevian, N. Lapointe and K.N. Drummond, Thyroid antigen-antibody nephritis, Clin. Immunol. Immunopathol. 6: 341 (1976).
8. D.W. Ploth, A. Fitz, D. Schnetzler, J. Seidenfeld and C.B. Wilson, Thyroglobulin-antithyroglobulin immune complex glomerulonephritis complicating radioiodine therapy. Clin. Immunol. Immunopathol. 9: 327 (1978).
9. M.F. Verger, B. Droz, and J. Venteloon, Maladies thyroidiennes autoimmune associées à une néphropathie glomérulaire. PresseMéd. 12: 83 (1983).
10. C. Garzelli, F.E. Taub, M.C. Jenkins, D.W. Drell, F. Ginsber-Fellner and A.L. Notkins, Human monoclonal autoantibodies that react with both pancreatic islets and thyroid, J. Clin. Invest. 77: 1627 (1986)

PERSISTENCE OF AUTOIMMUNE REACTIONS DURING

RECOVERY OF SUBACUTE THYROIDITIS

K.Bech, U.Feldt-Rasmussen, H.Bliddal, M.Høier-
Madsen, B. Thomsen, and H. Nielsen
Hvidöre Hospital, Med. dept. E, Frederiksberg
Hospital, Med. dept. TA, Rigshospitalet, State
Serum Institute, Copenhagen, Denmark

INTRODUCTION

Subacute thyroiditis (SAT) is a transitory inflammatory
thyroid lesion possibly of viral pathogenesis. We have recently studied the pattern of thyroid autoantibodies in patients
with SAT during and after recovery[1], but have now extended the
observation period with several years in order to see if the
humoral autoimmunity persists in these patients.

MATERIALS AND METHODS

Ten consecutive patients (4 men, 6 women, mean age 48 ±
12 years (SD)) were studied. The diagnosis was based as previously reported[1]. Recovery was obtained after median 6 months,
range 4-30 months, and the patients were followed for median 4
years, range 3-12 years after recovery. Thyroid function was
evaluated by routine radioimmunoassays and thyroglobulin (Tg)
determined as earlier described[2]. Thyroid stimulating antibodies were measured as TSH binding inhibition (TBII)[3] and
thyroid adenylate cyclase stimulation (TSAb)[4]. Thyroglobulin
antibodies (TgAb) were measured by radio-coprecipitation assay[5],
and thyroid microsomal antibodies (MAb) by immunofluorescence
technique[6]. Circulating immune complexes (CIC) were measured by
a complement consumption assay after precipitation with 2.5%
polyethylene glycol[7]. Tetanus toxoid anti-tetanus toxoid complexes were used as standards and the levels of CIC were expressed in terms of tetanus toxoid (TT) (µg/ml) in equivalent
amount of standard complexes with detection limit of 1.1 µg
TT/ml.

RESULTS

Eight patients were thyrotoxic at diagnosis but the hormone levels normalized spontaneously within 2 months through a
short phase of hypothyroidism with significantly increased TSH.
Tg was measurable in 4 patients and was high at diagnosis and
fell parallel to TSH and thyroid hormones. Presence of the different thyroid autoantibodies appears from table 1. Thyroid
stimulating antibodies (fig. 1) measured as TBII were present

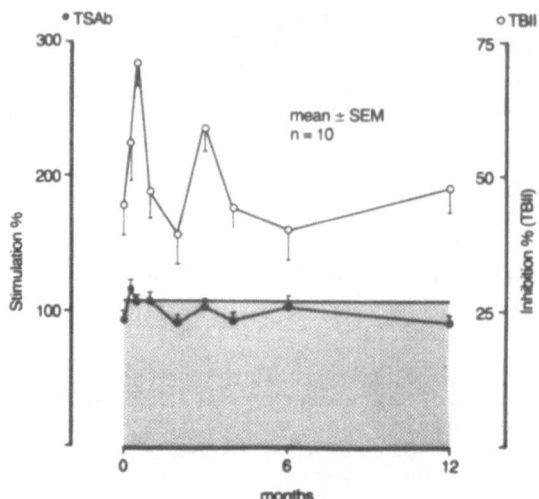

Fig. 1. The changes of thyroid stimulating antibodies (TSAb, ●) given as percentage stimulation by patient Ig of normal reference and TSH binding inhibiting immunoglobulins (TBII, o) given as per cent inhibition of ^{125}I-TSH binding by patient Ig compared to normal reference during the course of subacute thyroiditis. The hatched area indicates upper reference limit for both methods.

for some time in all patients during disease and remained detectable for up to 4 years in 6 patients. TSAb were only transitorily present in 3 patients (128%, 255%, 137%) without relation to the thyroid state. TgAb appeared in 4 and persisted in 3 patients, while MAb were negative. CIC were detected in all patients with maximal levels in the acute phase of SAT. CIC were still present up to 3 years but became after that time undetectable. Although there was no correlation between the thyroid antibodies and CIC, the changes in CIC during the course of SAT parallelled the changes of TBII.

DISCUSSION

The high levels of serum Tg coincident with thyrotoxicosis indicated acute damage of the thyroid with release of auto-antigenic components into circulation during the acute phase of SAT. This was also evidenced by low iodine uptake in the thyroid gland. Previously, anti-TSH receptor antibodies have been demonstrated in SAT[8]. As recently reported[1], TBII could be detected in all patients, while TSAb were negative in the majority. A remarkable finding was that CIC were present in all patients for very long time after the onset of the disease. This suggests that the self-limitation of the immune responses in SAT is a very slow process. Furthermore, immune complex formation seems to be a major feature in the regulatory mechanisms controlling the immune responses in SAT. Although there was no relation between CIC and thyroid autoantibodies, the resemblance between the changes in TBII and CIC suggests that idiotype-anti-idiotype interaction can be involved in the re-establishment of the immunological control.

Table 1. Presence of various thyroid antibodies during the course of subacute thyroiditis (SAT). The period was divided into an acute phase (diagnosis), an intermediary phase and a recovery phase lasting from 4 to 30 months (median 6 months). The number of positive patients/number of patients tested is indicated.

Presence of thyroid antibodies during the course of subacute thyroiditis

	Phase		
	Acute	Intermediary	Recovery
TgAb	2 / 6	4 / 10	2 / 10
TSAb	0 / 6	3 / 10	3 / 10
TBII	4 / 6	8 / 10	6 / 10
MAb	0 / 6	0 / 10	0 / 10

REFERENCES

1. H. Bliddal, K. Bech, U. Feldt-Rasmussen, M. Høier-Madsen, B. Thomsen and H. Nielsen, Humoral autoimmune manifestation in subacute thyroiditis. Allergy 40:559 (1985).
2. U. Feldt-Rasmussen, P.H. Petersen and J. Date, Sex and age correlated reference values of serum thyroglobulin measured by a modified radioimmunoassay. Acta Endocrinol 90:440 (1979).
3. H. Bliddal, A stable, reproducible radioreceptor assay for thyrotrophin binding inhibiting immunoglobulins (TBII). Scand J Clin Invest 41:441 (1981).
4. K. Bech and S.N. Madsen, thyroid adenylate cyclase stimulating immunoglobulins in thyroid diseases. Clin Endocrinol 11:47 (1979).
5. J. Date, U. Feldt-Rasmussen, P.H. Petersen, and K. Bech, An improved coprecipitation assay for determination of thyroglobulin antibodies. Scand J Clin Lab Invest 40:37 (1980).
6. T.H. Weller and A.H. Coons, Fluorescent antibody studies with agent of varicella and herpes propagated in vitro. Proc Soc Exp Biol 86:789 (1980).
7. I. Brandslund, H.C. Siersted, J.C. Jensenius and S.E. Svehag, Detection and quantitation of immune complexes with a rapid polyethylene glycol precipitation complement consumption method (PEG-CC). Methods Enzymol 74:551 (1981).
8. C.R. Strakosch, D. Joyner and J.R. Wall, Thyroid stimulating antibodies in patients with subacute thyroiditis. J Clin Endocrinol Metab 46:345 (1978).

PURIFIED PROTEIN DERIVATIVE REACTION AND URINARY IMMUNOSUPPRESSIVE ACIDIC PROTEIN IN PATIENTS WITH SUBACUTE THYROIDITIS

Hiroshi Fukazawa, Toshiro Sakurada, Keiji Tamura*, Katsumi
Yoshida, Makiko Yamamoto, and Shintaro Saito

The Second Department of Internal Medicine and *Bacteriology, Tohoku University School of Medicine, Sendai, Japan

INTRODUCTION

Recently we reported[1-2] that in acute phase of subacute thyroiditis (SAT) serum immunosuppressive acidic protein (IAP), a type of α_1-acid glycoprotein measured by single radial immunodiffusion method is increased, and peripheral K cell activity measured by the modified plaque-method of Biberfeld et al. was decreased and negatively correlated with serum IAP. Inhibition rate of K cells from a normal subject by sera of patients with SAT in acute phase was higher than that in recovery phase and those of normal control. Purified IAP inhibited K cell activity of normal subject in a dose-dependent manner. Circulating immune-complex measured by modified solid phase C1q-binding assay was almost normal and had no correlation with serum IAP in SAT. Trypsynization of K cells resulted in no change of K cells in both normal subjects and patients with SAT. From these results, it is conceivable that the K cell function is activated to destroy the affected cells probably by virus in the very early phase of SAT and that the K cell activity in SAT might be suppressed by IAP produced from macrophages as defense mechanism against the endless destruction of affected cells by K cells.

In the present study, we measured urinary IAP and purified protein derivative (PPD) reaction in patients with SAT to investigate the role of cellular immunity in SAT.

MATERIALS AND METHODS

Subjects The normal controls consisted of 16 women and 4 men, the patients with SAT 36 women and 8 men and the patients with Graves' disease 9 women and 4 men.

Serum IAP Serum IAP was measured with a single radial immunodiffusion method. Sera (30 μl) were added to microwells punched into Agarose gel plate containing 1-5% anti-IAP rabbit serum. After the reaction at 37°C for 48 hrs in a humid chamber, the diameter of the precipitin ring was measured. The mean normal values were 375 ± 70.3 (S.D.) μg/ml.

Urinary IAP For the quantitation of urinary IAP, passive hemagglutinin inhibition reaction method was[1] used. Twenty five microliters of anti-IAP rabbit sera were added into the two-times dilution series of 25 µl urine with phosphate buffer saline, pH 7.5, on microtiter plates, and then reaction mixtures were allowed to stand for 30 min at 22°C. After 50 µl of 0.4% IAP-coated sheep red blood cells suspension in phosphate buffer saline containing 1% bovine serum were added and mixed, the mixtures were allowed to stand at 22°C for 2 hrs. Urinary IAP per milliliters was calculated from final hemagglutinin inhibition titer, and then the concentration per 24 hrs was obtained. Mean normal value was 0.53 ± 0.39 mg/day. Upper limit of normal range was 1.50 mg/day.

PPD reaction For the measurement of PPD reaction, 0.1 ml of purified tuberculoprotein (Japan BCG Production Co.) as an indicater of established delayed hypersensitivity was injected intracutaneously. The test was evaluated by measuring maximal diameter of cutaneous reactions using customary guidelines at 48 hr. Negative value was less than 4 mm.

RESULTS

In 20 out of 42 patients with SAT in whom clinical courses were followed to complete recovery phase, mean PPD reaction in acute phase, 14.9 ± 12.8 (S.D.) mm, were lower than those in recovery phase, 30.4 ± 23.1 mm ($p < 0.01$, Fig. 1). Negative PPD reaction in three patients with SAT in acute phase became positive in recovery phase. Mean PPD reaction values in Graves' disease and controls were 10.9 ± 10.9 and 13.2 ± 7.0 mm, respectively, being not different from those of SAT in acute phase but lower than those in recovery ($p < 0.02$ and 0.02, respectively). In 5 patients with Graves' disease when their thyroid states were became euthyroid with the treatment, there was no change in PPD reaction values before and after the treatment, 8.6 ± 5.9 and 5.5 ± 3.6 mm, respectively (Fig. 2).

PPD reaction values in 44 patients with SAT in acute and in 18 pa-

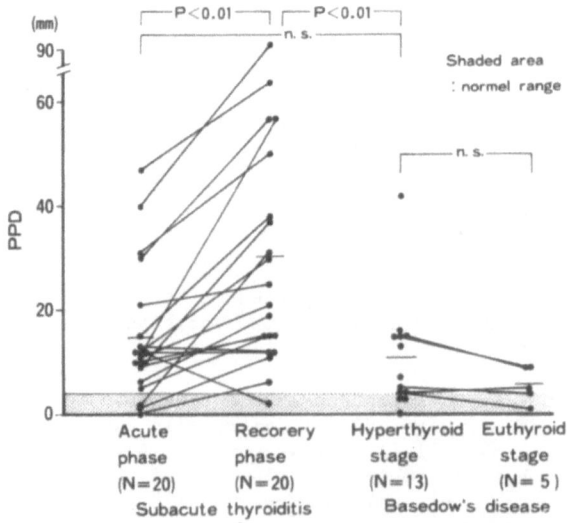

Fig. 1. PPD reaction values in patients with subacute thyroiditis and in hyperthyroidism treated with antithyroid drugs or [131]I.

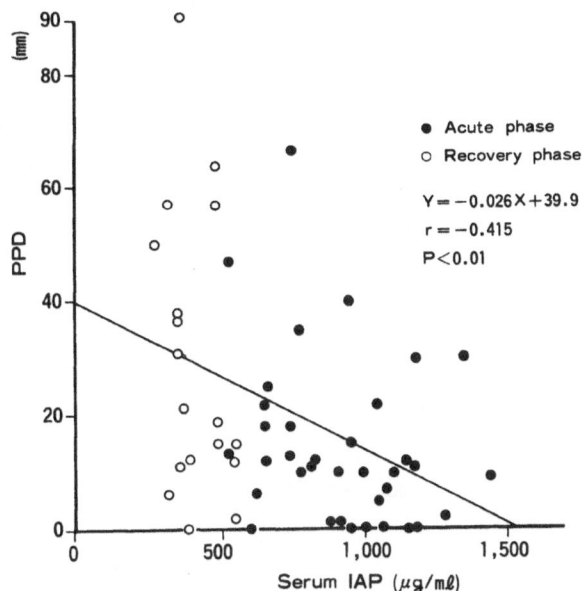

Fig. 2. Correlation between serum IAP and PPD reaction values in patients with subacute thyroiditis.

tients in recovery phases negatively correlated with serum IAP values
(Fig. 2), but not with urinary IAP in 20 patients with SAT. In acute
phase, 7 out of 20 patients with SAT showed urinary IAP above the upper
limit of normal and their urinary IAP values were decreased to normal in
accordance with the decrease of serum IAP. There was positive correlation between IAP values in serum and urine ($r = 0.35$, $p < 0.05$) in SAT.

DISCUSSION

In the present study PPD reaction, an expression of cellular immun-
nity, was decreased in acute phase of patients with SAT. It is suggested
that viral infection may cause the SAT. And negative PPD reaction is observed in viral diseases such as mumps and influenza. Though serum IAP
values are higher than normal in 100% of patients with SAT in acute
phase[1], high urinary IAP value was observed only 35% in the present study.
This may indicate that there is an accerelation of reabsorption or ca-
tabolism of IAP at renal tubule in patients with SAT.

REFERENCES

1. T. Sakurada, H. Fukazawa, K. Tamura, and K. Yoshinaga, Increased
level of immunosuppressive acidic protein in patients with subacute thyroiditis. In: Current Problems in Thyroid Research, N. Ui, K. Torizuka,
S. Nagataki, K. Miyai, eds., Excerpta Medica, Amsterdam, p453 (1982).
2. H. Fukazawa, T. Sakurada, K. Tamura, and K. Yoshinaga, Corela-
tion between peripheral K cells and circulating IgG immune complex of
immunosuppressive acidic protein in patients with subacute thyroiditis.
In: Abstract of 9th International Thyroid Congress, p188 (1985).

INTERFERENCES OF CIRCULATING ANTI-TSH ANTIBODIES IN METHODS FOR THYROTROPIN MEASUREMENT

Paolo Beck-Peccoz, Gabriella Medri, Cristina Rossi, and Giovanni Faglia

Department of Endocrinology, School of Medicine, University of Milan, Via F.Sforza 35, 20122-Milano, Italy

INTRODUCTION

Thyrotropin (TSH)immunometric assays may lose their peculiar specificity when heterophilic antibodies[1,2] or anti-TSH antibodies[3,4] are present in a given sample. In fact, both these kinds of antibodies may interfere in TSH immunometric assays, giving inappropriate hormone values, clearly inconsistent with other laboratory or clinical findings. In particular, circulating heterophilic antibodies, i.e. antibodies cross-reacting with immunoglobulins (Ig) of the animal in which the assay specific antibody has been raised, cause spuriously high values both in TSH radioimmunoassays (TSH-RIA) and in TSH immunoradiometric assays (TSH-IRMA).In TSH-RIA, the interference is usually due to an anti-rabbit Ig which neutralizes part of the rabbit anti-TSH antibody[1], while in TSH-IRMA it is due to an anti-mouse Ig which bridges both the labeled and solid-phased monoclonal antibodies, thus behaving as a complete TSH molecule[2]. On the contrary, the interference in TSH-RIA of circulating anti-TSH antibodies, i.e. antibodies induced by bovine TSH (bTSH) or impure pituitary extract injections, or occasionally found (autoantibodies?) in patients with Graves'disease[5], is mainly due to the sequestration of the tracer by the endogenous antibodies. Using second antibody (2nd Ab) separation methods or solid-phase techniques, spuriously high TSH-RIA levels are usually found[3,4],since the radioactivity either precipitated with 2nd Ab or bound to the solid-phased antibody decreases, giving TSH values higher than the actual ones, when extrapolated from the standard curve.

The aim of the present study is to investigate the possible interference of anti-TSH antibodies in the recently available ultrasensitive TSH-IRMA methods in which the specificity is of great importance in view of their alleged use as first line test of thyroid function.

MATERIALS AND METHODS

Patients. Five subjects (3 euthyroid and 2 hyperthyroid) showing discrepancies between free thyroid hormone and TSH-RIA levels were studied. Diagnosis, previous treatments and hormone measurements are reported in Table 1.

Table 1. Patients, hormone measurements and detection of anti-TSH antibodies

Case	Diagnosis	Previous treatment	FT4	FT3	TSH-RIA	TSH-IRMA	NSB*
			(pmol/l)		(mU/l)		%
1.	Pit.tumor	Bovine TSH, pit.extracts	14.5	20.2	4.5	< 0.07	69.1°
2.	Graves'	None	18.5	22.4	2.6	< 0.07	30.1
3.	Pit.tumor	Pit.extracts	13.6	--	48.0	< 0.07	71.9
4.	Chranioph.	Bovine TSH, pit.extracts	14.7	8.1	46.5	< 0.07	23.0°
5.	Normal	None	13.7	--	60.5	42.6	19.3°
NORMAL CONTROLS (n = 56)			9-20	4-8	<0.3-4.5	0.15-6.0	7-11

* NSB = nonspecific binding of ^{125}I-hTSH (see text for details).
° Similar % NSB was recorded using ^{125}I-bTSH.

Detection and cross-reaction of anti-TSH antibodies. The presence of
anti-TSH antibodies was documented measuring the percent of radioactivity
precipitated by polyethylene glycol (PEG) after incubation of diluted sera
with ^{125}I-hTSH (20,000 cpm) for 24 hours at room temperature. The cross-
reaction of endogenous antibody with bovine TSH was tested using the same
procedure but ^{125}I-bTSH.
TSH immunometric assays. Serum TSH was measured by an "in-house" RIA using
TSH-free serum in the standard curve, 72 hours preincubation with rabbit
anti-TSH antibody followed by 48 hours incubation with tracer and separation with 2nd Ab. The sensitivity was 0.3 mU/l. Serum TSH was also measured
by a two-site IRMA method using a commercial kit (Sucrosep TSH-IRMA, Boots-
Celltech, Slough, UK), showing a sensitivity of 0.07 mU/l.
TSH recovery tests in IRMA method. These tests were carried out measuring
TSH levels after 24 hours incubation of diluted sera (1:16) with TSH standard at various concentrations, in the absence or presence of bovine TSH (
55,000 mU/l), in order to saturate the endogenous antibody with a cross-
reacting molecule not recognized in the TSH-IRMA method (Table 2).

RESULTS AND DISCUSSION

In all patients the presence of anti-TSH antibodies was suspected on
the basis of discrepancies between TSH-RIA and free thyroid hormone circulating levels[3,4] and definitely documented by the finding of increased
nonspecific binding of labeled TSH to patients'immunoglobulins after precipitation with PEG (Table 1). In 3 patients the appearance of the anti-TSH
antibodies had been presumably induced by previous bovine TSH or impure
pituitary extract injections, while in the remaining two no previous treatment was recorded, thus confirming the possibility of a spontaneous occurrence of anti-TSH antibodies (autoantibodies?)[5]. Spuriously high serum
TSH-RIA values (Table 1) were recorded in all patients: in 3 of them the
TSH values were in the primary hypothyroid range in spite of normal free
thyroid hormone levels, and in 2 patients were clearly detectable in spite
of elevated free thyroid hormone concentration, a situation that could have
been confused with an inappropriate secretion of TSH (IST). However, when

Table 2. TSH recovery tests (see text for details). Data are
expressed in mU/l

hTSH standard		Case no. 1		Case no. 4		Case no. 5	
– bTSH	+ bTSH	– bTSH	+ bTSH	– bTSH	+ bTSH	– bTSH	+ bTSH
0.0	0.0	0.0	0.0	0.0	0.0	3.0	2.9
0.5	0.6	0.2	0.6	0.4	0.6	3.6	3.8
1.8	1.7	1.1	1.8	1.4	1.8	5.0	4.8
7.4	7.5	3.6	7.9	6.9	7.6	10.5	10.3
29.5	29.1	15.7	29.3	23.8	31.0	32.0	31.4
60.6	61.5	45.3	60.0	51.2	61.4	64.2	64.5
124.0	127.0	93.8	128.0	110.0	125.3	120.0	118.0

measured by IRMA, TSH values were undetectable in all cases with one exception
(case no.5) (Table 1). In the 2 hyperthyroid patients, these findings, along
with the positivity of the thyroid stimulating antibodies, indicated the existence of Graves'disease and not of IST. Furthermore, these data demonstate
that, contrary to TSH-RIA, TSH-IRMA is not affected by circulating anti-TSH
antibodies when TSH secretion is fully suppressed. On the contrary, the finding of undetectable TSH-IRMA levels in 2 euthyroid patients (no.3 & 4) suggest a possible interference of endogenous anti-TSH antibody yielding spuriously low TSH values. This hypothesis was confirmed by TSH recovery tests
in which a clear underestimation of the actual TSH levels both in eu- and
hyperthyroid sera was found (Table 2). Nevertheless, when the endogenous
antibody was saturated with high amount of bTSH (Table 2) the interference
completely disappeared. Therefore, it is possible to infer from these findings that circulating anti-TSH antibodies bind at least one of the TSH epitopes recognized by IRMA monoclonal antibodies, thus preventing the formation
of the "sandwich" (labeled monoclonal Ab = TSH = solid-phased monoclonal Ab)
and eventually causing the underestimation of the actual TSH concentrations.
A completely different situation seems to exist in case no. 5, in whom an
overestimation of TSH levels was observed using TSH-IRMA. In fact, TSH recovery tests carried out with or without bTSH were definitely normal (Table 2),
thus suggesting that this spontaneously occurring antibody may bind epitopes
different from those recognized by IRMA monoclonals. Therefore, TSH-IRMA
method in this case measures all the TSH molecules present in the sample,
i.e. both the "free" TSH and TSH bound to the endogenous antibody, giving
high TSH values, as actually they are, but inconsistent with the thyroid
status of the subject. In conclusion, the presence of circulating anti-TSH
antibodies should be carefully considered, even in patients never treated
with bovine TSH or impure pituitary hormone preparations, whenever discrepancies between TSH-RIA and TSH-IRMA values or between these measurements
and other laboratory or clinical findings are observed in order to avoid
misdiagnosis and consequently unnecessary treatments.

REFERENCES

1. P. J. Howanitz, H. V. Lamberson, and K. M. Ennis, Incidence and mechanism of spurious increases in serum thyrotropin, <u>Clin.Chem</u>. 28:427
   (1982).
2. C. F. Cusick, K. Mistry, G. M. Addison, Interference in a two-site
   immunoradiometric assay for thyrotropin ina child, <u>Clin.Chem</u>. 31:
   348 (1985).
3. L. A. Frohman, M. A. Baron, and A. B. Schneider, Plasma immunoreactive
   TSH: spurious elevation due to antibodies to bovine TSH which cross-
   react with human TSH, <u>Metabolism</u> 31:834 (1982).
4. P. Beck-Peccoz, G. Piscitelli, G. Medri, M. Ballabio, and G. Faglia,
   Thyroid test strategy, <u>Lancet</u> i:1456 (1985).
5. G. N. Beall, and S. R. Kruger, Binding of   I-human TSH by gamma-
   globulins of sera containing thyroid-stimulating immunoglobulin (TSI),
   <u>Life Sci</u>. 32:77 (1983).

INDEX

Amiodarone
   and thyroid autoantibodies, 599
Anti-alpha galactosyl antibodies
   antigen to, 297
   in various thyroid disorders,
      297
Antithyroid drug therapy adverse
   reaction to, 501
   and thyroid autoantibodies in
      Graves' disease, 453
   clinical outcome after, 221, 513
   high doses in Graves' disease,
      457
   immunosuppressive effect of,
      481
   predictive value of TSH receptor
      antibodies after, 517
Anti-TSH antibodies
   interference in TSH
   measurement, 631
   ATRA 1
   in thyroid autoimmune
   disorders, 45
Autoantigenic determinants
   in thyroid autoimmunity, 275
Autonomous toxic goiter
   and thyroid autoimmunity, 221

Bacterial antigens
   and thyroid autoimmunity, 35
Breast cancer
   and thyroid autoantibodies, 603

Cell-mediated immunity
   in endemic goiter, 579
   in Graves' ophthalmopathy, 125
Complement activity
   in Graves' disease and
      Hashimoto's thyroiditis,
      607
Congenital hypothyroidism
   and growth blocking antibodies,
      425
   and HLA gene involvement, 477
   and thyroid autoimmunity, 421
   thyroid autoantibodies in, 397

Endemic goiter
   and lymphocytic thyroiditis,
      583
   cell-mediated immunity in, 579
   immunological features of, 549
   iodine intake and autoimmune
   factors in, 559
   TGSAb in, 359
Exophthalmos see Graves'
   ophthalmopathy
Experimental thyroiditis
   in mice, genetics of, 191
   in rat, characterization of
   lymphocytes, 331

Forbidden clone theory
   somatic mutation in, 4
   autoantigen for TSAb and, 5

Genes
   encoding for thyroglobulin and
   TSH receptor auto- antibodies,
      175
Genetics
   and experimental autoimmune
      thyroiditis, 191
   and Graves' disease, 6
   and spontaneous autoimmune
      thyroiditis, 199
Graves' disease
   and antithyroid drug therapy,
      513
   autoimmune phenomena in, 1
   blocking antibodies in, 433
   complement activities in, 607
   effect of methimazole on
   gamma-interferon in, 445
   HLA-DR gene analysis in,
      489
   IgG subclass distribution of
   thyroid autoantibodies in, 301
   immune complexes in, 607
   immunogenetics of, 74, 153
   immunohistochemica studies in,
      355
   immunosuppressive action of

635

carbimazole in, 481
LATS protector in, 2
light chain restriction in, 335
natural killer cell activity in ,
    339
pathogenic autoimmunity in, 1
polyamine modulation of IgG in,
    367
post-partum onset of, 231
predictive value of TBII and
TSAb in, 413
prevalence in Dublin, 587
prognostic value of TSAb and
    thyroglobulin during
    antithyroid drug therapy,
    449
prognostic value of TSH
    receptor antibodies after
    antithyroid drug therapy in,
    517
specific DNA polymorphism in,
    469
thyroid autoantibodies during
    anti-thyroid drug treatment
    of, 453
thyroid suppressibility in, 505
TSH receptor antibodies in, 69,
    429
Graves' ophthalmopathy
    autoantibodies to eye muscle
        antigens in, 533
    cellular mechanisms in, 125
    cross-reactivity between
        thyroglobulin autoantibodies
        and torpedo acetylcholin-
        esterase in, 271
    humoral factors in, 99, 525, 529
    immunosuppressive treatment
        of, 541
    natural history of, 537
    natural killer cell cytotoxicity
        in, 127, 339
    orbital antigen purification by
        monoclonal antibodies in,
        521
    pathogenesis and treatment of,
        263
    results of treatment of,263,537
    retrobulbar corticosteroids and
        orbital radiotherapy in, 545

Hashimoto's thyroiditis
    and ageing, 555
    and dietary iodine intake, 555
    and endemic goiter, 583
    and kidney diseases, 619
    complement activities in, 607
    frequency of HLA-DR 5 in, 437
    immune complexes in, 607
    in obese subjects, 591

interferon gamma-producing T
    cells in, 309
natural killer cell activity in,
    337
specific DNA polymorphism in,
    469
T cell clones producing
    lymphokines in, 313
TGSAb in, 409
thyroid infiltrating lymphocytes
    in, 135
    TSH activity blocking
        antibodies in, 393

Histocompatibility antigens
    expression in thyroid
        autoimmune disorders, 11,
        497
    gene involvement in congenital
        hypothyroidism, 477
    in human thyroid cells
        transfected with SV-40,
        465
    in post-partum thyroid
        dysfunction, 211, 441
    in thyroid tumors, 567
HLA-DR
    expression by RHS cells, 485
    expression in thyroid
        autoimmune disorders, 110,
        497
    gene analysis in Graves' disease,
        489
    in Hashimoto's thyroiditis, 437
    in post-partum thyroiditis, 437

Idiopathic myxedema
    and ageing, 555
    and dietary iodine intake, 555
    in obese subjects, 591
    TSH activity blocking antibodies
        in, 393
Immune complexes
    in Graves' disease and
        Hashimoto's thyroiditis, 607
Immunogenetics of Graves' disease,
    74, 153
Interleukin-1
    effects on human thyroid cells,
        327
Intrathyroidal lymphocytes
    and thyroid autoantibodies, 117
    and thyroid destruction, 117
    in Hashimoto's thyroiditis, 135
Iodine intake
    and thyroid autoimmunity, 563

LATS
    studies on, 63
LATS protector
    in Graves' disease, 2

Monoclonal antibodies
    and thyroid autoantigens, 53
    to microsomal antigen, 30, 279
    to TSH receptor, 11

Natural killer activity
    influence of lymphokines and
        thyroid hormones on, 509
Neonatal hyperthyroidism
    TSH receptor antibodies in, 417
Nude mice
    use in human autoimmunity, 207

Pathogenic autoimmunity
    in Graves' disease, 1
Post-partum thyroid dysfunction
    and HLA status, 441
    and thyroid microsomal
        autoantibodies, 473
    Graves' disease as, 221
    immune status in, 211
Post-partum thyroiditis
    frequency of HLA-DR 5 in, 437

Retroorbital fibroblasts
    role in Graves' ophthalmopathy
        of, 99

Sjögren's syndrome
    thyroid function in, 611
Skin fibroblasts
    stimulation by immunoglobulins,
        401
Spontaneous thyroiditis
    failure of endocrine responses
        by immune signals in, 493
    in animals, 199
Subacute thyroiditis
    autoimmune reactions in, 623
    immunosuppressive protein in,
        627
Suppressor T cell
    activation by thyroglobulin, 315
    defect in thyroid autoimmunity,
        109, 323

TBII
    and outcome of therapy of
        Graves' disease, 413
    in primary hypothyroidism, 241
    relationship to TSAb, 244
TGSAb see Thyroid Growth
        Stimulating Antibody
Thymic endocrine activity
        and thyroid function in low
        birth-weight infants, 461
Thyroglobulin
    and TSAb during antithyroid
        drug treatment of Graves'
        disease, 449, 505

autoantigenicity of, 181
    role of iodination in, 185
    thyroid and renal amyloidosis
        after immunization with,
        615
Thyroglobulin autoantibody
    cross-reactivity with torpedo
        acetylcholinesterase, 271
    gene encoding for, 175
    IgG subclass distribution of,
        189
    regulation by T cells of IgG
        subclasses of, 319
Thyroid autoantibodies
    and congenital hypothyroidism,
        397
    and intrathyroidal lymphocytes,
        117
    during antithyroid drug
        treatment of Graves'
        disease, 453
    during chronic amiodarone
        administration, 599
    in children with insulin
        dependent diabetes mellitus,
        595
    in breast cancer patients, 603
    in general population, 551
    in Sjögren's syndrome, 611
    in thyroid cancer patients, 571,
        575
Thyroid autoantigens
    characterization by monoclonal
        antibodies, 53
    and TSH receptor, 11
Thyroid autoimmunity
    in autonomous toxic goiter, 221
    in vitro model for, 145
    theories on, 159
Thyroid cancer
    and thyroid autoantibodies, 571,
        575
Thyroid Growth Stimulating
        Antibodies
    and goiter, 257
    and FRTL-5 cells, 379, 385
    in Graves' disease, 87, 375, 385
    in Hashimoto's thyroiditis, 409
    intrathyroidal production of,
        371
Thyroid hormone
    autoantibodies to, 305
Thyroid microsomal antigen
    characterization of, 27, 279,
        285, 293
    proteolytic digestion of, 27
Thyroid peroxidase
    and thyroid microsomal antigen,
        28, 285, 293
    measurement of antibody to, 289

molecular cloning of, 283
Thyroid Stimulating Antibody *see* TSAb
Thyrotropin see TSH
TRAb see TSH receptor antibodies
TSAb
   and outcome of therapy of Graves' disease, 413
   and thyroglobulin during antithyroid drug treatment of Graves' disease, 449, 505
   effect on thyroid cyclic AMP, 351
   in non-thyroid autoimmune diseases, 347
   physiopathological relevance of, 77, 83
   studies on, 65
TSH
   interference of anti-TSH in the measurement of, 631
TSH binding inhibitor IgG see TBII
TSH blocking antibodies
   in Graves' disease, 433

TSH receptor
   antibodies to, 69
   characterization on thyroid plasma membranes, 405
   interaction of purified Graves' IgG with, 343
   monoclonal antibodies to, 11
   structure and signal transmission of, 12
TSH receptor antibodies
   and antiidiotypic blocking biologic activity, 389
   after antithyroid drug therapy of Graves' disease, 517
   and thyroid cell function, 83
   and thyroid cell growth, 363
   genes encoding for, 175
   in Graves' disease, 69, 429
   in neonatal hyperthyroidism, 417
   pathophysiological relevance, 91

Yersinia enterocolitica
   and thyroid autoimmunity, 35